PRODUCT SAFETY
EVALUATION HANDBOOK

PRODUCT SAFETY EVALUATION HANDBOOK

Second Edition, Revised and Expanded

edited by
Shayne Cox Gad

Gad Consulting Services
Raleigh, North Carolina

MARCEL DEKKER, INC.　　　　　　NEW YORK · BASEL

Library of Congress Cataloging-in-Publication Data

Product safety evaluation handbook / edited by Shayne Cox Gad. — 2nd
   ed., rev. and expanded.
        p.   cm.
   Includes bibliographical references and index.
   ISBN 0-8247-1971-9 (alk. paper)
      1. Toxicity testing Handbooks, manuals, etc.   2. Product safety
   Handbooks, manuals, etc.   I. Gad, Shayne C.
   RA1199.P77   1999
   615.9′07—dc21   99-30388
                                                              CIP

This book is printed on acid-free paper.

Headquarters
Marcel Dekker, Inc.
270 Madison Avenue, New York, NY 10016
tel: 212-696-9000; fax: 212-685-4540

Eastern Hemisphere Distribution
Marcel Dekker AG
Hutgasse 4, Postfach 812, CH-4001 Basel, Switzerland
tel: 41-61-261-8482; fax: 41-61-261-8896

World Wide Web
http://www.dekker.com

The publisher offers discounts on this book when ordered in bulk quantities. For more information, write to Special Sales/Professional Marketing at the headquarters address above.

Current printing (last digit):
10 9 8 7 6 5 4 3 2 1

PRINTED IN THE UNITED STATES OF AMERICA

Preface to the Second Edition

This new edition of the *Handbook* has been expanded and thoroughly revised to reflect the changes both in the science/practice of toxicology and in regulatory and statutory requirements that have occurred since the first edition was published over ten years ago. The objective remains the same—to provide a single volume, practical handbook that will meet the everyday needs of those involved in or responsible for ensuring the biologic safety of products other than drugs and medical devices.

To meet this objective, significant attention has been paid to reviewing relevant U.S. and international guidelines that are applicable to the performance of each category of tests. Additionally, wherever possible alternative testing schemes that involve fewer or no intact higher animals have been introduced and incorporated. The entirely new chapter on pharmaco- and toxicokinetics was likewise added to reflect the fact that in many cases such studies are now essential to allow a meaningful assessment of potential harm and the relevance to humans of findings in animal test models.

Shayne Cox Gad

Preface to the First Edition

This handbook has been prepared with a single objective—to present a practical guide for those professionals who are (or are planning to be) responsible for ensuring the biological safety of products for consumers and workers in fields where there are no detailed, regulatorily prescribed, test methods.

As a practical guide (and not just a workbook), this handbook has been written by professionals who are experienced and currently active in the field. Its chapters clearly set forth the nature of the hazards and the methods for their evaluation. The problems with toxicological methods are clearly delineated, followed by the solutions that have been utilized and a presentation of the scientific and philosophical basis for such guidance. Rigorous development of theoretical concepts or mathematical methods has been avoided. Furthermore, data on specific materials are not presented except to explain or amplify the topic of regulation.

The volume is, by design, aimed at the nonpharmaceutical industries, where there is some regulatory guidance, although it is not of a lockstep nature. It is hoped that the methodologies (though meeting such regulatory requirements as exist in their particular area) provide a flexible and truly scientific approach to evaluation and problem solving.

Shayne Cox Gad

Contents

Contributors

Carol S. Auletta, D.A.B.T.   Toxicology Department, Huntingdon Life Sciences, East Millstone, New Jersey

Paul T. Bailey, Ph.D.   Mobil Business Resources Corporation, Paulsboro, New Jersey

Joan M. Chapdelaine, Ph.D.   Immunology Department, Chrysalis Preclinical Services Corporation, Olyphant, Pennsylvania

Christopher P. Chengelis, Ph.D.   WIL Research Laboratories, Inc., Ashland, Ohio

Shayne Cox Gad, Ph.D.   Gad Consulting Services, Raleigh, North Carolina

Julia D. George, Ph.D.   Center for Life Sciences and Toxicology, Research Triangle Institute, Research Triangle Park, North Carolina

Richard A. Hiles, Ph.D.   Preclinical Development, Amylin Pharmaceuticals, Inc., San Diego, California

Robert W. Kapp, Jr., Ph.D.   BioTox, Richmond, Virginia

Victor T. Mallory, B.S., R.L.A.T.   Toxicology Department, Chrysalis Preclinical Services Corporation, Olyphant, Pennsylvania

Ann D. Mitchell, Ph.D.   Genesys Research, Inc., Research Triangle Park, North Carolina

Paul E. Newton, Ph.D., D.A.B.T.   MPI Research, Inc., Mattawan, Michigan

John L. Orr, Ph.D., D.A.B.T.   Drug Safety Evaluation, Purdue Pharma L.P., Ardsley, New York

Vincent J. Piccirillo, Ph.D., D.A.B.T.   NPC, Inc., Sterling, Virginia

James L. Schardein, M.S., A.T.S.   WIL Research Laboratories, Inc., Ashland, Ohio

Walter G. Switzer, M.S.   Consultant, San Antonio, Texas

1

Defining the Objective
Product Safety Assessment Program Design and Scheduling

Shayne Cox Gad
Gad Consulting Services, Raleigh, North Carolina

I. INTRODUCTION

The practical aspects of toxicology testing (biological safety assessment) for commercial products not regulated primarily by the Food and Drug Admnistration (FDA) is the subject of this book. Aspects include industrial and agricultural chemicals, consumer products, and cosmetics, and polymers. The most important part of a product safety evaluation program for such products is the initial overall process of defining and developing adequate data on the potential hazards associated with the manufacture, sale, and use of a product. This calls for asking a series of questions, and is a very interactive process, with many of the questions designed to identify and/or modify their successors. In fact, this volume should serve as a companion in such a process. This chapter is a step-by-step guide or map to this question-asking process.

In the product safety evaluation process, we must first determine what information is needed. This calls for an understanding of the way the product is to be made and to be used, and the potential health and safety risks posed by exposure of humans who will be associated with these processes. This is the basis of a hazard and toxicity profile (see Table 1). Next, a search of the available literature (as presented in Chapter 2) is made to determine what is already known. Taking the literature into consideration and the previously defined exposure potential, a tier approach (Table 2) is used to generate a list of tests or studies to be performed. What goes into a tier system is determined by both regulatory requirements imposed by government agencies and the philosophy of

Table 1 Mixture Toxicity Data Matrix

	Mixture	Component 1	Component 2	Component 3	Component 4	Intermediate A	Waste Material B
1. Literature review							
2. Physiochemical properties (includes quantity present)							
3. Use/exposure potential							
4. Oral lethality (rat) (mouse)							
5. Inhalation lethality (rat) (mouse)							
6. Dermal irritation							
7. Ocular irritation							
8. Skin sensitization/Immunotoxicity							
9. Genotoxicity							
10. Teratology							
11. Reproduction							
12. Repeated exposure studies							
13. Carcinogenicity							
14. Absorption/Distribution/Metabolism/Evaluation (ADME)							

Table 2 Tier Testing

Tier Testing	Mammalian Toxicology	Genetic Toxicology	Remarks
0	Literature review	Literature review	Upon initial identification of a problem data base of existing information and particulars of use of materials are established
1	Primary dermal irritation Eye irritation Dermal sensitization Acute systemic toxicity Lethality screens	Ames test In vitro SCE In vitro cytogenics Forward mutation/CHO	R&D materials and low volume chemicals with severely limited exposure
2	Subacute studies ADME	In vivo SCE In vivo cytogenetics *Drosophila*	Medium volume materials and/or those with limited exposure
3	Subchronic studies Immunotoxicity Reproduction Teratology Chronic studies Specialty studies		Any material with a high volume or a potential for widespread human exposure or one which gives indications of specific long-term effects

the parent organization. How such tests actually are performed is determined on one of two bases. The first (and most common) is the menu approach: selecting a series of standard design tests as "modules" of data. The second, which will also be covered in this chapter, is an interactive approach, where studies are designed (or designs are selected) based on both needs and what we have learned about the product. The test designs and approaches presented in the bulk of this text address these identified testing needs.

II. DEFINING THE OBJECTIVE

The initial and most important aspect of a product safety evaluation program is the series of steps that leads to an actual statement of problems or of objectives of any testing and research program. This definition of objectives is essential and, as proposed here, consists of five steps: defining product or material use, quantitating or estimating exposure potential, identifying potential hazards, gathering baseline data, and finally, designing and defining the actual research program. Each of these steps is presented and discussed in detail below.

A. Product/Material Use

Identifying how a material is to be used, what it is to be used for, and how it is to be made are the essential first three questions to be answered before a meaningful assessment program can be performed. These determine, to a large extent, how many people are potentially exposed, to what extent and by what routes they are exposed, and what benefits are perceived or gained from product use. The answers to these questions are generally categorized or qualitative, and become quantitative (as will be reviewed in the next section) at a later step (frequently long after acute data has been generated).

Starting with an examination of how a material is to be made (or how it is already being made), it generally occurs that there are several process segments, each representing separate problems. Commonly, much of a manufacturing process is "closed" (that is, occurs in sealed airtight systems) limiting exposures to leaks with (generally) low-level inhalation and dermal exposures to significant portions of a plant work force and to maintenance and repair workers (generally short-term higher level inhalation and dermal exposures to small numbers of personnel). Smaller segments of the process almost invariably will not be closed. These segments are most common either where some form of manual manipulation is required, or where the segment requires a large volume of space (such as when fibers or other objects are spun or formed or individually coated with something), or where the product is packaged (such as powders being put into bags or polymers being removed from molds). The exact manner and quantity of each segment of the manufacturing process, given the development of a exposure categories for each of these segments, will then serve to help quantitate the identified categories.

Likewise, consideration of a product's use and how to use it should be of help in identifying who outside of the manufacturing process potentially will be exposed, by what routes, and to what extent.

The answers to these questions, again, will generate a categorized set of answers, but will also serve to identify which particular acts of regular toxicity testing may be operative (such as those for the Department of Transportation or Consumer Product Safety Commission). If a product is to be worn (such as clothing or jewelry) or used on or as an environmental surface (such as household carpeting or wall covering), the potential for the exposure of a large number of people (albeit at low levels in the case of most materials) is very large, while uses such as exterior portions of building would have much lower potentials for the number of individuals exposed. Likewise, the nature of the intended use (say as a true consumer product vs. as an industrial product) determines potential for extent and degree of exposure in overt and subtle manners. For example, a finish for carpets to be used in the home has a much greater potential for dermal and even oral (in the case of infants) exposure than such a product used only for carpeting in offices. Likewise, in general, true consumer products (such as household cleaners) have a greater potential for both accidental exposure and misuse.

B. Exposure Potential

The next problem (or step) is quantitating the exposure of the human population, both in terms of how many people are exposed by what routes (or means) and what quantities of an agent they are exposed to.

This process of identifying and quantitating exposure groups within the human population is beyond the scope of this chapter, except for some key points. Classification methods are the key tools for identifying and properly delimiting human populations at risk.

Classification is both a basic concept and a collection of techniques that are necessary prerequisites for further analysis of data when the members of a set of data are (or can be) each described by several variables. At least some degree of classification (which is broadly defined as the dividing of the members of a group into smaller groups in accordance with a set of decision rules) is necessary prior to any data collection. Whether formally or informally, an investigator has to decide which things are similar enough to be counted as the same and to develop rules governing collection procedures. Such rules can be as simple as "measure and record exposures only of production workers," or as complex as that demonstrated by the expanded classification presented in Example 1. Such a classification also demonstrates that the selection of which variables to measure will determine the final classification of data.

Example 1.

1. Which groups are potentially exposed?
2. What are segments of groups? Consumers, production workers, etc.
3. What are routes of potential exposure?
4. Which group does each route occur in?
5. Which sex is exposed?
6. Which age groups are potentially exposed?

Data classification serves two purposes: data simplification (also called a descriptive function) and prediction. Simplification is necessary because there is a limit to both the volume and complexity of data that the human mind can comprehend and deal with conceptually. Classification allows us to attach a label (or name) to each group of data, to summarize the data (that is, assign individual elements of data to groups and to characterize the population of the group), and to define the relationships between groups (that is, develop a taxonomy).

Prediction, meanwhile, is the use of summaries of data and knowledge of the relationships between groups to develop hypotheses as to what will happen when further data are collected (as when production or market segments are expanded) and as to the mechanisms which cause such relationships to develop. Indeed, classification is the prime device for the discovery of mechanisms in all of science. A classic example of this was Darwin's realization that there were reasons (the mechanisms of evolution) behind the differences and similarities in species which had caused Linaeus to earlier develop his initial modern classification scheme (or taxonomy) for animals.

To develop a classification, one first sets bounds wide enough to encompass the entire range of data to be considered, but not unnecessarily wide. This is typically done by selecting some global variables (variables all data have in common) and limiting the range of each so that it just encompasses all the cases on hand. One then selects a set of local variables characteristics which only some of the cases have, e.g., the occurrence of certain tumor types, enzyme activity levels, or dietary preferences, and which thus serve to differentiate between groups. Data are then collected, and a system for measuring differences and similarities is developed. Such measurements are based on some form of measurement of distance between two cases (x and y) in terms of each single variable scale. If the variable is a continuous one, then the simplest measure of distance between two pieces of data is the Euclidean distance, (d[x,y]) defined as:

$$d(x, y) = (x_i - y_i)^2$$

For categorical or discontinuous data, the simplest distance measure is the matching distance, defined as:

$$d(x, y) = \text{number of times } x_i \neq y_i$$

After we have developed a table of such distance measurements for each of the local variables, some weighing factor is assigned to each variable. A weighting factor seeks to give greater importance to those variables that are believed to have more relevance or predictive value. The weighted variables then are used to assign each piece of data to a group. The actual act of developing numerically based classifications and assigning data members to them is the realm of cluster analysis. Classification of biological data based on qualitative factors has been well discussed by Glass (3) and Gordon (2) who do an excellent job of introducing the entire field and mathematical concepts. Many biological data are qualitative, with the best schemes for classification based on objectively determinable differences with a biological basis.

An investigator must first understand the process involved in making, shipping, using, and disposing of a material. The Environmental Protection Agency (EPA) recently proposed guidelines for such identification and exposure quantitation (6). The exposure groups can be very large or relatively small populations, each with a markedly different potential for exposure. For (di-2-ethyl-hexyl) phthalate (DEHP), for example, the following at-risk populations have been identified:

IV route	3,000,000 receiving blood trans- fusions	50 mg/year
	50,000 dialysis patients	4,500 mg/year
	10,000 hemophiliacs	760 mg/year
Oral route	10,800,000 children under 3 years of age	434 mg/year
	220,000,000 adults	dietary contamination 1.1 mg/year

Not quantitated for DEHP were possible inhalation and dermal exposure. The question of routes of potential exposure is a very important one to be resolved, not only because the routes (oral, dermal, and inhalation being the major routes for environmental exposures) each represent different potentials for degree of absorption, but also because the routes dictate potential target organ differences (such as the lung for inhalation exposures) and special toxicity problems (such as delayed contact dermal or respiratory sensitization). These route-specific concerns are addressed in individual chapters in this book.

All such estimates of exposure in humans (and of the number of humans exposed) are subject to a large degree of uncertainty.

C. Potential Hazard

Once the types of exposures have been identified and the quantities approximated, one can develop a toxicity matrix by identifying the potential hazards. Such an identification can proceed by one of three major approaches:

1. Analogy from data reported in the literature
2. Structure–activity relationships
3. Predictive testing

Each of these is addressed by one or more chapters elsewhere in this volume. Chapter 2 details how to perform both rapid and detailed literature reviews (both hard and electronic). Such reviews can be performed either on the actual compounds of interest or on compounds that are similar by structure and/or use. Either way, it is uncommon that the information from a literature review will exactly match our current interests (that is, the same compounds being produced and used the same ways), but an analogous relationship can frequently be developed.

The use of structure–activity relationships (SARs) is addressed in Chapter 13, covering the current state-of-the-art in mathematical SAR methods and models. There are, however, nonmathematical analogy methods that are still used effectively. These methods are really forms of pattern recognition, starting with a knowledge of the hazards associated with similar or related structures. An example of such a scheme is that of Cramner and Ford (7), where a decision tree based on structural features (or lack of them) is used to categorize potential hazards.

The third approach, which is the main focus of this volume, is actual predictive testing. The following section sets forth a philosophy for test and test program design.

It should be noted, however, that each of these approaches has the potential to evaluate hazards in one of two ways: the first is to identify and/or classify existing types of hazards. If the potential for a hazard is unacceptable for the desired use of the material (such as a carcinogen would be for a food additive), then this level of answer is quite sufficient. The second manner in which (or degree to which) a category of potential toxicity may be addressed is quantitatively. In general, quantitative (as opposed to categorical or qualitative) toxicity assessment requires more work and is more expensive. This principle will be stressed in the section on test and program design. In general, it should be recognized that the literature approach can really only categorize potential hazards, and that SAR approaches are most effective as screens to classify potential hazards. Only predictive testing is really effective at quantitating toxicities and hazards and testing also may be designed (either purposely or by oversight) so that it serves to screen or classify toxicities.

It should be noted that there is a major area of weakness in all three approaches. This is the question of mixtures. For neither the literature, nor SAR methods, nor our present testing methods are really effective at evaluating other than pure compounds. There are now promising approaches to testing mixtures with limited numbers of components.

III. SELECTING AND DESIGNING TESTING PROGRAMS

Most of this book is devoted to the conduct and interpretation of actual tests and studies in toxicology. There are, however, general principles for the design of these tests and before any tests are conducted at all, a program must be designed so that resources are employed in an efficient manner at the same time as all required information is generated.

Finally, there are techniques and guidelines that are necessary to allow scheduling and control of testing programs, whether they be at external contract labs or at an internal facility.

A. Program Design

As pointed out earlier, there are three approaches to selecting which tests will be included in a safety evaluation: package-battery testing, tier testing, and the special case of SAR approaches to designing programs to test series of compounds. For all three approaches, one must first perform a review of existing data ("prior art" as outlined in Chapter 2) and then decide whether or not to repeat any of the tests so reported. If the judgment is made that the literature data is too unreliable or incomplete, then a repeat may be in order.

The battery-testing approach, which is not generally recommended or favored by the author, calls for performing all of a set of tests from an existing list. This approach has two advantages: First, it is the most practical and easiest to control for a "factory"-type operation where an overriding concern is completing testing on as many compounds as possible. Second, the results of such test packages are easy to compare to those of other compounds evaluated in identical packages. The main disadvantages are more compelling, however. First, battery programs use up more of every resource (animals, manpower, and test material, for example) except calendar time. Second, the questions asked and answered by the battery approach are not as sharply focused, as the test designs employed cannot be modified in light of data from lower (earlier) tier tests.

The tier approach, as previously exemplified by the scheme shown in Table 2, arose in the 1970s when concern about health effects broadened in scope and there were insufficient testing capabilities available to do every test on every material of concern. These schemes are proposed as a means of arriving at and performing an appropriate level and efficient course of testing. The levels of testing, or information generation, are arranged in a hierarchical system. Each tier contains a number of suggested tests that can appropriate information necessary for safe use or disposal of the material. *It is emphasized that a tier or level of testing does not contain mandatory tests, but that judgment is used, both in moving from one level of testing to another and in selecting the appropriate tests.* Lu (9) has proposed one such scheme. Beck et al. (10) have also developed and published a tier approach type system aimed to include the broader scope questions of environmental effects testing. They provide some valuable points of guidance as to criteria for proceeding to the higher (and more expensive) tier levels.

The last approach is for the special case when one is faced with evaluating a large series of materials that have closely related chemical structures, and desires to be able to rank them as to relative hazard. Frequently, time is a concern in completing such a program for these purposes, and efficiency in use of assets is very much desired. The SAR matrix approach calls for first identifying and classifying the structured features of the compounds. These features frequently vary on a simple basis (for example, length of carbon chain or number of substituent nitrogens). One can select the compounds at either end of such a linear series (for example, the compounds with 5 and 18 carbon chains) and evaluate them in a tier one (as per Table 2) series of tests. From this, one should determine the endpoints (say, sensitization potential and dermal irritation) that are of the greatest concern for the compounds in their intended use. Each compound in the series can then be tested for these endpoints specifically. Those that are then selected for use or further development based on such a methodology should be evaluated fully in a tier approach system.

B. Study Design

The most important step in designing an actual study is to firmly determine the objective(s) behind it. Based on the broadest classification of tests, there are generally two major sets of objectives. The first leads to what can be called single endpoint tests. Single endpoint tests are those for which only one restricted question is being asked. As will be shown below, such studies are generally straightforward and generate relatively simple data.

Such tests and their objectives (the questions they ask) are detailed below.

Primary dermal irritation (PDI). Evaluate potential of a single dermal exposure to cause skin irritation.

Primary eye irritation. Evaluate potential of a single ocular exposure to cause eye irritation.

Dermal corrosivity. Determine if a single 4-hr dermal exposure will result in skin corrosion.

Dermal sensitization. Evaluate the potential of a material to cause delayed contact hypersensitivity.

Photosensitization. Evaluate the potential of a material to cause a sunlight-activated delayed contact hypersensitivity.

Lethality screen. Determine if a single dose of a material, at a predetermined level, is lethal.

Genotoxicity. Determine if the material has potential to cause undesirable genetic events.

The second category contains the shotgun tests. The name "shotgun" suggests itself for these studies because it is not known in advance what endpoints are being aimed at. Rather, the purpose of the study is to identify and quantitate all potential systemic effects resulting from a single exposure to a compound. Once known, specific target organ effects can then be studied in detail if so desired. Accordingly, the generalized design of these studies is to expose groups of animals to controlled amounts or concentrations of the material of interest, then to observe for and measure as many parameters as practical over a period past or during the exposure. Further classification of tests within this category is defined either by the route by which test animals are exposed/dosed (generally oral, dermal, or inhalation are the options here) or by the length of dosing. Acutes, for example, imply a single exposure interval (of 24 hr or less) or dosing of test material or a small number of doses (say three) over a single 24-hr period. Using this second (length of dosing) scheme, objectives of shotgun studies could be defined as below.

Philosophy for What We Want Our Studies to Do (Objectives)

Acute

1. Set doses for next studies
2. Identify very or unusually toxic agents
3. Estimate lethality potential
4. Identify organ system affected

Two-week

1. Set doses for next studies
2. Identify organ toxicity
3. Identify very or unusually toxic agents
4. Estimate lethality potential
5. Evaluate potential for accumulation of effects
6. Get estimate of kinetic properties (blood sampling/urine sampling)

Four-week

1. Set doses for next studies
2. Identify organ toxicity
3. Identify very or unusually toxic agents
4. Estimate lethality potential
5. Evaluate potential for accumulation of effects
6. Get estimate of kinetic properties (blood sampling/urine sampling)
7. Elucidate nature of specific types of target organ toxicities induced by repeated exposure

Thirteen-week

1. Set doses for next studies
2. Identify organ toxicity
3. Identify very or unusually toxic agents
4. Evaluate potential for accumulation of effects
5. Evaluate pharmacokinetic properties
6. Elucidate nature of specific types of target organ toxicities induced by repeated exposure
7. Evaluate reversibility of toxic effects

"Lifetime studies"

1. Identify potential carcinogens
2. Elucidate nature of specific types of target organ toxicities induced by prolonged repeated exposure

There is also a special group of tests that focuses on broad groups of endpoints and that do not fit into either the route or length of exposure categories. These are the reproductive and developmental toxicology studies, each of which is the subject of a separate chapter in this volume.

The other objective in designing studies is to meet various regulatory requirements. A complete review of this objective is beyond the intent of this chapter. As it pertains to various test types, it is addressed in a number of other chapters, and a short overview of regulatory considerations and their complications was provided earlier.

The approach to the design and conduct of systemic toxicity studies, at least in common practice, has become very rigid and has not been subject to the sort of critical review which is commonly focused on proposed new study designs or test types. The changes made in the last 25 years have been largely restricted to using more animals, making more measurements on each, and rigidly following a standard protocol. The first of these changes, in an attempt to increase the value of the information from such studies by increasing statistical power, is a crude approach to improving study design. The second change is meant to insure the integrity of the data trail and documentation, but by its nature makes sensitive and efficient conduct of investigations more difficult. Clearly, use of some of the approaches described in Gad et al. (12) or Chapter 13 (and more to the point, adoption of the underlying philosophy) has significantly reduced animal usage while increasing both the quantity and quality of information gained.

There is one special case problem that calls for extra thought on the design and conduct of each of the study types discussed. This is the evaluation of the effects of mixtures. As the components of a mixture may have very different physiochemical characteristics (solubility, vapor pressure, density, etc.), great care must be taken in preparing and administering the mixture so that what is actually tested is the mixture of interest. Examples of such procedures are making dilutions (components of the mixture may not be equally soluble or miscible with the vehicle) and generating either vapors or respirable aerosols (components may not have equivalent volatility or surface tension leading to a test atmosphere that contains only a portion of the components of the mixture).

A second problem/concern with evaluating mixtures arises when (as is often the case) one is asked to extrapolate from a set of data on one mixture system (say, one with 79% of A, 8% of B, 7% of C, and 6% of D) to another with the same components in different prevalence (say, 40% of A, 8% of B,

40% of C, and 12% of D). Because of the highly interactive nature of biological systems, without a basis of understanding the actions and interactions of the components in a biological system, one cannot generally make such extrapolations. The exception, of course, is when either one component is much more toxic than all others or when toxicities aren't very different. One component constitutes a vast majority of many of the mixtures (95+%) in commerce.

The vehicle for translating a study design into the finished product is the protocol. A good protocol details who will do what, when, where, and how. As such, it might well be considered to be like the itinerary for a long and complicated trip. Gralla (13) has provided excellent guidance as to the dos and don'ts of protocol preparation.

IV. PROGRAM AND STUDY SCHEDULING

The problem of scheduling and sequencing of toxicology studies and of entire testing programs has been minimally addressed in print. Though there are several books and many articles available that address the question of scheduling of multiple tasks in a service organization (e.g., Ref. 14) and there is an extremely large literature on project management (15–17), no literature specific to a research testing organization exists (though various operational aspects are now addressed—see Arnold et al. (18). Project management approaches are a set of principles, methods, and techniques for establishing a sound basis for scheduling and controlling a multitask project (or indeed, a multiproject operation) in the face of complex labor, skill and facility requirement, and of modifying such plans and schedules as external requirements change. These techniques also serve to allow one to reverse the process and give project (study) requirements and time frames and to determine both manpower and facilities requirements. This is accomplished by identifying and quantifying networks and the critical paths within them.

For all the literature on project management, a review will quickly establish that these do not address the rather numerous details that affect study/program scheduling and management. There is, in fact, to my knowledge, only a single article (19) in the literature, and it describes a computerized scheduling system for single studies.

There are available commercial computer packages for handling the network construction, interactions, and calculations involved in what, as will be shown below, is a complicated process. These packages are available both on mainframe and microcomputer systems.

The single study case for scheduling is relatively simple. One begins with the length of the actual study. Then you factor in that before the study is actually started, several resources must be ensured.

Animals must be on-hand and properly acclimated (usually for at least two weeks prior to the start of the study).

Vivarium space, caging, and animal care support must be available.

Technical support for any special measurements such as necropsy, hematology, urinalysis, and clinical chemistry must be available on the dates specified in the protocol.

Necessary and sufficient test material must be on hand.

A formal written protocol suitable to fill regulatory requirements must be on hand and signed.

The actual study (from first dosing or exposure of animals to the last observation and termination of the animals) is called the in-life phase, and many people assume that the length of the in-life phase defines the time until a study is done. Rather, a study is not truly completed until any samples (blood, urine, and tissue) are analyzed, and a report written, proofed, and signed off. Roll all of this together, and if you are conducting a single study under contract in an outside laboratory, an estimate of the least time involved in its completion should be

$$L + 6 \text{ weeks} + \frac{1}{2} L$$

where L is the length of the study. If the study is a single end-point study and does not involve pathology, then the least time can be shortened to $L + 6$ weeks.

When one is scheduling out an entire testing program on contract, it should be noted that, if multiple tiers of tests are to be performed (such as an acute, 2-week, 13-week, and lifetime studies), then these must be conducted sequentially, as the answer from each study in the series defines the design and sets the doses for the following study.

If, instead of contracting out, one is concerned with managing a testing laboratory, then the situation is considerably more complex. The factors and activities involved are outlined below. Within these steps are rate-limiting factors that are invariably due to some critical point or pathway. Identification of such critical factors is one of the first steps for a manager to take to establish effective control over either a facility or program.

A. Prestudy Activities

Before any studies actually start, all of the following must occur (and, therefore, these activities are underway currently, to one extent or another, for the studies not yet underway but already authorized or planned this year).

Sample Procurement

Development of formulation and dosage forms for study

If inhalation study, development of generation and analysis methodology, chamber trials and verification of proper chamber distribution

Development and implementation of necessary safety steps to protect involved laboratory personnel

Arrangement for waste disposal

Scheduling to assure availability of animal rooms, manpower, equipment, and support services (pathology and clinical)

Preparation of protocols

Animal procurement, health surveillance, and quarantine

Preparation of data forms and books

Conduct of prestudy measurements on study animals to set baselines as to rates of body

weight gain and clinical chemistry values

B. Designs of Studies Commonly Performed

90-Day Oral Study. Groups of animals are given different measured doses of test compound formulation by stomach tube once a day, 5 days a week for 13–14 weeks. Every animal is observed in detail for clinical signs twice a day, 7 days a week); weighed at least once a week; has blood and urine collected at least twice during the study (with detailed clinical chemistries and hematology being performed on each sample); has a detailed necropsy performed on it (10 to 12 organs are weight; 40+ tissues are collected, slides prepared, and a detailed microscopic examination is performed); detailed special measures (renal function, neurologic function, etc.) may also be performed. A minimum of 220,000 pieces of data are collected on a minimum of 240 animals.

90-Day Inhalation Study. As above, however, instead of oral dosing, the animal groups are exposed in chambers to gases, vapors, or aerosols of very tightly controlled concentration and nature for six hours a day. Performing a 90-day study by this route adds no animals but does add at least 1,200 additional pieces of information.

Reproduction Study. Groups of animals are dosed with, fed with, or exposed to (by inhalation) several levels of a test compound and to a positive control material. Pairs of animals are mated and the resulting pregnant females are allowed to go to term. The resulting offspring are assessed as to their development. All aspects of reproductive performance and of viability of the offspring are assessed in detail. Selected members of the offspring generation continue to be dosed and are also mated. The reproductive performance of this generation of animals and the viability of the resulting offspring are assessed. Histopathology is performed on reproductive organs and tissues. At least 320 animals are involved in breedings and at least 185,000 pieces of data are generated.

Special Target Organ Studies (e.g., a renal toxicity study). Route and length of dosing/exposure of animals is variable, dependent on the particular problem being evaluated. Renal function is assessed by histopathology, clinical chemistry, specialized biochemical studies, and by a series of studies requiring microsurgical manipulations. These studies can involve some 700 animals and can produce some 210,000 pieces of data.

Two-Week Oral. The design is the same as that for the 90-day oral study; however, animal group sizes are smaller and dosing is once a day, 5 days a week for 2 weeks. This study will involve at least 80 animals and 70,000 pieces of data.

Two-Week Inhalation. This, too, is the same as the 90-day inhalation study; however, animal group sizes are smaller and exposure is 6 hr a day, 5 days a week, for 2 weeks. This study will involve at least 80 animals and 70,300 pieces of data.

Acute Inhalation. Separate groups of animals are exposed for (depending on the design 2,4, or 6 hours (four is most common) to different concentrations of a test gas, vapor, or aerosol; the animals are then observed over 2 weeks for effects before being terminated and necropsied. Detailed clinical observations are performed twice daily on every animal. Each animal is weighed at least seven times during the study. A detailed necropsy and microscopic examination of tissues is performed, organ weights are determined, and special observations or tests may also be performed. If at all possible, an LC_{50} is determined. Between 20–70 animals are utilized, generating on the average 13,000 pieces of data.

Acute Oral Study. This procedure is the same as that for the acute inhalation study; however, instead of exposure to an atmosphere containing the test compound, the animals are given a single dose of the formulation by stomach tube.

Acute Dermal Study. This follows the same procedure as the acute inhalation study; however, instead of exposure to an atmosphere containing the test compound, the animals have a portion of their back shaved. Measured amounts of the test material are applied to these shaved areas and covered with an occlusive patch for 24 hr, after which times the patches are removed and any remaining test material is washed off.

Primary Dermal Irritation Study. A group of six animals each have separate large areas of their backs shaved, onto which a 0.5 g or 0.5 ml portion of test material is placed. The test substance is then covered by an occlusive patch and removed 4 hr later, at which time excess test material is washed off. Separate regions of the back are also used for positive and vehicle control sites. The different skin regions that had been exposed are then evaluated for irritation (erythema and edema) at 24, 48, and 72 hr after the patch is removed. If significant irritation is observed, additional observations are made up to one week after the removal of the patch. Six animals are utilized to generate from 108 to 252 pieces of data.

Primary Eye Irritation Study. This test is only performed if a material has a pH of 3.1–10.9 and has proven not to be a severe skin irritant. The primary dermal irritation study for a particular skin compound is therefore always conducted first. Nine rabbits are used to evaluate the potential of test substance to irritate or damage the eye and to determine what value water may have in reducing damage. For 6 of the rabbits, the material is instilled into the eye and left for a period before being washed out. For the other 3 rabbits, 20 sec after the material is instilled into the eye, the eye is vigorously rinsed with a stream of water. The eyes are then examined every other day with an ophthalmoscope, with all observations being scored on the Draize system. Nine rabbits generate some 126 pieces of data.

Guinea Pig Sensitization Study. A group of guinea pigs have patches of their skin shaved regularly, patched with test and control materials, and read for edema and erythema over a period of 6–7 weeks (a negative test result requires an additional week of testing). A separate group of animals is always concurrently exposed to a similar positive control substance.

The laboratory should always run batteries of these tests together to achieve an economy of mass by sharing one control group of animals for all of the studies. A group of 13–21 animals are used to generate 648 pieces of data.

Guinea Pig Maximization Study. A group of guinea pigs (larger than the number used in the preceding study) have test substance and immunological adjutant solution subcutaneously injected repeatedly during the induction phase. They are then exposed via patching to the above test substance during the challenge phase. Skin regions are evaluated for edema and erythema as above over a period of 6–7 weeks. A separate concurrent positive control group is also always used here. As many as 20–40 animals are used to generate 1,200 pieces of data.

1. Poststudy Activities

After completion of the in-life phase (that is, the period during which live animals are used) of any study, significant additional effort is still required to complete the research. This effort includes the following:

Preparation of tissue slides and microscopic evaluation of these slides
Preparation of data tables
Statistical analysis of data
Preparation of reports

There are a number of devices available to a manager to help improve/optimize the performance of a laboratory involved in these activities. Four such devices (or principles) are general enough to be particularly attractive.

Cross Training. Identification of rate-limiting steps in a toxicology laboratory over a period of time usually reveals that at least some of these are variable (almost with the season). At times, there is too much work of one kind (say, inhalation studies) and too little of another (say, dietary studies). The available staff for inhalation studies cannot handle this peak load and as the skills between these two groups are somewhat different, the dietary staff (which is now not fully occupied) cannot simply relocate down the hall and help out. However, if early on one identifies low and medium skill aspects of the work involved in inhalation studies, one could cross-train the dietary staff at a convenient time so that staff could be redeployed to meet peak loads.

Economy of Mass. Especially for acute studies, much of the effort involved in study preparation, conduct, and completion is baseline. That is, whereas it takes hours to set up for a single irritation study, it takes only 7 to set up for two, 8 for three, and so on. Such studies are most efficiently performed in groups or batteries.

Flexibility and Prioritization. All too many laboratories let themselves be caught up in bulky systems for study startup, such that any change in schedule means going back to the beginning and losing substantial effort along the way. Systems for study preparation should be studied to insure that they are flexible enough to allow for changes in priority that frequently occur. Likewise, prioritization of studies should be performed so that the results of planning efforts are as stable as possible.

Shared Controls. Acute studies frequently include a control group receiving either vehicle to guard against "background noise") or a positive control (to ensure system sensitivity). If such studies are performed in battery (that is, two or three guinea pig sensitization studies at a time), one can legitimately use one common ("shared") control group of animals for the entire battery of studies. This will both save labor and reduce the number of animals employed.

Chapter 14 should be consulted for detailed guidance as to contracting out studies. When doing so, it should be kept in mind that comparative shopping for toxicology studies is very tricky. A detailed examination of protocols is essential to ensure that the different prices are for two different things (apples and oranges) that are called the same thing. Small variations in such factors as numbers of animals used and length of postdosing observational period can make large differences in both the cost and information value of a study.

V. RISK AND HAZARD ASSESSMENT

Once one has the complete package of information resulting from a testing program, and must determine what it means in terms of the potential sales packaging and use of the project, a risk or hazard assessment is called for. Chapter 15 has addressed the nonmathematical aspects of such efforts. For guidance on the special case of mathematical risk assessment, one should refer to Gad (20). Beginning a meaningful risk or hazard assessment, however, must start with an understanding of what is acceptable in the case of the use for which a product is intended.

VI. GREAT DISASTERS IN PRODUCT SAFETY ASSESSMENT

No attempt to address the topic this chapter (or, indeed, this entire volume) is aimed at would be complete without providing the reader with some guidance as to common pitfalls to avoid.

Indeed, there are a number of common mistakes (in both the design and conduct of studies and in how such information is used) that have led to unfortunate results, ranging from losses in time and money and the discarding of perfectly good potential products to serious threats to people's health. Such outcomes are indeed the great disasters in product safety assessment, especially since many of them are avoidable if attention is paid to a few basic principles.

VII. FALLACIES AND FAILURES

A. Program Design

1. All too many people believe that if a material is polymer based, that no toxicities can be associated with it. Based on this assumption, polymers then may not be evaluated at all for safety. The basis for this assumption is the premise that molecules of greater than approximately 10,000 MW cannot gain entry to the body by traditional routes of exposure.

The errors in this assumption are that very few polymers are the products of reactions that have gone to completion (and therefore contain contaminants of lower molecular weight that may gain entry to the body) and that polymers may burn (therefore decomposing into smaller and more reactive molecules).

2. A generalization of the above "molecular weight rule" holds that monomers are more toxic than dimers, which in turn, are more toxic than the trimers, and so on. This is not true; dicyclopentadiene, for example, is much more toxic than cyclopentadiene. Another way of saying this is that SAR models

provide guidance as to trends in effects within structural series, but not hard and fast rules.

3. It has also been assumed by a number of people that if a material is handled only within a closed system, there is no product safety concern because there is no exposure potential. This assumption has always been fallacious; dosed systems must be opened up to be cleaned and maintained. And they leak, sometimes disastrously, as at Bophal.

4. The best model for studying effects of materials in humans is the human itself. What is seen in animal models should never be expected to be exactly the same in humans, and seeing nothing adverse in tightly controlled animal studies does not guarantee that the same material will be "safe" in the hands of humans.

B. Study Design

It is quite possible to design a study for failure. Common shortfalls include:

1. Wrong animal model.
2. Wrong route.
3. Wrong vehicle or form of test material.
4. In studies where several dose levels are studied, the worst thing that can happen is to have an effect at the lowest level tested (not telling you what dosage is safe in animals much less in humans). The next worst thing is to not have an effect at the highest dose tested (generally meaning, you won't know what the signs of toxicity are and invalidating the study in the eyes of many regulatory agencies).
5. Making leaps of faith. An example is to set dosage levels based on others' data and to then dose all your test animals. At the end of the day, all animals in all dose levels are dead. The study is over, the problem remains.
6. Using the wrong concentration of test material in a study. Many effects (including both dermal and gastrointestinal irritation, for example) are very concentration dependent.
7. Failure to include a recovery group. If you find an effect in a 90-day study (say, gastric hyperplasia), how do you interpret it? How does one respond to the regulatory question, "Will it progress to cancer?" If an additional group of animals was included in dosing, then was maintained for a month after dosing had been completed, recovery (reversibility) of such observations could be both evaluated and (if present) demonstrated.

REFERENCES

1. Hartigan, J.A. (1983). Classification. In *Encyclopedia of Statistical Sciences*, Vol. 2. Edited by S. Katz and N.L. Johnson. New York, John Wiley.
2. Gordon, A.D. (1981). *Classification*. New York, Chapman and Hall.

3. Glass, L. (1975). Classification of biological networks by their qualitative dynamics. *J. Theor. Biol.* 85–107.
4. Schaper, M., Thompson, R.D., and Alarie, Y. (1985). A method to classify airborne chemicals which alter the normal ventilatory response induced by CO_2. *Toxicol. Appl. Pharmacol.* 79:332–341.
5. Kowalksi, B.R. and Bender, C.F. (1972). Pattern recognition. A powerful approach to interpreting chemical data. *J. Am. Chem. Soc.* 94:5632–5639.
6. EPA (1984). *Proposed Guidelines for Exposure Assessment*, F R 49 No. 227, November 23, 46304–46312.
7. Cramner, C.M., Ford, R.A., and Hall, R.L. (1978). Estimation of toxic hazard-a decision tree approach. *Food. Cosmet. Toxicol.* 16:255–276.
8. Hisham, A.F.M., Reardon, K.F. and Yang, R.S.H. (1997). Integral approach for the analysis of toxicologic interactions of thermal mixtures. *Ent Rev. Toxicology.* 267: 175–198.
9. Lu, Frank C. (1985). *Basic Toxicology.* New York, Hemisphere Publishing Corp., pp. 68–95.
10. Beck, L.W., Maki, A.W., Artman, N.R., and Wilson, E.R. (1981). Outline and criteria for evaluating the safety of new chemicals. *Reg. Toxicol. Pharmacol.* 1: 19–58.
11. Page, N.P. (1986). International harmonization of toxicity testing. In *Safety Evaluation of Drugs and Chemicals.* Edited by W.E. Lloyd. New York, Hemisphere Publishing, Inc., pp. 455–467.
12. Gad, S.C., Smith, A.C., Cramp, A.L., Gavigan, F.A., and Derelanko, M.J. (1984). Innovative designs and practices for acute systemic toxicity studies. *Drug Chem. Tox.* (5):423–434.
13. Gralla, E.J. (1981). Protocol preparation design and objectives. In *Scientific Considerations in Monitoring and Evaluating Toxicological Research.* (Edited by E. J. Gralla.) New York, Hemisphere Publishing Corporation, pp. 1–26.
14. French, S. (1982). *Sequencing and Scheduling.* New York, Halsted Press.
15. Kaufman, A. and Desbazeille, G. (1969). *The Critical Path Method.* Gordon and Breach Science Publishers.
16. Martin, C.C. (1976). *Project Management: How to Make It Work.* New York, Animal Management Association.
17. Kerzner, H. (1979). Project Management: *A Systems Approach to Planning, Scheduling and Controlling.* New York, Van Nostrand Reinhold Company.
18. Arnold, D.L., Derice, H.C. and Kerewski, D.R. (1990) *Handbook of In Vivo Toxicity Testing.* San Diego, Academic Press.
19. Levy, A.E., Simon, R.C., Beerman, T.H., and Fold, R.M. (1977). Scheduling of toxicity protocol studies. *Comput. Biomed. Res.* 10:139–151.
20. Gad, S.C. (1997). *Statistics and Experimental Design for Toxicologists, 3rd Edition,* Boca Raton, FL, CRC Press.

2
Toxicology Information Sources and Their Use

Robert W. Kapp, Jr.
BioTox, Richmond, Virginia

Searching for information on toxic chemicals can be complex. One critical stumbling block is the fact that key information is frequently spread throughout books, journals, electronic databases, company files, and state, federal, and local documents. There is no single source where one can go to acquire these data. It also may be that a considerable amount of data are simply in a company file somewhere and are not available to any outside source. One must be diligent in trying to obtain these data from all available sources in order to get a focused and accurate toxicological profile of any chemical.

The science of toxicology, as with all scientific disciplines, is predicated upon documented research of prior toxicological studies. In other words, the work of all previous toxicologists is considered before one can make a well-founded judgment about the characteristics of a chemical. Hence, the appropriate starting place in the review of the toxicity of a compound is the determination of what is known about the material and its analogs. Access to these data is absolutely critical to the accurate assessment of the toxicological potential of any material. With the ever-increasing number of data sources, it is particularly important that the toxicologist be familiar with how to locate relevant reference data. To further complicate the picture, some of the existing toxicological data is not available either in published form or in electronic databases because it is considered proprietary. It becomes difficult to obtain some information depending upon the nature of the material. Informal acquisition of some of these unpublished data from colleagues in the field can be another mechanism by which one can obtain this information. Frequently these unpublished data are negative and are not submitted to any journal nor made available to electronic databases simply because there appears to be no publication interest. There are some journals that refuse negative studies in lieu of more "interesting" positive findings, so the lack of pursuit of publishing negative data has some basis in fact. This is unfortunate since there is considerable effort and use of resources wasted in pursuit of these data that could be used elsewhere. Because of the difficulties in locating some unpublished data, it is important that one knows how to obtain as much available published and electronic data as possible.

This chapter is divided into 4 sections. The purpose of the first section is to outline the types of information that should be gathered out the outset in order to get the most out of a search of the literature. It is a starting point that should help the reader accumulate some necessary information prior to initiating a literature search. These basic data can be found in reference books, company records (if attainable) and manuals as well as databases such as CHEMID, Chemical Abstract Service, CS ChemFinder and ChemInfo. The MSDS databases can also be useful in obtaining basic physical and biological information.

The second section provides a list of the more common published literature sources and general traditional information sources. This would include sources such as textbooks and published reference books, abstracts and indices, handbooks and toxicology journals. Generally, after identifying the material and obtaining the basic information as described above, one should locate what data are well established. This includes general toxicology textbooks, toxicology handbooks, and reference books.

The third section provides online data sources such as university, private, and government web sites, the National Library of Medicine, and MSDS information systems. Considerable toxicological data are now available online. One has to be able to determine which data are validated and which data are of questionable origin. The National Library of Medicine Databases are the best place to start. They have the most information and are reliable. There are numerous government web sites now available. Some do have toxicological information while others have limited data. There are several web sites that provide online resources. These are very helpful in seeking various additional toxicological data sources after one exhausts the NLM databases.

The fourth section provides miscellaneous online sources such as search engines, listservs, and organization sites. The search engines are very useful in locating general information on many subjects. They are more limited in their usefulness in seeking specific chemical data per se. The listservs are mailing lists where various topics are discussed based upon topics thrown out by the listserv participants. The EPA has various unidirectional listservs that simply distribute regulatory information as it appears in the Code of Federal Regulations. These are helpful in keeping up with the very latest from Washington, but cannot be searched for specific chemicals. The organizational sites are even less helpful; however, the Society of Toxicology has several excellent subsites that present up-to-date online data sources as well as narrative about regulatory activities in Washington.

URLs (Uniform Resource Locators) for the Internet Sites that have been mentioned in this chapter have been provided. Because of the constantly changing nature of the World Wide Web, some of these URLs may have changed or been discontinued by the time this chapter goes to press. In that case, you should seek a search engine (see Section III) and search for the topic in question.

I. GETTING STARTED

Prior to reviewing the literature, it is critical to collect as much of the compositional and exposure information as possible. These data might include the following:

Chemical Abstracts Service Registry Number (CAS). This information is usually available from various sources. One can access this from Chemical Abstract Service (STN or STN Easy) directly on the Internet: http://www.cas.org/. The NLM's CHEMID is an excellent source of basic information that also provides synonyms and the location of other material on the chemical in question. Another service that can provide basic chemical information is CS ChemFinder: http://chemfinder.camsoft.com/.

Molecular formula/molecular weight. This basic information is available at the ChemFinder site noted above as well as at the National Institute of Standards and Technology web site: http://webbook.nist.gov/chemistry/; see also NLM's CHEMID.

Common synonyms. General search of World Wide Web via search engines, the NLM's CHEMID and CS ChemFinder: http://chemfinder.camsoft.com/.

Trade names. General Search of World Wide Web and the NLM's CHEMID.

Structural diagram. CS ChemFinder: http://chemfinder.camsoft.com/ or ChemInfo: http://accounts.camsoft.com/cheminfo/.

Chemical composition and major impurities. Manufacturer's MSDSs; various MSDS systems (See Section III below) and ChemInfo: http://accounts.camsoft.com/cheminfo/.

Production and use information. Available from manufacturer; sometimes available on NLM's TRI (Toxic Chemical Release Inventory).

Physical properties. See ChemFinder, ChemInfo, and NIST databases above.

Chemical analogs/SAR information. ChemInfo, STN (Scientific and Technical Information Network): http://www.cas.org.stn.html; Dialog: http://www.dialogweb.com/ and Health Designs Inc. (see below).

Known pharmacological/toxicological properties. NLM's TOXLINE, HSDB (Hazardous Substance Data Bank), IRIS (Integrated Risk Information System), STN, Dialog, and MSDS Databases (see below).

The purpose of collecting this information at the outset is twofold. First, as noted above, even though there are a myriad of places one can locate toxicological information, much data are unavailable due to the proprietary nature of the material in question and there are few journals that will publish uninteresting or completely negative data on a routine basis. Secondly, these data can provide a broader perspective on hazard assessment and possible information sources. For instance, a low pH would indicate a high irritation potential while a particular use pattern might indicate numerous databases where toxicological information might be available (i.e., a pesticide could have several EPA databases with toxicological data because of the fact that it is a pesticide).

The National Library of Medicine (see Section III) has an online Chemical Identification file (CHEMID) that is available on the Medical Literature Analysis and Retrieval System (MEDLARS®) for a fee. It serves as a mechanism to identify all 335,000 substances cited in all NLM databases. In addition, CHEMID contains SUPERLIST, providing regulatory information maintained by federal and state regulatory agencies on the chemical in question.

A good starting point can be one of the numerous MSDS systems that are described in Section III. These systems usually contain basic information about the physical–chemical nature of the material and they frequently have references to the source of the stated information. From this point, one can access the National Library of Medicine's CHEMID to locate any data within the NLM system as well as to determine whether or not the chemical is present on any federal or state regulatory list.

II. PRINTED GENERAL TEXTBOOKS AND REFERENCE MANUALS

The most obvious sources of information are conventionally published toxicology textbooks and general toxicology reference manuals. These publications provide the well-documented picture of the data the material. These books rarely speculate on the findings and generally do not provide undocumented facts regarding the chemical's toxicity. It should also be pointed out that much of latest research is not included in these texts because of the nature of the publishing time involved in a textbook. While these data are substantiated, they are usually 2 to 3 years behind the current research. However, the basics and generally recognized toxicological data are usually presented in these types of texts. This generally provides a sound starting point in the quest for toxicological data sources.

A. General Search Techniques

There are several sources that provide guidance on how to search the Internet. Among the more useful ones is the following:

Safety & Health on the Internet, Ralph B. Stuart, ISBN: 0865875235, Government Institutes, Inc., December 1996.

While these appear to be dated, the concept and approach to the search remain the same:

Information Resources in Toxicology, Philip Wexler, Elvelsier, June 1988.
Available Toxicology Information Sources and Their Use, In: Product Safety Evaluation Handbook, S.C. Gad (ed.), ISBN: 0824778294, Marcel Dekker, June 1988.
Information Sources and Support Networks in Toxicology, K.S. Sidhu, T.M. Stewart, and E.W. Netton, Amer. Coll. Toxicol. 8:1011–1026, 1989.

B. General Toxicology Textbooks

The following is a list the most common printed sources of information in the field of toxicology at this writing:

Animal Clinical Chemistry; A Primer for Toxicologists, G.O. Evans (ed.), ISBN: 0748403515, Taylor & Francis, Inc., April 1996.
Annual Review of Pharmacology & Toxicology, Vol. 37, Reviews, Incorporated Annual, ISBN: 0824304373, Annual Reviews, April 1997.
Basic Guide to Pesticides; Their Characteristics and Hazards, Shirley A. Briggs, ISBN: 1560322535, Taylor & Francis, Inc., August 1992.
Basic Toxicology: Fundamentals, Target Organ & Risk Assessment, Frank C. Lu, ISBN: 1560323809, Taylor & Francis, Inc., January 1996.
Casarett & Doull's Toxicology: The Basic Science of Poisons, Curtis D. Klaasen (ed.), ISBN: 0071054766, McGraw-Hill, November 1995.
Chemical Exposure & Toxic Responses, Stephen K. Hall, Joanna Chakraborty, and Randall J. Ruch, ISBN: 1566702399, Lewis Publishers, October 1996.
Comprehensive Toxicology, I. Sipes, Charlene A. McQueen, A. Gandolfi (eds.), ISBN: 0080423019, Elsevier Science, August 1997.
Food Safety & Toxicity, Vries De, ISBN: 0849394880, CRC Press, Inc., July 1995.
Handbook of Toxicology, Michael J. Derelanko, Mannfred A. Hollinger (eds.), ISBN: 0849386683, CRC Press, Inc., July 1995.
Industrial Toxicology (Industrial Health & Safety), Phillip L. Williams, ISBN: 047128887X, Wiley/VNR, December 1989.
Introduction to Toxicology, John A. Timbrell, ISBN: 0748402411, Taylor & Francis, Inc., January 1995.
Loomis's Essentials of Toxicology, 4th Edition, Ted A. Loomis, A. Wallace Hayes, ISBN: 0124556256, Academic Press, April 1996.
Occupational Toxicology, Neill H. Stacey (ed.), ISBN: 085066831X, Taylor & Francis, Inc., January 1993.
Patty's Industrial Hygiene & Toxicology: General Principles, George D. Clayton and

Florence E. Clayton (eds.), ISBN: 0471501964, John Wiley & Sons, Inc., due in January 2000.

Principles of Toxicology, Karen E. Stine and Thomas M. Brown, ISBN: 873716841, Lewis Publishers, June 1996.

Regulatory Toxicology, Shayne C. Gad, Joseph F. Holson, and Christopher P. Chengelis, ISBN: 0781701910, Lippincott, January 1995.

Textbook of Toxicology: Principles & Applications, Raymond J. Niesink, John De Vries, and Mannfred A. Hollinger, ISBN: 0849392322, CRC Press, Inc., January 1996.

The TSCA Compliance Handbook, Ginger L. Griffin, ISBN: 0471162272, John Wiley & Sons, Inc., August 1996.

Toxicology, Osweiler & Osweiler, ISBN: 0683066641, Williams & Wilkins, October 1995.

Toxicology of Industrial Compounds, Helmut Thomas, Robert Hess, Felix Waechter (eds.), ISBN: 074840239X, Taylor & Francis, Inc., November 1995.

Toxicology of Pesticides in Animals, T.S.S. Dikshith, ISBN: 084936907X, January 1991.

C. Reference Materials

The following books and manuals contain mostly tables of data and toxicological assessments of specific chemicals rather than general concepts:

A Comprehensive Guide to the Hazardous Properties of Chemical Substances (Industrial Health & Safety), Pradyot Patnaik, ISBN: 0471283932, Wiley/VNR, December 1992.

Catalog of Teratogenic Agents, 8th Edition, Thomas H. Shapard, ISBN: 0801851823, Johns Hopkins University Press, September 1995.

Chemical Information Manual, OSHA Staff, ISBN: 0865874697, Government Institutes, Inc., August 1995.

Chemical Safety Data Sheets: Toxic Chemicals, Royal Society of Chemistry—Staff, ISBN: 0851863213, CRC Press, January 1992.

Chemical Ranking & Scoring: Guidelines for Relative Assessments of Chemicals, SETAC, Adam Socha; Foundation for Environmental Education, Mary Swanson, ISBN: 1880611120, SETAC, November 1997.

Dangerous Properties of Industrial and Consumer Chemicals, Nicholas P. Cheremisinoff, John Allison King, and Randi Boyko, ISBN: 0824791835, Marcel Dekker Inc., January 1994.

Dictionary of Toxicology, Ernest Hodgson, Janice E. Chambers, and Richard B. Mailman, ISBN: 1561592161, Groves Dic, August 1997.

Encyclopedia of Toxicology Chemicals and Concepts, Philip Wexler, ISBN: 012227220-X, Academic Press, March 1998.

Essentials of Environmental Toxicology: Environmentally Hazardous Substances and Human Health, W. Hughes, ISBN: 1560324708, Taylor & Francis, Inc., September 1996.

Handbook of Data on Pesticides, George W.A. Milne, ISBN: 0849324475, CRC Press, Inc., January 1995.

Handbook of Chemical Toxicity Profiles of Biological Species: Aquatic Species, Vol. 1, Sub Ramamoorthy, Earle Gerard, Yantdeo Baddaloo, ISBN: 1566700132, Lewis Publishers, June 1995.

Health Effects of Hazardous Materials, Vol. 3, Neil Ostler, Thomas Byrne, and M.J. Malachowski, ISBN: 0023895519, Prentice Hall, May 1996.

Medical Toxicology: Diagnosis & Treatment of Human Poisoning, Matthew J. Ellenhorn and Donald G. Barceloux, ISBN: 0683300318, Williams and Wilkins, September 1996.

NIOSH Pocket Guide to Chemical Hazards, Henry Chan (ed.), DHHS (NIOSH), Publication No. 97-140, US Government Printing Office, June 1997.

National Toxicology Program's Chemical Database, Vol. 1: Chemical Names & Synonyms, Edward J. Calabrese and Linda Baldwin, ISBN: 0873717031, Lewis Publishers, September 1993.

Patty's Industrial Hygiene & Toxicology: Health Effects of Hazardous Materials, Lewis J. Cralley, Lester V. Cralley, and Robert L. Harris, ISBN: 0471586773, John Wiley & Sons, Inc., May 1993.

Sax's Dangerous Properties of Industrial Materials: 1993 Update, Richard J. Lewis and N. Irving Sax, ISBN: 0442016751, Van Nostrand Reinhold, January 1994.

Toxicology Desk Reference: The Toxic Exposure and Medical Monitoring Index 4th Ed., Robert Ryan, Claude E. Terry, ISBN: 1560326158, Hemisphere Publishing Corp., April 1997.

Toxicology & Environmental Health Information Resources: The Role of the National Library of Medicine, Catharyn T. Liverman, Carolyn E. Fulco, Carrie Ingalls, and Howard Kipen (eds.), ISBN: 0309056861, National Academy of Social Insurance, February 1997.

Toxicology Handbook of Hazardous Chemicals, N. Howard (ed.), ISBN: 0873713958, Lewis Publishers, October 1996.

D. Abstracts and Indices

These print indices are rarely used; however, they are available in many libraries. Most of the data contained in these printed indices are available through the National Library of Medicine.

Biological Abstracts.   1926 to date. Comprehensive coverage of biological research literature. Animal toxicology of toxic substances covered.

Index Medicus.   1879 to date. Comprehensive coverage of worldwide biomedical literature.

Industrial Hygiene Digest.   1980 to date. Coverage of industrial medicine, chemical and physical hazards, environmental and safety issues, and accident prevention.

Pollution Abstracts.   1970 to date. Coverage of air, marine, freshwater, noise, and land pollution, sewage treatment, and pesticide and chemical contaminants.

E. Journals

The following is a partial listing of some representative journals that are commonly referenced in the field of toxicology.

> American Industrial Hygiene Association Journal
> Environmental Health Perspectives
> Environmental Science and Technology
> Environmental and Molecular Mutagenesis
> Fundamental and Applied Toxicology
> International Journal of Toxicology
> Journal of Occupational and Environmental Medicine
> Journal of Applied Toxicology
> Journal of Toxicology and Environmental Health
> Pesticide and Toxic Chemical News
> Regulatory Toxicology and Pharmacology
> Toxicology and Applied Pharmacology
> Toxicology and Industrial Health
> Toxicology Letters
> Toxicology

III. ONLINE DATA SOURCES

The number of online data sources has expanded considerably over the last few years. New web sites go online every day. So, by the time this book goes to press, there will be a host of new sites that have been omitted and some of the ones mentioned will no longer be operating. Perhaps some will have new URLs or addresses. Most will probably be out there on the World Wide Web somewhere.

Some of the more important online data sources are outlined below. The purpose here is to familiarize the reader with what is available and not to be a line-by-line flowchart as to how to access or search the data.

A. National Library of Medicine

The National Library of Medicine (NLM) is probably the most critical source of information for toxicologists. It is the world's largest medical library and supports a large network of regional and medical libraries. MEDLARS® is the information retrieval system for the NLM. It provides access to over 40 online databases that contain over 18 million citations. One needs an NLM User ID code to search all of these files except PubMed and Internet Grateful Med (IGM) (see below). MEDLINE® database contains more than 9 million reference articles dating back to 1966 published in 3,900 biomedical journals in the United States and in over 70 countries worldwide. 88% of the citations are in English and 76% have English abstracts. MEDLINE® contains all of the Index Medicus citations. Over 30,000 new citations are added each month.

In June of 1997, NLM announced that this MEDLINE® database could be accessed for free over the World Wide Web. The systems that provide this access are PubMed and Internet Grateful Med. If the reader desires more information about these free online databases, more information can be obtained at the following URL: http://www.nlm.nih.gov/databases/freemedl.html.

Of particular interest to the toxicologist are the following databases:

CHEMID (Chemical Identification) serves as an authority file for the identification of chemicals in the NLM databases. It contains basic information on over 335,000 substances found in the NLM databases. The data elements provided in CHEMID include: Registry Numbers, Molecular Formulas, Systematic Names, Synonyms, Name and Formula Fragments, and List and File Locator Designations. CHEMID also provides directory assistance for the chemical in question as to where it has been identified. This feature is termed SUPERLIST and it is a collection of federal and state regulatory agencies as well as selected scientific organizations concerned with health and environmental hazards of chemical substances.

TOXLINE (Toxicology Information Online) is the NLM's extensive collection of online bibliographic information covering the pharmacological, biochemical, physiological and toxicological effects of chemicals. It contains over 2.5 million citations, most of which have abstracts, index terms, and Chemical Abstract Service (CAS) Registry Numbers. Citations with a publication year 1980 or older are located in the backfiles. (TOXLINE65) Information in TOXLINE is taken from 19 secondary subfile sources list in Table 1.

TOXNET (Toxicology Data Network) is a computerized network of files oriented primarily toward toxicology and related areas. The system contains modules for building and reviewing records as well as providing sophisticated search and retrieval features. The following 11 files are currently available on the TOXNET system:

1. HSDB (Hazardous Substances Data Bank) is a toxicology databank containing information on over 4,500 hazardous chemicals. The files contain toxicology, emergency handling procedures, environmental fate, human exposure, detection methods, and regulatory requirements. The file is referenced and peer-reviewed by a Scientific Review Panel.

2. TRI (Toxic Chemical Release Inventory) contains information from private companies on the annual estimated releases of toxic chemi-

Table 1   Secondary Subfiles Utilized in the TOXLINE Database

Acronym	Information and/or Citation Source
ANEUPL	Aneuploidy
CA	Chemical-Biological Activities
DART	Developmental and Reprodcutive Toxicology
EMIC	Environmental Mutagen Information Center File
ETIC	Environmental Teratology Information Center File
EPIDEM	Epidemiology Information System
FEDRIP	Federal Research in Progress
HMTC	Hazardous Materials Technical Center
IPA	International Pharmaceutical Abstracts
NIOSHTIC	National Institute of Occupational Safety and Health Technical Information Center
PESTAB	Pesticides Abstracts
PPBIB	Poisonous Plants Bibliography
RISKLINE	Swedish National Chemicals Inspectorate
TSCATS	Toxic Substances Control Act Submissions
TOXBIB	Toxicity Bibliography
BIOSIS	Toxicology Aspects of Environmental Health
NTIS	Toxicology Document and Data Depository
CRISP	Toxicology Research Projects

cals to the environment. This information is mandated by the Right-to-Know Act and is collected by the EPA. These data have been collected since 1991 and include approximately 300 chemicals.

3. IRIS (Integrated Risk Information System contains EPA carcinogenic and noncarcinogenic health risk and regulatory information on over 600 chemicals. IRIS contains EPA Drinking Water Health Advisories and references. The risk assessment data have been reviewed by EPA and represent EPA consensus opinion.

4. RTECS® (Registry of Toxic Effects of Chemical Substances) contains acute, chronic eye, skin, carcinogenicity, mutagenicity, reproductive, and multiple dose study effects data on over 135,000 chemicals. These data are maintained by NIOSH and are not peer-reviewed.

5. CCRIS (Chemical Carcinogenesis Research Information System) contains peer-reviewed data derived from carcinogenicity, mutagenicity, tumor promotion, and tumor inhibition tests on over 7,000 chemicals.

6. GENE-TOX (Genetic Toxicology) is a data bank maintained by EPA

containing genetic toxicology data on over 3,000 chemicals. The test systems and data are peer-reviewed.

7. DART® (Developmental and Reproductive Toxicology) is a database covering teratology and reproductive literature published since 1989. It contains over 30,000 citations and is a continuation of ETIC-BACK.

8. ETICBACK (Environmental Teratology Information Center Back-file) is a database covering teratology and reproductive literature published from 1950 to 1989. It contains 49,000 citations and is continued by DART® above.

9. EMIC (Environmental Mutagen Information Center) is a database containing over 15,000 citations to literature on chemical, biological, and physical agents that have been tested for genotoxic activity since 1991.

10. EMICBACK (Environmental Mutagen Information Center Backfile) is a database containing over 75,000 citations on chemical, biological, and physical agents published from 1950 to 1991.

11. TRIFACTS (Toxic Chemical Release Inventory Facts) is a supplemental database to the TRI file noted above containing information related to health, ecological, safety, and handling of these chemicals.

B. Other Government Web Sites

For a complete directory of online Government Information resources see Official Federal Government Web Sites: http://lcweb.loc.gov/global/ncp/ncp.html.

Below are some of the more common government sites that may have toxicology information:

EPA Homepage: http://www.epa.gov/epahome.
National Archives and Records Administration: http://www.access.gpo.gov/.
Agency for Toxic Substances and Disease Registry (ATSDR): http://atsdr1.atsdr.cdc.gov/.
OSHA Computerized Information System—Homepage: http://www.osha.gov/.
NIOSH Homepage: http://www.cdc.gov/niosh/homepage.html.
NIOSH AgCenter: http://agcenter.ucdavis.edu/agcenter/niosh.html.
FedWorld Information Network: http://www.fedworld.gov/.
National Institute of Environmental Health Sciences: http://www.niehs.nih.gov/.
NTP (National Toxicology Program)—Homepage: http://ntp-server.niehs.nih.gov/.
National Institutes of Health—Homepage: http://www.nih.gov/.

National Cancer Institute, Division of Cancer Epidemiology and Genetics—Homepage: http://www-dceg.ims.nci.nih.gov/.

Army IH Program Regulation and Summary Index: http://chppm-www.
apgea.army.mil/Armyih/rundex.htm.

New Jersey—Occupational Disease & Injury Services: http://www.state.
nj.us/health/eoh/odisweb/odishome.htm.

California EPA Homepage: http://www.calepa.cahwnet.gov/.

ATSDR Science Corner: http://atsdr1.atsdr.cdc.gov:8080/cx.html see also:
http://atsdr1.atsdr.cdc/gov:8080/popdocs.html.

CDC National Center for Environmental Health (NCEH): http://www.cdc.
gov/nceh/ncehhome.htm.

Comprehensive Epidemiologic Data Resource: http://cedr.lbl.gov/.

EPA—Overview—Office of Pesticide Products Databases: http://www.
epa.gov/opppmsd1/PPISdata/index.html.

U.S. Environmental Protection Agency/OPP Pesticide Products Database
Overview: http://www.cdpr.ca.gov/docs/epa/m2.htm.

U.S. Environmental Protection Agency/Registered and Cancelled Pesticide
Product Information: http://www.cdpr.ca.gov/docs/epa/epachem.htm.

U.S. Environmental Protection Agency Registration Information: http://
www.cdpr.ca.gov/docs/epa/regnum.htm.

U.S. Environmental Protection Agency—National Pesticide Telecommunications Network: http://ace.orst.edu/info/nptn/.

Environ$enSe: http://es.epa.gov/index.html.

EMCI Chemical Reference Index: http://www.epa.gov/enviro/html/emci/
chemref/index.html.

FDA Homepage: http://www.fda.gov.

Organisation for Economic Co-operation and Development (OECD):
http://www.oecd.org/.

C. Miscellaneous Web Sites

1. General Information

The following sites generally summarize what is available on the Internet at the
time of the request. These are excellent places to start an Internet search. Frequently they have up-to-date information and still can provide the person new
to the Internet many of the more well-known sites that contain toxicology information.

A Guide to Medical Information and Support on the Internet: http://www.
geocities.com/HotSprings/1505.

Basic Information Resources for Toxicology: http://libweb.sdsu.edu/
scidir/toxicologyblr.html.

Biology and Toxicology Resources on the Internet: http://www. ashland.edu/~bweiss/biotox.html.

Doctor's Guide to the Internet—Doctor's Guide HomePage: http://www. pslgroup.com/docguide.htm.

Duke's Occupational and Environmental Medicine Resource Index: http:// occ-env-med.mc.duke.edu/oem/index2.htm.

EnviroLink: http://envirolink.org/.

EXTOXNET (The EXTension TOXicology NETwork) Pesticide toxicology information: http://ace.orst.edu/info/extoxnet/.

Internet Environmental Resources: http://www.lff.org/advocacy/environment/environet.html.

List of Occupational Medicine and Toxicology Resources: http://www. pitt.edu/~martint/pages/omtoxres.htm.

MedWeb Electronic Publications: Toxicology: http://www.gen.emoryedu/ MEDWEB/keyword/electronic_publications/tox.html.

Merck & Company—Merck Manual: http://www.merck.com.

National Pesticide Telecommunications Network: http://ace.orst.edu/info/ ntpn/index.htm.

Occupational Medicine & Toxicology Resources: http://www.pitt.edu/ ~martint/pages/omtoxres.htm.

Pharmaceutical and Chemical Information: http://ulisse.etoit.eudra.org/.

SciCentral: Best Toxicology Online Resources: http://www.scicentral. com/H-toxico.html.

The Chemical Industry Homepage: http://www.neis.com/index.html.

The National Library for the Environment: http://www.cnie.org/.

The Virtual Library: Environment: http://earthsystems.org/Environment. shtml.

Toxicology Basic Information Resources: http://libweb.sdsu.edu/scidiv/ toxicologyblr.html.

Toxicology Internet URL's: http://tigger.uic.edu/~crockett/toxlinks.html.

U.K. World Wide Resources—Toxicology: http://uky.edu/Subject/toxicology.html.

University of Edinburgh—Health, Environment and Work, Environmental and Occupational Health Resource: http://www.med.ed.ac.uk.hew/.

University of Kentucky—Electronic Information Resources: http://www. uky.edu/Libraries/elec.html.

2. Nongovernment Organizations

American College of Toxicology: http://landaus.com/toxicology/.

American Industrial Hygiene Association (AIHC)—Homepage: http:// www.aiha.org.

American National Standards Institute (ANSI) Homepage: http://web.ansi-org/default.htm.

Chemical Industry Institute of Toxicology (CIIT)—Homepage: http://www.ciit.org/CIIT.html.

Chemical Manufacturers Association (CMA)—Homepage: http://www.cmahq.com/body.html.

International Society of Regulatory Toxicology and Pharmacology: http://www.isrtp.org.

Society of Environmental Toxicology and Chemistry (SETAC): http://www.setac.org.

Society of Toxicology—Homepage: http://www.toxicology.org/.

3. Online Journals

While most of the following journals claim to be "online" they are usually not searchable. The "online" capabilities do permit one to see the table of contents and sometimes the abstracts to determine whether or not there are articles of interest. It is cumbersome if one has no idea whether or not an article on the chemical in question exists.

Archives of Environmental Contamination and Toxicology: Table of Contents and Abstracts: http://link.springer.de/link/service/journals/0244/index.htm.

Archives of Toxicology: Table of Contents and Abstracts: http://link.springer.de/link/service/journals/0204/index.htm.

Chemical & Engineering News—The Newsmagazine of the Chemical World: Table of Contents:http://acsinfo.acs.org/cen/.

Toxicological Sciences (formerly Fundamental and Applied Toxicology): an official journal of the Society of Toxicology—Table of Contents and Abstracts:http://www.apnet.com/www/journal/fa.htm.

Environmental Health Perspectives Journals: http://ehpnet1.niehs.nih.gov/ehp.html.

Hazardous Substances & Public Health: newsletter published by ATSDR: http://atsdr1.atsdr.cdc.gov:8080/HEC/hsphhome.html.

Human and Experimental Toxicology: The Official Journal of the British Toxicology Society: Table of Contents: http://www.stockton-press.co.uk/het/index.html.

Journal of the American Medical Association (JAMA): http://www.ama-assn.org/public/journals/jama/jamahome.htm.

Journal of Biochemical Toxicology: Table of Contents and Abstracts: http://journal.wiley.com/0887-2082.

Mutation Research: Table of Contents: http://www.elsevier.nl/inca/publications/store/5/2/2/8/2/0/.

The New England Journal of Medicine: http://www.nejm.org/.

Poison Review: http://tigger.uic.edu/~crockett/Gusso.html.

Regulatory Toxicology and Pharmacology: Official Journal of the International Society for Regulatory Toxicology and Pharmacology: Table of Contents and Abstracts: http://www.apnet.com/www/journal/rt.htm.

Reproductive Toxicology: Table of Contents: http://www.elsevier.com/inca/publications/store/5/2/5/4/8/9/.

Toxicology and Applied Pharmacology: Table of Contents and Abstracts: http://www.apnet.com/www/journal/to.htm.

Toxicology and Ecotoxicology News: Table of Contents and Abstracts: http://www.bdt.org.br/bioline/te.

Toxicology Update: Table of Contents: http://www.toxupdate.com/.

4. Regulatory Information

Chemical Abstracts Registry File—STN or STN Easy: http://www.cas.org/.

Chemicals on Reporting Rules: http://www.epa.gov/docs/opptintr/CORR/index.html.

DOE Technical Standards Home Page: http://apollo.osti.gov/html/tech stds/techstds.htm.

EPA Federal Register Environmental Documents: http://www.epa.gov/fedrgstr/.

European Regulations: H & H Scientific Consultants LTD: http://ds-pace.dial.pipex.com/hhsc.

EXTOXNET—The EXTension TOXicology NETwork—Pesticide toxicology information: http://ace.orst.edu/info/extoxnet/.

Federal Register Subscription Information: http://www.epa.gov/fedrgstr/subscribe.htm.

HAZMAT: http://www.text-trieve.com/dotrspa/.

NFPA Codes & Standards Server Page: http://www.nfpa.org/.

Organisation for Economic Co-operation and Development (OECD): http://www.oecd.org/.

OSHA Standards & Related Documents: http://www.osha-slc.gov/.

Proposition 65—List of Chemicals: http://www.cdpr.ca.gov/docs/regulate/prop65/prop65.htm.

The APPA Regulatory Reporter: http://appa1.appa.org/pubpol/regrep.htm.

The Prop 65 Page: http://members.aol.com/calprop65/index.html.

5. MSDS Systems

With the advent of federal and state requirements for Material Safety Data Sheets (MSDSs) to be available on all hazardous chemicals in the workplace, a number of databases have been developed that contain toxicological as well as health and safety information. These databases are derived from secondary sources, therefore, they may not be entirely sufficient for determining health determinations. They do provide a good starting point and can provide generally good basic information. These are available from the manufacturer, from private sources that can provide printed or electronic documents, or directly from the Internet.

There are several well-known services that provide MSDS information offline such as:

Genium Publishing Corporation, 1145 Catalyn Street, Schenectady, NY.
Hazardous Materials Information Service, Department of Defense, Government Printing Office, Washington, DC.
Information Handling Services, 15 Inverness Way East, Englewood, CO.
Occupational Health Services, Inc. (OHS), 400 Plaza Drive, Secaucus, NJ.
VCH Publishers, 303 NW 12th Avenue, Deerfield Beach, FL.

MSDSs sources found directly on the Internet:

The University of Kentucky provides many links to various sources of MSDSs: http://www.chem.uky.edu/resources/msds.html.

Additional MSDS Sites: Listed below are the largest and most frequently used MSDS sources as of this writing:

Canada: MSDS: number of MSDSs available unknown: http://www. hc-sc.ca/main/lcdc/web/bmb/msds/index.html#2.

ChemExper-Search: 12,000 MSDSs available: http://www.chemex per.be.

Cornell University: 325,000 MSDSs available: http://www.pdc. cornell.edu/ISSEARCH/MSDSsrch.HTM.

Eastman Kodak: 1500 MSDSs available: http://www.kodak.com/ US/en/hse/prodSearchMSDS.shtml.

ECDIN (Environmental Chemicals Data and Information Network): 125,000 MSDSs available: http://ulisse.etiot.eudra.org/Ecdin/E_ hinfo.html.

Fisher, Acros, Curtin Matheson: 60,000 MSDSs available: http:// www.fisher1.com/catalogs/index.html.

International Chemical Safety Cards: 900 MSDSs available: http:// www.cdc.gov/niosh/ipsc/icstart.html.

New Jersey Hazardous Chemical Fact Sheets: 700 MSDSs available: http://www.alternatives.com/libs/envchemh.htm.

Oxford University MSDSs: number of MSDSs available unknown: http://physchem.ox.ac.uk/MSDS/.

Rhone-Poulenc: 5000 MSDSs available: http://rhone-poulenc.esi.be/norp.htm.

Sigma, Aldrich, Fluka, Supelco: 100,000 MSDSs available: http://www.sigma.sial.com/.

The Vermont SIRI MSDS Collection: 180,000 MSDSs available: http://hazard.com/msds/index.html.

The National Toxicology Program (fee based): 2000 MSDSs available: http://ehis.niesh.nih.gov/ntp/docs/chem_hs.html.

VWR Scientific Products: http://www.vwrsp.com/catalog.

Worksafe Australia: 2700 MSDSs available: http://allette.com.au/worksafe/wsa/wksafe22.htm.

W.W. Grainger: 6000 MSDSs available: http://www.grainger.com/index.htm.

IV. MISCELLANEOUS DATA SOURCES

There are several other powerful sources of information which must be described. First are the numerous search engines which are available on the Internet.

A. Search Engines

An Internet Search Engine is a remotely accessible program that performs keyword and/or concept searches for information on the Internet. The engine searches a database of information collected from the Internet based upon specific characteristics. The information is gathered primarily by software programs called robots or spiders that serach thruough the Internet files and subsequently downloads them into a searchable database. These search engines can search through hundreds of millions of pieces of information in seconds to provide the requester with relevant infromation. One problem with seraching the Internet is that unless you carefully word your terms, you will frequently get back thousands of useless data sites. Another problem is that there is no way to be able to verify data. Some will be obvious, such as an article from the Journal of the American Medical Association (JAMA). However, there are many unsubstantiated web sites on the web that have information that may or may not be accurate. Validation of the open web data is important particularly if the writer is writing a scientific document.

Below are listed some of the more common search engines. One site to obtain full details on these and many other search engines is Danny Sullivan's Search Engine Watch: http://searchenginewatch.internet.com/.

Common search engines:

Altavista	http://www.altavista.digital.com/
Excite	http://excite.com/
Infoseek	http://www.infoseek.com
Lycos	http://www.lycos.com/
Magellan	http://www.mckinley.com/
OSHA Search	http://www.osha-slc.gov/
Open Text	http://www.opentext.com/
Snap	http://www.snap.com
Starting Point	http://www.stpt.com/
Webcrawler	http://www.webcrawler.com/
Yahoo	http://www.yahoo.com/

B. Listservs

A listserv is an automatic mailing list server that redistributes e-mail to names on a mailing list. When e-mail is sent to a listserv mailing list, it is automatically redistributed to everyone on the lsit. Generally, users can subscribe to a mailing list by sending an e-mail to the mailing list to which they have interest. The listserv program adds the e-mail address and automatically distributes future e-mail postings to every e-mail subscriber. While listserv specifically refers to a commercial product marketed by L-Soft International, the term is frequently incorrectly applied to any mailing list such as Majordomo which is termed freeware. To get more information about listservs in general, one can access the L-Soft web site: http://www.lsoft.com/.

The EPA has about 20 of its own automatic e-mail lists. These distribute everything from EPA press releases to Federal Register documents. These can be quite useful. Rather than try to list and define them in this chapter, the reader is referred to the EPA Homepage, specifically the listserv information: http://www.epa.gov/epahome/listserv.htm.

There are several toxicology lists to which one can subscribe. Each list has a different procedure to follow to join. One can get a current listing of all applicable lists in toxicology at the Liszt Search: http://www.liszt.com/.

Ecotoxicology	Ecotoxicology discussion list
FIRETOX	Fire toxicology list
NBTOX-L	Neurobehavioral toxicology discussion list
PSST	Graduate student disc in pharmacology and toxicology
tox	Integrated toxicology program list
Toxlink	An open forum for the exchange of information related to toxicology

C. Other Mailing Lists of Interest

SAFETY	list general discussion of environmental health and safety

LEPC	list planning for hazardous materials emergencies
LAB-XL	list performance oriented environmental regulation of laboratories
	To obtain more information about the above lists, e-mail Ralph Stuart, at the following address: rstuart@esf.uvm.edu.
Canadian Centre for Occupational Health and Safety (CCOHS) list	general discussion of Canadian health and safety issues. To obtain more information, contact the technical moderator, Chris Moore at the following address: chrism@ccohs.ca.
Doctor's Guide E-Mail Edition	weekly update of the latest developments in medicine—searchable. To obtain more information, go to the primary website at: http://www.docguide.com.
InteliHealth Online	home to Johns Hopkins Health Information— daily update of medical research. To obtain more information, go to the primary website at: http://www.intelihealth.com/signup

D. CD-ROM Data Sources

ATSDR's Toxicological Profiles on CD-ROM: Agency for Toxic Substances & Disease Registry, Lewis Publishers (ed.), Lewis Publishers, December 1996.

U.S. Code of Federal Regulations—Titles 1 through 50, EPA Compliance Sector Guides, Solutions Software Corporation, Enterprise, FL, http://www.env-sol.com.

TSCA Chemical Inventory + DSL/NDSL, PMN, SARA Title II requirements, CORR, and ELINCS data; MSDS Databases: 200,000 products; MSDS Solvent Database: 8000 solvents; OSHA Chemical Safety Database, Solutions Software Corporation, Enterprise, FL, http://www.env-sol.com.

E. Other Miscellaneous Data Sources

Health Designs Inc. (HDI), 183 E. Main Street, Rochester, NY 14604, (716) 546-1464.

HDI performs computational toxicology based upon molecular structure. This service can be valuable when trying to identify which materials might be bad actors and which materials are structurally closely related to the chemical in question.

The Bureau of National Affairs, 1231 25th Street NW, Washington, D.C. 20037, (202) 452-4615.

Chemical Regulation Reporter: A weekly review of activity affecting chemical users and manufacturers. The review is available both on CD-ROM and in print form by subscription. This is searchable and very complete.

Pardalis Software, Inc., 324 S. Husband, Stillwater, OK 74074, web Site: http://www.pardalis.com.

The Pardalis EnviroSafe eLetter is a fee-based electronic letter sent twice a week that provides a complete review of regulations effecting environmental regulations.

ACKNOWLEDGMENTS

The author wishes to thank Susan Byrd and Susan Henry for their valuable input and critical review of this manuscript.

3

Acute Systemic Toxicity Testing

Carol S. Auletta
Huntingdon Life Sciences, East Millstone, New Jersey

I. INTRODUCTION

Acute systemic toxicity studies evaluate the biological effects of a single exposure to a material, generally in a large amount, and most frequently as a result of an accident. Exposure can occur as a result of an industrial accident, a shipping mishap (train derailment, tank car leak, etc.), a chemical spill, misuse of a household product, a faulty container, a curious child left unsupervised for a moment, a wide variety of other accidents, or, occasionally, as a result of intentional ingestion (suicide attempt). It is the responsibility of the manufacturer and supplier of a material to adequately characterize the nature of the hazards likely to result from such exposures and to use this information to (1) assure that appropriate precautions are taken to prevent accidental exposures and (2) make available all appropriate information for use in providing first aid and treatment for persons exposed to the material. Likewise, if a material is essentially nonhazardous, it is important that this information be available to prevent needless concern.

Acute systemic toxicity studies are designed to provide this information. Acute (accidental) exposures are generally oral (by mouth), dermal (through the skin), or by inhalation. This chapter discusses methods for the evaluation of acute oral and dermal toxicity; inhalation toxicity testing is discussed in a separate chapter.

II. REGULATIONS, GUIDELINES, AND REGULATORY AGENCIES

Manufacture, distribution, packaging, labeling, and use of chemicals and other materials are regulated or monitored on the basis of acute toxicity data by a diverse and frequently confusing number of agencies, guidelines, and regulations.

Currently these regulations vary from country to country and from agency to agency within the same country, depending on the nature of the chemical. These discrepancies among labeling and classification criteria for different countries create difficulties in labeling and transporting materials intended for international use and cause confusion among handlers and users. Clearly, consistent criteria would be more cost-effective and would lead to safer handling practices and a better understanding of hazards.

An international effort to address these concerns is currently in progress, with a goal of achieving global harmonization by the year 2000. The Globally Harmonized System (GHS) for the classification and labeling of hazardous chemicals, coordinated by the Organization for International Cooperation and Development (OECD), is being developed by several countries in order to "promote common, consistent criteria for classifying chemicals according to their health, physical and environmental hazards, and to develop compatible labeling, material safety data sheets for workers, and other information based on the resulting classifications." (1) Three key components of the GHS, being coordinated by different groups, are 1) development of health and environmental hazard classification criteria, 2) establishment of criteria for physical hazards and 3) hazard communication through label warning statements and modifications of material safety data sheets.

The first initiative, development of health hazard classification criteria, is likely to influence the number of acute toxicity tests performed and the nature of such tests. Although no testing requirements will be included in the new system, changes in health hazard criteria may result in changes in the waytest results are used to classify materials. The intent of the new system is to serve as a mechanism to promote consistency. Although it will have no regulatory weight in the U.S. and will not supersede any U.S. laws and regulations, it will certainly influence future regulations and may lead to modifications of current ones. The United States Environmental Protection Agency (EPA) has taken the lead for several key federal agencies with domestic and international responsibility for regulation based on health, safety, and environmental issues. The major impact will be on the chemical industry. Pharmaceuticals and food additives are covered by these regulations only in terms of worker exposure and labeling for transport if warranted by potential exposure.

As of preparation of this book, the proposed international hazard and labeling criteria are those summarized in Table 1. (2) The major disagreement in finalizing these criteria is the question of whether the criterion for a Class 3 hazard based on acute oral toxicity should be 200 or 500 milligrams per kilogram of body weight (mg/kg bw). This issue is more political than scientific, since the difference between these two numbers is not significant from a toxico-

Table 1 GHS Criteria for Classification of Substances Based on Acute Toxicity LD_{50}

Route of Exposure (mg/kg)	Class 1	Class 2	Class 3	Class 4	Class 5
Oral	5	50	200 or 500	2000	2000+
Dermal	50	200	1000	2000	2000+

logical perspective. A difference of this magnitude can easily result from experimental or biological variability. However, such differences currently can result in the same material being labeled as extremely hazardous in one country and moderately hazardous in another, with consequent differences in the expense of packaging and transportation.

Other issues of discussion that appear to be resolved but could be reopened and lead to future changes are the issues of proportionality and the need for Class 5 (low toxicity but potentially hazardous to vulnerable populations). The proportionality issue arises from concerns that criteria for the same classes should provide the same level of protection for various routes of exposure (oral and dermal, discussed in this chapter, and inhalation, covered elsewhere). The principle of proportionality assumes that absorption and, therefore, exposure is similar for different routes or that a constant factor should be used for extrapolation among routes. There is general agreement that dermal exposure is less than oral exposure for the same material, because of the barrier provided by the skin. However, proponents of proportionality point out that current classifications for dermal hazards vary from 2 to 10 times those for oral exposure.

The inclusion of Class 5 in the current scheme indicates general acceptance, although discussion still continues on whether the criteria should be greater than 2000 mg/kg bw or greater than 5,000 mg/kg bw. The current proposal (2) indicates that a material would be placed in this category if 1) reliable evidence is already available that the LD_{50} value is in this range or other animal studies or human experience indicate a concern for human health of an acute nature or 2) assignment to a lower class is not warranted, based on a number of criteria including animal studies and/or human exposure experience. Although animal testing at doses up to 5,000 mg/kg bw for acute oral toxicity has been common in the past and is still a criterion for EPA labeling, new guidelines generally consider 2,000 mg/kg bw to be an appropriate limit dose. Some European countries have adopted animal testing policies which forbid administering doses of this magnitude.

These criteria, of course, have been developed for single chemical entities. The issue of mixtures is also a topic of discussion. Various work groups have been convened to discuss this issue but little consensus has been reached to date. Several current regulations are discussed below.

A. United States

1. Consumer Product Safety Commission (CPSC)

This group is responsible for assuring that the consumer is not exposed to any unduly hazardous products and that any potentially hazardous products are labeled appropriately.

The CPSC administers the Federal Hazardous Substances Act (FHSA), passed in 1967, which replaced the earlier Federal Hazardous Substances Labeling Act (FHSLA). The current law, found in the Code of Federal Regulations as 16 CFR 1500, defines "hazardous substances" based on several characteristics, including toxicity, and applies to a wide range of consumer products. Some exemptions are made for substances regulated by other laws: economic poisons subject to the Federal Insecticide, Fungicide and Rodenticide Act; food, drugs, and cosmetics subject to the Federal Food, Drug, and Cosmetic Act; substances intended for use as fuels when stored in containers and used in the heating, cooking, or refrigeration system of a house; and radioactive materials, which are regulated under the Atomic Energy Act.

A substance is considered "toxic" under the FHSA if it "has the capacity to produce personal injury or illness to man through ingestion, inhalation, or absorption through any body surface." A material is defined as "highly toxic" by ingestion or dermal absorption, on the basis of acute toxicity tests, if it: "produces death within 14 days in half or more than half of a group of 10 more laboratory white rats each weighing between 200 and 300 grams, at a single dose of 50 milligrams or less per kilogram of body weight [mg/kg] when orally administered" or "produces death within 14 days in half or more than half of a group of 10 or more rabbits tested in a dosage of 200 milligrams or less per kilogram of body weight, when administered by continuous contact with the bare skin for 24 hours or less."

"Toxic" substances are defined similarly except that death must be produced in half or more than half of animals receiving oral doses between 50 and 5,000 mg/kg or dermal doses between 200 and 2000 mg/kg. A further provision "to provide flexibility in the number of animals tested" deletes the specific number of animals per dose (10), but states that the number "should be sufficient to give a statistically significant result and shall be in conformity with good pharmacological practices."

Substances defined as highly toxic must be labeled as poisons and carry a "DANGER" label. Other hazardous substances must carry "WARNING" or "CAUTION" labels and comply with additional labeling requirements as defined in the FHSA regulations. Exemptions to labeling requirements for orally toxic substances may be made if it can be demonstrated that such labeling is not necessary because of "the physical form of the substance (solid, thick plastic, emulsion, etc.), the size or closure of the container, human experience with the article or any other relevant factors."

It should be noted that this is a labeling act only. The CPSC does not register materials, and there is no requirement for submission of toxicity data to the commission. The manufacturer or distributor's sole obligation is to comply with the labeling regulations.

2. Department of Transportation (DOT)

Materials transported on U.S. roadways, railways, or airways must be shipped in appropriately labeled vessels. Regulations for labeling, packaging, transporting, and storing materials are presented in 49 CFR 173 and are based on the hazard classification of a material, also defined in this regulation. Class A poisons, "extremely dangerous poisons," represent inhalation hazards and are defined (in 49 CFR 173, Section 173.326) as "poisonous gases or liquids of such nature that a very small amount of the gas, or vapor of the liquid, mixed with air is dangerous to life." They include such materials as phosgenes and cyanogenic materials. Class B poisons are classified based on hazards resulting from ingestion or dermal absorption as well as by inhalation. Based on acute oral and dermal toxicity, a material is considered by the DOT to be a Class "B" poison (and thus subject to specific shipping and packaging regulations) if it "produces death within 48 hours in half or more than half of a group of 10 or more white laboratory rats weighing 200 to 300 grams at a single dose of 50 milligrams or less per kilogram of body weight when administered orally" or "produces death within 48 hours in half or more than half of a group of 10 or more rabbits tested at a dosage of 200 milligrams or less per kilogram body weight, when administered by continuous contact with the bare skin for 24 hours or less" (49 CFR 173.343).

Exemptions to this classification can be made "if the physical characteristics or the probable hazards to humans as shown by experience indicate that the substances will not cause serious sickness or death."

3. Environmental Protection Agency (EPA)

The Environmental Protection Agency has responsibility for registration and labeling of pesticides under the Federal Insecticide, Fungicide, and Rodenticide Act (FIFRA) and for regulation of chemicals and other potentially hazardous materials under the Toxic Substances Control Act (TSCA).

   a. Labeling. Labeling and packaging standards for pesticides are established on the basis of toxicity categories and are detailed in 40 CFR, Part 156: Labeling Requirements for Pesticides and Devices. Categories range from IV (no significant toxicity) to I (very toxic) and are defined on the basis of results of acute toxicity and irritation testing.

Toxicity category criteria for acute oral and dermal toxicity are presented in Table 2.

b. Testing Guidelines.

1. U.S. EPA, Office of Prevention, Pesticides, and Toxic Substances (OPPTS). This office has developed a set of testing guidelines, including acute toxicity testing guidelines, for use in the testing of pesticides and toxic substances and developing test data for submission to the agency for review. These guidelines, first submitted for comment in June of 1996, were issued on August 5, 1998 (*Federal Register* 63 (150)) as Health Effects Test Guidelines OPPTS 870.1100 (Acute Oral Toxicity) and OPPTS 870.1200 (Acute Dermal Toxicity). They are intended to be harmonized with international guidelines (OECD) and supersede previous FIFRA and TSCA guidelines. Previous guidelines were published by the EPA under FIFRA (*Pesticide Assessment Guidelines*, Subdivision F: Hazard Evaluation: Human and Domestic Animals; Office of Pesticide Programs, United States Environmental Protection Agency, Office of Pesticide and Toxic Substances, October 1982) and TSCA (*Health Effects Test Guidelines*; Office of Toxic Substances; Office of Pesticides and Toxic Substances, United States Environmental Protection Agency, August 1982). Guidelines for acute oral and dermal toxicity were updated in October 1984 to address public concern about the LD_{50} test and to clarify the agency's policy in this area.

In contrast to previously-cited regulations that provide minimal specifications (generally species, weight, dose, and duration of exposure and observation periods), the FIFRA, TSCA, and OPPTS guidelines provide several pages of detailed information and testing procedures. The advantage of this approach is the increased consistency of studies performed in a variety of laboratories. However, because materials and circumstances differ, it is important to keep in mind that these are guidelines only (not rules), and regulators should be careful not to assume that studies which do not adhere to every detail of the guidelines are flawed. (EPA guidance on adherence to guidelines is discussed in Section III.) Major provisions of these testing guidelines are summarized in Tables 3 and 4 and discussed in more detail below. A number of specialized regulations and guidelines are also administered by the EPA.

2. Biorational Pesticides. The new generation of "biological" pesticides, which rely on specific pathogens, presumably hazardous only to the target species, are also regulated under FIFRA regulations. The August 5, 1998 Federal Register notice discusses these as follows: Biochemical pest control agents are tested in a special tiered progression. The technical grade biochemical pest control agent is always characterized by acute toxicity tests. However, because of their nontoxic mode of action against the target pest, further testing of the bio-

Table 2 Toxicity Category Criteria for Pesticide Labeling—EPA (FIFRA)[a]

Hazard indicator	Category I	Category II	Category III	Category IV
Oral LD_{50}	Up to and including 50 mg/kg	50–500 mg/kg	500–5,000 mg/kg	>5,000 mg/kg
Dermal LD_{50}	Up to and including 200 mg/kg	>200–2,000 mg/kg	2,000–5,000 mg/kg	>5,000 mg/kg
Human hazard signal word(s)	Danger, poison	Warning	Caution	Caution

[a]U.S. Environmental Protection Agency: Federal Insecticide, Fungicide and Rodenticide Act; *Federal Register*, 63(150): August 5, 1998: OPPTS 870,1000, Health Effects Test Guidelines, Acute Toxicity Testing-Background.

Table 3 Summary of Testing Guidelines/Regulations: Acute Oral Toxicity Tests

	FHSA	DOT	OPPTS	OECD	J MAFF
Test Animals					
Species	Rat	Rat	Rat[a]	Rat[a]	Rat plus on other
Age	NS	NS	Young adult (8–12 wks old)	Young adult	Young adult
Weight (g) 200–300	200–300	200–300	NS	Ns[b]	NS
Limit test					
Amount (mg/kg)	5000[c]	50[d]	2000	2000	5000
Acceptable mortality	Less than half	Less than half	None	None	None
LD_{50} *determination*					
Minimum no. Animals per group	10	10	5[e]	5[e]	10[e]
No. of groups	NA	NA	3	At least 3	5
Vehicle control	NR	NR	No[g]	No[g]	No[g]
Dosing solution					
Volume	NS	NS	Constant	Constant	NS
Concentration	NS	NS	Variable	Variable	NS

Observations

Observation period	14 Days	48 hr	14 Days[h]	14 Days[h]	14 Days[h]
Body weights	NS	NS	Weekly[i]	Weekly[i]	Weekly[i]
Necropsy	NR	NR	Yes	Yes	Optional[l]
Histopathology	NR	NR	Optional[k]	Optional[k]	Optional[k]

[a]Preferred species (several mammalian species acceptable but must be justified).

[b]Weight not specified, but weight variation not to exceed ±20% of the mean weight for each sex.

[c]To be considered not "toxic."

[d]To define Class B poison.

[e]10 = 5 males and 5 females; 5 = 5 animals of the same sex are tested initially. 5 animals of the other sex are tested at one dose to assure that no marked differences in sensitivity between sexes are present.

[f]Required unless historical data are available to determine acute toxicity of vehicle.

[g]The toxic characteristics of the vehicle should be know.

[h]14 Days is minimum duration; study may be extended if delayed mortality is seen.

[i]Body weights pretest, weekly and at death.

[j]Should be considered where indicated.

[s]Should be considered for animals surviving more than 24 hours.

[l]Clinical chemistry studies should also be considered.

Abbreviations: FHSA = Federal Hazardous Substances Act; DOT = Department of Transportation Regulations; TSCA = Toxic Substances Control Act (EPA); FIFRA = Federal Insecticide, Fungicide and Rodenticide Act (EPA); OPPTS = Office of Prevention, Pesticides and Toxic Substances Health Effects Test Guidelines (EPA: OPPTS 870.1100 (Oral) and OPPTS 870.1200 (Dermal); OECD = Organization for Economic Cooperation and Development—Toxicity Testing Guidelines 401 (Oral) and 402 (Dermal); J MAFF = Japanese Ministry of Agriculture, Forestry and Fisheries—Requirements for Safety Evaluation of Agricultural Chemicals; NS = not specified; NR = not required; NA = not applicable.

Table 4 Summary of Testing Guidelines/Regulations-Acute Dermal Toxicity Tests

	FHSA	DOT	OPPTS	OECD	J MAFF
Test Animals					
Species	Rabbit	Rabbit	Rat, rabbit, or guinea pig[a]	Rat, rabbit, or guinea pig	One mammalian species, (rat, rabbit, guinea pig, etc.)
Age	NS	NS	Young Adult[aa]	Adult	Adult
Weight (g) 200–300					
Rat (g)	NA	NA	NS	200–300	200–300
Rabbit (kg)	2.3–3	NA	NS	2–3	2–3
Guinea pig (g)	NA	NA	NS	350–450	350–450
Limit test					
Amount (mg/kg)	2000[b]	200[c]	2000	2000	2000
Acceptable mortality	Less than half	Less than half	None	None	None
LD_{50} determination					
Minimum no. Animals per group	10	10	5[d]	5[d]	5[d]
No. of groups	NA	NA	3	At least 3	At least 3
Vehicle control	NR	NR	No[g]	No[g]	No[g]

Observations

Observation period	14 Days	48 hr	14 Days[h]	14 Days[h]	14 Days[h]
Body weights	NS	NS	Weekly[i]	Weekly[i]	Weekly[i]
Necropsy	NR	NR	Yes	Yes	Optional[j]
Histopathology	NR	NR	Optional[k]	Optional[k]	Optional[k]

[a]Rabbit is preferred.

[aa]Young adult: Rate: 8–12 weeks; Rabbit: at least 12 weeks; Guinea pig: 5–6 weeks.

[b]To be considered not "toxic."

[c]To define Class B poison.

[d]10 = 5 males and 5 females; 5 = 5 animals of the same sex are tested initially. 5 animals of the other sex are tested at one dose to assure that no marked differences in sensitivity between sexes are present.

[e]Smaller numbers may be used, especially in the case of the rabbit.

[f]Required unless historical data are available to determine acute toxicity of vehicle.

[g]The toxic characteristics of the vehicle should be know.

[h]14 Days is minimum duration; study may be extended if delayed mortality is seen.

[i]Body weights pretest, weekly and at death.

[j]Should be considered where indicated.

[k]Should be considered for animals surviving more than 24 hours.

[l]Clinical chemistry studies should also be considered.

Abbreviations: See Table 3.

chemical pest control agent is normally not required. Microbial pest control agents are tested using the OPPTS Harmonized Test Guidelines Series 885, Microbial Pesticide Test Guidelines, for pathogenicity/infectivity. In addition, all formulations of microbial pest control agents are tested for precautionary labeling using acute toxicity tests in the OPPTS Harmonized Test Guidelines Series 870, Health Effects Test Guidelines.

　　　　3.　Hazardous Waste. CFR 4-(Protection of Environment, Environmental Protection Agency), Subpart B, 261.11: Criteria for Listing Hazardous Waste, presents criteria for listing hazardous waste, based in part on acute toxicity data. Section (a) (2) of this paragraph states that:

> The Administrator shall list a solid waste as a hazardous waste only if it has been found to be fatal to humans in low doses or, in the absence of data on human toxicity, it has been shown in studies to have an oral LD_{50} toxicity (rat) of less than 50 milligrams per kilogram . . . or a dermal LD_{50} (rabbit) of less than 200 milligrams per kilogram or is otherwise capable of causing or significantly contributing to an increase in serious irreversible, or incapacitating reversible, illness. (Waste listed in accordance with these criteria will be designated Acute Hazardous Waste.)

　　　　4.　United States Forest Service (USFS). This group has established its own set of testing protocols for flame retardants used in combating forest fires. These protocols generally follow FIFRA guidelines, but the Forest Service requires a more direct involvement in testing than other agencies, by actually providing materials directly to the testing laboratory for evaluation and requesting that reports to be submitted directly to the agency by the testing laboratory.

4.　Department of Health, Education, and Welfare (HEW) Food and Drug Administration (FDA)

In addition to regulating pharmaceuticals, which are not within the scope of this book, the FDA is responsible, through its Bureau of Foods, for the safety of direct food additives and color additives used in food. Materials that are to be directly added to foods and are not considered to meet GRAS criteria (generally recognized as safe) must be approved by the FDA. Under the Food, Drug, and Cosmetic Act, the safety of a food or color additive must be established prior to marketing. (Natural foods are not regulated.) Indirect food additives (materials that leach through packaging, pesticide residues, residues of animal feed additives) are regulated separately by the FDA (packaging components), the EPA (pesticide residues), the U.S. Department of Agriculture (animal feed additives), and other agencies. The safety of food and color additives is defined in the Code of Federal Regulations (21 CFR 170.3) as a reasonable certainty that a substance is not harmful under the intended conditions of use. Safety evaluation by the FDA includes estimates of probable consumer exposure and evaluation of appropriate toxicological information. In 1982 the FDA Bureau of Foods published "Toxicological Principles for the Safety Assessment of Direct Food Additives and Color Additives used in Foods." This document, which has a red cover and has come to be known as "the Redbook," was developed to provide guidelines for use by FDA personnel in evaluating food additive petitions submitted for review.

One of the premises of this document is that, because additives are substances that people ingest intentionally, the agency should possess at least some toxicological or other biological safety information for each additive intended for addition to the food supply. Although an acute oral toxicity study is not required for safety evaluation of direct food additives, guidelines for this study are presented in the "Redbook" for use when the acute toxicity of an additive is of concern or when acute toxicity data are required for the design of longer-term studies.

5. United States Pharmacopeia (USP)

The USP XX specifies certain biological testes "designed to test the suitability of plastic materials intended for use in fabricating containers or accessories thereto, for parenteral preparations, and to test the suitability of polymers for medical use in implants, devices and other systems." One of the required tests is a "systemic injection test," which is performed by intravenously injecting extracts of the test plastic in various vehicles into mice (ten per group) and comparing response over 72 hours with that of mice injected with vehicle alone.

B. International

1. Organization for Economic Cooperation and Development (OECD)

Member nations include the United States and much of the European Economic Community. OECD has formed expert groups on short-term and long-term toxicology to review toxicity testing requirements of the member nations and formulate testing guidelines which would be acceptable to all members. "Test Guidelines for Toxicity Testing" were issued in draft form in December 1979 by prominent member countries (United States and the United Kingdom). Most acute toxicity testing for products to be registered, sold, or distributed in Europe is performed according to these guidelines, whose aim was stated as follows:

> The aim of the present work has been to produce a framework for each toxicity test which is sufficiently well-defined to enable it to be carried out in a similar manner in different countries and to produce results that will be fully acceptable to various regulatory bodies. The growing demands for testing and evaluating the toxicity of chemical substances will place increasing pressure on personnel and laboratory resources. A harmonized approach, promoting the scientific aspects of toxicity testing and ensuring a

wide acceptability of test data for regulatory purposes, will avoid wasteful duplication or repetition and contribute to the efficient use of laboratory facilities and skilled personnel.

On February 24, 1987 the OECD published guidelines for acute oral and dermal toxicity testing (Guidelines 401 and 402, respectively). These guidelines incorporate some procedures that are designed to reduce numbers of animals used in experiments and limit the amount of pain to which they are subjected. Subsequent guidelines for acute oral toxicity testing have developed these procedures further. On July 17, 1992, Guideline 420, Acute Oral Toxicity—Fixed Dose Method, was published. This guideline suggests a set of doses, utilizes a very small range-find ("sighting") study, and incorporates the concept of "evident toxicity," rather than mortality, as an endpoint. Evident toxicity is defined as "a general term describing clear signs of toxicity following administration of a test substance." The definition further states that "These should be sufficient for hazard assessment and, in relation to the fixed dose procedure, should be such that an increase in the dose administered can be expected to result in the development of severe toxic signs and probable mortality." Interpretation of results and toxicity classification is performed as detailed in Table 5.

The most recently published OECD guideline for acute oral toxicity testing is Guideline 423, Acute Oral Toxicity—Acute Toxic Class Method, published on March 22, 1996. Studies performed using this procedure are conducted at predefined doses in small numbers of animals (3 per dose) and the guideline advocates killing of moribund animals. ("Test animals in obvious pain and showing signs of severe and enduring distress should be humanely killed.") The procedures were based on biometric evaluations and validated by the German government, both in an independent study and in an international validation study carried out under the patronage of OECD. A comparison of the three OECD guidelines for acute oral toxicity testing is presented in Table 6.

Although additional guidelines for acute dermal toxicity studies have not yet been promulgated by the OECD, a biometric evaluation similar to that performed to develop the Acute Toxic Class method for acute oral toxicity has been completed by the German government and was presented at the March 1998 Society of Toxicology meeting (3). It is likely that this will become an accepted OECD guideline in the near future.

2. Japan

In Japan, regulations exist for toxicity testing of medicinal products and for agricultural chemicals. Agricultural chemicals are regulated by the Japanese Ministry of Agriculture, Forestry and Fisheries (MAFF), which updated its requirements and testing guidelines, effective April 1, 1985. "Requirements for Safety Evaluation of Agricultural Chemicals" states that acute oral toxicity testing in at least two species and acute dermal toxicity testing in at least one

Table 5 OECD Guideline 420: Acute Oral Toxicity—Fixed Dose. Annex 2: Interpretation of Results

Dose	Results	Interpretation
5 mg/kg[a]	Less than 100% survival[b]	Compounds that may be very toxic (i.e. with LD_0 values of ca 25 mg/kg or less) if swallowed
	100% survival, but evident toxicity	Compounds that may be toxic (i.e. with LD_{50} values between ca 25 mg/kg and ca 200 mg/kg) if swallowed
	100% survival, no evident toxicity	Test at 50 mg/kg if not already tested at that dose.
50 mg/kg	Less than 100% survival[b]	Compounds that may be toxic or very toxic if swallowed. Test at 5 mg/kg if not already tested at that dose level.
	100% survival, but evident toxicity	Compounds that may be harmful (i.e. with LD_{50} values between ca 200 mg/kg and 2000 mg/kg) if swallowed.
	100% survival, no evident toxicity	Test at 500 mg/kg if not already tested at that dose level.
500 mg/kg	Less than 100% survival[b]	Compounds that may be toxic or harmful if swallowed. Test at 50 mg/kg if not already tested at that dose level.
	100% survival, but evident toxicity	Compounds with LD_{50} values above ca 2000 mg/kg but which may be of some concern due to the nature of the toxic effects.
	100% survival, no evident toxicity	Test at 2000 mg/kg if not already tested at that dose level.
2,000 mg/kg	Less than 100% survival[b]	Compounds that may be of some concern if swallowed. Test at 500 mg/kg if not already tested at that dose level.
	100% survival, with or without evident toxicity	Compounds that do not present a significant acute toxic risk if swallowed.

[a]Where a dose of 5 mg/kg produces significant mortality, or where a sighting study suggests that mortality will result at that dose level, the substance should be investigated at a lower dose level. The level chosen should be that which is likely to produce evident toxicity by no mortality.

[b]Includes compound related mortality and humane kills but not accidental deaths.

Note. Interpretation has been given with respect to the data obtained in the extensive validation studies of the method and related to approximate LD_{50} values in the range below 25 mg/kg, 25–200 mg/kg, 200–2,000 mg/kg and 2,000 mg/kg/. The results can however be used for other ranges by consideration of both the data from the sighting study and the main study, with judgment as to whether the interpretation given here is adequate (bearing in mind the natural variability in the LD_{50} value and the slope of the dose-response curve) or whether any adjustment is necessary.

Table 6 OECD Acute Oral Toxicity Testing Guidelines

Guideline No.:	401	420	423
Date Adopted:	24 Feb 1987	17 July 1992	22 March 1996
Method:	Traditional	Fixed Dose	Acute Toxic Class
Endpoint:	Mortality[a]	Evident Toxicity[b]	Mortality[a]
Limit Test:	2000 mg/kg	2000 mg/kg	2000 mg/kg
	(5 rats per sex)	(5 rats per sex)	(3 rats per sex)
Toxicity Study: Range-Find	Optional	None	Yes (3–6 animals)
LD_{50}	Defined	Approximate	Approximate
Doses	Not Specified	5, 50, 500, 2000	25, 200, 2000
			(optional: 5, 50, 500)
No. of Animals per Group	5[c]	5[c]	3[c]
Normal No. of Animals per Test	20–30	20–30	6–12

[a] However "Animals showing severe and enduring signs of distress and pain may need to be humanely killed."
[b] Evident toxicity—a general term describing clear signs of toxicity following administration of test substance. These should be sufficient for hazard assessment and, in relation to the fixed dose procedure, should be such that an increase in the dose administered can be expected to result in the development of severe toxic signs and probable mortality.
[c] Animals of one sex are tested initially. An equal number of animals of the opposite sex are tested subsequently at one or more doses.

species, using both the end-use product and the technical grade of the active ingredient, are required for registration of agricultural chemicals used on either food or nonfood crops. "Testing Guidelines for Toxicology Studies" state that if limit tests (10 animals) demonstrate no compound-related mortality at an oral dose of 5000 mg/kg or a dermal dose of 2000 mg/kg, "no further testing might be necessary.

III. CONDUCT OF ACUTE TOXICITY TESTS

After the applicable regulations and/or guidelines have been established, one must then design and conduct appropriate studies, interpret the results and submit them to the appropriate agency for consideration. Although most agencies keep details of their reviews internal, the EPA has in recent years worked with industry to clarify key issues and in September of 1997 published a guidance document for the conduct of acute toxicity studies for registration of pesticides (4). This document, published by the Registration Division of the EPA Office of Pesticide Programs, was preceded by a "rejection rate" analysis performed by the agency in 1993. This analysis indicated that 11 percent of acute oral toxicity studies and 10 percent of acute dermal toxicity studies submitted for registration had been rejected for various deficiencies considered significant enough to disqualify the studies. Based on a number of questions from industry about the criteria for rejection, the Registration Division met in 1995 with representatives from industry and from Health Canada and the California Department of Pesticide Regulation to discuss acceptable procedures and methods. The published document presents decisions made as a result of this meeting. Its stated intent is to serve as a supplement to the (FIFRA) Subdivision F Guidelines "so that there will be a reduction in the number of studies rejected or flawed due to insufficient reporting or incorrect methodology" and "to insure that the correct procedures are followed for acute toxicity studies. Guidance presented in this document (referred to as the EPA Guidance Document) is included in the OPPTS guidelines (August, 1998) and has been incorporated where applicable into the following discussions.

A. Study Protocols

Study protocols, specifying materials and methods to be used in performing toxicity evaluations, can be obtained from testing laboratories or may be designed by the manufacturer of the material to be tested. Fortunately, it is not necessary to perform separate tests for each regulatory agency, since requirements are essentially similar, and one test can be designed which satisfies all of the requirements. If cost is critical and only one of the less comprehensive regulations is applicable, a smaller, less expensive study design will frequently suffice. However, one cannot later attempt to apply the limited information obtained for purposes other than those for which it was originally intended. Thus, some forethought may result in a slightly higher initial expenditures but can ultimately save time, money, and animals.

Major provisions of several of the testing guidelines presented above are summarized in Tables 3, 4, and 6 and discussed below, along with other factors to be considered in establishing protocols for acute toxicity studies.

B. Study Design/Number of Animals: Alternatives

Use of animals for acute toxicity testing has undergone considerable scrutiny over the past two decades. A number of changes reflecting two of the "Three R's" of the alternatives credo (Reduction and Refinement) have been incorporated into industry practice and are becoming components of regulatory guidelines. (The third R, Replacement, has progressed more slowly and is discussed below, under "Nonanimal Tests").

Use of the limit test and conduct of LD_{50} studies with as few as three dose groups have been in common use for several years. More recent refinements include testing with small group sizes, testing in one sex only (the more sensitive sex), killing of moribund animals and the establishment of evident toxicity, rather than mortality, as an endpoint. Use of all available information on similar materials, structure-activity-relationships and previous studies is also encouraged/required to eliminate duplication of work and minimize additional animal testing. These study designs and refinements are "alternatives" to the "traditional" LD_{50} study, which has long been criticized by a number of responsible toxicologists (5,6) as requiring an unnecessary degree of precision for its use in evaluating relative toxicity and assigning hazard classifications. The OECD expert group on short-term testing states "The numerical value of the median lethal dose (LD_{50}) is widely used in toxicity classification systems, but it should not be regarded as an absolute number identifying the toxicity of a chemical substance. LD_{50} values for the same chemical may vary from study to study and between species or within a species because acute toxicity is influenced by both internal and external factors." (7) The consensus among toxicologists is that a precise (but frequently nonreproducible) LD_{50} value is of limited usefulness and that significant information can be obtained by using fewer animals treated at doses producing little or no lethality (5,6,8,9). The OPPTS guidelines have taken the position that any of these alternatives that provide an estimate of the LD_{50} are acceptable in lieu of a "conventional" acute toxicity study.

Study designs incorporating these refinements, as well as the "traditional" LD_{50} study, are discussed below.

1. Limit Test

Virtually all regulatory and labeling guidelines accept the concept of the limit test, a study in which a large amount of the test product is administered to several laboratory animals, generally 5 males and 5 females. If no mortality is seen at this "limit" dose, then no further testing is required. Some confusion exists, however, about interpretation of the limit test when some mortality is seen but less than half of the animals die; in other words, the apparent median lethal dose (LD_{50}) is greater than the amount administered.

The EPA Guidance Document states that when mortality of more than one animal per sex occurs in a limit test, then additional doses should be tested to determine the LD_{50}. The OPPTS guidelines suggest that any compound-related mortality in the limit test may result in the need for additional testing. However, the Agency agreed with an industry comment that additional doses should be administered as necessary to determine the label category, not necessarily the LD_{50}.

2. "Bracketing"

The Agency's agreement with this comment is indicative of a clear trend toward testing schemes designed to "bracket" a material by placing it in an appropriate toxicity category through the use of minimal testing rather than reliance on the "traditional" LD_{50} study.

Care is needed, however, to select doses appropriately. The EPA Guidance Document states that "An acute . . . study where one or more test concentrations are tested that do not allow LD_{50} determination or bracketing will be rejected" and cites two examples of insufficient information for classifying a material. One example is an acute oral toxicity test at doses of 50 and 300 mg/kg and no mortality, which could place the material in EPA category II, III, or IV. The second is a limit test with complete mortality (10 of 10 animals) which would place the material in category I or II. Clearly, the data provided must enable the regulator to make a judgment about relative toxicity.

3. Fixed Doses

Both the OECD Fixed Dose Method and Acute Toxic Class Method for acute oral toxicity testing (Guidelines 420 and 423, respectively) employ a procedure in which doses to be used are established (fixed) by the guideline and testing is performed using the minimum number of doses necessary to rank the tested materials in regulatory agency-specified classification systems. The Fixed Dose Method uses a more traditional approach to numbers of animals (5 per sex per group) but uses evident toxicity, rather than mortality, as an endpoint.

The design of the Fixed Dose Method is based on an approach to acute toxicity testing proposed by the British Society of Toxicology in 1984 (9). The concept of using fewer animals to approximate toxicity is not new.As early as 1943 (10,11), procedures for determining an approximate lethal dose (ALD) using as few as six animals were suggested. The "up-and-down" study, designed by R. Bruce (12) in 1985 incorporates similar principles and allows for a calculation of an approximate LD_{50} value. (This procedure is proposed in an additional draft OECD guideline (No. 425) and is discussed below, in Section III.B.4.) The concept of staggering doses, or observing for effects in animals dosed initially prior to administering doses to additional groups of animals, is also an integral part of several approaches proposed to reduce laboratory animal use (8,13). The practice of performing most testing in a single sex is supported by studies demonstrating that sex-related differences in acute toxicity are relatively rare (14–16).

Studies performed using the Fixed Dose Method are generally preceded by a preliminary "sighting" (range-finding) study in which various doses are administered to single animals of the same sex in a sequential fashion. Results are used to estimate a dose response and to select the starting dose for the main study. A dose just below that expected to produce mortality is selected from one of the four fixed dosed (5, 50, 500, and 2,000 mg/kg of body weight) and administered to five male and five female animals. Animals are then observed for evident toxicity (defined in Section II.B.1). If no toxicity is evident, the next higher dose is administered to ten additional animals (five per sex). If severe toxicity or mortality occurs, the next lower dose is administered to ten additional animals (five per sex).

The Acute Toxic Class method refines this procedure further by using fewer animals (3 to 6 per dose). As stated in the guideline, "the method is not intended to allow the calculation of a precise LD_{50}, but does allow for the determination of a range of exposures where lethality is expected since death of a proportion of the animals is still the major endpoint of this test. The results of the test should allow for classification according to any of the commonly used systems." The fixed doses in this method are 25, 200, and 2,000 mg/kg of body weight with an option to administer additional fixed doses of 5, 50, and 500 mg/kg. A starting dose that is likely to produce mortality is selected, based on all available information, and administered to three animals of one sex. Based on results of this dose, three subsequent options are to 1) discontinue testing, 2) administer the same dose to three animals of the other sex or 3) administer a higher or lower dose to three additional animals of the same sex. Annex 1 and Annex 3 of this guideline, presented as Figures 1 and 2, describe the test procedure and interpretation of results.

Some qualifications to the outlined testing schemes in order to avoid "false positive and false negative" projections are noted in the preface to Annex 1. When only one animal of the second sex dies after a dose of 25 or 200 mg/ kg body weight, testing is normally discontinued. However, when this results in a total mortality of only one of the six animals and no toxic signs are evident in the other five animals, consideration should be given to the possibility that the single death may not have been related to the test substance and dosing at the next higher level should be considered. Conversely, while the death of only one of three animals that receive the 2,000 mg/kg body weight dose would indicate that the LD_{50} value is greater than 2,000 mg/kg (and indicate that no further testing is required), the presence of signs of marked toxicity in the two surviving animals would suggest that the LD_{50} value may be 2,000 mg/kg or less and would justify further testing (at the 20 mg/kg dose in three animals of the other sex).

4. Up-and-Down Procedure

This procedure is described in the OECD draft proposal for a new guideline (Guideline 425: Acute Oral Toxicity: Up-and-Down Procedure), which was submitted by the United States and accepted by the OECD in June, 1998. The study design, first proposed for use in acute toxicity testing by Bruce in 1985 (12) and adopted by the ASTM in 1987 (16a), begins with a single animal that receives a dose close to the estimated LD_{50} value. Based on the survival in this animal, a second animal is dosed 24 hours later with a higher or lower dose. Dosing in individual animals continues until the point at which the response

TEST PROCEDURE WITH A STARTING DOSE OF 25 MG/KG BODY WEIGHT

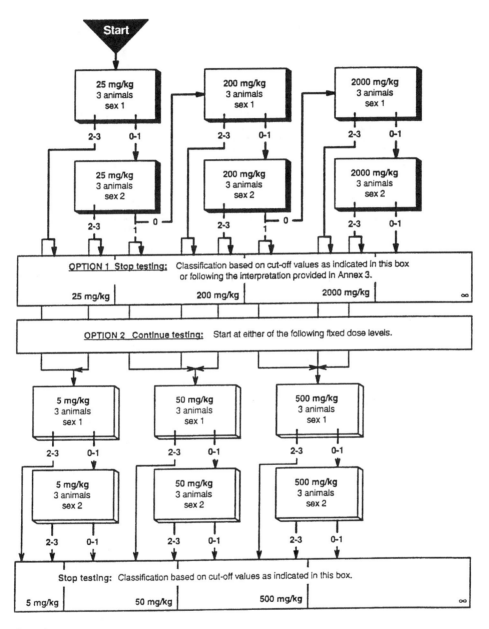

Figure 1 Acute oral toxicity, acute toxic class method (OECD Guideline 423) testing procedure.

TEST PROCEDURE WITH A STARTING DOSE OF 200 MG/KG BODY WEIGHT

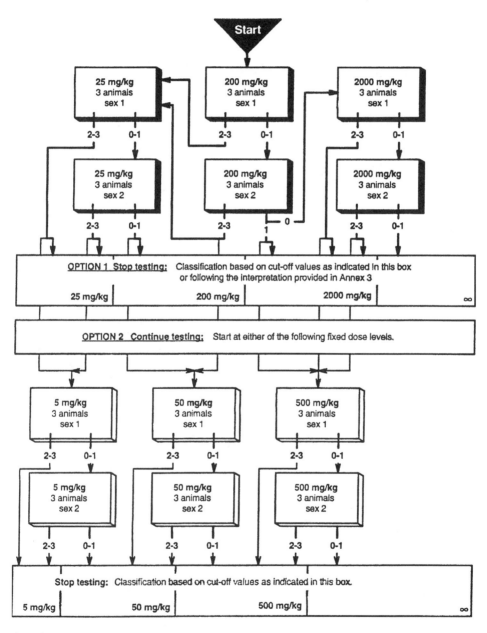

Figure 1 Continued.

TEST PROCEDURE WITH A STARTING DOSE OF 2000 MG/KG BODY WEIGHT

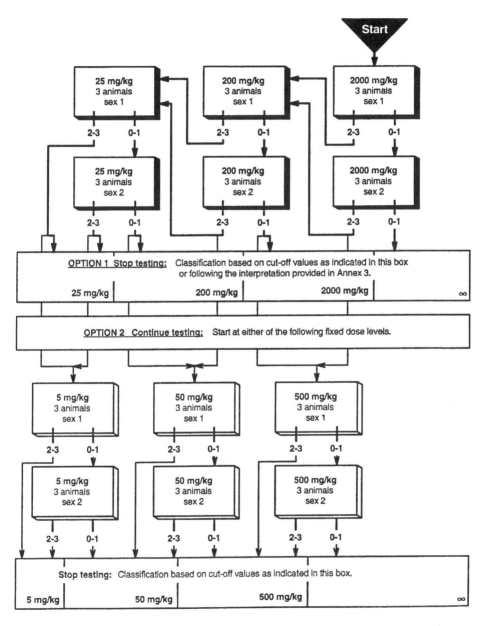

Legend:
0,1,2,3: Number of moribund or dead animals of each sex

Figure 1 Continued.

Starting dose: 25 mg/kg body weight

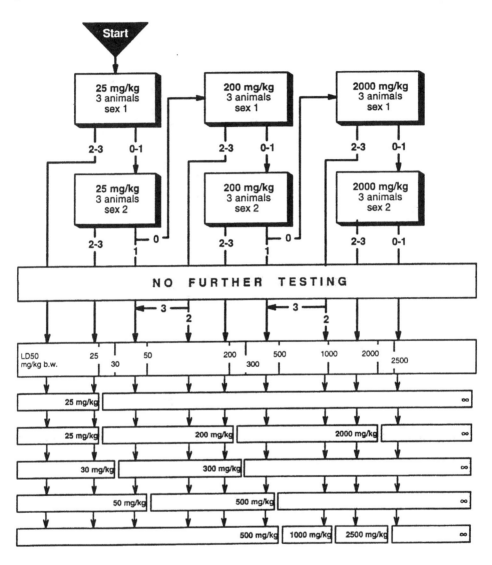

Figure 2 Acute oral toxicity, acute toxic class method (OECD Guideline 423) interpretation of results.

Starting dose: 200 mg/kg body weight

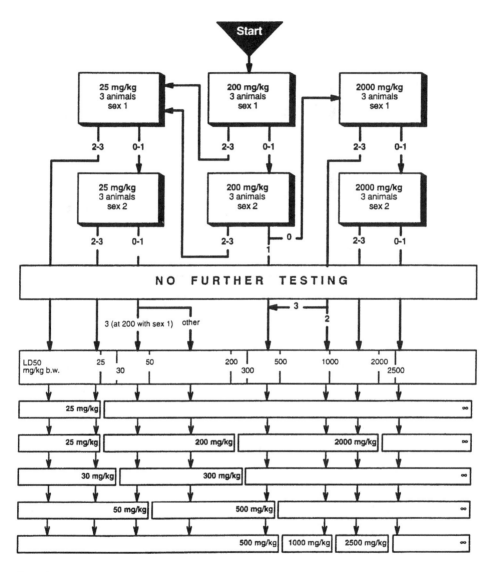

Legend:
0,1,2,3: Number of moribund or dead animals of each sex.

Figure 2 Continued.

Starting dose: 2000 mg/kg body weight

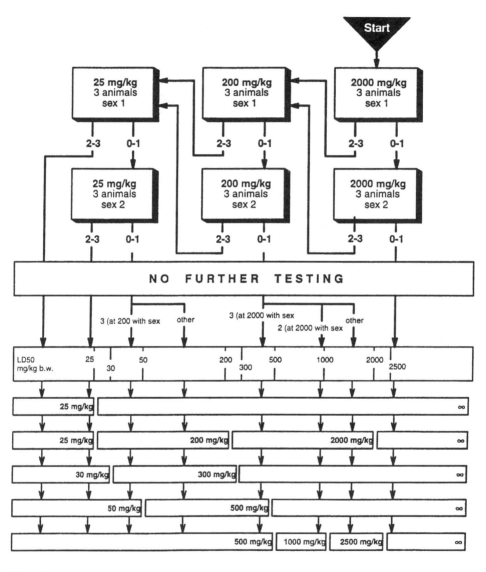

Legend:
0,1,2,3: Number of moribund or dead animals of each

Figure 2 Continued.

changes (the point at which two successive doses result in death in one animal and survival in the other). At this point, four additional animals are dosed at one of the two doses, alternating in the up-and-down pattern based on response, and the test is considered complete. Testing is performed in only one sex (females unless there is information suggesting that males are more sensitive to effects of a specific test material). Testing in the opposite sex, when information on one sex is considered inadequate, is included as an option in this procedure. A limit test, with 3 males and 3 females dosed at 2000 mg/kg, is also an option.

The advantage of this method is that it appears to be the one that potentially produces the most accurate estimate of the LD_{50} value with the smallest number of animals (6 to 10 animals of one sex), based on a comparative study published in 1995 (16b). One potential disadvantage is the limited usefulness and logistical difficulty in using this procedure for a material which produces delayed deaths. In fact, the guideline does not recommend this procedure for materials which are expected to produce considerable delays (5 days or more) in death.

It should also be noted that, even though fewer animals are tested than in other study designs, the work involved in performing a study of this type is generally greater than that in tests using larger numbers of animals with more compressed, defined timelines. Because dosing is performed over several days and the dose concentration may change with each dose, it may be necessary to prepare dose solutions on several different occasions. Any "economies of scale" from performing evaluations of several animals concurrently are also lost. Data records become more complicated and, if a study is spread over too long an interval, it may not be possible to use animals from the same shipment due to rapid body weight changes which render the study population non-homogeneous.

5. (LD_{50}) Determination

If a material produces mortality in the limit test, additional doses are usually administered to determine the approximate median lethal dose (LD_{50}), or the dose that will kill approximately half of the animals. If only one animal dies after receiving the amount specified for the limit test, no further testing is necessary.

For material of unknown toxicity or for those with an anticipated LD_{50} value below the limit test, it is often useful to perform a preliminary range-finding test to provide guidance in selecting dose levels. Four or more different dosage levels are generally administered to two animals (one male and one female) per level. If no information is available, a wide range of doses, for example from 450 to 5,000 mg/kg should be selected. It is usually possible to select doses for LD_{50} determination based on one range-finding study, although, occasionally, additional studies are necessary. Animals used for range-finding studies are generally observed for mortality only and are held for 7 days after dosing. Clinical observations may provide useful information about anticipated effects in the definitive study.

Based on results of range-finding, doses are selected for the LD_{50} study. An attempt should be made to select one dose which will produce little or no mortality, one dose which will produce mortality of approximately 50%, and one dose which will be lethal to most of the animals. Traditionally, five or more dosage levels have been used for LD_{50} studies; however, current regulations generally specify three dosage levels, and attempts are usually made to use as small a number of animals as possible. However, dose selection based on a small group size (2 animals) is not always accurate. The 2 animals in the range-finding study may represent either end of the spectrum of effects. Therefore, mortality of 50% (1 of 2) in the range-finding study may represent mortality of 10% (1/10) or 90% (9/10) in a study with a larger group size. It is sometimes necessary to add additional groups if an appropriate mortality range is not achieved initially. Care should be taken to maintain conditions of the additional doses as close as possible to those of the initial doses. Variables in body weights, age, environmental conditions, test material conditions/preparation, etc. may produce confusing results and present difficulties in data interpretation. Thus, while this stepwise approach decreases the total number of animals used in LD_{50} studies, it can sometimes lead to variable results and must be administered carefully. The judgment and experience of the laboratory are important factors in determining the initial and total numbers of dosage levels to be used for LD_{50} determination. For rabbits, a stepwise approach, giving one dose at a time to 5 or 10 animals, will usually produce a reasonable LD_{50} estimate with three doses.

Currently, the Fixed Dose, Acute Toxic Class, and Up-and-Down procedures are contained in guidelines for acute toxicity evaluations by the oral route. However, the same principles can be applied to studies using the dermal route, and guidelines specific to dermal studies will undoubtedly be published in the near future.

A variety of methods can be used to calculate the actual LD_{50} value (the dose which is lethal to half of the animals) with 95% confidence limits, that is, the range of doses that would be expected to include the LD_{50} value 95% of the time (17–22). The precision of the LD_{50} value and the extent of the 95% confidence limits vary with the method used and the number of animals tested.

a. Nonanimal Tests. The search for "alternatives" includes, in addition to the alternative approaches to classical study designs discussed above, investigations of nonanimal systems that might replace animal testing or reduce the number of animals uses. A wide and fascinating variety of approaches have been suggested.

Evaluation of existing data may sometimes be used to avoid or minimize animal testing. The OPPTS guidelines state:

> EPA recommends the following means to reduce the number of animals used to evaluate acute effects of chemical exposure while preserving its ability to make reasonable judgements about safety:
>   Use of data from structurally related substances or mixtures. In order to minimize the need for animal testing for acute effects, the Agency encourages the review of existing acute-toxicity information on chemical substances that are structurally related to the agent under investigation. In certain cases, it may be possible to obtain enough information to make preliminary hazard evaluations that may reduce the need for further animal testing for acute effects. Similarly, mixtures or formulated products that are substantially similar to well-characterized mixtures or products may not need additional testing if there are sufficient bridging data available for meaningful extrapolation. In those cases, classification would be extrapolated from the mixture already tested.

In vitro methods using various types of cells and organs in culture and evaluating a variety of effects on growth, viability, and metabolism abound. Studies using lower organisms (bacteria, algae, fungi, plants, insects, lower vertebrates) have also been developed. Mathematical models, based on structure-activity relationships and computer modeling are available as well. The major difficulty with these alternatives is the problem of validation, a term on which there is still much disagreement among toxicologists. Validation of a procedure should include some comparison to currently accepted in vivo methods and some agreement that results generated by the new procedure can provide information that is reasonably equivalent to that provided by current methods. Most methods currently under development have not reached this stage of validation.

Thus, while much research continues into alternative methods, the consensus among toxicologists and regulatory agencies is that currently no acceptable methods exist that will eliminate entirely the need for whole animal testing.

C. Test Animals

1. Species/Strain

a. Acute Oral Toxicity. The rat is the animal used most commonly for acute oral toxicity testing. If a second species is required, the mouse is generally selected. Rabbits and hamsters are used occasionally, but such studies are relatively rare. If data on a large animal species are required, generally by special request of certain agencies and usually to provide preliminary information for longer-term studies, dogs and (rarely) nonhuman primates may be tested. (Guidelines generally state that they may be adapted for nonrodents). Such studies would almost always be done using the up-and-down method (12), which requires only a small number of animals, usually 6–10.

The three commonly used stocks or strains of albino rat are the Sprague-Dawley–derived, the Fisher 344, and the Wistar. The hooded (Long-Evans) rat is also used occasionally, but one of the three albino strains is more likely to be selected. Most laboratories have a stock/strain and animal supplier(s) that they use routinely and, thus, have historical experience with specific strain. Because stock/strain-related differences in response to various materials have been demonstrated, it is generally best to test the one with which the laboratory has had experience.

   a. Acute Dermal Toxicity.   The New Zealand White (albino) rabbit has historically been the species of choice for acute dermal toxicity testing, although use of albino rats or guinea pigs has become increasingly accepted. Because of their size, rats and guinea pigs are easier (and less expensive) to test. However, they are also generally less sensitive to topically administered material than are rabbits, and there is no significant historical data base available for comparison with other materials. Thus, based on the extensive database available and its superior skin permeability, the rabbit continues to be the species of choice for acute dermal toxicity evaluations and the EPA Guidance Document confirms that the rabbit is the preferred species, followed by the rat and the guinea pig. (It also states that justification for use of other species *must* be provided for the study to be acceptable.) In our laboratory, use of the rat for acute dermal toxicity studies has increased over recent years and the rat is currently used more commonly than the rabbit, especially for materials intended for European registration.

2. Husbandry/Housing

Guidelines exist that define facilities and environmental conditions appropriate for standard laboratory species (23). Laboratories accredited by the American Association for Laboratory Animal Care (AALAC) are inspected periodically and must adhere to appropriate standards to maintain accreditation. Facilities in the United States housing rabbits, guinea pigs, and hamsters must adhere to specifications of the Animal Welfare Act and are subject to periodic inspection by the U.S. Department of Agriculture (USDA). (Rats and mice are not regulated.) Cage sizes are specified based on the size and activity patterns of each species. Temperature ranges of 18–26°C (64–79°F) for rats and 16–21°C (61–70°F) for rabbits are specified; desired relative humidity values are usually in the range of 30–70%. OPPTS and OECD guidelines specify slightly different temperature ranges (19–25°C for rodents and 17–23°C for rabbits). Light cycles (for artifical lighting) of 12 hours light, 12 hours dark are specified in the OPPTS guidelines.

The intent of husbandry guidelines is to assure that standard conditions are maintained and to minimize environmental stress that might complicate interpretation of study results. Newer facilities are designed to adhere to these standards. However, one must keep in mind that acute toxicity studies have been performed for several decades and that many older facilities cannot always maintain the exact environmental conditions specified in some of the guidelines. Temperature and humidity variations are only two of the multiple variables that may influence results of acute toxicity studies (5,6). Thus, while reasonable care should be exercised, deviations from desired environmental conditions are likely to occur and, unless they are severe and sustained over a long period, they will not generally compromise an acute toxicity study or preclude meaningful interpretation of results. Rodents and guinea pigs may be housed as a group or individually. However, animals treated dermally should be housed individually to prevent disturbance of the dose site and ingestion of test material by cagemates. Individual caging provides easier identification and observation of animals and prevents loss by cannibalism of animals that die. Rabbits are generally housed individually.

3. Age, Sex, and Weight

Most current guidelines specify the use of adult or young adult animals; some also suggest weight ranges (200–300 g for rats, 2–3 kg for rabbits). OPPTS guidelines and the EPA Guidance Document specify that rats should be 8 to 12 weeks of age and rabbits should be at least 12 weeks of age at study initiation. The guidance document further states that body weights should be within "normal" ranges for animals of the given age and that the laboratory should be able to document this fact (using growth curves from the supplier and/or historical control data) in order to demonstrate acceptable health of the animals.

Because there is a sex-related size difference in rats, males and females of the same weight will be of different ages. Thus, one or the other will be variable. Young adult male and female rabbits are generally comparable in size; a weight range of approximately 2–3 or 3.5 kg is appropriate. Most current guidelines specify that females should be nulliparous and nonpregnant. Guidelines generally specify that weight variations among animals of the same sex should not exceed 20 percent of the mean weight for that sex. This is not a problem when doses are administered concurrently or within a similar time frame. However, when dosing is staggered, this recommendation must be kept in mind, since the weight range of animals from the same shipment will become greater over time and it may be necessary to obtain additional animals to complete the study while adhering to this criterion.

4. Animal Health

Healthy laboratory animals are generally readily available, and maintaining healthy animals for acute toxicity studies is usually not a problem. However, monitoring health and assuring that animals are healthy at the beginning of a study is obviously critical to performing a successful evaluation of acute toxicity. The use of unhealthy animals is specifically cited as a reason for rejection of acute studies by the EPA Guidance Document, which states that "40 CFR 160.90 states that at the beginning of a study, test systems shall be free of any disease or conditions that might interfere with the purpose or conduct of study." Animals should be observed carefully during the quarantine/acclimation period to assure acceptable health. In our laboratory, we acclimate rats for a minimum of one week and rabbits for a minimum of two weeks and require a physical examination to confirm appropriate health prior to assignment to study. The EPA Guidance Document specifically requires a minimum quarantine time of five days and considers a shorter period to be sufficient reason for rejection of a study. Health problems which are sometimes seen during quarantine/acclimation include sialodacryoadenitis virus in rats and respiratory or intestinal disorders in rabbits.

Sialodacryoadenitis virus (SDAV) is a disease characterized by enlargement of the salivary glands with resultant cervical swelling and often accompanied by ocular abnormalities (drying of the cornea) (24). This disease is acute, self-limiting, and seldom fatal. However, it frequently appears just as animals are completing quarantine and are ready to be tested and may create delays in initiating studies. Serological surveillance and strict quarantine procedures will help to reduce the incidence of SDAV infections. Diseases commonly found in laboratory rabbits include respiratory problems (sniffles) or intestinal disease generally associated with pasteurellosis or coccidiosis (25). It is important to monitor carefully for such diseases and assure that animals placed on acute toxicity studies are free of any abnormal clinical signs. Based on the recommendation of our rabbit supplier, we have found that a practice of feed restriction in rabbits helps to reduce the incidence of intestinal disorders (primarily mucoid enteritis) that commonly occur in rabbits. We do not feed rabbits on the day of arrival and gradually introduce them to a ration of 125 grams of standard laboratory diet per day that we feed during study. Because nutritional requirements are met at this amount of food, this program does not restrict growth rates.

It is not uncommon, however, for animals harboring diseases subclinically to exhibit signs of illness after the stress of test material administration. Experience in observing clinical and morphological manifestations of common rabbit diseases is useful in deciding whether or not death of an animal is a toxic response to the test material.

D. Administration of Materials

The following definitions relevant to dose administration have been provided in the OECD and OPPTS guidelines for acute oral and dermal toxicity studies.

It would be useful to be cognizant of these when communicating with these agencies.

> Dose: the amount of test substance administered. Dose is expressed as weight (milligrams or grams) per unit weight of test animal (e.g., milligrams per kilogram or mg/kg).
>
> Dosage: a general term comprising the dose, its frequency and the duration of testing.
>
> Dose-response: the relationship between the dose and the proportion of a population sample showing a defined effect.
>
> Dose-effect: the relationship between the dose and the magnitude of a defined biological effect, either in an individual or in a population sample.

1. Oral Administration

Oral administration of materials is generally performed by using a syringe fitted with a ball-tipped intubation needle or a flexible rubber of tygon tube. This delivery technique, known as oral intubation or gavage, requires practice and skill; it is important that well-trained, experienced technicians perform this procedure. However, even experienced technicians sometimes have "dosing accidents" (intratracheal delivery of material or perforation of the esophagus), especially when administering viscous materials. It is standard procedure in our laboratory to prepare one additional rat per sex per dose level to be used as a replacement in case of dosing accidents. Such accidents are usually apparent immediately by the animal's response, but may take several hours (or, occasionally, a few days) to produce death. It is important, therefore, to carefully examine animals that die for evidence of injuries sustained during dosing. Animals in which the cause of death is determined to be accidental should be replaced, if possible, and excluded from mortality estimates and calculations.

The EPA Guidance Document accepts the concept of replacing animals for which deaths have occurred as a result of dosing accidents or other unrelated events, but states that necropsy should be conducted to prove the cause of death. If death is delayed, it is frequently not possible or practical to dose a replacement animal because the dosing solution and suitable animals are no longer available and the replacement animal(s) would be on a different time schedule than those dosed originally.

The physical form of a material designated for oral administration often presents unique challenges. Liquids can be administered as supplied or diluted with an appropriate vehicle, and powders or particulates can often be dissolved or suspended in an appropriate vehicle.

Dilution of the test material for oral administration is a key concern for the EPA. Their Guidance Document cites "unnecessary or improper dilution of the test material" as an "error in study conduct" and a cause for rejection of a study. EPA guidance is that liquids should be administered undiluted when possible and that the "highest workable concentration" should be used for solids and viscous materials. (A note of caution: very viscous materials are difficult to administer and the possibility of a dosing accident increases under these conditions). This is consistent with early guidance from the U.S. government that liquids should be tested in the form to which the consumer or worker will be exposed (28). The reason given by the EPA for the current mandate is concern that "dilution of caustic test materials may reduce their corrosive effects, thus giving an inaccurate representation of their potential threats." Minimal dilution of the administered material is required. It is worth noting that the OPPTS guideline for acute oral toxicity testing (OPTS Guideline No. 870.1100) states that "dosing test substances in a way known to cause marked pain and distress due to corrosive or irritating properties need not be carried out."

Based on the above philosophy, and confirmed in the Guidance Document, the EPA is, therefore, recommending that doses of the same material be administered at the same (a constant) concentration and that the dose volume be varied. This is in contrast to OECD Guideline 401 which states "Variability in test volume should be [sic] by adjusting the concentration to ensure a constant dose volume at all levels." (Subsequent OECD protocols for acute oral toxicity do not address this issue.) The rationale for use of a constant volume is that this procedure minimizes variability in gastric absorption related to differences in administered volume. Industry's attempt to clarify this by proposing the following guidance was found acceptable by the EPA and represents a reasonable compromise. This proposal, incorporated into the OPPTS guideline, is: either constant volume or constant concentration administration is acceptable, provided that the following guidance on dilutions is employed: When possible, liquid materials should be dosed neat. If dosing with neat material is not possible, due to high viscosity or toxicity that would preclude accurate low dose volumes, or if constant volume has been deemed to be the more appropriate method, the test material may be diluted. The highest concentration possible should be administered. Solid materials should be suspended or dissolved in the minimum amount of vehicle and dosed at the highest concentration possible.

Selection of an appropriate vehicle is often difficult. Water and oil (usually a vegetable oil, such as corn or peanut oil) are used most commonly. Materials which are not readily soluble in water or oil can frequently be suspended in a 1% aqueous mixture of methylcellulose, which is essentially nontoxic. Occasionally a more concentrated methylcellulose suspension (up to 5%) may be necessary. Materials for which appropriate solutions/suspensions cannot be prepared using one of these three vehicles often present major difficulties.

Limited solubility/suspendability of materials often dictates preparation of dilute mixtures, which require large volumes to be administered and are cause for concern as discussed above. The total volume of liquid dosing solution or suspension that can be administered to a rat is limited to the size of its stomach. However, because a rodent lacks a gagging reflex and has no emetic mechanism, material administered will generally be retained, although aspiration has been known to occur for very high volumes. Current guidelines state that the maximum volume that can be administered to a rodent is 20 ml/kg of body weight for aqueous solutions and 10 ml/kg for other vehicles (oils), although some references have indicated that volumes of aqueous solutions as high as 50 to 64 ml/kg can be given (26,27). We have administered volumes of up to 30–35 ml/ kg of aqueous suspensions of methylcellulose to control rats in our laboratory with no adverse effects and feel this is a reasonable maximum volume for aqueous mixtures. Although similar volumes of oil mixtures can be physically administered, a maximum volume of 10 ml/kg appears reasonable because of the cathartic effect of oils. Dose volumes of 10 and 20 ml/kg are equivalent to total volumes of 2–3.5 ml and 4–7 ml for rats in the 200–350 g weight range.

Limitations on total volume, therefore, present difficulties for materials which cannot easily be dissolved or suspended. The most dilute solutions that can be administered for a limit test (5000 mg/kg), using the maximum volume discussed above, are 25% for aqueous mixtures and 50% for oils. In cases where it is necessary to administer larger volumes, two or more small doses can be given over a period of up to 24 hours.

Administration of very low volumes, for materials with high toxicity, can also present problems. The lowest dose suggested in the EPA Guidance Document is 0.5 ml per animal, although lower dose volumes are considered acceptable if they can be administered accurately. None of the published guidelines address analytical confirmation of dose solutions/suspensions for acute toxicity studies. However, the EPA Guidance Document specifically states that analytical confirmation of dosing solutions is not a requirement.

Although vehicle control animals are not required for commonly used vehicles (water, oil, methylcellulose), most regulations require that the toxic characteristics should be known and/or that historical data be available. Our laboratory periodically generates control data by selecting 10 animals (5 of each sex) from shipments of rats used for acute oral toxicity studies. These animals are dosed with 1.0% methylcellulose (the vehicle most commonly used in acute oral studies) at a volume of 20 ml/kg (the maximum volume administered in any study) and observed following a standard protocol. Data are used for reference in preparing the final report and are appended to the report if applicable. Unfortunately, the best solvents are generally toxic and, thus, cannot be used as vehicles. Ethanol and acetone can be tolerated in relatively high doses but produce effects that may complicate interpretation of toxicity associated with the test material alone. It is sometimes possible to dissolve a material in a small amount of one of these vehicles and then dilute the solution in oil. Gels and resins often present problems because of their viscosity at room temperature. Warming these materials in a water bath to a temperature of up to 50°C will frequently facilitate mixing and dosing. However, it is important to ascertain that no thermal degradation occurs.

Another possibility for insoluble materials and granular materials that cannot be suspended is to mix the desired amount of material with a small amount of the animal's diet. The difficulty with this approach is the likelihood that the animal will not consume all of the treated diet or that it may selectively not consume chunks of test material. In some cases, if all of these approaches fail, it may not be possible to test a material by oral administration.

Rats are usually fasted overnight prior to oral dosing in order to assure an empty stomach. Mice, because of a more rapid metabolic rate, may be fasted for a shorter interval. This has been the traditional procedure and represents the most conservative approach and the one specified in testing guidelines and mandated in the EPA Guidance Document. Doses are calculated using weights obtained after fasting.

2. Dermal Administration

Materials administered dermally are applied to the skin of the back and sides. Fur is usually removed using a veterinary clipper on the day prior to dosing. Care should be taken to avoid nicks, cuts, or "clipper burns," which would disrupt the integrity of the skin and could alter permeability or enhance irritation. Clipping rats and guinea pigs is relatively easy, but rabbits require additional care because of their larger size, long fine hair, and delicate skin. A band extending from the scapulae (shoulders) to the wing of the ilium (hipbone) and halfway down the flank on each side of the animal comprises approximately 600^2 cm in an average-sized (3 kg) rabbit and represents approximately 10% of the body surface.

The EPA Guidance Document has confirmed that this is the appropriate exposure area and has rejected studies because the size of the exposure area was incorrect. However, the OPPTS guideline for acute dermal toxicity testing does acknowledge that administration of a material at a low dose volume (i.e., a highly toxic material) may not expose this entire area.

Dermal administration presents fewer logistic difficulties than oral administration. However, the EPA has expressed some concerns and provided guidance in this area as well, citing dilution of materials or over-moistening of dry test materials as "errors in study conduct" and reasons for rejection of studies. The Guidance Document states that liquids should be administered undiluted. (The only potential concern in this area is the use of small volumes that do not cover the entire exposure site. However, the EPA has acknowledged that this is acceptable and in keeping with their desire to use undiluted products. In cases where the entire site is not covered, measurement of the area of exposure is required.) The EPA Guidance Document specifies that dry materials must be moistened "in a beaker or other suitable vessel" only to the point necessary to assure proper contact with the skin. The "paste" thus formed should not be "runny" and should be applied directly to the skin (the dorsum). The OPPTS guidelines merely state that the test substance should be moistened sufficiently to ensure good contact with the skin. Although water and saline are the preferred vehicles for moistening test materials, the EPA will accept other materials as long as they are nontoxic, nonirritating and do not substantially change the properties of the test material or affect its permeability. Acceptable alternative vehicles include gum arabic, ethanol and water, carboxymethyl cellulose, glycerol, propylene glycol, PEG vegetable oil, and mineral oil. The inability to use water or saline must be justified in the report.

Liquids, pastes, and solid materials (sheets of plastic, fabric, etc.) are usually applied directly to the skin, taking care to cover the entire exposure site (or as large an area as possible), covered with a sheet of gauze and held in place with a semi-occlusive or occlusive dressing (covering). Technique is important here. The EPA has rejected studies because of "improper occlusion, covering, and wrapping of the test site" and has provided specific guidance for these procedures. A preference for application of materials directly to the skin is stated. However, the Agency has indicated a willingness to accept the following wording suggested by industry: "When possible the test substance should be applied directly to the skin, otherwise it may be applied directly to a porous gauze dressing that is immediately placed in contact with the animal's skin." This flexibility allows for judgment on the scientist's part and appropriate administration of materials that are not amenable to direct application to the dorsum. For example, materials that are not readily absorbed and may run off the skin are more appropriately applied to the gauze or applied to the back while a gauze is held on the back to catch any excess material. Administration of a dry material to the gauze, with water or saline added to form a dry paste at the time of application, also allows for a more precise measurement of the dose than mixing a paste in a container in which significant loss of material may occur. The procedure generally used in our laboratory is to weigh the dose of powder required for each animal, place this on the gauze strip, moisten it with physiological saline (one milliliter per gram of material) so that it adheres to the gauze, and apply the gauze to the dorsum.

The amount and thickness of gauze used has been reviewed extensively. The EPA confirms that the purpose of the gauze covering is to act as a reservoir for the test material and to keep the material localized and expresses concern that too many layers of gauze may absorb the material or the water used to moisten it and minimize the amount of material available to the skin. The following wording, proposed by industry, is considered acceptable to the EPA; "The test site must be covered in a suitable manner to retain the test material in contact with the skin, avoid wicking of the material from the skin surface, and to ensure that the animal cannot ingest the material. To minimize wicking, the gauze should be no more than 8-ply; fewer layers of gauze may be needed for small test volumes." Further covering with an occlusive material (such as plastic sheeting) or a semi-occlusive covering (such as perforated plastic) to prevent evaporation of liquids and ingestion of the test material is then required. Although both types of covering are acceptable, the semi-occlusive one is preferred. The final OPPTS guideline merely states: The test substance should be held in contact with the skin with a porous gauze dressing (<8 ply) and nonirritating tape throughout a 24-h exposure period. The test site should be further covered in a suitable manner to retain the gauze dressing and test substance and ensure that the animals cannot ingest the test substance. Restrainers may be used to prevent the ingestion of the test substance, but complete immobilization is not a recommended method. Although a semiocclusive dressing is preferred, an occlusive dressing will also be acceptable.

In our laboratory, a plastic sleeve, consisting of a rectangle cut from a sheet of plastic, folded and reinforced with masking tape on both ends, is used. This rectangular band is wrapped (overlapped) over the gauze band and secured in place by athletic tape. Application is performed by two technicians. One applies the material and secures the gauze and plastic covering; the second grasps the rabbit by the shoulders and pelvis and lifts it to allow the wrapping procedure. Other types of covering used are Saran Wrap, athletic bandages, or other surgical wrapping materials.

Most guidelines specify a 24-hr exposure period. Although animals may be immobilized (restrained in stocks) during this exposure period to prevent ingestion of test material or disturbance of the wrapping, it is preferable not to inhibit mobility. This can be accomplished by using Elizabethan-type collars. These can be purchased commercially from veterinary suppliers. We use collars fabricated from plastic (approximately 1/4-inch thick) and consisting of two semicircular pieces drilled with several holes in each end. The two pieces are secured with wing nuts: the holes allow the collars to be adjusted to fit each individual rabbit. These lightweight collars are tolerated well, allow free access to food and water, and serve their purpose by preventing the rabbits from disturbing the test site. They are generally worn throughout the exposure period and for the entire postdose period.

Although excess test material is wiped or washed after termination of the exposure, it is not uncommon for residual material to remain. The collars remove the possibility of ingestion. Materials administered dermally to rats and guinea pigs are generally secured by a flexible overlapping adhesive bandage (Elastoplast).

Doses are administered on the basis of animal body weight, although some toxicologists feel that dosing based on amount of skin surface covered is a more scientifically sound procedure.

E. Experimental Evaluation

Acute toxicity testing is generally the first, and frequently the only, evaluation of mammalian systemic toxicity performed on a product. Therefore, studies should be designed to obtain the maximum amount of information possible. Most acute toxicity studies attempt to provide some characterization of the nature and extent of the hazard of accidental exposure in addition to estimates of lethality.

1. Clinical Signs

Animals should be observed for mortality and unusual signs several times on the day of dosing and at least once daily thereafter (twice daily for mortality). Animals that appear to be moribund (close to death) should be checked frequently. Historically, moribund animals have generally not been killed in acute toxicity studies. Because mortality is one of the major endpoints and because some animals that appear to be moribund do recover, animals were held until death or recovery was seen. However, current testing guidelines (OECD, OPPTS) allow (or mandate) killing, for humane reasons, of animals that show "severe and enduring signs of distress and pain." OECD guideline 420 uses "evident toxicity" rather than mortality as an endpoint. These changes may result in slightly lower LD_{50} values than those obtained from previous tests but should not alter the ability to evaluate the relative toxicity of materials.

Observations are usually made for up to 14 days after dosing, but this interval may be extended if necessary to better characterize response. In our laboratory, we generally extend studies, if needed, in one-week intervals for logistic/scheduling reasons. It is important to make complete and appropriate observations, as detailed in the applicable test guidelines. One of the reasons for EPA's rejection of acute toxicity studies has been failure to conduct sufficient observations of the test animals.

Animals should be observed for effects on behavior (increased or decreased activity, etc.), neurologic function (tremors, convulsions, ataxia), respiratory parameters (alteration in rate or character, secretions), secretory and excretory functions (salivation, lacrimation, diarrhea, urination, fecal or urinary staining of the fur), physiologic state (hypothermia, etc.), and any other unusual signs. Although food consumption is generally not measured in acute toxicity tests, animals that are not eating or are eating poorly can be identified and these observations noted. OPPTS guidelines specifically state:

Observations should be detailed and carefully recorded, preferably using explicitly defined scales. Observations should include, but not be limited to, evaluation of skin and fur, eyes and mucous membranes, respiratory and circulatory effects, autonomic effects such as salivation, central nervous system effects, including tremors and convulsions, changes in the level of activity, gait and posture, reactivity to handling or sensory stimuli, altered strength, and stereotypes or bizarre behavior (e.g., self-mutilation, walking backwards).

"Cage-side" observations will detect mortality and extreme abnormalities. However, detailed observations generally require that the animal be handled, observed closely for behavioral/locomotor changes, and evaluated for such abnormalities as unusual respiratory sounds (rales). Recording forms or systems that provide the previous observations for each animal are preferable; this allows the technician to ascertain if unusual signs seen previously are still present and helps prevent oversights and data inconsistencies. Each laboratory develops a set of terminology and definitions that are used to describe unusual signs. Some observations are fairly unambiguous (convulsions), while others are more likely to vary from laboratory to laboratory. Such terms as lethargy, hypoactivity, depression and (possibly) sedation, and prostration are probably describing the same essential observation. It is important, therefore, to obtain a general sense of the types of abnormalities seen and not to attempt to make too fine a distinction between individual terminologies.

Neurologic effects may be seen for some materials. Specific regulatory guidelines (Neurotoxicology Screening Battery OPPTS Health Effects Test Guidelines 870.6200, August 1998), exist for evaluation of neurotoxic effects, generally for repeated-dose studies. However, for materials that may only be subjected to acute testing some toxicologists (8) suggest the inclusion of a neurologic screen (29). One must be careful, however, to distinguish true neurotoxic effects from manifestations of the overwhelming general toxic effects of a lethal or near-lethal dose of a material.

Some indication of severe dermal effects (necrosis, eschar formation) is warranted for dermal studies, although the systemic, rather than the local, effects are of primary importance in this type of study. EPA guidelines and their Guidance Document are unclear on the extent of dermal observations that should be made. The Guidance Document states that "Evaluations of . . . local irritation should be made frequently on the day of application and daily thereafter." However, unless the study is intended to support dermal irritation labeling, i.e., a waiver of a dermal irritation study, it does not appear that specific scoring of dermal responses is necessary. The OPPTS guideline includes skin among organs to be evaluated and states a preference for "defined scales" for observations. However, no specific requirement for scoring of dermal observations is included.

Assignment of dermal scores (30) can be done, but this may be misleading because of the large surface area covered and the possible variability from area to area. Materials that are severely irritating and/or corrosive may produce such severe skin damage that alterations in activity, locomotion, and food consumption are seen. In extremely severe cases, secondary septicemia of damaged skin may intervene. If such severe local tissue damage is seen, it is generally advisable to sacrifice the animals, not only for humane reasons, but also because any systemic toxic manifestations would be secondary to the skin destruction and evaluation of the hazard should be made based on the irritant, rather than the toxic potential of this type of material.

2. Body Weights

Most guidelines recommend that body weights be obtained at least weekly as well as at the time of death. More frequent weighing may help to distinguish between levels of toxicity and speed of recovery for different materials or for different doses of the same material. Animals that die generally exhibit antemortem weight losses. Weight changes are usually not calculated for animals that die during the first 24 hr, since these animals were fasted prior to dosing and probably did not consume any food after dosing. Recovery of weight to pretest values or higher is usually apparent after the first week or, occasionally after two weeks in survivor rats. Failure to recover weight, especially when accompanied by continuing signs of toxicity, may indicate a delayed effect. In such cases, the postdose observation period should be extended for one or more weeks to characterize the nature and time course of toxic effects and recovery.

Weight changes in rabbits are not as marked as those in rats, and it is not unusual to see little or no weight change (± 0.2 kg) in untreated rabbits over a 1- or 2-week interval. However, some materials do produce marked weight decreases indicative of systemic toxicity.

3. Clinical Laboratory Studies

Previous EPA, FIFRA, and TSCA guidelines suggested that clinical laboratory studies should be considered. However, this suggestion does not appear in the OPPTS guidelines. Although such studies increase the cost of acute toxicity evaluations, they may provide important information about possible target organs and the nature of the hazards. Certain classes of materials with known effects would be likely candidates for such studies, for example, cholinesterase evaluations for pesticides; methemoglobin determinations for anilines; hematology studies for benzenes; liver and kidney function studies for some solvents. Correlation of blood effects with lethal and nonlethal dosage levels can provide useful information for personnel monitoring and other industrial hygiene considerations.

4. Postmortem Examinations

Mose guidelines suggest or require that gross postmortem examinations be considered, and these are generally performed, although the usefulness of information obtained is sometimes questionable. It is seldom possible to determine a specific cause of death (except in the case of intubation accidents). Examination of animals found dead is usually complicated by postmortem autolytic changes (discoloration of several organs). Severe gastrointestinal damage may be indicated by red or black discoloration of the stomach and intestinal walls and the presence of red or black material in the gastrointestinal tract. However, similar changes can be seen with advanced autolysis. A common finding in male rats found dead in our laboratory is the presence of one or both testes in the body cavity. No relationship to specific types of materials has been evident, and we have concluded that this represents a nonspecific response to antemortem stress rather than an effect on the reproductive system.

Animals surviving to study termination (usually 14 days) have generally recovered from any acute toxic effects and seldom exhibit any remarkable postmortem findings. Adhesion of abdominal viscera sometimes provides evidence of severe gastrointestinal irritation. The presence of historical control data is useful in interpreting postmortem observations. It is important to distinguish changes resulting from the method of killing the animals (i.e., red foci in the lungs as a result of carbon dioxide asphyxiation) from true toxic effects.

In some cases, obtaining organ weights may provide useful information on target organ toxicity. However, unless concurrent control values are available, it may be difficult to interpret these data. Obtaining weights of spleen and thymus as a measure of immunotoxic effect has been suggested, and accumulation of such data would probably provide useful information in this relatively new area of toxicology.

Microscopic pathology is seldom performed for acute toxicity studies and tissues are rarely saved. In some cases, histopathological examination of target organs is suggested and may provide useful information however, and this option should be considered. Treated skin from animals used for acute dermal toxicity tests is sometimes preserved for possible microscopic examination. Such examinations are not likely to provide information on the acute systemic toxicity of a material.

F. Reporting

Guidelines are generally specific in the types of information required for reports and should be reviewed carefully. Detailed information describing all aspects of the study is expected. Inadequate reporting has been a cause for rejection of large numbers of studies submitted to the EPA. Fortunately, such errors and oversights can be corrected (as long as the data exist). The unnecessary delays this creates are reason to report studies completely the first time.

ACKNOWLEDGMENT

Grateful acknowledgment is given to Ms. Donna L. Blaszcak for editorial comments, reality checks and helpful suggestions.

REFERENCES

1. United States State Department. Harmonization of hazard classification and labeling, questions and answers. December 14, 1997.
2. OECD (Organization for Economic Cooperation and Development). Classification of substances based on acute toxicity. Sixth meeting of the advisory group on harmonization of classification and labeling systems, 22nd–24th April, 1998. ENV/MC/CHEM/HCL(98)1. March 1998.
3. Diener, W. and E. Schlede, Federal Institute for Health Protection of Consumers and Veterinary Medicine (BgVV), Berlin, Germany (1998). The dermal acute toxic class method as an alternative to the dermal LD_{50} test. The Toxicologist. 42: 1-S, p. 219 (Abstract 1078).
4. U.S. Environmental Protection Agency, Technical Review Branch, Registration Division, Office of Pesticide Programs. Conduct of acute toxicity studies for registration. September 1997.
5. Acute Toxicity Texts, LD_{50} (LC_{50}) Determinations and Alternatives. European Chemical Industry Ecology and Toxicology Centre (ECETOC) Monograph No. 6, May 1985.
6. Steelman, R.L. (1965). Factors Influencing Acute Toxicity Values. Presented at the East$_2$ Subcommittee Meeting, Pharmaceutical Manufacturers Association Drug Safety Evaluation Committee, New York City, February 11, 1965.
7. OECD (Organization for Economic Cooperation and Development). Guidelines for testing of chemicals, Section 4: Health effects, short term toxicology, p. 3, 1993.
8. Gad, S.C., Smith, A.C., Cram, A.L., Gavigan, F.A., and Derelanko, M.J. (1984). Innovative designs and practices for acute systemic toxicity studies. *Drug Chem. Toxicol.* 7(5):423–434.
9. A New Approach to the Classification of Substances and Preparations on the Basis of their Acute Toxicity. A Report by the British Toxicology Society Working Party on Toxicity. Human Toxicol. 3:85–92, 1984.
10. Deichmann, W.B. and Leblane, T.J. (1943). Determination of the approximate lethal dose with about six animals. J. Indust. Hyg. Toxicol. 25:415–417.
11. Smyth, Jr., H.F. and Carpenter, C.P. (1944). The place of the range finding test in the industrial laboratory. J. Ind. Hyg. Toxicol. 26:269.
12. Bruce, R.D. (1985). An up-and-down procedure for acute toxicity testing. Fund. Appl. Toxicol. 5:151–157.

13. LeBeau, J.E. (1983). The role of the LD_{50} determination in drug safety evaluation. Reg. Toxicol. Pharmacol. 3:71–74.

14. Depass, L.R., Myers, R.C., Weaver, E.V., and Weil, C.S. (1984). Alternative Methods in Toxicology, Vol. 2. Acute Toxicity Testing: Alternative Approaches. New York, Mary Ann Liebert Inc., publishers.

15. Schultz, F. and Fuchs, H. (1982). A new approach to minimising the number of animals used in acute toxicity testing and optimising the information of test results. Arch. Toxical. 51:197.

16. Tattersall, M.C. (1982). Statistics and the LD_{50} study. Arch. Toxicol. (Suppl.) 5: 267.

16a. ASTM E-1163-87. Standard Test Method for Estimating Acute Oral Toxicity in Rats. American Society for Testing and Materials, Philadelphia, PA, 1987.

16b. Lipnik, R.L., Contruvo, J.A., Hill, R.N., Bruce, R.D., Stitzel, K.A., Walker, A.P., Chiu, I., Goddard, M., Segal, L., Springer, J.A., and Myers, R.C. (1995). Comparison of the up-and-down, conventional LD_{50} and fixed dose acute toxicity procedures. Fd. Chem. Toxicol. 33, 223–231.

17. Bliss, C.I. (1938). Quart. J. Pharm. Pharmacol. 11:192–216.

18. Finney, D.G. (1971). Probit Analysis, 3rd ed. London, Cambridge University Press.

19. Litchfield, J.T. and Wilcoxon, F. (1949). J. Pharmacol. Exp. Ther. 96:99–113.

20. Miller, L.C. and Tainer, M.L. (1944). Proc. Soc. Exp. Biol. Med. NY 57:261–264.

21. Thompson, W. (1947). Bact. Rev. 11:115–141.

22. Weil, C.S. (1952). Biometrics 8:249–263.

23. Guide for the Care and use of Laboratory Animals, Institute of Laboratory Animal Resources, Commission on Life Sciences, National Research Council, National Academy Press, Washington, DC, 1996.

24. Baker, H.J., Lindsey, J.R., and Weisbroth, S.H. (Eds.). (1979). The Laboratory Rat. New York, Academic Press.

25. Weisbroth, S.H., Flatt, R.E., and Kraus, A.L. (Eds.). (1974). The Biology of the Laboratory Rabbit. New York, Academic Press.

26. Auletta, C.S. Acute, Subchronic and Chronic Toxicology, CRC Handbook of Toxicology, M.J. Delelanko and M.A. Hollinger, eds. CRC Press, 1995 p. 79

27. Appraisal of the Safety of Chemicals in Foods, Drugs and Cosmetics. (1959). Association of Food and Drug Officials of the United States.

28. Principles and Procedures for Evaluating the Toxicity of Household Substances. (1977). Washington, D.C. National Academy of Science.

29. Gad, S.C. (1982). A neuromuscular screen for use in industrial toxicology. J. Toxicol. Env. Health 9:691–704.

30. Draize, J.H. (1959). The Appraisal of Chemical in Foods, Drugs, and Cosmetics. Austin, TX, Association of Food and Drug Officials of the United States.

4

Evaluating Products for Their Potential to Cause Dermal and Ocular Irritation and Corrosion

Shayne Cox Gad
Gad Consulting Services, Raleigh, North Carolina

I. INTRODUCTION

Among the most fundamental assessments of the safety of a product or, indeed, of any material that has the potential to be in contact with a significant number of people in our society, are tests in animals that seek to predict potential eye and skin irritation or corrosion (that is, local tolerance to chemicals in the most common body regions of exposure). As in all the other tests in what is called range-finding, tier I, or acute battery studies, the tests used here are both among the oldest designs and are currently undergoing the greatest degree of scrutiny and change. All currently established test methods for these endpoints use the same model—the rabbit (almost exclusively the New Zealand White). These tests have become the first focus point of concern and protest by those concerned with the humane treatment and rights of animals. Because of this, the design and technique used in these tests have been modified. Also, alternatives have been developed that use models other than the rabbit or other mammals, and await regulatory recognition.

II. DERMAL TESTING

Virtually all man-made chemicals have the potential to come into contact with human skin. In fact, many (cosmetics and shampoos, for example) are intended for skin contact. The greatest number of industry-related medical problems are skin conditions, indicating the large extent of dermal exposure where none is intended. The testing procedures that are currently used are basically those proposed by Draize et al. (1), and have changed little since their initial use in 1944.

Testing is performed to evaluate the potential occurrence of two different, yet related endpoints. The broadest application of these is an evaluation of the potential to cause skin irritation,characterized by erythema (redness) and edema (swelling). Severity of irritation is measured in terms of both the degree and duration of these two parameters. There are three types of irritation tests, each designed to address a different concern.

1. Primary (or acute) irritation, a localized reversible dermal response resulting from a single application of or exposure to a chemical without the involvement of the immune system
2. Cumulative irritation, a reversible dermal response caused by repeated exposure to a substance (each individual exposure not being capable of causing acute primary irritation)
3. Photochemically induced irritation, which is a primary irritation resulting from light-induced molecular changes in the chemical to which the skin has been exposed

Though most regulations and common practice characterize an irritation that persists 14 days past the end of exposure as other than reversible, the second endpoint of concern with dermal exposure corrosion is assessed in separate test designs. These tests start with a shorter exposure period (4 hours or less) to the material of concern, and then evaluates simply whether tissue has been killed or not (or, in other words, if necrosis is present or not).

It should be clear that, if a material is found to have less than severe dermal irritation potential, it will not be corrosive and therefore need not be tested separately for the corrosion endpoint.

A. Objectives

The first step in undertaking a dermal testing program is developing a clear statement of objective, that is, understanding exactly what question is being asked for what purpose. The three major objectives for such testing are presented below.

1. Providing Regulator Required Baseline Data. Any product now in commerce must both be labeled appropriately for shipping (2) and accompanied by a material safety data sheet (MSDS) which clearly states potential hazards associated with handling it. Department of Transportation (DOT) regulations also prescribe different levels of packaging on materials found to constitute hazards as specified in the regulations. These requirements demand absolute identification of severe irritants or corrosives and adherence to the basics of test

methods promulgated by the regulations. False positives (type I errors) are to be avoided in these usages.

2. Hazard Assessment for Accidents. For most materials, dermal exposure is not intended to occur, yet will in cases of accidental spillage or mishandling. Here we need to correctly identify the hazard associated with such exposures, being equally concerned with false positives or false negatives.

3. Assessment of Safety for Use. The materials at issue here are the full range of products for which dermal exposure will occur in the normal course of use. These range from cosmetics and hand soaps to bleaches, laundry detergents, and paint removers. No manufacturer desires to market a product which cannot be used safely and will lead to extensive liability if entered in the market place. Accordingly, the desire here is to accurately predict the potential hazards in humans, that is, to have neither false positives nor false negatives.

Table 1 sets forth the regulatory mandated test designs, that form the basis of all currently employed test procedures.

All of these methods use the same scoring scale: the Draize scale (1,3), which is presented in Table 2. However, although the regulations prescribe these

Table 1 Regulatory-Mandated Test Designs

Agency	Test Material		Exposure time (r)	Number of rabbits	Sites per animal (intact/ abraded)
	Solid	Liquid			
Department of Transportation (DOT)	Not specified	Not specified	4[b]	6	1/0
Environmental Protection Agency (EPA)[a]	Moisten	Undiluted	24	6	2/0
Consumer Product Safety Commission (CPSC)	Dissolve in appropriate vehicle	Neat	24	6	1/1
Organization for Economic Cooperation and Development (OECD)	Moisten	Undiluted	4[b]	3[b]	1/0

[a]Most recent EPA guidelines are the same as OECD.
[b]But additional animals may be required to clarify equivocal results.

Table 2 Evaluation of Skin Reactions

Skin reaction	Value
Erythema and eschar formation:	
No erythema	0
Very slight erythema (barely perceptible)	1
Well-defined erythema	2
Moderate to severe erythema	3
Severe erythema (beet redness) to slight eschar formation	
(injuries in depth)	4
Necrosis (death of tissue)	+N
Eschar (sloughing)	+E
Edema formation:	
No edema	0
Very slight edema (barely perceptible)	1
Slight edema (edges of area well defined by definite raising)	2
Moderate edema (raised approximately one millimeter)	3
Severe edema (raised more than one millimeter and extending	
beyond the area of exposure)	4
Total possible score for primary irritation	8

different test methods, most laboratories actually perform some modified methods. Below are two recommended modifications (one for irritation, the other for corrosion) that reflect laboratory experience by the author.

B. Primary Dermal Irritation Test

1. Rabbit Screening Procedure

    1. A group of at least 8–12 New Zealand White rabbits are screened for the study.

    2. All rabbits selected for the study must be in good health; any rabbit exhibiting sniffles, hair loss, loose stools, or apparent weight loss is rejected and replaced.

    3. One day (at least 18 hr) prior to application of the test substance, each rabbit is prepared by clipping the hair from the back and sides using a small animal clipper. A size No. 10 blade is used to remove the long hair and then a size No. 40 blade is used to remove the remaining hair.

    4. Six animals with skin sites that are free of hyperemia or abrasion (due to shaving) are selected. Skin sites that are in the telogen phase (resting stage of hair growth) are used; those skin sites that are in the anagen phase (stage of active growth) are not used.

2. Study Procedure

1. As many as four areas of skin, two on each side of the rabbit's back, can be utilized for sites of administration.

2. Separate animals are not required for an untreated control group. Each animals serves as its own control.

3. Besides the test substance, a positive control substance (a known skin irritant, 1% sodium lauryl sulfate) and a negative control (untreated patch) are applied to the skin. When a vehicle is used for diluting, suspending, or moistening the test substance, a vehicle control patch is required, especially if the vehicle is known to cause any toxic dermal reactions or if there is insufficient information about the dermal effects of the vehicle.

At end of exposure	Scoring intervals postexposure	Note	References
Skin washed with appropriate vehicle	4 and 48 hr	Endpoint is corrosion in 2 of 6 animals	(3)
Skin wiped but not washed	24 and 72 hr; may continue until irritation fades or is judged irreversible	Toxic Substance Act test	(4)
Not specified	24 and 72 hr	Federal Hazardous Substances Act (FHSA)	(5)
Wash with water or solvent	30–60 min, 24, 48, 72 hr or until judged irreversible	European Common Market	(6)

4. The four intact (free of abrasion) sites of administration are assigned a code number:

1   Test substance
2   Negative control
3   Positive control
4   Vehicle control (if required)

5. The following diagram illustrates the pattern of administration used in each study. This pattern of administration makes certain that the test substances and controls are applied to each position at least once.

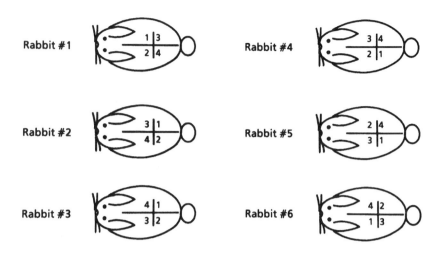

6.   Each test or control substance is held in place with a 1 × 1 inch square 12-ply surgical gauze patch. The gauze patch is applied to the appropriate skin site and secured with 1 in.-wide strips of surgical tape at the four edges, leaving the center of the gauze patch nonoccluded.

7.   If the test substance is a solid or semisolid, a 0.5 g portion is weighed and placed on the gauze patch. The test substance patch is placed on the appropriate skin site and secured. The patch is subsequently moistened with 0.5 ml of physiological saline.

8.   When the test substance is in flake, granule, powder, or other particulate form, the weight of the test substance that has a volume of 0.5 ml (after compacting as much as possible without crushing or altering the individual particles, such as by tapping the measuring container) is used whenever this volume weighs less than 0.5 g.

When applying powders, granules, and so on, the gauze patch designed for the test sample is secured to the appropriate skin site with one of the four strips of tape at the most ventral position of the animal. With one hand, the appropriate amount of sample measuring 0.5 ml is carefully poured from a glycine weighting paper onto the gauze patch which is held in a horizontal (level) position with the other hand. The patch containing the test sample is then placed carefully in position on the skin by raising the remaining three edges with tape dorsally until they are completely secured. The patch is subsequently moistened with 0.5 ml of physiological saline.

9.   If the test substance is a liquid, a patch is applied and secured to the appropriate skin site. A 1 ml tuberculin syringe is used to measure and apply 0.5 ml of test substance to the patch.

10. If the test substance is a fabric, a 1 × 1 in. square sample is cut and placed on a patch. The test substance patch is placed on the appropriate skin site and secured. The patch is subsequently moistened with 0.5 ml of physiological saline.

11. The negative control site is covered with an untreated 12 ply surgical gauze patch (1 × 1 in.).

12. The positive control substance and vehicle control substance are applied to the gauze patch in the same manner as a liquid test substance.

13. The entire trunk of the animal is covered with an impervious material (such as Saran wrap) for a 24-hr period of exposure. The Saran wrap is secured by wrapping several long strips of athletic adhesive tape around the trunk of the animal. The impervious material aids in maintaining the position of the patches and retards evaporation of volatile test substances.

14. An Elizabethan collar is fitted and fastened around the neck of each test animal. The collar remains in place for the 24-hr exposure period. The collars are utilized to prevent removal of wrappings and patches by the animals, while allowing the animals food and water ad libitum.

15. The wrapping is removed at the end of the 24-hr exposure period. The test substance skin site is wiped to remove any test substance still remaining. When colored test substances (such as dyes) are used, it may be necessary to wash the test substance from the test site with an appropriate solvent or vehicle (one that is suitable for the substance being tested). This is done to clean the test site to facilitate accurate evaluation for skin irritation.

16. Immediately after removal of the patches, each 1 × 1 in. square test or control site is outlined with an indelible marker by dotting each of the four corners. This procedure delineates the site for identification.

3. Observations

1. Observations are made of the test and control skin sites 1 hr after removal of the patches (25 hr post-initiation of application). Erythema and edema are evaluated and scored on the basis of the designated values presented earlier in Table 2.

2. Observations again are performed 48 and 72 hr after application and scores are recorded.

3. If necrosis is present or the dermal reaction needs description, this should be done. Necrosis should receive the maximum score for erythema and eschar formation (4) and a (+N) to designate necrosis.

4. When a test substance produces dermal irritation that persists 72 hr postapplication, daily observations of test and control sites are continued on all animals until all irritation caused by the test substance resolves or until day 14 postapplication.

4. Evaluation of Results

1. A subtotal irritation value for erythema or eschar formation is determined for each rabbit by adding the values observed at 25, 48, and 72 hr postapplication.

2. A subtotal irritation value for edema formation is determined for each rabbit by adding the values observed at 25, 48, and 72 hr postapplication.

3. A total irritation score is calculated for each rabbit by adding the subtotal irritation value for erythema or eschar formation to the subtotal irritation value for edema formation.

4. The primary dermal irritation index is calculated for the test substance or control substance by dividing the sum of total irritation scores by the number of observations, 18 (3 days × 6 animals = 18 observations).

5. A test/control substance producing a primary dermal irritation index (PDII) of 0.0 is a nonirritant: >0.0–0.5 is a negligible irritant; >0.5–2.0 is a mild irritant; >2.0–5.0 is a moderate irritant; and >5.0–8.0 is a severe irritant. This categorization of dermal irritation is a modification of the original classification described by Draize.

PDII = 0.0	Nonirritant
>0.0–0.5	Negligible irritant
>0.5–2.0	Mild irritant
>2.0–5.0	Moderate irritant
>5.0–8.0	Severe irritant

5. Limitation of the Test

The results of this test are subject to considerable variability due to the relatively small differences in technique, such as how snuggly the occlusive wrap is applied. Weil and Scala (7) arranged and reported on an intralaboratory study (by 25 laboratories) which clearly established this fact. However, the method outlined above has proven to give reproducible results in the hands of the same technicians over a period of years (8) and contains some internal controls (the positive and vehicle controls) against large variabilities in results or the occurrence of false negatives or false positives. However, it should be recognized that the test is designed with a bias to preclude false negatives, and therefore tends to exaggerate results in relation to what would happen in humans. Findings of negligible (or even very low range mild) irritancy should therefore not be of concern unless the product under test is to have large-scale and prolonged dermal contact.

   a. Factors Affecting Irritation Responses and Test Outcome.   The results of local tissue irritation tests are subject to considerable variability due to relatively small differences in test design or technique. Weil and Scala (7) arranged and reported on the best known of several intralaboratory studies to clearly establish this fact. Though the methods presented above have proven to give reproducible results in the hands of the same technicians over a period of years (8) and contain some internal controls (the positive and vehicle controls in the PDI) against large variabilities in results or the occurrence of either false positives or negatives, it is still essential to be aware of those factors that may systematically alter test results. These factors are summarized below.

1. In general, any factor that increases absorption through the stratum corneum or mucous membrane will also increase the severity of an intrinsic response. Unless this factor mirrors potential exposure conditions, it may, in turn, adversely affect the relevance of test results.

2. The physical nature of solids must be carefully considered both before testing and in interpreting results. Shape (sharp edges), size (small particles may abrade the skin due to being rubbed back and forth under the occlusive wrap), and rigidity (stiff fibers or very hard particles will be physically irritating) of solids may all enhance an irritation response.

3. Solids frequently give different results when they are tested dry than if wetted for the test. As a general rule, solids are more irritating if moistened (going back to Item A, wetting is a factor that tends to enhance absorption). Care should also be taken as to selecting a moistening agent—some (few) batches of U.S. Pharmacopeia physiological saline (used to simulate sweat) have proven to be mildly irritating to the skin and mucous membrane on their own. Liquids other than water or saline should not be used.

4. If the treated region on potential human patients will be a compromised skin surface barrier (e.g., if it is cut or burned) some test animals should likewise have their application sites compromised. This procedure is based on the assumption that abraded skin is uniformly more sensitive to irritation. Experiments, however, have shown that this is not necessarily true; some materials produce more irritation on abraded skin, while others produce less (8,29).

5. The degree of occlusion (in fact, the tightness of the wrap over the test site) also alters percutaneous absorption and therefore irritation. One important quality control issue in the laboratory is achieving a reproducible degree of occlusion in dermal wrappings.

6. Both the age of the test animal and the application site (saddle of the back, vs. flank) can markedly alter test outcome. Both of these factors are also operative in humans, of course (Mathias, 1983), but in dermal irritation tests, the objective is to remove all such sources of variability. In general, as an animal ages, sensitivity to irritation decreases. For the dermal test, the skin on the middle of the back (other than directly over the spine) tends to be thicker (and therefore less sensitive to irritations) than that on the flanks.

7. The sex of the test animals can also alter study results, because both regional skin thickness and surface blood flow vary between males and females.

8. Finally, the single most important (yet also most frequently overlooked) factor that influences the results and outcome of these (and, in fact, most) acute studies is the training of the staff. In determining how test materials are prepared and applied and in how results are "read" against a subjective scale, both accuracy and precision are extremely dependent on the technicians involved. To achieve the desired results, initial training must be careful and all-inclusive. As important, some form of regular refresher training must be exercised, particularly in the area of scoring of results. Use of a set of color photographic standards as a training and reference tool is strongly recommended; such standards should clearly demonstrate each of the grades in the Draize dermal scale.

9. It should be recognized that the dermal irritancy test is designed with a bias to preclude false negatives and, therefore, tends to exaggerate results in relation to what would happen in humans. Findings of negligible irritancy (or even in the very low mild irritant range) should therefore be of no concern unless the product under test is to have large-scale and prolonged dermal contact.

b. Problems in Testing (and Their Resolutions). Some materials, by either their physicochemical or toxicological natures, generate difficulties in the performance and evaluation of dermal irritation tests. The most commonly encountered of these problems are presented below.

1. Compound volatility. One is sometimes required or requested to evaluate the potential irritancy of a liquid that has a boiling point between room temperature and the body temperature of the test animal. As a result, the liquid portion of the material will evaporate off before the end of the testing period. There is no real way around the problem; one can only make clear in the report on the test that the traditional test requirements were not met, though an evaluation of potential irritant hazard was probably achieved (for the liquid phase would also have evaporated from a human that it was spilled on).

2. Pigmented. material. Some materials are strongly colored or discolor the skin at the application site. This makes the traditional scoring process difficult or impossible. One can try to remove the pigmentation with a solvent; if successful, the erythema can then be evaluated. If use of a solvent fails or is unacceptable, one can (wearing thin latex gloves) feel the skin to determine if there is warmth, swelling, and/or rigidity—all secondary indicators of the irritation response.

3. Systemic toxicity. On rare occasions, the dermal irritation study is begun only to have the animals die very rapidly after test material is applied.

C. Dermal Corrosivity Test

This procedure is based on the Department of Transportation "Method of Testing Corrosion to Skin" (9).

1. Rabbit Screening Procedure

1.   A group of at least 8–12 New Zealand White rabbits are screened for the study.

2.   All rabbits selected for the study must be in good health; any rabbit exhibiting sniffles, hair loss, loose stools, or apparent weight loss is rejected and replaced.

3.   One day (at least 18 hr) prior to application of the test substance, each rabbit is prepared by clipping the hair from the back and sides using a small animal clipper. A size No. 10 blade is used to remove the long hair and then a size No. 40 blade is used to remove the remaining hair.

4.   Six animals with skin sites that are free of hyperemia or abrasion (due to shaving) are selected. Skin sites that are in the telogen phase (resting stage of hair growth) are used; those skin sites that are in the anagen phase (stage of active growth) are not used.

2. Study Procedure

1.   Separate animals are not required for an untreated control group. Each animals serves as its own control.

2.   In addition to the test substance, a negative control (untreated patch) is applied to the skin.

    a.   If the test substance is a liquid, it is applied undiluted.

    b.   If the test substance is a solid or a semisolid, it is applied as such.

    c.   If information about the effects of moistening a solid or semisolid test substance is required, a third optional site can be added to that test.

3.   The intact (free of abrasion) sites of administration are assigned a code number:

1	Test substance
2	Negative control
3	(Optional) test substance moistened with 0.5 ml of physiological saline

4.   The following diagram illustrates the pattern of administration used in each study.

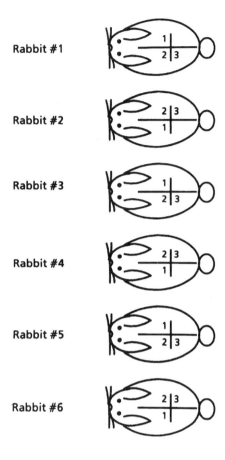

5. Each test or control substance is held in place with a 1 × 1 in. square 12-ply surgical gauze patch. The gauze patch is applied to the appropriate skin site and secured with 1 in.-wide strips of surgical tape at the four edges, leaving the center of the gauze patch nonoccluded.

6. If the test substance is a solid or semisolid, a 0.5 g portion is weighed and placed on the gauze patch. The test substance patch is placed on the appropriate skin site and secured.

a. When the test substance is in flake, granule, powder, or other particulate form, the weight of the test substance that has a volume of 0.5 ml (after compacting as much as possible without crushing or altering the individual particles, such as by tapping the measuring container) is used whenever this volume weighs less than 0.5 g.

b. When applying powders, granules, and so on, the gauze patch designed for the test sample is secured to the appropriate skin site with one of the four strips of tape at the most ventral position of the animal. With one hand, the appropriate amount of sample measuring 0.5 ml is carefully poured from a glycine weighting paper onto the gauze patch which is held in a horizontal (level) position with the other hand. The patch containing the test sample is then placed carefully in position on the skin by raising the remaining three edges with tape dorsally until they are completely secured.

7.   As an option, the effects of moistening a solid or semisolid can be investigated. If this is done the test substance is applied to site 3 (as described above) and the patch holding the test substance is subsequently moistened with 0.5 ml of physiological saline.

8.   If the test substance is a liquid, a patch is applied and secured to the appropriate skin site. A 1 ml tuberculin syringe is used to measure and apply 0.5 ml of test substance to the patch.

9.   The negative control site 2 is covered with an untreated 12-ply surgical gauze patch.

10.   The entire trunk of the animal is covered with an impervious material (such as Saran wrap) for a 24-hr period of exposure. The Saran wrap is secured by wrapping several long strips of athletic adhesive tape around the trunk of the animal. The impervious material aids in maintaining the position of the patches and retards evaporation of volatile test substances.

11.   An Elizabethan collar is fitted and fastened around the neck of each test animal. The collar remains in place for the 4-hr exposure period. The collars are utilized to prevent removal of wrappings and patches by the animals, while allowing the animals food and water ad libitum.

12.   The wrapping is removed at the end of the 4-hr exposure period. The test substance skin site is wiped to remove any test substance still remaining. When colored test substances (such as dyes) are used, it may be necessary to wash the test substance from the test site with an appropriate solvent or vehicle (one that is suitable for the substance being tested). This is done to clean the test site to facilitate accurate evaluation.

13.   Immediately after removal of the patches, each 1 × 1 inch square test or control site is outlined with an indelible marker by dotting each of the four corners. This procedure delineates the site for identification.

3. Observations

1.   After 4 hr of exposure, observations of the test and control sites are described. Observations are made again at the end of a total of 48 hr (44 hr after the first reading).

2.   In addition, the Draize grading system (3) for evaluation of skin reactions was used to score the skin sites at 4 and 48 hr after dosing (Table 2).

4. Evaluation of Results

1.   Corrosion would be considered to have resulted if the test substance caused destruction or irreversible alteration of the tissue on at least 2 of the 6

rabbits tested. Ulceration or necrosis of the tissue at either 4 or 48 hr postexposure would be considered permanent tissue damage (i.e., tissue destruction does not include merely sloughing of the superficial epidermis, or erythema, edema, or fissuring) (9).

2. If a conclusive assessment of the extent of damage to the skin can not be made after 48 hr (it is difficult to determine whether or not permanent, irreversible damage is present) daily observations of the skin sites will be made and recorded, either until a determination can be made about the extent of skin damage or until day 14 after exposure. Photographs will be taken at those time intervals after exposure that are most meaningful for documentation purposes.

3. If the test continues to day 14 after exposure, a final evaluation of the skin is made, resulting in a conclusive assessment of the test substance's potential to cause corrosion to skin. Scar tissue formation at this time is indicative of permanent tissue damage.

5. Limitation of the Test

Unlike the primary dermal irritancy test, the results from the corrosivity test should be taken at face value. There is some lab-to-lab variability and the test does produce some false positives (though these are almost always at least severely irritating compounds), but does not produce false negatives.

Extensive progress has been made in devising alternative (*in vitro*) systems for evaluating the dermal irritation potential of chemicals. This is an effort that extends back to the early 1960s, but which saw little progress until the 1990s. Table 3 overviews 20 proposed systems constituting five very different approaches (40).

The first set of approaches (I) uses patches of excised human or animal skin maintained in some modification of a glass diffusion cell that maintains the moisture, temperature, oxygenation, and electrolyte balance of the skin section. In this approach, after the skin section has been allowed to equilibrate for some time, the material of concern is placed on the exterior surface and wetted (if not liquid). Irritation is evaluated either by swelling of the skin (a crude and relatively insensitive method for mild and moderate irritants), by evaluation of inhibition of uptake of radiolabeled nutrients or by measurement of leakage of enzymes through damaged membranes.

The second set of approaches (II) utilizes a form of surrogate skin culture comprising a mix of skin cells which closely mirror key aspects of the architecture and function of the intact organ. These systems seemingly offer a real potential advantage but, to date, the "damage markers" employed (or proposed) as predictors of dermal irritation have been limited to cytotoxicity.

The third set of approaches (III) is to use some form of cultured cell (either primary or transformed), with primary human epidermal keratinocytes (HEKs) preferred. The cell cultures are exposed to the material of interest, then

Table 3 In Vitro Dermal Irritation Test Systems (40)

System	End-point	Validation data?*
I. SKIN PATCHES		
Excised patch of perfused skin	Swelling	No
Mouse skin organ culture	Inhibition of incorporation of $[^3\text{H}]$-thymidine and $[^{14}\text{C}]$-leucine labels	No
Mouse skin organ culture	Leakage of LDH and GOT	Yes
II. SURROGATE SKIN		
Testskin—cultured surrogate skin patch	Morphological evaluation	No
Cultured surrogate skin patch	Cytotoxicity	No
III. CULTURED CELLS		
Human epidermal keratinocytes (HEKs)	Release of labeled arachidonic acid	Yes
Fibroblasts	Acid release	
HEKs	Cytotoxicity	Yes
HEKs	Cytotoxicity (MIT)	Yes
HEKs, dermal fibroblasts	Cytotoxicity	Yes
HEKs	Inflammation mediator release	No
Cultured Chinese hamster ovary	Increases in β-hexosaminidase levels in the media	No
Cultured C_3 H10T$_{1/4}$ and HEK cells	Lipid metabolism inhibition	No
Cultured cells		
BHK21/C13		
BHK21/C13		
primary rat thymocytes	Cell detachment	Yes
	Growth inhibition	
	Increased membrane permeability	
Rat periodontal mast cells	Inflammation mediator release	Yes (surfactants)
IV. MISCELLANEOUS BIOLOGICAL SYSTEMS		
Hen's egg	Morphological examination	
Skintex—protein mixture	Protein coagulation	Yes
V. MATHEMATICAL MODELS		
Structure-activity relationship (SAR) model	NA	Yes
SAR model	NA	No

*Evaluated by comparison of predictive accuracy for a range of compounds compared with animal test results.
NA = not applicable.

either ectotoxicity, release of inflammation markers or decrease of some indicator of functionality (lipid metabolism, membrane permeability, or cell detachment) is measured.

The fourth group (IV) contains two miscellaneous approaches—the use of a membrane from the hen's egg with morphological evaluation of damage being the predictor of end-point (Reinhardt *et al.*, 1987), and the SKINTEX system, which utilizes the coagulation of a mixture of soluble proteins to predict dermal response.

Finally, in group V there are two structure–activity relationship models which use mathematical extensions of past animal results correlated with structure to predict the effects of new structures.

Many of these systems are in the process of evaluation of their performance against various small groups of compounds for which the dermal irritation potential is known. Evaluation by multiple laboratories of a wider range of structures will be essential before any of these systems can be generally utilized.

4. Alternatives. The major attempts to modify the actual test designs themselves centered on the use of abrasion as a means of increasing sensitivity and therefore further precluding false negatives. However, the results of comparative studies of materials on both abraded and unabraded skin have not established that abrasions consistently increase sensitivity (8).

III. OCULAR TESTING

Evaluating chemicals for their potential to cause eye irritation in animals and extrapolating to potential results in humans did not start with, as is popularly believed, Draize et al. (1). Animal models had been utilized and the results reported prior to this 1944 publication.

In 1942, Mann and Pullinger (10) reported on the use of a rabbit model to predict eye irritation in humans. No specific scoring system was presented to grade the results, and the use of animals with pigmented eyes (as opposed to albinos) was advocated. Early in 1944, Friedenwald et al. (11) published a method using albino rabbits in a manner very similar to that of the original Draize publication, but still prescribing description of the individual animal response as the means of evaluating and reporting the results though a scoring method provided.

What the method developed and published in 1944 by Draize, Woodward, and Calvery did was to provide a new numerical scoring system for the observations resulting from the test. This scoring system provided a basis for classification of agents as to their potential to cause ocular irritation and it became widely accepted. This scoring system, shown in Table 4, gives the greatest weight to

Table 4 Scale of Weighted Scores for Grading the Severity of Ocular Lesions

I. Cornea
    A. Opacity: Degree of density (area which is most dense is taken for
        reading)
        Scattered or diffuse area-details of iris clearly visible   1
        Easily discernible translucent areas, details of iris slightly obscured   2
        Opalescent areas, no details of iris visible, size of pupil barely dis-
        cernible   3
        Opaque, iris visible   4
    B. Area of cornea involved
        One quarter (or less), but not zero   1
        Greater than one-quarter, less than one-half   2
        Greater than one-half, less than three-quarters   3
        Greater than three-quarters, up to whole area   4
            Scoring equals A × B × 5 Total maximum = 80

II. Iris
    A. Values
        Folds above normal, congestion, swelling, circumcorneal injection
        (any one or all of these or combination of any thereof), iris still re-
        acting to light (sluggish reaction is positive)   1
        No reaction to light, hemorrhage; gross destruction (any one or all
        of these)   2
            Scoring equals A × B Total maximum = 10

III. Conjunctivae
    A. Redness (refers to palpebral conjunctivae only)
        Vessels definitely injected above normal   1
        More diffuse, deeper crimson red, individual vessels not easily dis-
        cernible   2
        Diffuse beefy red   3
    B. Chemosis
        Any swelling above normal (includes nictitating membrane)   1
        Obvious swelling with partial eversion of the lids   2
        Swelling with lids about half closed   3
        Swelling with lids about half closed to completely closed   4
    C. Discharge
        Any amount different from normal (does not include small amount
        observed in inner canthus of normal animals)   1
        Discharge with moistening of the lids and hair just adjacent to the
        lids   2
        Discharge with moistening of the lids and considerable area around
        the eye   3
            Scoring (A + B + C) × 2 total maximum = 20

The maximum total score it the sum of all scores obtained for the cornea, iris, and conjunctivae.

corneal changes (80 out of 110 points), and is based on observations at 24, 48, and 72 hr. Both of these points are weaknesses of the original test method, as will be discussed later.

Since the introduction of the Draize test, ocular irritation testing in rabbits has both developed and diverged. Indeed, clearly there is no longer a single test design that is used and there are different objectives that are pursued by different groups using the same test. This lack of standardization has been recognized for some time and attempts have been made to address standardization of at least the methodological, if not the design aspects of the test.

The common core design of the test calls for instilling either 0.1 ml of a liquid or 0.1 g of a powder (or other solid) into one eye of each of 6 rabbits. The material is not washed out, and both eyes of each animal (the nontreated eye acting as a control) are graded according to the Draize scale at 24, 48, and 72 hr. The resulting scores are summed for each animal.

Although the major objective of the Draize scale was to standardize scoring, it was recognized early on this was not happening and that different people were reading the same response differently. To address this, two sets of standards using the modified Draize scale (to provide guidance by comparison) have been published. In 1965 the Food and Drug Administration (FDA) published a guide featuring color illustrations as standards (12). The quality of the color in their prints was fair to begin with, and the prints have since faded with age. In 1974 the Consumer Product Safety Commission (CPSC) published a second illustrated guide (13) that provided 20 color photographic slides as standards. The color quality on these is better and the slides have retained their original color quality well through time.

A second course of methodological variability has been in the procedure utilized to instill test materials into the eyes. There is now consensus that the substance should be dropped into the cul de sac formed by pulling the lower eye lid gently away from the eye, then allowing the animal to blink and spread the material across the entire corneal surface.

There are also variations in the design of the "standard" test. Most laboratories observe animals until at least 7 days after instillation and may extend the test to 21 days after instillation if any irritation persists. These prolonged postexposure observation periods are designed to allow for evaluation of the true severity of damage and for assessing the ability of the ocular damage to be repaired. The results of these tests are evaluated by a descriptive classification scale (Table 5) such as that described in NAS publication 1138 (14), which was derived from that reported by Green et al. (15).

This classification is based on the most severe response observed in a group of 6 nonirritated eyes and data from all observation periods are used for this evaluation.

Table 5   Severity and Persistence (14)

Inconsequential or complete lack of irritation. Exposure of the eyes to a material under the specified conditions caused no significant ocular changes. No staining with fluorescein can be observed. Any changes that did occur clear within 24 hr and are no greater than those caused by normal saline under the same conditions.

Moderate irritation. Exposure of the eye to the material under the specified conditions causes minor, superficial, and transient changes of the cornea, iris, or conjunctivae as determined by external or slit-lamp or subsequent grading of any of the following changes is sufficient to characterize a response as moderate irritation: opacity of the cornea (other than a slight dulling of the normal luster), hyperemia of the iris, or swelling of the conjunctivae. Any changes that are seen to clear within 7 days.

Substantial irritation. Exposure of the eye to the material under the specified conditions causes significant injury to the eye, such as loss of the corneal epithelia, corneal opacity, iritis (other than a slight injection) conjunctivitis, pannus, or bullae. The effects clear within 21 days.

Severe irritation or corrosion. Exposure of the eye to the material under the specified conditions results in the same types of injury as in the previous category and in significant necrosis or other injuries that adversely affect the visual process. Injuries persist for 21 days or more.

Different regulatory agencies within the United States have prescribed slightly different procedures for different perceived regulatory needs (37). These are looked at in more depth in the text.

A. Objectives

Any discussion of current test protocols must begin with a review of why the tests are done. What are the objectives of those causing eye irritation testing to occur and how are these different objectives reflected not only in test design and interpretation, but also in the regulations prescribing testing and in the ways that test results are utilized?

There are four major groups of organizations (in terms of their products) that require eye irritation studies to be performed. These can be generally (thought not absolutely, as for all such classifications) classified as the pharmaceutical, cosmetic, consumer product, and industrial/agricultural chemical groups.

For the pharmaceutical industry, eye irritation testing is performed when the test material is intended for use in the eye, as a matter of course. There are a number of special tests applicable to pharmaceutical or medical device applications. In general, however, it is desired that an eye irritation test that is utilized by this group be both sensitive and accurate in predicting the potential to cause irritation in humans. Failure to identify irritants (lack of sensitivity) is to be avoided, but of equal concern is the occurrence of false positives. The products here have a real value and benefit to the user in terms of better health and alleviation of discomfort, and prohibiting their use based on a faulty identification as significant irritants, would be an error with unacceptably high costs to society. Rather, a cost/benefit analysis based on an accurate prediction of human hazard is desired.

Similarly, in the cosmetics industry, products of interest are frequently intended for direct contact with the eye or at least to be used in a manner that such contact is unavoidable. At the same time, the benefit to the user is not as clear. In this case the objective is a test that is as sensitive as possible, even if this results in a low incidence of false positives. Even a moderate irritant would not be desirable.

Consumer products (such as soaps, detergents, and shampoos) have a different perspective. These products are not intended to be used in a manner that causes them to get into eyes, but because they are used by a large population and since their modes of use do not include active measures to prevent eye contact (such as the use of goggles and face shields), and the benefit derived from using the products is relatively moderate, accurate identification of severe eye irritants is desirable. A mild or moderate eye irritant would still be a viable product—a severe irritant would not. Only in the case of children's shampoos would there be major interest in identifying mild irritants to preclude their use.

Finally, there are industrial chemicals. These are handled by (relative to consumer products) a smaller population. Eye contact is never intended, and in fact, active measures are taken to prevent it. The use of eye irritation data in these cases is to fulfill labeling requirements for shipping and to provide hazard assessment information for accidental exposures and their treatment. The results of such tests do not directly affect the economic future of a material or product. It is desirable to identify accurately moderate and severe irritants (particularly those with irreversible effects) and to determine if rinsing of the eyes after exposure will improve or aggravate the consequences of exposure. False negatives for mild reversible irritation are acceptable.

To fulfill these objectives, a number of basic test protocols have been developed and mandated by different regulatory groups. Table 6 gives an overview of these.

The philosophy underlying these test designs, almost universally, equates maximization of the biological response with production of the most sensitive test. As our review of objectives has shown, the greatest sensitivity (especially at the expense of false positive findings which is an unavoidable consequence) is not what is universally desired, and, as we shall see later, maximizing the response in rabbits does not *guarantee* sensitive prediction of the results in humans.

Table 6 Regulatory Guidelines for Ocular Irritation Test Methods

Reference	Draize et al., 1944	FHSA* 1972, 1979	NAS* 1977	OECD* 1981	IRLG* 1981	CFR*16, 1981(CPSC*)	TOSCA* 1982	FIFRA*, 1982**	Japan (MAFF, 1985)
Test Species	Albino rabbit	Same	Same	Same	Same	Same	Same	Same	Same
Age/Wt.	NSb	NS	Sexually mature/ less than 2 yrs. old	NS	Young adult/2.0	NS	NS	NS	Young adult
Sex	NS	NS	Either	NS	Either	NS	NS	NS	NS
No. of Animals/ Group	9	6	4 (min.)	3 (min.)	3 (prelim. test)c; 6	6–18	6	6	At least 6
Test Agent Vol. and Method of In- stillation Liquids	0.1 ml on the eye	Same as Draize	Liquids and solid; two or more dif- ferent doses within the proba- bly range of hu- man exposuredd	Same as Draize	Same as Draize	Same as Draize	Sme as FHSA	Same as FHSA	Same as OECD
Solids	0.1 g	100 mg or 0.1 ml equivalent when this vol. weighs less than 100 mg; direct instillation into conjunctival sac	Manner of appli- cation should re- flect probable route of acciden- tal exposure	Same as FHSA	Same as FHSA	Same as FHSA	Same as FHSA	Same as FHSA	Same as OECD
Aerosols	NS	NS	Short burst of dis- tance approxi- mating self-in- duced eye exposure	1 sec burst sprayed at 10 cm	1 sec burst sprayed at ap- prox. 4 in.	NS	As OECD	As OECD	As OECD

(Continued)

Table 6 Continued

Irrigation Schedule	At 1 sec (3 animals) and at 4 sec (3 animals) following instillation of test agent (3 animals remain nonirrigated)	Eyes may be washed after 24-hr reading	May be conducted with separate experimental groups	Same as FHSA; in addition for substances found to be irritating; wash at 4 sec (3 animals) and at 30 sec	Same as FHSA	Same as FHSA	As FHSA	As FHSA	Similar to OECD; if irritation does not disappear at 72 hr after dosing
Irrigation Treatment	Sodium chloride solution (USP or equivalent)	20 ml tap water (body temp.)	NS	Wash with water for 5 min. Using vol. And velocity of flow which will not cause injury	Tap water or sodium chloride solution (USP or equivalent)	Same as FHSA	NS	NS	As OECD
Examination Times (postinstillation)	24 hr 48 hr 72 hr 4 days 7 days	24 hr. 48 hr. 72 hr.	1 day 3 days 7 days 14 days 21 days	1 hour 24 hr. 48 hr. 72 hr.	24 hr 48 hr 72 hr	24 hr 48 hr 72 hr	As OECD	As OECD	As OECD
Use of Fluorescein	NS	NS	NS	May be used	May be used	NS	May be used	May be used	Same as FHSA
Use of Anesthetics	NS	NS	NS	May be used	May be used	NS	May be used	May be used	NS

| Scoring and Evaluation | Draize et al., 1944 (Table 4) | Modified Draize et al., 1944 or a slit lamp scoring system based on CPSC, 1976 | CPSC, 1976 | CPSC, 1976 | CPSC, 1976 | CPSC, 1976 | CPSC, 1976 | CPSC, 1976 | As FHSA |

*FHSA = Federal Hazard Substance Act; NAS = National Academy of Sciences; OECD = Organization for Economic Cooperation and Development; IRLG = Interagency Regulatory Liaison Group; CFR = Code of Federal Regulations.

**Office Pesticide Assessment

ªTests should be conducted on monkeys when confirmatory data are required.

ᵇNot specified.

ᶜIf the substance produces corrosion, severe irritation or no irritation in a preliminary test with 3 animals, no further testing is necessary. If equivocal responses occur, testing on at least 3 additional animals should be performed.

ᵈSuggested doses are 0.1 and 0.05 ml for liquids.

ᵉCurrently no testing guidelines exist for gases or vapors.

ᶠEyes may also be examined at 1 hr, 7, 14, and 21 days (at the option of the investigator).

B. Ocular Irritation Test

1.   Test Article Screening Procedure

1.   Each test substance will be screened in order to eliminate potentially corrosive or severely irritating materials from being studied for eye irritation in the rabbit.

2.   If possible, the pH of the test substance will be measured.

3.   A primary dermal irritation study will be performed prior to the study.

4.   The test substance will not be studied for eye irritation, if it is a strong acid (pH is 2.0 or less) or strong alkali (pH 11.0 or greater), and/or if the test substance is a severe dermal irritant (with a primary dermal irritation index of 5 to 8) or causes corrosion of the skin.

5.   If it is predicted that the test substance does not have the potential to be severely irritating or corrosive to the eye, continue to Rabbit Screening Procedure.

2.   Rabbit Screening Procedure

1.   A group of at least 12 New Zealand White rabbits of either sex are screened for the study. The animals are removed from their cages and placed in rabbit restraints. Care should be taken not to accidentally cause mechanical damage to the eye during this procedure.

2.   All rabbits selected for the study must be in good health; any rabbit exhibiting sniffles, hair loss, loose stools, or apparent weight loss is rejected and replaced.

3.   One hour prior to instillation of the test substance, both eyes of each rabbit are examined for signs of irritation and corneal defects with a hand-held slit lamp. All eyes are stained with 2.0% sodium fluorescein and examined to confirm the absence of corneal lesions.

   a.   Fluorescein Staining.   Cup the lower lid of the eye to be tested and instill one drop of a 2% sodium fluorescein solution onto the surface of the cornea. After 15 seconds, the eye is thoroughly rinsed with physiological saline. The eye is examined employing a hand-held long wave ultraviolet illuminatory in a darkened room. Corneal lesions, if present, appear as bright yellowish-green fluorescent areas.

4.   Only 9 of the 12 animals are selected for the study. These 9 rabbits must not show any signs of eye irritation and must show either a negative or minimum fluorescein reaction (due to normal epithelial desquamation).

3.   Study Procedure

1.   At least 1 hour after fluorescein staining, the test substance is placed on one eye of each animal by gently pulling the lower lid away from the eyeball

to form a cup (conjunctival cul de sac) into which the test material is dropped. The upper and lower lids are then gently held together for 1 sec to prevent immediate loss of material.

2.   The other eye remains untreated and serves as a control.

3.   For testing liquids, 0.1 ml of the test substance is used.

4.   For solids or pastes, 100 mg of the test substance is used.

5.   When the test substance is in flake, granular, powder, or other particulate form, the amount that has a volume of 0.1 ml (after gently compacting the particles by tapping the measuring container in a way that will not alter their individual form) is used whenever this volume weighs less than 100 mg.

6.   For aerosol products, the eye should be held open and the substance administered in a single, short burst for about one second at a distance of about 4 inches directly in front of the eye. The velocity of the ejected material should not traumatize the eye. The dose should be approximated by weighing the aerosol can before and after each treatment. For other liquids, propelled under pressure, such as substances delivered by pump sprays, an aliquot of 0.1 ml should be collected and instilled in the eye as for liquids.

7.   The treated eyes of 6 rabbits are not washed following instillation of the test substance.

8.   The treated eyes of the remaining 3 rabbits are irrigated for 1 min with room temperature tap water, starting 20 sec after instillation.

9.   In order to prevent self-inflicted trauma by the animals immediately after instillation of the test substance the animals are not immediately returned to their cages. After the tests and control eyes are examined and graded at 1 hr post-exposure, the animals are returned carefully to their respective cages.

4.   Observations

1.   The eyes are observed for any immediate signs of discomfort after instilling the test substance. Blepharospasm and/or excessive tearing are indicative of irritating sensations caused by the test substance and the duration should be noted. Blepharospasm does not necessarily indicate that the eye will show signs of ocular irritation.

2.   Grading and scoring of ocular irritation are performed in accordance with modified Draize's scale (1) (Table 3). The eyes are examined and grades of ocular reactions are recorded.

3.   If signs of irritation persist at 7 days, readings are continued on day 10; and if the toxic effects are not resolved after 10 days, readings are made on day 14.

4.   In addition to the required observations of the cornea, iris, and conjunctiva, serious effects (such as pannus, rupture of the globe, or blistering of the conjunctivae) indicative of a corrosive action are reported.

5.   Whether or not toxic effects are reversible depends on the nature,

extent, and intensity of damage. Most lesions, if reversible, will heal or clear within 21 days. Therefore, if ocular irritation is present at the 14-day reading, a 21-day reading is required to determine whether the ocular damage is reversible or nonreversible.

5. Evaluation of Results

The results are evaluated by the following two methods

1.   Federal Hazardous Substances Act (FHSA) Regulations (12): Interpretation of data is made from the 6 test eyes which are not irrigated with water. Only data from days 1, 2, and 3 are used for this evaluation; data from the 1 hr observation and days 4, 7, 10, 14, and 21 are not used. An animal shall be considered as exhibiting a positive reaction if the test substance produces at any of the readings ulceration of the cornea (other than fine stippling) (grade 1), or opacity of the cornea (other than a slight dulling of the normal luster) (grade 1), or inflammation of the iris (other than a slight deepening of the rugae or a slight circumcorneal injection of the blood vessels) (grade 1), or if such substance produces in the conjunctivae (excluding the cornea and iris) an obvious swelling with partial eversion of the lids (grade 2) or a diffuse crimson red color with individual vessels not easily discernible (grade 2).

The test shall be considered *positive* if four or more of the animals in the test group exhibit a positive reaction.

If only one animal exhibits a positive reaction, the test shall be regarded as *negative*.

If two or three animals exhibit a positive reaction, the test is repeated using a different group of 6 animals. The second test shall be considered positive if 3 or more of the animals exhibit a positive reaction.

If only 1 or 2 animals in the second test exhibit a positive reaction, the test shall be repeated with a different group of 6 animals. Should a third test be needed, the substance will be regarded as an irritant if any animal exhibits a positive response.

2.   A modified Classification Scale of Ocular Responses is based on severity and persistence [derived from NAS, 1977 (4) and Green (15)]. The most severe response seen in a group of 6 test animals is used for classification.

  a.   Inconsequential or nonirritation.   Exposure of the eye to the material under the specified conditions caused no significant ocular changes. No tissue staining with fluorescein was observed. Any changes that did occur cleared within 24 hr.*

---

*Slight conjunctival injection (grade 1, some vessels definitely injected) that does not clear within 24 hr is not considered a significant change. This level of change is inconsequential as far as representing physical damage to the eye and can be seen to occur naturally for unexplained reasons in otherwise normal rabbits.

b. Moderate Irritation. Exposure of the eye to material under the specified conditions caused minor, superficial, and transient changes of the cornea, iris, or conjunctivae as determined by external or slit-lamp examination with fluorescein staining. The appearance at any grading interval of any of the following changes was sufficient to characterize a response as irritation: opacity of the cornea (other than a slight dulling of the normal luster), hyperemia of the iris, or swelling of the conjunctivae. Any changes that were seen cleared within 7 days.

c. Substantial Irritation. Exposure of the eye to the material under the specified conditions caused significant injury to the eye, such as loss of the corneal epithelium, corneal opacity, iritis (other than a slight injection), conjunctivitis, pannus, or bullae. The effects healed or cleared within 21 days.

d. Severe Irritation or Corrosion. Exposure of the eye to the material under the specified conditions resulted in the types of injury described in the former category and resulted in significant tissue destruction (necrosis) or injuries that probably adversely affected the visual process. The effects of the injuries persisted for 21 days or more.

Figure 1 gives a diagrammatic presentation of the prescreening step incorporated into this test to preclude undue discomfort on the part of the test animals.

6. Limitations

Commonly used methodological variations to improve the sensitivity and accuracy of describing damage in these tests are inspection of the eyes with a slit lamp and instillation of the eyes with a vital dye (very commonly, fluorescein) as an indicator of increases in permeability of the corneal barrier. These techniques and an alternative scoring system which is more comprehensive than the Draize scale are reviewed well by Ballantyne and Swanston (19) and Chan and Hayes (20).

To assess the adequacy of the currently employed eye irritation tests to fulfill the objectives behind their use, we must evaluate them in terms of (a) their accuracy (how well do they predict the hazard to humans) and (b) can comparable results be obtained by different technicians and laboratories, and finally (c) what methods and designs have been developed and are being employed as alternatives to rabbit eye irritation tests.

Assessing the accuracy of rabbit eye irritation tests—or indeed, of any predictive test of eye irritation—requires that the results of such tests be compared to what happens in humans. Unfortunately, the human database for making comparisons is not large. The concerns, however, have been present almost as long as the tests have been performed (21).

There are substantial differences between the eye of humans and rabbits,

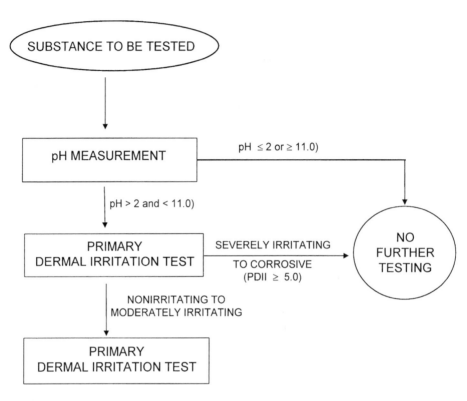

Figure 1 Tier approach for eye irritation testing.

and indeed, other species that have also been considered as test models. Beckley (22) presented the following comparison of corneal thickness and area (as a percentage of the total area of the globe) of four species, as shown in Table 7.

The aqueous humor of the rabbit also has a different pH (7.6 vs. 7.1–7.3 for humans), a less effective tearing mechanism, and a nictitating membrane.

Table 7 Corneal Thickness and Area

Species	Thickness	Area (%)
Humans	0.53–0.54	7
Rabbit	0.4	25
Mouse	0.1	50
Rat	?	50

Calabrese (23) presents a comprehensive review of the anatomical and biochemical differences between the ocular systems of humans and rabbits.

Some have claimed that the rabbit, as the test is currently performed, is more sensitive than man. Anionic formulations, for example, are severe irritants to rabbit eyes, but are nonirritants in humans. However, generally the rabbit is no more sensitive than man. Rather, the relative sensitivities vary from class to class of chemical. Alexander (1965) and Calabrese (23) have provided reviews of materials for which rabbits are more sensitive than humans. MacDonald et al. (24) published a review of materials that were either more or less irritant in rabbits than in humans. Swanston (25) has also published a comparative review of seven different species, including humans.

It should be noted, however, that rabbit eye tests do not detect ocular toxicities associated with some ocular anesthetics and eye drops (26).

A second long-standing concern regarding the adequacy of the rabbit tests is its reproducibility. Weil and Scala (7) published the most frequently cited study, in which 25 labs evaluated a common battery of 12 materials. The results did show variability between laboratories, with a number of labs reporting consistently either more or less severe results than the other labs. The causes and cures for such variability are multiple, but we have already mentioned differences in protocols and methodologies (to name just two major sources).

Since the Weil and Scala study (7) a number of authors have published comparative studies that have shown a greater degree of reproducibility. Some of these are summarized in Table 8.

Several authors have made the point that reproducible predictability of nonirritants and strong irritants is easier to achieve. For other materials, several

Table 8 Summary of Rabbit Eye Studies

Study	Results	Reference
1. Three materials by 3 readers under two separate conditions	90% Reproducibility of irritant/ nonirritant classification	(27)
2. 7 Materials evaluated in duplicate	Tests results reproducible	(28)
3. 56 Materials evaluated in three separate protocols	Each protocol reproducible— variations between tests by different protocols	(29,30)
4. 29 Materials (detergents) evaluated in 2 rabbit, 2 monkey and 1 human test	Results for all tests more severe than human but low volume rabbit test data were rank comparable to human data	(31)

authors have made the point that the use of concurrent reference materials (32) or semiannual refresher training of readers versus a set of standards (24) improves reproducibility of results and gives a set of standard results against which we can evaluate a drift in test or reading practices.

C. Alternatives

The alternatives, which have been proposed and adapted for the performance of rabbit eye irritation tests themselves, should be reviewed. These alternatives have been directed at the twin objectives of making the tests more accurate in predicting human responses and at reducing both the use of animals and the degree of discomfort or suffering experienced by those that are used.

1. Alternative Species

Dogs, monkeys, and mice (25) have all been suggested as alternatives to rabbits that would be more representative of humans. Each of these, however, also has shown differences in responses compared to those seen in humans, and pose additional problems in terms of cost, handling, lack of database, etc.

2. Use of Anesthetics

Over the years, a number of authors have proposed that topical anesthetics be administered to the eyes of rabbits prior to their use in the test. Both OECD and IRLG regulations provide for such usage. However, numerous published [such as Falahee et al. (16)] and unpublished studies have shown that such use of anesthetics interfere with test results usually by increasing the severity of eye irritation findings.

3. Decrease Volume of Test Material

An alternative proposal (one in which a survey showed has been adopted by a number of labs) is to use a reduced volume/weight of test material.

In 1982, Williams et al. (28) reported a study in which they evaluated 21 different chemicals at volumes of 0.1, 0.03, 0.01, and 0.003 ml. These are materials on which there was human data already available. It was found that the volume reduction did not change the rank order of responses, and that 0.01 ml (10μl) gave results that best mirrored those seen in humans.

In 1984, Freeberg et al. (31) published a study of 29 detergents (for which human data was available), each evaluated at both 0.1 and 0.01 ml test volumes in rabbits. The results of the 0.01 ml tests were reported to be more reflective of results in humans.

In 1985 Walker (33) reported an evaluation of the low volume (0.01 ml) test which assessed its results for correlation with those in humans based on the number of days until clearing of injury, and reported that 0.01 ml gave better correlation than did 0.1 ml.

While it must be pointed out that there may be some classes of chemicals for which low volume tests may give results less representative of those seen in humans, it seems clear that this approach should be seriously considered by those performing such testing.

4. Use of Prescreens

This alternative may also be considered a tier approach. Its objective is to avoid testing severely irritating or corrosive materials in many (or, in some cases, any) rabbits. This approach entails a number of steps that should be considered independently.

First is a screen based on physiochemical properties. This usually means pH, but also should be extended to materials with high oxidation or reduction potentials (hexavalent chromium salts, for example).

Though the correlation between low pHs (acids) and eye damage in the rabbit has not been found to be excellent, all alkalis (pH 11.5 or above) tested have been reported to produce opacities and ocular damage (34). Many laboratories now use pH cutoffs for testing of 2.0 or lower and 11.5 or 12.0 and higher. If a material falls outside of these cutoffs (or is so identified due to other physiochemical parameters), then it is either (a) not tested in the rabbit eye and assumed to be corrosive, or (b) evaluated in a secondary screen such as an in vitro cytotoxicity test or primary dermal irritation test (35), or (c) evaluated in a single rabbit before a full-scale eye irritation test is performed. It should be kept in mind that the correlation of all the physiochemical screen parameters with acute eye test results is very concentration dependent, being good at high concentrations and marginal at lower concentrations (where various buffering systems present in the eye are meaningful).

The second commonly used type of level of prescreen is the use of primary dermal irritation (PDI) test results. In this approach the PDI study is performed before the eye irritation study, and if the score from that study (called the primary dermal irritation index (PDII) and ranging from 0 to 8) is above a certain level (usually 5.0 or greater), the same options already outlined for physiochemical parameters can be exercised. There is no universal agreement on the value of this prescreen. Gilman et al. (37) did not find the PDII a good predictor, but made this judgment based on a relatively small data set and a cutoff PDII of 3.0 or above. In 1984 and 1985, Williams (38, 39) reported that severe PDII scores (5.0 or greater) predicted severe eye irritation responses in 39 of 60 cases. He attributed the false positives to possible overprediction by current PDI test procedures. On the other hand, Guillot et al. (29, 30) reported good prediction of eye irritation based on skin irritation in 56 materials and Gad

Table 9   In Vitro Alternatives for Eye Irritation Tests (40)

I. MORPHOLOGY
    A. Enucleated superfused rabbit eye system
    B. Balb/c 3T3 cells/morphological assays (HTD)

II. CELL TOXICITY
    A. Adhesion/cell proliferation
        1. BHK cells/growth inhibition
        2. BHK cells/colony formation efficiency
        3. BHK cells/cell detachment
        4. SIRC cells/colony forming assay
        5. Balbe/c 3T3 cells/total protein
        6. BCL/D1 cells/total protein
        7. Primary rabbit corneal cells/colony forming assay
    B. Membrane integrity
        1. LS cells/dual dye staining
        2. Thymocytes/dual fluorescent dye staining
        3. LS cells/dual dye staining
        4. RCE-SIRC-P815-YAC-1/Cr release
        5. L929 cells/cell variability
        6. Bovine red blood cell/hemolysis
        7. Mouse L929 fibroblasts-erythrocin C staining
        8. Rabbit corneal epithelial and endothelial cells/membrane leakage
        9. Agarose diffusion
    C. Cell metabolism
        1. Rabbit corneal cell cultures/plasminogen activator
        2. LS cells/ATP assay
        3. Balb/c 3T3 cells/neutral red uptake
        4. Balb/c 3T3 uridine uptake inhibition assay
        5. HeLa cells/metabolic inhibition test (MIT-24)
        6. MDCK cells/dye diffusion

III. CELL AND TISSUE PHYSIOLOGY
    A. Epidermal slice/electrical conductivity
    B. Rabbit ileum/contraction inhibition
    C. Bovine cornea/corneal opacity
    D. Proposed mouse eye/permeability test

IV. INFLAMMATION/IMMUNITY
    A. Chorioallantoic membrane (CAM)
        1. CAM
        2. HET-CAM
    B. Bovine corneal cup model/leukocyte chemotactic factors
    C. Rat peritoneal mast cells/histamine release
    D. Rat peritoneal mast cells/serotonin release
    E. Rat vaginal explant/prostaglandin release
    F. Bovine eye cup/histamine (Hm) and leukotriene C4 (LtC4) release

Table 9 Continued

V.   RECOVERY/REPAIR
A.   Rabbit corneal epithelial cells-wound healing
VI.   OTHER
A.   EYTEX assay
B.   Computer-based structure-activity (SAR)

et al. (8) reported good prediction of severe eye irritation results based on PDIIs of 72 test materials.

5.   Staggered Study Starts

Another approach, which is a form of screen, calls for starting the eye test in 1 or 2 animals, then offsetting the dosing of the additional animals in the test group for 4 hr a day. During this offset period, if a severe result is seen in the first 1 or 2 animals, the remainder of the test may be canceled. This staggered start allows one to both limit testing severe eye irritants to a few animals and yet have confidence that a moderate irritant would be detected.

6.   Alternative Models

Intensive work has been conducted to develop models which are either in vitro or use lower order living organisms. Table 9 presents a short list of methods as previously presented elsewhere by this author (40).

REFERENCES

1.   Draize, J.H., Woodard, G., and Calvery, H.O. (1944). Methods for the study of irritation and toxicity of substances applied topically to the skin and mucous membranes. *J. Pharmacol. Exp. Ther.* 82:377–390.
2.   Department of Transportation Code of Federal Regulations. Title 49, 173.240.
3.   Draize, J.H. (1959). Dermal toxicity. In *Appraisal of the Safety of Chemicals in Foods, Drugs and Cosmetics.* Austin, TX, Association of Food and Drug Officials of the U.S.
4.   Environmental Protection Agency. (1979). *Acute Toxicity Testing Criteria for New Chemical Substances.* Washington D.C., Office of Toxic Substances, EPA 560/13-79-009.
5.   Consumer Product Safety Commission. (1980). Federal Hazardous Substances Act Regulations. CFR 1500. 41.
6.   Organization for Economic Cooperation and Development. *OECD Guidelines for Testing of Chemicals*, Sect. 404, Acute Dermal Irritation/Corrosion, Paris.
7.   Weil, C.S., and Scala, R.A. (1971). Study of intra- and interlaboratory variability

in the results of rabbit eye and skin irritation tests. *Toxicol. Appl. Pharmacol.* 19: 276–360.

8. Gad, S.C., Walsh, R.D., and Dunn, B.J. (1986). Correlation of ocular and dermal irritancy of industrial chemicals. *Ocular Dermal Toxicol.* 5(3):195–213.

9. Code of Federal Regulations, Transportation, Title 49: Part 173, Appendix A-Method of Testing Corrosion to skin, Revised; November 1, 1984.

10. Mann, I., and Pullinger, B.D. (1942). A study of mustard gas lesions of the eye of rabbits and men. *Proc. R. Soc. Med.* 35:229–244.

11. Friedenwald, J.S., Huges, W.F., and Hermann, H. (1944). *Arch Ophthalmol.* 31: 279.

12. *Illustrated Guide for Grading Eye Irritation by Hazardous Substance.* (1965). Washington, D.C., Food and Drug Administration.

13. CPCS. (1976). *Illustrated Guide for Grading Eye Irritation Caused by Hazardous Substances.* 16 CFR 1500.

14. National Academy of Sciences. (1977). *Principles and Procedures for Evaluating the Toxicity of Household Substances.* NAS Publication 1138. Washington, D.C., National Academy of Sciences.

15. Green, W.R., Sullivan, J.B., Hehir, R.M. Scharpf, L.F., and Dickinson, A.W. (1978). *A Systematic Comparison of Chemically Induced Eye Injury in the Albino Rabbit and the Rhesus Monkey.* New York, The Soap and Detergent Association.

16. Falahee, K.J., Rose, C.S., Siefried, H.F., and Sawhney, D. (1982). Alternatives in toxicity testing. *Product Safety Evaluation.* Edited by A.M. Goldberg. New York, Mary Ann Lieber, pp. 137–162.

17. Interagency Regulatory Liaison Group (Jan. 1981). Testing Standards and Guidelines Work Group. Recommended Guideline for Acute Eye Irritation Testing.

18. Environmental Protection Agency. (1981). *Eye Irritation Testing.* EPA-560/11-82-001.

19. Ballantyne, B., and Wanston, D.W. (1977). The scope and limitations of acute eye irritation tests. *Current Approaches in Toxicology.* Edited by B. Ballantyne. Bristol, John Wright & Sons, pp. 139–157.

20. Chan, P.K., and Hayes, A.W. (1985). Assessment of chemically induced ocular toxicity; a survey of methods. *Toxicology of the Eye, Ear, and Other Special Senses.* Edited by A.W. Hayes. New York, Raven Press, pp. 103–143.

21. McLaughlin, R.S. (1946). Chemical burns of the human cornea. *Am. J. Ophthalmol.* 29:1355–1362.

22. Beckley, J.H. (1965). Comparative eye testing: Man vs. Animal. *Toxicol. Appl. Pharmacol.* 7:93–101.

23. Calabrese, E.J. (1984). *Principles of Animal Extrapolation.* New York, John Wiley & Sons, pp. 391–402.

24. McDonald, T.O., Seabaugh, V., Shadduck, J.A., and Edelhauser, H.F. (1983). Eye irritation. *Dermatoxicology.* Edited by F.N. Marzulli and H.I. Maibach. New York, Hemisphere Publishing, pp. 555–610.

25. Swanston, D.W. (1985). Assessment of the validity of animal techniques in eye irritation testing. *Food Chem. Toxicol.* 23:169–173.

26. Andermann, G., and Erhart, M. (1983). *Meth. Find. Exptl. Clin. Pharmacol.* 321–333.

27. Bayard, S., and Hehir, R.M. (1976). Evaluation of proposed changes in the modified Draize rabbit irritation test. *Toxicol. Appl. Pharmacol.* 37(1):186.

28. Williams, S.J., Graepel, G.J., and Kennedy, G.L. (1982). Evaluation of ocular irritancy potential: Intralaboratory variability and effect of dosage volume. *Toxicol. Letters* 12:235–241.

29. Guillot, J.P., Gonnet, J.F., Clement, C., Caillard, L., and Truhaut, R. (1982). Evaluation of the cutaneous-irritation potential of 56 compounds. *Food Chem. Toxicol.* 201:563–572.

30. Guillot, J.P., Gonnet, J.F., Clement, C., Caillard, L., and Truhaut, R. (1982). Evaluation of the ocular-irritation potential of 56 compounds. *Food Chem. Toxicol.* 20: 573–582.

31. Freeberg, F.E., Griffith, J.F., Bruce, R.D., and Bay, P.H.S. (1984). Correlation of animal test methods with human experience for household products. *J. Toxicol. Cut. Ocular Toxicol.* 1:53.6.

32. Gloxhuber, C.H. (1985). Modification of the Draize eye test for the safety testing of cosmetics. *Food Chem. Toxicol.* 23:187–188.

33. Walker, A.P. (1985). A more realistic animal technique for predicting human eye responses. *Food Chem. Toxicol.* 23:175–178.

34. Murphy, J.C., Osterberg, R.E., Seabaugh, V.M., and Bierbower (1982). Ocular irritancy response to various pHs of acids and bases with and without irrigation. *Toxicology* 23:281–291.

35. Jackson, J., and Rutty, D.A. (1985). Ocular tolerance assessment-integrated tier policy. *Food Chem. Toxicol.* 23:309–310.

36. *Federal Register.* (1973). *Federal Hazardous Substances Act.* 38 No. 187, Section 1500, September 27.

37. Gilman, M.R., Jackson, E.M., Cerven, D.B., and Moreno, M.T. (1985). Relationship between the primary dermal irritation index and ocular irritation. *J. Toxicol. Cut Ocular Toxicol.* 2:107–117.

38. Williams, S.J. (1984). Prediction of ocular irritancy potential from dermal irritation test results. *Food Chem. Toxicol.* 2:157–161.

39. Williams, S.J. (1985). Changing concepts of ocular irritation evaluation: Pitfalls and progress. *Food Chem. Toxicol.* 23:189–193.

40. Gad, S.C. and Chengelis, C.P. (1997). *Acute Toxicology,* 2nd Ed., Academic Press, San Diego, CA.

5
Predicting Dermal Hypersensitivity Responses

Richard A. Hiles
Amylin Pharmaceuticals, Inc., San Diego, California

Paul T. Bailey
Mobil Business Resources Corporation, Paulsboro, New Jersey

Joan M. Chapdelaine and Victor T. Mallory
Chrysalis Preclinical Services Corporation, Olyphant, Pennsylvania

I. INTRODUCTION

Delayed contact hypersensitivity is the expression of the ability of a chemical to cause a greater dermal response than would have been anticipated based on simple irritancy. Unlike the inflammatory response in irritation, the responsiveness to an allergen is highly variable within a population. As Jackson (1) stated, irritation tells us about how we are similar while sensitivity tells us about how we are different. That is, everyone is irritated by strong acids, alkalis, and solvents, but only a select number of people respond to 3-pentadecylcatechol in poison ivy. Sensitization responses can be very undesirable in humans, the allergens difficult to avoid, and in the case of persistent sunlight-activated reactions, can be totally disabling.

The outward expression of irritation and sensitization are often similar (erythema, edema, heat, etc.) but the mechanisms leading to these two inflammatory responses are very different (2). Skin sensitization and dermal photosensitization are delayed humoral immune responses mediated by T cells. A chemical hapten or incomplete allergen passes into the dermis and complexes with dermis protein to form a hapten–protein complex. The Langerhans' cells in the area interact with this allergen as if it were a completely foreign protein. The Langerhans' cells migrate to the thymus gland to "educate" the naïve T cells about the allergen. The now educated T cells proliferate and leave the thymus as sensitized cells. With the proper stimulus they can initiate the inflammatory process through the release of lymphokines.

All assays for delayed contact hypersensitivity have common elements: irritation/toxicity screens, induction phase, primary challenge phase, and rechallenge phase. All assays require knowledge of the dermal irritancy and systemic toxicity of the test material(s) to be used in the induction, challenge, and rechallenge. These properties are defined in the *irritation/toxicity screen*. Most assays will allow mild irritation in the induction phase, but no systemic toxicity. Generally, a nonirritating concentration is required for the challenge and the rechallenge. As will be discussed in the sections on the individual assays, even a carefully designed screen does not always provide the desired guidance in selecting workable concentrations.

The *induction phase* involves exposing the test animals to the test material several times over a period of days or weeks. A number of events must be accomplished during this phase if a sensitization response is to be elicited. The test material must penetrate through the epidermis and into the dermis. There it must interact with dermis protein. The protein test material complex must be perceived by the immune system as an allergen. Finally, the production of sensitized T cells must be accomplished. Some assays enhance the sensitivity of the induction phase by compromising the natural ability of the epidermis to act as a barrier. These enhancement techniques include irritation of the induction site, intradermal injection, skin stripping, and occlusive dressings. In contrast, events such as the development of a scab over the induction site can reduce penetration. Light is used in the photosensitization assays to produce a chemically active species for interaction with the dermis protein. The attention of the immune system can be drawn to the induction site by the intradermal injection of oil-coated bacteria (Freund's complete adjuvant).

The *primary challenge phase* consists of exposing laboratory animals to a concentration of the test material that would normally not be expected to cause a response (usually an irritation-type response). The responses in the test animals and of the control animals are then measured.

A *rechallenge phase* is a repeat of the challenge phase and can be a very valuable tool if used properly. Sensitized animals (with the exception of one of the assays presented in this chapter where the final evaluation requires that the animals be euthanized) can be rechallenged with the same test material at the same concentration used in the challenge in order to assist in confirming sensitization. Sensitized animals can be rechallenged with different concentrations of the allergen to evaluate dose versus response relationships. Animals sensitized to an ingredient can be challenged to a formulation containing the ingredient to evaluate the potential of the formulated product to elicit a sensitization response under adverse conditions. Conversely, animals that responded (sometimes unexpectedly) to a final formulation can be challenged with formulation without the suspected sensitizer or to the ingredient that is suspected to be the allergen. Cross reactivity can be evaluated, that is, the ability of one test material to elicit a sensitization response following exposure in the induction phase to a different test material. A well-designed rechallenge is important and should be considered at the same time that the sensitization evaluation is being designed, since the rechallenge must be run within 1 to 2 weeks after the primary challenge. Unless plans have been made for a possible rechallenge, one may have to reformulate a test material or obtain additional pure ingredient and perhaps run additional irritation/toxicity screens before the rechallenge can be run. The ability of the sensitized animals to respond at a rechallenge can fade with time, thus the necessity that the rechallenge be run shortly after the challenge. In addition, some assays use sham-treated controls and these must be procured while the induction phase is in progress. One additional piece of information must be kept in mind when evaluating a rechallenge. The animal does not differentiate between an induction exposure and a challenge exposure. If one is using an assay involving three induction exposures and one challenge exposure, then at the rechallenge the animal has received four induction exposures. Thus, this "extra" induction may actually serve to strengthen a sensitization response.

And what does one do with the results of the assay for delayed contact hypersensitivity? The plan of action depends on the nature of the material, how it will be used, and how conservative a risk factor the investigator is using. The author has seen companies use of the results ranging from refusal to use any ingredient that gave any positive results, to one that does not worry unless all test animals exhibit strong (+2) reactions. One can use the percentage of the animals responding as a guide:

% Responding	Classification
0–10	Nonsensitizer
11–30	Weak to mild
31–60	Moderate
61–90	Strong
91–100	Extreme

A "responding animal" is one that exhibits a response at the challenge that is definitely greater than that observed in the controls. This system denotes the ease with which the test material can elicit a sensitization response in a population, but not the strength of the response. As previously discussed, the responsiveness of the animals can be a function of the particular assay used, solvents, vehicles, and concentration. In cases where human exposure is not intended or expected, then a warning to avoid dermal contact may be sufficient. (It is interesting that the EPA labeling guidelines (3) do not address sensitizers.)

In situations where human contact is probable or desirable, then even weak sensitizers require careful consideration: human patch testing may be in order, but this subject is beyond the scope of this discussion.

Positive controls are available for each assay for delayed contact hypersensitivity. A good positive control is one giving predictable positive results only when the assay is run properly. A control that yields 100% strong responders is not impressive, as the assay may be run in a flawed manner and still yield 100% responders. Each laboratory should consider running control assays every 6 months, if not with each assay, and qualify every technician. If a company places a significant amount of work at outside contract testing laboratories, then the sponsoring company would be wise to send "blind" positive controls on a regular basis. Some companies take the conservative approach of running a positive control with every assay. If the testing laboratory has a collection of historical data generated with a consistent source of animals as well as data generated within the last 6 months, then the running of a positive control with each assay is not necessary. Experience would indicate that regulatory agencies do not require that a positive control be run with each evaluation and will accept historical data.

Over the past 50 years, a number of investigators have evaluated the usefulness of different animal models and assays for predicting dermal hypersensitivity responses in humans. To the credit of each investigator, and almost without exception, the method devised by each investigator worked better for the investigator's purpose than did the method devised by someone else. Some of these assays have never become popular while others are used frequently and some are preferred by regulators. In some cases, the lack of popularity may have more to do with lack of a strong champion for the assay rather than lack of scientific merit. Because of the desire to have more rapid assays, which cost less and use fewer animals, and because the perfect assay for predicting human responses has not been found, research into modified or new approaches continues. This presentation will provide insight into the Buehler Test (4) and the Guinea Pig Maximization Test (GPMT) (5) for detecting dermal sensitizers in the guinea pig, the Armstrong Test (6) for detecting photosensitizers in guinea pigs, as well as two assays that do not use the traditional guinea pig, the Mouse Ear Swelling Test (MEST) (7) and the Local Lymph Node Test (LLNT) in mice (8).

II. REGULATORY OVERVIEW

In the hazard assessment of new chemicals, it is prudent to determine the potential for skin sensitization before incorporating the chemical into products/formulations whose use involves frequent and prolonged skin contact. Many countries understand this and have regulatory requirements that include premarket testing of new chemicals for skin sensitization potential. This section discusses the skin sensitization testing procedures required to meet these regulatory requirements.*

A. European Union

The notification procedure for new chemicals in the European Union requires a skin sensitization test when the amount of a new chemical is expected to exceed a production volume of 100 kg/yr. The recommended skin sensitization testing procedures and detail descriptions of these test methods are cited in the OECD Guidelines for Testing of Chemicals (9). Predictive sensitization test procedures in the guinea pig are the most acceptable. Regulatory preference is given to studies that are conducted according to the Guinea Pig Maximization Test (GPMT) of Magnusson and Kligman, which uses an adjuvant (5,10), and the nonadjuvant Buehler Test (4,11). Other adjuvant and nonadjuvant guinea pig assays are also acceptable with proper scientific justification and validation. It has been our experience to obtain prior approval from the Competent Authority/ Regulatory Agency before use of another predictive sensitization test procedure. This would eliminate the need for extensive scientific justification and validation of the alternative test procedure to the Regulatory Agency and demands for testing in accordance with the preferred methods. Although various sensitization methods are provided in the OECD guidelines, the European Communities favor the adjuvant-type testing procedures (viz., GPMT) that are considered to be more accurate in predicting probable skin sensitizing effect of a new chemical in humans than nonadjuvant methods (10,12). In the event the Buehler test is used in place of the GPMT, scientific justification is often required.

Other assays that have recently gained acceptance by OECD (9) and the European Communities (12) are the mouse ear swelling test (MEST) and the mouse local lymph node assay (LLNA). These methods are recognized screening tests in the assessment of skin sensitization potential of new chemicals. If a positive sensitization response is observed in either of these assays, the test substance may be designated as a potential sensitizer without further guinea pig testing. However, a negative sensitization response in these assays would require further testing in guinea pigs as described in the OECD guidelines.

B. United States

The Environmental Protection Agency (EPA) has regulatory responsibility for chemicals under the Toxic Substances Control Act (TSCA) and the Federal Insecticide, Fungicide, and Rodenticide Act (FIFRA). The EPA's Office of Pes-

---

Science 282 (1998), p. 39, reports the U.S. Interagency Coordinating Committee on Validation of Alternative Methods has endorsed the Local Lymph Node Test in mice.

ticide Programs (OPP) has issued testing guidelines that include skin sensitization tests. Skin sensitization testing is a requirement for registration of pesticides under FIFRA, Subdivision F Guidelines. However, testing can be omitted with the necessary scientific rationale (e.g., dermal exposure is not likely to occur) and approval from the EPA.

Under the TSCA, there are no requirements for the determination of the skin sensitization potential of a new chemical for Premanufacture Notification (PMN). However, the manufacture is obligated to submit any toxicological data (e.g., sensitization) for the chemical that was performed prior to the submission of the PMN or initiated during the 90-day review period. The EPA can request sensitization testing for a PMN under a Section 4 test rule. EPA testing standards or generic methodology guidelines must be followed. These generic guidelines allows sensitization testing according to FIFRA, TSCA, or OECD protocols. Chemicals can also be tested by other sensitization procedures with the prior approval of the EPA. Currently, the EPA has designated seven guinea pig sensitization methods as satisfactory to meet the needs of FIFRA and TSCA. References providing background information are provided in 40 CFR 798.4100(7-1-97 Edition).

C. Pacific Rim and Australia

Notification procedures for new chemicals in most Pacific Rim countries include a health hazard determination for skin sensitization potential modeled after European and Canadian requirements. New Zealand, South Korea, and other Pacific Rim countries are developing guidelines for the evaluation of skin sensitization potential of new chemicals based on the results of the harmonization activity currently underway in the OECD and other international organizations. However, the notification procedures for new chemicals in Australia allow for some flexibility in the assessment of the potential occupational health and safety, public health, and environmental hazards of the substance. If a substance has been shown to be a skin sensitizer in humans, then a skin sensitization test in animals is not required. If this information is not available, then the methods cited in the OECD Guidelines for the Testing of Chemicals should be used. These are mentioned in the Australian Handbook for Notifiers (Part *C*; 1.6 Skin Sensitization) as TG 406 or Equivalent.

D. Mexico

In Mexico, the employer has the responsibility to inform workers of the risk involved in handling corrosives, irritants, sensitizers, and toxic substances. Also the employer is responsible for the implementation of adequate measures to prevent occupational illnesses. Currently, there are no specific testing guidelines for the evaluation of skin sensitization potential of chemicals in Mexico. Although knowledge of skin sensitization potential of a chemical is a requirement for the prevention of occupational illness, any sensitization method that is recommended by OECD or the United States is considered acceptable.

E. Canada

The Canadian Hazardous Products Act and pursuant regulations deal with three types of hazardous products identified as prohibited, restricted, and controlled. Certain substances under the Controlled Products Regulations are subject to the Workplace Hazardous Materials Information System (WHMIS) information requirements. In order to determine the skin sensitization potential of a substance or product in Canada, the OECD Test Guideline No. 406 (May 12, 1981) is recommended. This particular OECD Guideline No. 406 lists seven methods for evaluation that are considered acceptable. The revised OECD Guideline No. 406 (1997) will probably be implemented shortly. The Canadian regulations also have a criteria to include any evidence that shows that a chemical and/or product that causes skin sensitization in persons following occupational exposure.

III. BUEHLER METHOD FOR DETECTING DERMAL ALLERGENS

A. Background

The Buehler Test using guinea pigs has been used for over 30 years and has demonstrated its ability to detect chemicals that can be strong, moderate, and in most cases, weak topical sensitizers in humans. The Buehler Test, originally published in 1965, was developed to provide an exaggerated exposure time and in combination with occlusive conditions, in order to investigate the development of delayed contact hypersensitivity and predict human responses with a low degree of false negatives (4,11,13,14). There are several key elements that must be followed to properly evaluate the dermal sensitization potential of a chemical by the Buehler Test. These elements along with recent modifications of the original method as described Buehler (4,11,13) should be followed explicitly.

B. Guinea Pigs and Assignment to Study Groups

The Hartley outbred albino guinea pig is the animal of choice since there is a large body of background information on the effects of chemicals on their immune system. All animals should be randomly assigned to cages upon receipt and, therefore, randomly assigned to dose groups within the study. Animals in the treatment groups should have essentially identical body weight distributions.

Any guinea pig that becomes abnormal/unhealthy prior to dosing/patching may be replaced with one of the healthy animals that have not been assigned to a treatment group. After dosing begins, no animal should be replaced. Each animal should be individually housed in stainless steel wire mesh cages. Conventional guinea pig laboratory diets containing an adequate amount of ascorbic acid should be used. No differences between the responsiveness of either sex to known sensitizers has been documented, but as a matter of principle groups containing approximately equal numbers of males and females are normally used. Female animals should be nulliparous and nonpregnant. All test and untreated control animals should be healthy after an acclimation period of at least 5 days. At the commencement of induction, all test animals should weigh between 300 and 400 g. This weight range allows a workable size at the start of the study (i.e., large enough to obtain a good occlusive patching) and yet, still fit into the standard restrainer at challenge and rechallenge (i.e., 7 weeks later if a rechallenge is conducted). In addition, each animal should be observed daily for signs of illness and reweighed at weekly intervals (preferably before each treatment). An end-of-test body weight should also be taken. Test and untreated control animals should gain about the same amount of weight if they are healthy and if there is no systemic toxicity from the test material. Guinea pigs outside the weight range of 300–400 g can be assigned to the irritation screening group since it is acceptable if their body weights are over 400 g. Animals should not be identified by ear punch, top clip, ear tag, or tattoo, as all of these have the theoretical potential of compromising the assay. Therefore, identify animals with cage cards. When animals are removed from their cages and placed in the restrainers, the restrainers are identified with the animal number using a marking pen. A useful aid is to use colored stickers on the cage card when more than one test is being done in the same room and to use a matching colored marking pen to mark the hair on the nose of the test animals and the rump of the control animals when they are in the restrainers. However, some laboratories think they must use ear tags to be in compliance with Good Laboratory Practice (GLP), in which case, self-piercing ear tags of Monel stainless steel from Gay Band and Tag Company (Type NSPT 20101) work well.

C. Site Preparation

The appropriate test site on each animal must be prepared before each induction exposure, prior to the challenge or rechallenge, the irritation screens, and before grading. The hair is removed by electric clippers from the area designated to be patched 18–24 hr prior to the application of the test material or grading in order to provide time for any small surface injuries to the skin to close. Care should be taken to avoid injury (e.g., electric clipper burns, scratches, and abrasions) to the skin. The skin must be clear of any form of irritation or lesions. A No.

40 or No. 80 electric clipper blade provides for close removal of the hair. Clipping is necessary to provide a suitable surface for the adhesion of the patch-test system. Depilation of the induction sites is not required for a suitable surface for patch application and should be avoided since the active ingredient (viz., calcium thioglycolate) has been demonstrated to cause delayed contact hypersensitivity in guinea pigs. Therefore, depilation should only be used for complete removal of hair stubble prior to grading at challenge, rechallenge, or during the irritation screens. It is not advisable to depilate at any other time. Depilation is accomplished by the use of a depilatory such as Neet Cream Hair Remover (Reckitt & Colman, Wayne, NJ 07474). Since depilatories are irritants, they should not be left in contact with the skin for more than 15 minutes. It has been our experience that 5–10 minutes is adequate for complete removal of the hair stubble prior to grading. After the allowed period for depilation, the depilatory must be completely rinsed away with warm running water and immediately dried with a towel. If warm running water is not available in the testing room; animals can be wiped with a towel moistened from multiple containers of warm tap water. The containers of warm tap water should be frequently changed to assure an adequate temperature and relatively clean water. Before returning animals to their cages, the sides of the cage must be wiped clean of any depilatory and the animals held in the cage at least 2 hours before grading.

D. Patching

One of the most critical parameters in the performance of the Buehler Test is the application of the test material under occlusive patch testing conditions. Unlike some dermal guinea pig sensitization methods, the Buehler Test does not potentiate the penetration of material into the dermis by damaging the skin through the application of irritants (e.g., 10% sodium lauryl sulfate in petrolatum) or by stripping away the epidermis (e.g., tape stripping). Also, the response is not potentiated through the intradermal injection of experimental adjuvants (e.g., Freund's complete adjuvant) or test material. To assure proper occlusion of the patch-test system to the skin, the Buehler Test recommends the use of a special restrainer that is described in the original paper (4,11).

Figure 1 shows an animal properly situated in the restrainer with an induction patch in place. Restrainers can be custom fabricated or can be purchased (Suburban Equipment, Chicago, IL). Over the years, numerous investigators have modified the Buehler method by not using the special restrainer but utilizing various wrapping techniques (e.g. elastic bandage) to achieve occlusion. The Official Journal of the European Communities (12) indicates that if wrapping is used in place of the appropriate restrainer, additional exposures may be required. Although some of these wrapping techniques have been successful in the detection of potential skin sensitizers, this approach is considered to be inappropriate

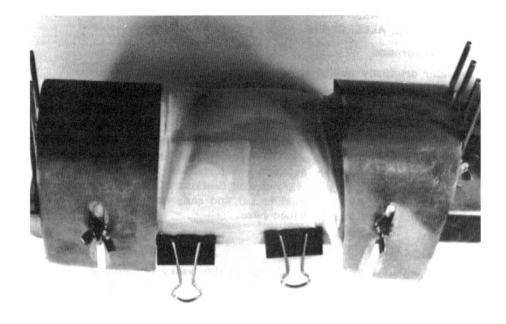

Figure 1 A guinea pig properly restrained, patched, and occluded for induction in a restrainer for the Buehler assay.

and a serious deviation from the intended Buehler method (13,14). The test material to be tested is applied to a patch-test system before being applied to the skin of the animal. A patch-test system utilizing a Webril pad is the preferred method for holding the test material in close contact with the skin. The size of the Webril pad is not that important but should be on the order of approximately 20×20 mm (or 4–6 cm^2 according to OECD Guidelines (9)). The Webril pad needs to be saturated with the test material to obtain maximum concentration at the interface of the patch with the skin and an adequate external reservoir of the test material for optimum penetration into the skin (13). A saturated Webril pad should not allow leakage of the test material from the pad onto the interface between tape and skin. Care should also be taken not to allow excessive evaporation of the test material or vehicle before patch application. If the test material is a grease or paste, a thin film of test material should be spread over the surface of the Webril pad that will contact skin.

        After the exposure period and removal of the patch-test system, the patch site should be gently wiped free of any excess test material with an appropriate solvent (e.g., water, saline) and gauze. This solvent should not compromise the response to the test material or alter the integrity of the epidermis. Two commercial patch-test systems that are commonly used are the so-called professional pad (a 20×20 mm Webril pad on Blenderm tape) and the Hill Top Chamber (25 mm Webril pad). Both of these patch-test systems can be purchased from Hill Top Research, Miamiville, OH. Investigators usually prefer the Hill Top Chamber because it is thought to provide better occlusion and less tape irritation. In addition, the rim of these chambers will leave a slight skin indentation that assures proper occlusion. A single challenge patch at challenge is preferred; however if more patches are required, one should not exceed two patches. At rechallenge, it is acceptable to use up to three patches per animal.

The occlusive material is a medium-weight rubber dental dam. The 6-in. wide roll cut into pieces of approximately 6 in. in length works well. It is convenient to clip one side of the dental dam to the bottom of the restrainer before placing the animal in it. The freshly prepared patch-test system with test material is applied to the prepared test site; the dam is pulled over the upper part of the animal and then clipped to the restraint on the opposite side. Adjustments are then made to give a firm restraint by the rubber without overstressing the animal. One should be able to just pinch a bit of the rubber on the back. If the dental dam squeezes the test material out from under the pad or if the animal begins to lachrimate during the exposure, the dental dam is too tight. The final adjustment is to snug the animal down with the steel restrainer straps. The dental dam must be secured under the restrainer straps to assure good occlusion. Animals should be checked frequently, especially the first time they are placed in the restrainer, to assure that they have not twisted into a position where the patch is no longer occluded. Repositioning of the animal in the restrainer may be required.

E. Grading/Scoring

Scoring of the skin reactions is based on the visual perception of redness or erythema by the investigator. This is a subjective process that requires careful training of the investigator/technician in order to assure accuracy and consistency. In order to reduce the level of subjectivity and uncertainty, it is advisable to have scoring conducted by two trained evaluators. All animals should be scored without the evaluators knowing the induction animals from naïve controls. However, if reactivity is observed in the treated naïve controls animals (baseline animals), the investigator may elect to score them first. The scoring system used in the Buehler Test is as follows:

0	No reaction
±0.5	Slight, patch erythema (barely perceptible or questionable)

1   Slight, but confluent or moderate but patchy erythema
2   Moderate erythema
3   Severe erythema with or without edema

Lighting in the laboratory animal room is usually inadequate for attempting to score skin reactions. Therefore, it is advisable to have an overhead fluorescent laboratory lamp [e.g., 40-W fluorescent-type lights (GE Watt-Miser 11, F4OLW P>S> WMI I Lite White or equivalent] above a flat-black background. One of the most critical scores in the performance of the procedure is the designation between a patchy erythema (±) and a score of "1," as a "±" is not considered a "positive responder" while a grade of "1" is often considered a positive response. The "±" designation covers a wide range of barely perceptible reactions from an effect due to hydration to a more substantive erythema that is still patchy (13). In situations where the majority of the test animals have "±" reactions when compared to naïve controls, a rechallenge is necessary to clarify the reactions. If the test animals at rechallenge continue to show a high incidence of "±" reactions compared to naïve controls, the test material is considered not to be a sensitizer. Rechallenge reactions that are greater than "±" in the test material animals should be counted as positive responses. The score of "1" is used to identify slight to moderate erythema reactions that are not observed in control animals. These dermal sensitization reactions are usually delayed in appearance and will persist longer than primary irritation. OECD Guidelines (9) also allows other procedures such as histopathological examination to clarify doubtful reactions. Scores of "0" (no reactions) or "2" (moderate erythema) or "3" (severe erythema) are easily discerned. Although Buehler (11,13,14) averaged the scores to obtain a relative indication of severity, the most important criteria is the number of "positive responders." Various regulatory agencies consider a "positive" response rate of 15% or more in a nonadjuvant guinea pig test method to be indicative of a dermal sensitizer [OECD Test Guideline 406 (9,12)]. Dermal responses that are not erythema (e.g., pin-point red spots, brown crusty surface, etc.) should not be used in determining the score but should be described in the final report.

OECD guidelines also requires the observation and recording of all skin reactions and any unusual findings during induction. Buehler (13) indicates that these data are not useful for interpretation of the sensitization potential of a chemical since "strong sensitizers" can be manifested during the second or third induction application. However, without the proper controls one cannot differentiate sensitization from cumulative irritation.

F. Vehicles

Test materials should be used undiluted whenever possible provided that they are not primary irritants. However, if the test material is only slightly irritating and is acceptable for induction treatment, the test material must be diluted to an appropriate concentration in a suitable solvent for challenge. Care must be exercised in the selection of a suitable solvent/vehicle and justified. The choice of solvent should be based on the physicochemical properties of the test material that allows for optimal percutaneous absorption. In some situations it may be appropriate to use the intended formulation that the test material is soluble in for evaluation, particularly if the formulation is nonirritating. If the test material is water-soluble, water is the most desirable solvent since there is no concern of the solvent causing a sensitization reaction. When a suitable solvent can not be located, Buehler (11,13) recommends the use of ethanol/water (80/20 v/v) for induction and acetone for challenge treatment. Other solvents/vehicles that have been used in certain cases are propylene glycol, a diluted nonirritating solution of surfactant, 95% ethanol, vegetable oils, pharmaceutical mineral oils (e.g., Squibb Mineral Oil), and petrolatum. Buehler (13) has reported that mineral oils and petrolatum are variable in their irritation potential and should be avoided if possible. With the exception of water, it is undesirable to use the same vehicle for the induction as is being used for the challenge, since it is possible to elicit a sensitization response to the vehicle or to impurities in the vehicle during the challenge phase, thereby causing a false positive reaction to the test material. In the event the same vehicle must be used during induction and challenge, a vehicle experimental group is recommended or a vehicle challenge patch should be included along with the test material during challenge treatment. This would indicate if the vehicle had the potential to cause sensitization. Solids that are not soluble in standard vehicles can be finely pulverized and suspended in petrolatum, mineral oil, or a blend of mineral oil and petrolatum (50/50 wt/wt.). Other solids, such as a plastic film, can be placed directly on the animal under a nonirritating tape or cut to an appropriate size for placement on the major portion of an aqueous saturated Webril pad. When deciding on a suitable solvent/vehicle, one should always keep in mind the effect the vehicle can have on the penetration of test material through the epidermis and how the results of the sensitization assay with a particular vehicle will relate to the intended final use.

G. Irritation Screens

A preliminary evaluation to determine the irritancy of the test material is often done prior to the actual evaluation of the sensitization potential. The concentration of the test material is generally one that is greater than the anticipated level of human exposure. The Buehler assay requires a concentration of test material for the induction that will not cause a level of irritation that will result in eschar formation and will not cause systemic toxicity. Therefore, pilot studies are performed in order to establish a suitable concentration for induction and challenge. Animals from a previous shipment at the laboratory or heavier animals in the current shipment (if requested, the animal supplier will provide 4–8 heavier animals) are used to establish an appropriate induction concentration prior to study initiation. A concentration that produces slight to mild irritation (grades of "±" or an occasional "1") is acceptable for induction. It has been our experience to rescore an acceptable induction concentration patch site 6–7 days later for a possible delayed irritant effect of the test material (e.g., a reaction that has been observed with gasoline). If all of the selected concentrations are too irritating, the pilot screen is repeated. The typical irritation screen uses 2–4 animals with 4 patches and up to 4 different concentrations on each animal. One of these concentrations should include the vehicle/solvent if its irritation is unknown. Three-to-four animals are also used to establish the challenge concentration; this screen can be performed later during the induction phase of the study. The concentration of the test material (if in a different vehicle or not) used at challenge should not produce more than the slightest irritation (i.e., not more than 50% grades "±" in the control animals). The locations of the various concentrations on the back of each animal are normally varied to correct for any site-to-site variations. This second pilot screen has been found to be an excellent predictor of the results that will be observed in the control animals at challenge and reduces the number of times that a rechallenge has to be run because of high background levels of irritation in the untreated controls. If any of the pilot screens are unsuccessful, then an additional irritation screen must be performed.

H. Performing the Buehler Test

The foregoing discussion has provided insight into the reasons for the details of many of the steps in the Buehler Test. The following scheme combines these into an evaluation:

1. Pre-induction Irritation/Toxicity Screen (2–4 Animals)
    a. Day −1: Hair is clipped from the entire back of the animals 18–24 hour prior treatment.
    b. Day 0: Prepare up to 4 different concentrations of test material. Patch each animal with occluded patches for 6 hours (±30 min).
    c. Day 1: Depilate the patched area 18–22 hr (OECD suggests 21 hr) after removal of the patches. Grade at least 2 hr (OECD suggests 3 hr and refer to this as the 30-hr grade) after depilation (24-hr grade).
    d. Day 2: Repeat the grading 24 hr later (48-hr grade). OECD suggests a 24 hr grade after the 30-hr observation for a 54-hr grade.

2. Induction (20 Test Material Animals + 10 Naïve Control Animals + Any Rechallenge Naïve Controls; and 10 Vehicle Control Animals + 10 Positive Control Animals and Respective Naïve Controls, if required by study design)
    a. Day −1: Weigh the all of the animals and remove hair 18–24 hour prior to the first exposure from the upper left quadrant (shoulder) with clippers of only animals receiving treatment.

b. Day 0: Patch treatment animals for approximately 6 hr (±30 min).

c. Weeks 2 and 3: Repeat the clipping and patching twice more on the treatment animals with a 5- to 9-day interval between patching. (OECD recommends intervals of 6–8 days for the second treatment and 13–15 days for the third treatment after the first treatment). Check the induction site during clipping for eschar formation; move patches to a new site if eschar is present.

3. Prechallenge Irritation Screen for Challenge Levels (4–8 Animals)

Perform this screen during the induction phase. Use the same procedure as the prestudy screen except use ≤4 patches per animal. The lowest concentration that caused slight irritation in the prestudy screen is used as the highest concentration in the prechallenge screen. If needed, include a prechallenge screen for vehicle control and positive control animals.

4. Challenge 12 to 16 Days (OECD requires 12 to 14 days) After the Last Induction (20 Test Material + 10 Naïve Control Animals; if required by study design, 10 Vehicle + 10 Naïve Control Animals, 10 Positive Control + 10 Naïve Control Animals)

a. Day −1: Weigh all of the animals, and remove hair from the rear quadrant to be patched with clippers 18–24 hr prior treatment. (Do not use the induction site for challenge).

b. Day 0: Challenge the experimental test animals and naïve control animals with a nonirritating concentration of the corresponding test material using an occluded patch and an exposure time of approximately 6 hr (±30 mm).

c. Day 1: Depilate and grade as in the irritation screens (24-hr grade). In certain situations, the investigator may elect to grade the naïve control animals first, particularly if reactivity or questionable dermal responses are present.

d. Day 2: Grade a second time as in the irritation screens (48-hr grade).

5. Rechallenge (6–10 Days After the Primary Challenge)

All or selected animals may be rechallenged with the same material used in the challenge at the same or a different concentration or a new test material may be used. Use 10 new control animals, naïve test sites on all induced animals, and the same procedures used in the challenge phase. (OECD allows rechallenge of the original control animals if new animals are not available, but this is not recommended.)

6. Report

Determine the number of positive responders (number of animals with a score ≥1 at *either* the 24- or 48-hr grading or with a score one unit higher than the highest score in the naïve control group). Determine the average score (scores at face value and with "±" = 0.5) at 24 hr and at 48 hr for the test and the control group (4 values).

I. Advantages, Disadvantages, and Problems

The Buehler Test has been used for over 30 years to predict the skin sensitization potential of chemicals prior to human exposure. Correctly performed, it has been demonstrated to detect chemicals that can be strong, moderate, and in most cases, weak topical sensitizers in humans (4,11,13,14). Ritz and Buehler (11) published the standard for the proper performance of the Buehler Test in *Current Concepts in Cutaneous Toxicity* in 1980. The original 1965 publication of the Buehler test (4) which required more than three induction applications in 10 experimental animals is not considered to represent the standardized procedure, even though it is still cited in various regulatory guidelines. The only indication of a possible modification of the standardized procedure (viz., additional exposures beyond the one pàtch/week for 3 weeks) is if wrapping is used in place of the appropriate restrainer (12).

As a topical "nonadjuvant" test, the Buehler test allows for the investigation of dose responses, cross reactivity between structurally related chemicals, and the sensitization potential of contaminants in raw material mixtures. It also provides an initial indication of the sensitization potential of the substance under relevant, but exaggerated, exposure conditions (14). When preformed according to the published methodology and the results properly interpreted the Buehler Test can accurately detect the sensitization potential of most chemicals that will come in contact with the skin. Although it is a sensitive procedure, it is generally considered to be less sensitive than the adjuvant guinea pig sensitization procedures (e.g., Guinea Pig Maximization Test). Therefore, it is not the preferred method (9,12) for predicting the sensitization potential of substances in most European countries and scientific justification must be given when the Buehler Test is used. It should be noted that since no adjuvant is used in the assay, far less stress on the animals is caused when compared to the Maximization Test.

J. Positive Control

In order to validate the occlusivity of the methodology, Buehler (15) recommends a single induction patch application of 2,4-dintro-1-chlorobenzene (DNCB) at a concentration of 0.3% w/v solution in ethanol/water 80:20 (v/v). Most induced animals should respond positively to a challenge of 0.2% (w/v)

DNCB in acetone and about half to a concentration of 0.02%, if you have had proper occlusion. More recently, Buehler (13) has recommended that laboratories performing the assay validate their procedure at least twice a year using DNCB as a standard sensitizer. Animals should be induced (i.e., one patch/week for 3 weeks) with 0.1% w/v DNCB in 80% ethanol/water and challenged with 0.1% (w/v) DNCB in acetone, and then rechallenged with concentrations of 0.1% (w/v) and 0.01% (w/v) DNCB in acetone. This is intended to produce a positive response rate of 80–100% at the 0.1% DNCB concentration and a rate of 40–50% at the 0.01% DNCB concentration. Similarly, the OECD guidelines (9, 12) recommend sensitivity and reliability checks of the assay every 6 months with a substance known to have mild-to-moderate skin sensitization properties. The preferred mild-to-moderate substances are hexyl cinnamic aldehyde (CAS No. 101-86-0), mercaptobenzothiazole (CAS No. 149-30-4) and benzocaine (CAS No. 94-09-7).

With adequate scientific justification, other substances that are considered mild/moderate sensitizers can be used. If the Buehler Test is properly conducted with a mild/moderate sensitizer, there should be a positive response rate of 15%.

IV. GUINEA PIG MAXIMIZATION TEST (GPMT) FOR DETECTING DERMAL ALLERGENS

A. Background

Magnusson and Kilgman published a procedure for evaluating the potential for chemicals to elicit a delayed contact hypersensitivity response (5). This procedure attempted to "maximize" the potential for a response through the use of Freund's complete adjuvant (FCA), intradermal injection of the test material, and the use of a pretreatment to produce irritation at the induction site. The epidermis was initially bypassed by intradermally injecting adjuvant, adjuvant mixed with test material, and test material in vehicle. The second phase consisted of irritating the skin over the injection sites with a surfactant when a nonirritating test material is being evaluated and then applying the test material to the skin under an occlusive patch. The stated purpose of the assay was to determine if a chemical has any potential as a dermal allergen. The GPMT was recommended for testing individual chemicals and not complex mixtures, finished products, or formulations. The GPMT tends to overestimate the risk to humans.

B. Induction

1. Site Preparation and Intradermal Induction Stage

The hair from an area over the shoulders of the guinea pigs is removed 24 to 48 hr prior to dosing using a small-animal clipper. The test article and vehicle control groups with and without FCA are injected in the shoulder region of each animal. A 1-cc syringe with a 1/4-in. 25 or 28 gauge needle works well. However, some test material preparations (especially suspension) may require a larger needle; leakage from the needle hole may occur. The vehicle controls receive adjuvant, vehicle, and adjuvant with vehicle but no test material. A row of three injections, on each side (i.e., 6 in all), are made as seen in Figure 2.

Injections 1 and 2 are given close to each other nearest to the head and injection 5 and 6 are given most caudally; injections 3 and 4 are given between injection sites 1 and 2 and 5 and 6. The injection sites *must* be just within the boundaries of a 2×4 cm patch, which will be applied one week later for the topical induction.

2. Topical Induction Stage

The test sites will be reclipped free of hair after a minimum of 7 days. The assay requires the use of concentration of irritating test material. If the test material is not irritating, then skin irritation should be induced by a surfactant prior to the application of the topical patch. The surfactant irritation step uses a 10% w/w preparation of sodium lauryl sulfate in petrolatum; test and vehicle control sites are pretreated on Day 7 (normally 0.3 mL). On Day 8 the test article in vehicle is spread over a 2×4 cm filter paper, saturated (normally 0.3 mL) with the test article, and applied to the injection site area and occluded

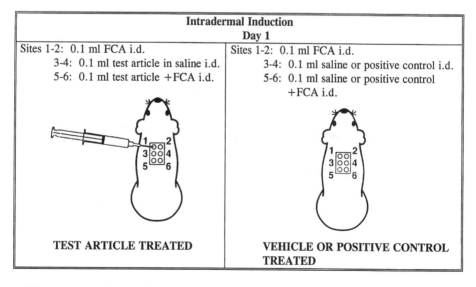

Figure 2 A diagram showing the injection sites for the intradermal (i.d.) induction phase of the guinea pig maximization test.

using Blenderm® tape. The Blenderm tape is held in place with an appropriate occlusive bandage. Forty-eight hr later (±30 min) the dressings are removed. This same procedure is employed with the vehicle, control article, and positive control animals.

3. Challenge Period

Two weeks after the topical induction the test-article treated and control animals are challenged with occluded patches for 24 hr on the right and left flanks. The hair will have been removed from these areas using a clipper 24 to 48 hrs before application of the patch. A 2×2 cm filter paper is saturated (normally 0.2 mL) with the test article and applied to the left flank. Another 2×2 cm filter paper is saturated (normally 0.2 mL) with the vehicle and applied to the right flank. The same occlusive technique as for topical induction is then employed. 24 hr later the wrapping is removed and the sites wiped clean. 21 hr (20 to 22 hr) after unwrapping, the sites are clipped if necessary. The use of a commercial depilatory is optional. Approximately 24, 48, and 72 hr (±1 hr) after removal of the bandages, individual animals are graded according to Table 1.

C. Grading

The grading system for dermal irritation and sensitization responses are presented below (Table 1). The first system was developed by Kligman while the second was developed by Draize. Depending on the regulatory requirements to be met, the appropriate grading system should be employed.

D. Classification for Ranking Substances

Kligman's classification scheme has been modified to reflect a treatment group of twenty animals being used for ranking the substances in order of their sensitization capacity.

Grades of ≥ 1 in the test group are required to be indicative of sensitization. If grades of ≥ 1 are seen on the vehicle animals, then the reactions of the test article group animals that exceed the most severe vehicle control reactions at the interval are considered to be positive scores (see Table 2).

E. Preliminary Screens

The GPMT involves two types of screens: one for the intradermal injections and one for dermal irritation. A concentration for the intradermal injections that does not cause systemic toxicity or necrosis is required. A concentration which is mildly irritating is preferred for topical induction while a nonirritating concentration is used for challenge.

Table 1 Individual Animal Scores

Score	Skin Reaction
0	No reaction
1	Slight patchy mild redness
2	Moderate and diffuse redness
3	Intense redness and swelling
4	Severe erythema and edema; skin damage

Reaction	Numerical Grading
Erythema	
No erythema	0
Slight erythema	1
Well-defined erythema	2
Moderate erythema	3
Severe erythema to slight eschlar formation	4
Edema	
No edema	0
Slight edema	1
Well-defined edema	2
Moderate edema	3
Severe edema	4

Note: Other adverse changes of the skin sites shall be recorded and reported.

Table 2 Maximization Grading

Sensitization Rate (%)	No. of Animals Responding	Grade	Class
0–8	1–2	I*	Weak
9–28	3–6	II	Mild
29–64	7–13	III	Moderate
65–80	14–16	IV	Strong
81–100	17–20	V	Extreme

*Magnusson and Kligman do not regard sensitization of Grade I as significant.

1.   Intradermal Dose Range-Finding

Prior to initiation of the induction, the irritation potential must be determined. Four naïve animals are exposed to several different concentrations (generally 1 to 5%) of the test article by the intradermal technique described in site preparation and intradermal induction stage. In this test, both sides of the animal are clipped and exposed to the various concentrations of the test article. These concentrations should be prepared in both vehicle and FCA. For grading of the response, the procedure described for primary challenge will be used, except that only 24-hr grades are obtained. The highest concentration to be used in the induction phase of the GPMT is one shown to be well tolerated systemically, and causing only mild to moderate skin irritation.

2.   Topical Dose Range-Finding

Four naïve guinea pigs are exposed to several different concentrations (generally 25, 50, 75, and 100%) of the test article. Solids are applied at the maximum attainable concentration suitable for topical application (up to a maximum concentration of 25% solution or suspension) plus three lower concentrations. The procedure described in topical induction period is employed except that the wrapping will be removed at 48 hours after dosing. Twenty-one hr (±15 min) after unwrapping the sites are clipped or depilated as necessary. Three hr later (±15 min) the sites are examined for skin reactions (24-hr grade). The location of each of the concentrations of the test article will differ in each of the four animals to compensate for any site-to-site variations.

   If the test material is suspected to be very irritating, or toxic by the dermal route, then lower concentrations may be investigated and/or fewer patches will be applied to each animal. The highest concentration producing only mild to moderate dermal irritation will be selected for the topical induction stage of the main study.

3.   Topical Challenge Dose Range-Finding

Four naïve guinea pigs will be exposed to several different concentrations of the test article. Information from the range-finding study for the topical induction dose should be reviewed before selecting doses for the challenge dose-range study. The highest concentration producing no evidence of skin irritation at the 24 and 48 hr observations (the maximum nonirritant concentration), and one lower concentration will be selected for the topical challenge stage of the main study.

4.   Discussion on Dose-Range Finding Studies

In recent years, many instances of significant irritating reactions have been seen at challenge in the vehicle control animals receiving the test material at a concentration previously determined in the irritation screen to be nonirritating. This has been explained as the "angry back" syndrome. Needless to say, this unexpected reaction can make grading difficult to understand. It is thought that "angry back" syndrome is a response to a previous high level of irritation, which in the case of the GPMT, is brought on by the use of both the FCA and the 10% sodium lauryl sulfate exposure (16).

In order to better prepare for this situation, minor changes can be made to the topical screening studies. The exact procedures for the topical-dose-range-finding studies will be utilized except the animals will have been injected previously (i.e., 1 week earlier) with FCA. Usually the reactions seen and the doses selected are more realistic to the model and have reduced the incidence of irritating responses in the vehicle animals receiving the test material at challenge.

F. Vehicles

The vehicles to be used in preparing the various concentrations of the test material must be given careful consideration. As many as three different vehicles may be required: one for the injection of test material in vehicle, one for the preparation of test material in adjuvant, and one for the dermal application. Water-soluble test materials present the least problem as this single vehicle can be used in all phases. When a water-soluble material is to be mixed with adjuvant, it is first dissolved in water and this solution is then mixed with an equal volume of adjuvant. Complete dispersion is accomplished by rapid stirring. One must observe that the mixing of the test material preparation with adjuvant has not disrupted the emulsion of the adjuvant. Oil soluble or insoluble test materials can often be dissolved or suspended directly in the adjuvant and then the mixture diluted with water to a final 1:1 dilution. In some cases, it has been found advantageous to first dissolve a test material in acetone or ethylacetate and then add up to 0.1 mL of the solution to the adjuvant. Under these conditions, the adjuvant should be stirred rapidly and the organic solution added in very small drops so as not to compromise the oil preparation of the FCA.

The injection of the test material in vehicle without adjuvant may use water, mineral oil, vegetable oil, or propylene glycol as the vehicle. The use of many organic solvents such as acetone or alcohol generally will cause an excess of tissue damage.

Test material is prepared for dermal application (topical patch, irritation screen, and challenge) by dissolving it in an appropriate solvent such as water, ethanol:water (80/20 v/v), or acetone or by dispersing it in petrolatum. If one must work with a suspended solid, the solid should be micronized before use.

G. Number of Animals

20   Test material

20   Vehicle controls
6   Positive control

Ten naïve animals may be maintained with the colony in the event of a rechallenge or better, carried with the vehicle control animals so that they have been exposed to all aspects of the study except test material.

The weight ranges, ages, strains, etc. are the same as discussed in the Buehler Test.

I. Running the Maximization Assay

The foregoing discussion has provided insight into the reasons for the details of many of the steps in the assay. The following scheme combines these into an evaluation:

1. Irritation/Toxicity Screen (16 animals)
    a. Intradermal Screen Concentration (8 animals)
        i.   Day 1: Prepare 4 concentrations of test material in vehicle and 4 concentrations in FCA. Clip the hair from the back over the shoulders. Inject 2 animals with each of the concentrations, i.e., 2 injections of one of the FCA concentrations and 2 injections of the corresponding concentration in vehicle.
        ii. Days 2 and 3: Evaluate the injection sites for gross irritation and necrosis and the animals for systemic toxicity.
    b. Dermal Irritation (4 animals)—Topical Concentration Screen Induction
        iii. Day −1: Remove the hair from the back using clippers.
        iv. Day 1: Patch each animal with 4 different concentrations of test material. Occlude the patches and wrap the animals.
        v.   Day 3: Remove the patches 48 hr (±30 min) after the start.
        vi. Day 4: Remove the hair with depilatory approximately 21 hr after removing the patches. Grade the test sites for irritation 24 hr (±1 hr) after removing the patches.
        vii. Day 5. Grade the test sites 48 hr (±2 hr) after removing the patches.
    c. Dermal Irritation (4 animals)—Challenge Concentration Screen
        viii. Day −1: Remove the hair from the back using clippers.
        ix. Day 0: Patch each animal with 4 different concentrations of test material. Occlude the patched and wrap the animals with elastic tape.
        x.   Day 2: Remove the patches 24 hr (±30 mm) after the start.
        xi. Day 3: Remove the hair with depilatory approximately 21

hr after removing the patches. Grade the test sites for irritation 24 hr (1± hr) after removing the patches.

    xii.   Day 4: Grade the test sites 48 hr (2 hr) after removing the
patches.

2.   Induction (20 Test, 20 Vehicle Control, and 6 Positive Control)

    i.   Day 1: Weigh the animals. Remove the hair from the shoul-
der region with clippers. Inject each test animal with 2 intradermal 0.1 mL each of diluted FCA, FCA, and test material in vehicle (6 injections per animal). Inject each vehicle
control animal and positive controls in a similar manner
except do not use test material for controls. Vehicle and
positive control animals should receive their respective
treatment.

    ii.   Day 7: If the test article concentration to be used for the
topical induction was not irritating in the screen, treat the
injection site area with 10% sodium lauryl sulfate in petrolatum. Remove the hair with clippers prior to the treatment.
If the test article was irritating, omit this step.

    iii.   Day 8: Remove the hair from the injection sites with clip-
pers if this was not done on day 7. If the test material is
a liquid, saturate the filter paper (20×40 mm filter patch
Whatman No. 4) or coat the paper with test material in
petrolatum if it is a solid. Place the paper over the injection
sites of the test animals, cover with Blenderm and wrap the
animal. Treat the controls with vehicle only. Positive controls will receive the positive test material.

    iv.   Day 10: Remove the patches 48 hr (±2 hr) after initiating
the patching.

3.   Challenge

    v.   Day 20: Remove the hair from the entire back of each test,
control, and positive control animals using an animal
clipper.

    vi.   Day 21: Patch each test and control animal with test mate-
rial on a 20×20 mm filter paper patch (Whatman No. 4)
on a naïve test site with a nonirritating concentration of test
material as determined in the irritation screen. Use a vehicle control patch if appropriate. The positive control group
should receive the positive control material. Occlude the
patches with Blenderm and wrap the animals.

    vii.   Day 22: Remove the patches and any excess test material
24 hr (±30 min) after application.

    viii.   Day 23: Remove any remaining hair with depilatory starting approximately 21 hr after the patches were removed. Grade the test sites 24 hr (±1 hr) after patches were removed (24-hr grade).

ix. Day 24: Grade the sites again 48 hr (±2 hr) after the patches were removed (48-hr grade).

x. Day 25: Grade the sites again 72 hr (±2 hr) after the patches were removed (72-hr grade). Weigh the animals.

4. Rechallenge

All or selected animals may be rechallenged with the same test material at the same or a different concentration or with a different test material within 7–30 days after the primary challenge. Use new control animals or the extra control animals carried with the main study and naïve test sites on all animals.

J. Advantages, Disadvantages, and Problems

Maximization assay provides a very sensitive determination of a test material having any potential to be a dermal sensitizer. Because of the use of FCA, intradermal injections, and skin irritants, all of which compromise the epidermal barrier, it is difficult to relate the results to potential danger in "normal" human exposure. On the other hand, a negative result tends to be very reassuring that there is little concern for sensitization in humans. If the investigator is interested in determining if a single component in a complex mixture that is a recognized sensitizer might elicit a sensitization response when in the mixture, then a group of animals can be sensitized to the pure component and challenged with the final formulation. As with any assay that involves the injection of adjuvant, there is often a problem with using the results of the irritation screen in naïve animals to accurately predict the results that will be seen in the sham controls at the challenge. If the material being tested is a nonirritant or if one selects a concentration of an irritant that is far below the irritating concentration, then the screen does an adequate job of predicting the background irritation level in the challenge controls. However, if a slightly nonirritating concentration of an irritant is used, the screen often underpredicts the response and a high background level of irritation is observed at the challenge in the sham-treated controls. The interpretation of the challenge results become difficult. If additional control animals have not been carried with the main study, it might be wise to do the initial challenge with 2 different concentrations of test material to adjust for possible "angry back" syndrome, but this will remove a possible rechallenge site. Thus, it is often necessary to rechallenge the test animals at a lower concentration; therefore additional sham-treated controls must be available. The possible need for rechallenge control animals adds additional cost to the assay. The use of adjuvant injections causes a significant increase in the stress to the animals.

K. Positive Control

The positive control will use six animals and induction exposures to 0.1% 1-chloro-2,4-dinitrobenzene (DNCB) in saline (intradermal exposure) and petrolatum (topical exposure), with a topical challenge exposure of 0.05 and 0.01% DNCB in petrolatum. Additional substances that are known to have mild to moderate skin sensitization properties are a-hexyl cinnamicaldehyde (CAS No. 10 1-86-0), mercaptobenzothiazole (CAS No. 119-304), and benzocaine (CAS No. 91-09-7). A sensitization response in at least 30% of animals tested is expected for these substances.

V. MOUSE EAR SWELLING TEST (MEST) ASSAY FOR DETECTING DERMAL ALLERGENS

A. Background

The guinea pig has historically been the animal of choice, and methods such as the Buehler Test and Guinea Pig Maximization Test have traditionally been used to evaluate the potential of a chemical or mixtures to elicit a sensitization response. Since, compared to mice, guinea pigs are relatively expensive to purchase and maintain and the guinea pig assays require weeks to complete, investigators have sought an alternative assay. Gad has presented an assay called the Mouse Ear Swelling Test (MEST) (7,17). The mouse was shown to exhibit the capability for delayed-type contact hypersensitivity in 1959 (18). Asherson and Ptak (19) developed the technique of quantitatively assessing contact delayed hypersensitivity by measuring the swelling of the mouse ear with a micrometer. Chapman et al. (20) demonstrated that an excellent correlation exists between ear swelling and histological changes. Gad's group performed an extensive evaluation using a variety of exposure conditions, animal strains, and test materials in order to elucidate the conditions for optimum response. The MEST results compared favorably with the results of maximization assay when 72 test materials were identified as sensitizers or nonsentizers. Several laboratories have participated in a validation of the procedure (21).

B. Animals

Female CF-1 mice are used in the assay. They should be 6–8 weeks of age when the study is initiated. The sex of the animal is not critical from a sensitization criterion. However, there is a cost advantage to group housing (5 per cage) and the use of females avoids the fighting problems often found with male mice. Both CF-1 and BALB/C mice respond well to known sensitizers while several other strains of mice are not sensitive responders; the CF-1 mice are much less expensive than the BALB/C strain. Animals less than 4 weeks old and greater than 13 weeks old are not as responsive as the 6–8-week-old animals. Animals are not given an ear tag or notch for identification as this would compromise the assay. Extra care must be taken not to confuse the test and control animals.

C. Induction Site Preparation

The abdominal region is used for the induction applications as it was found that very poor or no induction could be achieved when the back was used. An enhancement of responsiveness is obtained by the use of both Freund's complete adjuvant (FCA) (Calbiochem-Behring, San Diego, CA or Difco, Detroit, MI) and skin stripping. On the day of the first induction exposure (day 0), the hair is removed from the abdominal region using an animal clipper fitted with a No. 40 or 80 blade. An evaluation of the use of a depilatory to remove the last traces of hair has not been reported. Two intradermal injections of 20 μL each of undiluted FCA are made in the belly region using a 30-ga needle. It is important that these injections be intradermal. The epidermis is then compromised by tape stripping 10 times or until the skin is shiny using Dermiclear transparent tape (1 in. wide) (Johnson & Johnson Products, Inc., New Brunswick, NJ). The stripping is best accomplished with one person holding and supporting the mouse and a second person firmly pressing the tape to the belly region and quickly removing it. Both the test and control animals are stripped and injected.

D. Induction

Four exposures to the test material on four consecutive days constitute the induction. The concentration of the test material is one which, if possible, causes slight irritation but no systemic toxicity. The belly skin is tape stripped 10 times on day 0 after the injection of FCA and then 5 times or until shiny on days 1, 2, and 3, but no adjuvant is given. Test animals are dermally dosed with 100 μL of test material preparation and control animals are dosed with 100 μL of vehicle on each day of the induction. The dosed volume is spread over the stripped area with the side of the dosing needle. It is recommended that a blunt needle be used to assure avoidance of unscheduled skin damage. It is necessary to rapidly dry the induction site before returning the animal to the cage. This is readily accomplished by applying a hair dryer to vehicles of low volatility though care must be taken not to use heat, just air flow.

E. Challenge

The challenge is done on the seventh day after the last induction. Shorter or longer waiting periods do not provide as much sensitivity as the 7-day period. The challenge consists of applying 20 μL of vehicle to the right ear and 20 μL of test material to the left ear. The 20 μL dose is divided such that 10 μL is applied on the dorsal side of the ear and 10 μL is applied to the ventral side. The substances are carefully applied evenly over the ear from a microliter pipetter and dried in a stream of warm air. Both the test and control animals are dosed with test substance in vehicle and vehicle only.

F. Evaluation of Response

Unique to the MEST is the use of a thickness gauge rather than a subjective irritation response used in most other dermal allergen assays to measure the elicited sensitization response. The gage is an Oditest D-1000 Thickness Gage (Dryer Company, Lancaster, PA) equipped at the factory with a fixed 5-mm diameter contact surface. The thickness of both the left and right ears is determined 24 hr (±1 hr) and 48 hr (±2 hr) after the application of the challenge dose. It is important to measure the thickness of the ear toward the outer edge and not in the cartilage area. The spring load of the gage can cause a redistribution of edemic fluid in the ear. Thus, the animal is anesthetized lightly with ether or other volatile anesthetic, which easily facilitates a rapid and consist measurement of the ear thickness. The measurement at 48 hr is important, as some test materials exhibit a response at this time that is not fully developed at 24 hr. A responder is considered an animal having a test ear thickness 20% greater than the thickness of the control ear at either 24 or 48 hr after the challenge. Gad et al. (7) determined that the variation among ear thicknesses of any one animal was ≤4% and that low levels of simple irritation rarely caused a 10% increase in thickness (responses of >10% occurred at a frequency of approximately 0.5%). Thus, the 20% criteria is a strong indication of a sensitization response (i.e., a positive responder) (see Figure 3).

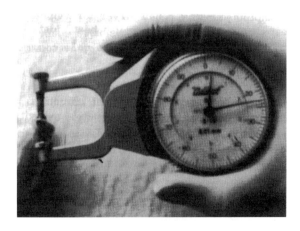

Figure 3   Measure of ear thickness in the MEST evaluation.

% ear change = [(test ear − control ear) ÷ (control ear thickness)] × 100

The measurement of the ears of the control animals is used as an indicator of background responses of a nonallergic nature. The swelling of the test ears of the animals compared to the control ears is also calculated as follows:

% Ear swelling = [(Σ test (left) ear thickness) ÷ (Σ control (right) ear thickness)] × 100

G. Rechallenge

The mice can be rechallenged to the same concentration of test material to confirm sensitization, to weaker concentrations to evaluate dose-versus-response relationships, to a finished product containing the allergen, or to a different material to evaluate cross reactivity. The mouse assay must rechallenge on a previously exposed skin site (the left ear), which could cause problems if previous exposures have compromised this site. One must plan for any rechallenges by providing 5 additional sham-treated control animals for each rechallenge. Rechallenges should be done approximately 7 days after the previous challenge. Since the induction of sensitization is relatively short for the MEST assay, it may be advisable to induce additional animals if one has absolute plans for rechallenges.

H. Prestudy Screens

Preliminary data must be obtained before starting the induction and challenge portion of the study. A screen must be run to determine a slightly irritating but nontoxic concentration for the induction and to determine a nonirritating level for application to the ear at the challenge. Two mice are used to test each concentration of test material; both the belly region and the ears of each animal are used. The hair is clipped from the belly region and tape stripped 10 times on day 0. A volume of 100 µL is applied to the belly and 20 µL of the same concentration is applied to the left ear. The right ear is dosed with 20 µL of vehicle. The thickness of the test ear and the control (right) ear are measured 24 hr (±1 hr) and 48 hr (±2 hr) after the application. The belly region skin is stripped 5 times on days 1, 2, and 3 and an additional 100 µL of test material applied after each stripping. At 24 hours after the last dose, the belly skin is observed for irritation. Animals are observed daily for signs of systemic toxicity. An acceptable level for the induction should cause no more than slight irritation while the challenge dose should cause less than a 10% increase in the test ear thickness when compared to the control ear.

I. Vehicles

Water is the ideal vehicle since it is neither irritating nor an allergen. Other acceptable vehicles that have been used successfully include acetone, ethanol/ water (70/30, 30/20 or 95/5 v/v), methyl ethyl ketone, propylene glycol, petrolatum, and vegetable oils. It is best, with the exception of water, to use different vehicles for the induction and the challenge in order to avoid any possible allergic responses due to impurities in the vehicle. It is also desirable to have the test material dissolved in the vehicle rather than suspended. One must keep in mind that some vehicles can have a dramatic effect on the penetration of an allergen and thus on the results of the assay.

J. Running the MEST Assay

1. Irritation/Toxicity Screen (8 Animals for 4 Concentrations)

Day 0.   Prepare 4 concentrations of test material in the vehicle(s) to be used in the induction and challenge phases. Remove the hair from the belly region of a pair of animals for each of the concentrations. Tape strip the belly region 10 times and apply 100 μL of one of the concentrations to a pair of the animals. Apply 20 μL of the same concentration (in the same or a different vehicle) to the left ear of the same pair or animals and vehicle to the right ear.

Day 1.   Measure the thickness of the left and right ears of each animal 24 hr (±1 hr) after the application. Tape strip the belly skin 5 times and apply 100 μL of test material in vehicle.

Day 2.   Measure the thickness of the left and right ear 48 hr (±2 hr) after application of the challenge dose. Tape strip the belly region 5 times and apply 100 μL of test material.

Day 3.   Tape strip the belly region 5 times and apply 100 μL of test material.

Day 4.   Evaluate the belly for irritation and necrosis and the animals for systemic toxicity.

2. Induction (15 Test + 5 Control + Rechallenge Control Animals)

Day 0.   Remove the hair from the belly of all animals with a clipper. Give each animal two, 20 μL intradermal injections in the belly region of FCA. Tape strip the region 10 times or until shiny. Apply 100 μL of test material in vehicle to the test animals and 100 μL of vehicle to the sham-controlled animals

Days 1, 2, 3.   Tape strip the animals until shiny and dose with test material or vehicle as on day 0.

3. Challenge (15 Test + Sham-Control)

Day 10.   Apply 20 μL of test material in vehicle to the left ear and 20 μL of vehicle to the right ear of both the test and control animals

Day 11. Determine the thickness of the left and right ears of each animal 24 hr (±1 hr) after the challenge application.

Day 12. Repeat the ear measurements 48 hr (±2 hr) after application of the challenge dose.

4. Rechallenge:

All or selected test animals and new sham-control animals may be rechallenged 7 days after the first challenge.

5. Report:

Report the number of positive responders (test animals with left ear thickness ≥20% of the right ear provided the left ear of the control animals is <10% thicker than the right ear of the control) and the % swelling for the test group.

K. Advantages/Disadvantages and Problems

The MEST assay offers a very economical means of rapidly screening materials for their potential to elicit a delayed contact-type hypersensitivity response. The assay requires relatively inexpensive animals, economy of vivarium space, a small amount of test material, and less time than any of the more commonly used guinea pig assays. The assay results have been shown to correlate well with known human sensitizers. It has an advantage over the more conventional assays in that an objective measurement (thickness) is used in the evaluation rather than the subjective measurement of degrees of irritation. The major problem with the assay is its lack of history. The procedure is relatively new and has not been fully accepted by all of the regulatory agencies as a substitute for the guinea pig assays and has not been tested in litigation. It should provide an efficient screening tool until such time as it has the appropriate patina to be acceptable to the toxicology community at large. The use of adjuvant often causes a hypersensitivity of the skin to irritation in the guinea pig assays and the effects of adjuvant on the responsiveness of the ear to swelling are unknown. Another possible problem in the assay is the need to reuse the test-skin (left ear) in rechallenges that was used in the challenge; some test materials may compromise the ear and lead to confusing results. An alternative for one rechallenge is to switch and use the ear which was used for the vehicle in the primary challenge.

L. Positive Control

Typical results using a 0.5% solution of 1-chloro-2,4-dinitrobenzene in 70% ethanol/water (v/v) for induction and a 1% preparation for the challenge are shown in Table 3.

Table 3

Left (test) Ear Thickness	Right (control) Ear Thickness
Test group	
30[a]	21
26	23
26[a]	21
24	22
29[a]	24
26[a]	20
30[a]	21
29[a]	23
29[a]	22
32[a]	21
38[a]	23
31[a]	22
31[a]	23
26[a]	24
34[a]	24
Sum: 441	334
Responders: 80%	
% Swelling: 132%	
Control group	
22	21
23	23
25	24
24	24
25	24

[a]Responder = test ear thicker than control ear.

VI. THE LOCAL LYMPH NODE TEST (LLNT)

A. Background

The desire for a faster, more economical assay for the detection of sensitizing agents also led to the development of the Local Lymph Node Test (LLNT) (8). The LLNT uses mice, which are less expensive than guinea pigs, and the assay is completed in 6 days.

The LLNT measures events occuring in the induction phase of sensitization. When an animal is exposed to a sensitizing agent, there is an activation and clonal expansion of the allergen-reactive T lymphocytes in the lymph nodes regional to the site of exposure. In addition, the vigor of the T cell proliferative response induced in the draining lymph nodes correlates directly with the extent to which the animal becomes sensitized (22). Kimber and his colleagues made use of these facts in developing the LLNT (23).

B. Animals

Several strains of mice have been evaluated in the LLNT (8). The strain of choice is the inbred strain CBA/Ca. Either males or females can be used; however, in a given study, a single sex is recommended. Young adult mice, 6–12 weeks of age are used. Each group normally consists of 4–6 mice. Mice should not be ear tagged since the ear is the site of sensitization.

C. Vehicles

Water is not considered to be a proper vehicle for the LLNT. However, several organic vehicles have been used successfully such as, 4/1 acetone/olive oil, methyl ethyl ketone, N,N-dimethylformamide, propylene glycol and dimethyl sulfoxide (24). The vehicle is normally selected based on the solubility of the test material.

D. Test Material Concentrations

Typically at least three concentrations of the test material are used. One approach is to use 50, 25, and 10% (w/v). However, solubility and potential toxicity may influence the concentrations that can be tested.

E. Sensitization

Mice receive an application of the potential sensitizing agent on the dorsal surface of both ears on 3 consecutive days. Comparative studies indicated that an increase of the number of exposures to 4 did not significantly influence the performance of the assay (25).

F. Evaluation

On Day 5 (two days after the last application of the test material), the mice are injected intravenously in the tail vein with ^{3}H-thymidine. Five hours later the mice are euthanized and the draining auricular lymph nodes are excised. The lymph nodes for each experimental group are pooled and a single cell suspension is prepared. Alternatively the lymph nodes from individual mice can be analyzed. Although this method allows for statistical evaluation and a small increase in sensitivity, it may be at the expense of some loss of selectivity (25). The cells are treated with trichloroacetic acid (TCA) overnight. The resulting precipitates are washed and added to scintillation fluid. ^{3}H-thymidine incorporation is measured by β-scintillation counting.

G. Running the LLNT

Day 1, 2, 3.   CBA/Ca mice are treated topically on the dorsum of both ears with 25 µl of the test material or the vehicle alone.

Day 5.   Mice are injected intravenously with 20 µCi ^{3}H-thymidine (specific activity 2 Ci/mmol) in 250 µl of phosphate-buffered saline (PBS). Five hours later the mice are euthanized and both draining auricular lymph nodes are removed from each mouse. The lymph nodes for each experimental group are pooled and a single cell suspension is prepared by gentle mechanical disaggregation through a 200-mesh stainless steel gauze, or by using a Teflon pestle in a 10 mL plastic round bottom test tube. Cells are washed twice with PBS and precipitated with 3 mL of 5% TCA at 4°C overnight.

Day 6.   Pellets are recovered by centrifugation, resuspended in 1 mL of 5% TCA and transferred to 10 mL of scintillation fluid. Samples are counted in a β-scintillation counter. The results are expressed as background-corrected disintegration per minute (dpm).

H. Reporting

Results are reported as total dpm per node and as a stimulation index when compared to the value for the vehicle control group. A test material is considered to be a sensitizer if one or more concentrations of the test material results in a stimulation index of 3 or greater.

I. Advantages and Disadvantages

As previously mentioned, the LLNT is cost effective and saves time. The cost for mice as well as their housing is much less than for guinea pigs. Also the results are obtained in 6 days.

Since mice are used in the LLNT, less test material is required. In addition, the color of the test material does not obscure the results. It also appears that irritants do not elicit a positive response in the LLNT and thus an irritation screen is not required. Also, higher concentrations of these materials can be used in the LLNT than can be used in the guinea pig assays provided that there is no systemic toxicity. One disadvantage of the LLNA is the use of radioactive material. Although the use of ^{3}H-thymidine allows for an objective and quantifiable end point, disposal of the radioactivity is costly and a Federal and State license for radiation is required. It should be noted that locating the proper lymph nodes may be difficult when there is no induction by the test material. It is suggested that inexperienced personnel practice with a known sensitizer until confidence is obtained.

J. Positive Control

Historical results with two positive controls are shown in Table 4.

VI. ARMSTRONG/HARBER TEST FOR DETECTING PHOTOALLERGENS

A. Background

The interaction of light [generally ultraviolet (UV)] with certain chemicals can lead to a reactive chemical species. Under the proper circumstances, some of these reactive chemicals can result in a sensitization response. Ichikawi and colleagues (6) published a testing method for evaluating the potential of a chemical to be a photosensitizer. Evaluating the potential for photosensitization has become of significant interest to the cosmetic industry since two widely used fragrance materials, musk ambrette and 6-methyl coumarin, have become recognized as photoallergens in humans. It is interesting that the EPA has not formally endorsed an evaluation for photoallergic potential since several pesticides have similar structures to the aforementioned fragrances and numerous pesticides are known to form reactive species in the presence of UV light. It should be noted that a "best method" to screen for chemicals for photoallergic potential has not been generally accepted and important aspects of the assay remain in flux (e.g., UVA compared to UVA + UVB light, adjuvant injections, skin stripping).

B. Lights

The Armstrong Test uses UVA light (320–400 nm) in the induction and challenge phase. UVA lights are commonly known as "black lights" and can be purchased as "BLB" fluorescence-type bulbs from major light manufacturers. However, the selection of the light source is critical since the range of wave lengths emitted by the bulb is controlled by the phosphor coating and different

Table 4

Treatment	dpm/node	Stimulation Index
Dimethylformamide (vehicle)	673	—
0.1% DNCB	10676	15.86
DMSO (vehicle)	300	—
0.5% p-phenylene diamine	2175	7.25
1.0% p-phenylene diamine	3733	12.44
2.5% p-phenylene diamine	13399	44.66

manufacturers use different phosphors to produce BLB lights. Sometimes different phosphors are used by the same manufacturer and there is no code on the bulbs to indicate which phosphor is being used. Cole et al. (26) reported an excellent study of this problem. Figure 4 shows the photoemission spectrum of General Electric and Sylvania BLB lights. General Electric bulbs emit effective energy only at wavelengths longer than 350 nm while the entire spectrum of the total energy emitted by the General Electric light is between 250 and 350 nm; 42% of the energy from the Sylvania light falls in this range. There are known photoallergens that require the energy contained in the spectrum below 345 nm for activation and thus give a false negative if the incorrect light source is used. The best precaution is to determine the emission spectrum of the lights in the assay using a photoradiometer. As an alternative, it should be possible to obtain the emission spectrum data from the manufacturer.

It is necessary to determine the total energy being emitted by the lights in order to calculate the proper J/cm^2 exposure. An international Light Model 760 provides a relatively inexpensive means of measuring the light energy when fitted with a cosine-corrected UVA detector (W150s quartz diffuser, UVA-pass filter SEE015 detector). The device has a peak sensitivity of 360 nm with a

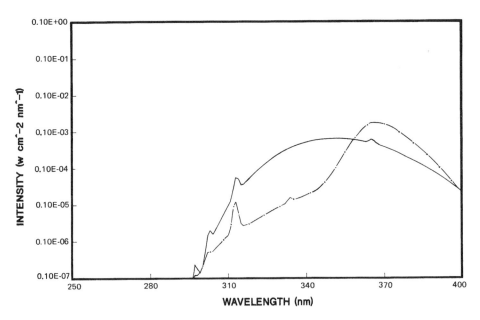

Figure 4 Energy spectra of Sylvania F40 BLB lights (solid line) and GE F40 BLB lights (dashed line). Spectra were measured with an Optronics Model 742, dual holographic grating, spectral radiometer fitted with a Teflon™ diffuser.

bandwidth of 50 nm. A bank of 8 bulbs is readily prepared by bolting together two industrial 4-bulb (48 in. long) reflectors. Two sets of these will allow 40 animals to be treated at one time. The lights are allowed to warm 30 minutes before use. They are turned off just before the animals are placed under them and then turned back on. The light intensity is measured at several locations at the level of the top of the backs of the animals and the correct exposure time then calculated. The lights are adjusted to 4–6 in. above the back. 10 J/cm^2 is the proper exposure.

C. Patching

The Hill Top Chamber provides a good patching system in this assay. A volume of 0.3 mL/patch is used. The animal restrainers described in the Buehler Test work well for holding the animals during the patching and the exposure to the light as well as assisting in providing excellent occlusion.

D. Induction Site Preparation

The majority of hair is removed from the intended patching site with small animal clippers fitted with a #80 blade. The assay has a frequent requirement for the complete removal of hair using a depilatory. Neet® (Whitehall Laboratories, New York, NY) cream or lotion is applied and left in contact with the skin for no more than 15 minutes. It must be washed away completely with a stream of warm running water. The animals are towel-dried and the inside of the cages wiped clean of any depilatory before returning the guinea pigs to the cages.

When required, the epidermis is partially removed with transparent adhesive tape [3M brand (Company, St. Paul, MN) or similar]. The skin must be completely dry or the stripping will be ineffective. A length of tape approximately 8 in. long is used. Starting at one end, the tape is placed against the skin and rubbed with the finger a few times to cause good adhesion. It is then peeled away, taking with it some dry epidermis cells. A new section of the tape is then applied to the skin and the procedure is repeated 4 or 5 times. The skin will have a shiny appearance due to the leakage of moisture from the dermis. The tape should not be jerked away from the skin as this can cause rupture to dermal capillaries.

The potential of the animal to respond to a sensitizer is enhanced by the injection of Freund's Complete Adjuvant (FCA) (Calbiochem-Behring, San Diego, CA or Difco, Detroit, MI). The adjuvant is diluted 1 : 1 with sterile water before using. The injections *must* be intradermal. In the Armstrong assay, a pattern of four 0.1 mL injections are given just prior to the first induction patching in the nuchal area. All 4 injections should fit under the edge of the area to be covered by the Hill Top chamber. It is advisable to perform the skin-stripping operation before the injections, since adjuvant can leak onto the skin and prevent good stripping.

The occlusion of the patches is done in the same manner as described in the Buehler Test. The test site(s) is exposed to the UVA light after 2 hours of occlusion. The animal is left in the restrainer and the dental dam above the test site to be exposed is cut and the patch removed. Sites not to be exposed are left patched. Excess material is wiped from the site of exposure and the remaining parts of the animal are covered with aluminum foil. All patches are removed after the light exposure step, the patched areas wiped free of excess material, and the animal returned to the cage.

E. Grading

Grading is the same as in the Buehler Test.

F. Vehicles

With the exception of water, it is desirable to use a vehicle for the inductions different from the one used at the challenge (see Buehler Test). Since the control animals in the Armstrong Test are sham treated (including any vehicle), one can patch the test and control animals with vehicle at the challenge if the same vehicle must be used for both the induction and the challenge. It is advantageous to use a vehicle that dissolves the test material, though suspensions may not be avoided in all cases.

G. Irritation Screens

The irritation screen is used to determine acceptable concentrations for the induction phase (i.e., should not produce eschar with repeated exposures or systemic toxicity) and the challenge phase (no more than slightly irritating). Each concentration must be tested with and without exposure to UVA light, as both conditions are used in the challenge. Thus, to evaluate 4 concentrations requires that 8 animals be used. Each animal receives a pair of patches with each pair being a different concentration (i.e., each concentration is patched on 4 animals). One of each pair of patches is placed on the left side and the corresponding concentration on the remaining patch is placed on the right side. The hair is removed by depilation on the day of patching. The patches on the right side are removed after 2 hours of occlusion, the remaining parts of the animal covered with foil, and the right side exposed to 10 J/cm^2 of UVA light. Animals are returned to the their cages after the exposure. If different solvents are being used in the induction and challenge phase, then two separate screens need to be run. Because of the use of FCA, there is a potential for a heightened irritation response at the challenge; one may want to use animals previously exposed to FCA during the irritation screen (see Guinea Pig Maximization Test).

H. Animals

The animals (guinea pigs) are the same as described in the Buehler Test.

I. Running the Armstrong Assay

Combining the discussed techniques in a specific regimen yields the assay as follows:

1. Irritation/Toxicity Screen (8 animals)

Day 0. Remove the hair from the lumbar region by clipping and depilation. Apply 2 concentrations on each animal on adjacent left-side/right-side locations for a total of 4 dose concentrations. Occlude the patches for 2 hours (± 15 min). Expose the right side to 10 J/cm^2 of UVA light after removing the patches on the right side. Remove the remaining patches and excess material after the exposure.

Day 1. Grade all test sites 24 hr (± 1 hr) after removal of all patches (24-hr grade).

Day 2. Repeat the grading 48 hr (± 2 hr) after removing the patches (48-hr grade).

2. Induction (20 Test + 10 Sham Controls + Any Rechallenge Controls)

Day 0. Weigh all test and control animals. Remove the hair from the nuchal area with clippers and depilatory. Remove the epidermis by stripping 4 to 5 times with tape. Make four 0.01 mL injections of a 1:1 dilution of FCA in an area to be covered by the patch. Cover this area on the test animals with a Hill Top Chamber, which has 0.3 mL of test material preparation. Patch the sham controls with water or solvent on the patch. Occlude with dental dam and restrain the animal in a holder for 2 hr (+15 min). Remove the patches, cover with the nonpatched areas with foil, and expose to 10 J/cm^2 of UVA light.

Day 2, 4, 7, 9, 11. Repeat the activities of day 0 with the following exceptions: do not weigh animals and do not inject adjuvant. Move the patch back when the original induction site becomes too damaged but remain in the nuchal area. Dipilation may not be needed at each induction.

3. Challenge (20 Test + 10 Sham Control Animals 9–13 Days After Last Induction Exposure)

Day 0. Weigh all animals, clip the lumbar region free of hair, and dipilate. Do not strip the skin. Patch each animal with a pair of adjacent patches (one on the left side and one on the right side) containing 0.3 mL of nonirritating concentration of test material on a Hill Top chamber. Occlude the patches and restrain the animal for 2 hr (± 15 min). Remove the patches from the right side and cover the rest of the animal with foil. Expose the right side to 10 J/cm^2 of UVA light. Remove the remaining patch and any excess material.

Day 1.   Grade all challenge sites keeping separate the grades of the sites exposed to light and those not exposed to light 24 hr (±1 hr) after removal of the patches (24-hr grade).

Day 2.   Repeat the grading 48 hr (±2 hr) after removal of the patches (49-hr grade).

4.   Rechallenge

All or selected animals may be rechallenged with the same or a different test material 7–12 days after the challenge. Use 10 new sham-treated controls and naïve test sites on all animals following the same procedure as used in the challenge.

5.   Report

Determine the number of positive responders (number of animals with a score 1 at either the 24- or 48-hr grading or with a score one unit higher than the highest score in the control). Determine the average score at 24 and at 48 hr for the test and control groups using face values and $\pm = 0.5$. Keep the data for the sites exposed to light separate from the data for sites not exposed to light.

J.   Advantages, Disadvantages, and Problems

The Armstrong assay was found to give responses in the guinea pig that were consistent with what has been observed in humans: positive responses for 6-methyl coumerin and musk ambrett. One major disadvantage is that the procedure is time consuming with six induction exposures; additional work might demonstrate that fewer exposures will yield the same results. The procedure is very stressful on the animals because of the injection of adjuvant and the multiple skin strippings and depilations. As with any assay involving the intradermal injection of adjuvant, there is often a problem with using the results of the irritation screen in naïve animals to accurately predict the results that will be seen in the sham controls at the challenge. If the material being tested is a nonirritant or if one selects a concentration of an irritant far below the irritating concentration, then the screen does an adequate job of predicting the background irritation level in the challenge controls. However, if a slightly nonirritating concentration of an irritant is used, then the screen often underpredicts the irritation response and a high background level of irritation is observed at the challenge in the sham controls. The interpretation of the results of the challenge becomes difficult. The use of animals in the irritation screen that have had a prior injection of adjuvant might provide a viable alternative and reduce the number of times that rechallenges must be run because of high background levels of irritation. The Armstrong Test was designed to evaluate materials for their photoactivated sensitization potential and not their potential to be nonpho-

Table 5

Group	Challenge Level	Incidence[a]	Severity 24 hr	Severity 48 hr	Maximum Score 24 hr	Maximum Score 48 hr
Test						
No UV light	0.1%	0/20	0.0	0.0	0	0
UV light		17/20	2.0	1.8	3	3
No UV light	0.01%	0/20	0.0	0.0	0	0
UV light		17/20	0.6	0.4	2	1
Control						
No UV light	0.1%	0/10	0.0	0.0	0	0
UV light		0/10	0.0	0.0	0	0
No UV light	0.01%	0/10	0.1	0.0	±	0
UV light		0/10	0.1	0.0	±	0

[a]Animals with a score ≥ 1 at 24 or 48 hr.

toactivated dermal sensitizers. At this time, there is no background data that will allow for properly positioning results of the Armstrong Test with regard to human risk if the assay indicates that a test material is a sensitizer or that a material is both a sensitizer and a photoallergen. Thus, it is highly recommended that a "standard" sensitization assay that can be related to humans be run before or in conjunction with the photosensitization assay. The use of a subjective grading system can be a source of significant variation.

K. Positive Control

The recommended positive control is musk ambrett. TCSA (3,3,4,5-tetrachlorasalicylanilide) will also give positive results, but this material has been reported to be an allergen without UV light activation. Animals are induced with a 10% w/v solution of musk ambrett in acetone and sham controls are patched with acetone alone. The Hill Top chamber is used for all patchings. The challenge is also done in acetone. A note of warning: Both types of UVA lights yield the same results. Typical results are in Table 5.

REFERENCES

1. Jackson, E.M. (1985). Difference between irritation and sensitization. J. Toxicol. Cut. Ocular Toxicol. 4:1.
2. Jackson, E.M. (1984). Cellular and molecular events of inflammation. 1. Toxicol. Cut. Ocular Toxicol. 3:847.

3. Labeling Requirements for Pesticides and Devices. Fed. Reg. (49 CFR Parts 156 and 167) September 26, 1984.

4. Buehler, E.V. (1965). Delayed contact hypersensitivity in the guinea pig. Arch. Dermatoi. 91:171.

5. Magnusson, B. and Kligman, A.M. (1964). The identification of contact allergens by animal assay. The maximization test. J. Invest. Dermatol. 52:268.

6. Ichikawa, H., Armstrong, R.B., and Harber, L.C. (1981). Photoallergic contact dermatitis in guinea pigs: Improved induction technique using Freund's complete adjuvant. J. Invest. Dermatol. 76:498.

7. Gad, S.C., Dunn, B.J., and Dobbs, D.W. (1985). Development of an alternative dermal sensitization test: mouse ear swelling test (MEST). In Alternative Methods in Toxicology vol. 3. New York, Mary Ann Liebert, Inc., p. 539.

8. Kimber I. and Weisenberger C. (1989). The murine local lymph node assay for identification of contact allergens: assay development and results of an initial validation study. Arch. Toxicol. 63:274–282.

9. Organization for Economic Cooperation and Development—OECD guidelines for the testing of chemicals. TO 406 Skin sensitization. (Updated Guideline, adopted 17th July 1997.

10. Schlede F. and Eppler R. (1995). Testing for skin sensitization according to the notification procedure for new chemicals: the Magnusson and Kligman test. Contact Dermatitis 32:1–4

11. Ritz, H.L. and Buehler, F.V. (1980). Planning, conduct and interpretation of guinea pig sensitization patch test. In Current Concepts in Cutaneous Toxicology. New York, Academic Press, p. 25.9.

12. B.6 Skin Sensitization. Official Journal of the European Communities. No. L 248/206-212.30. 9.96. Annex IV C.

13. Buehler, E.V. (1994). Occlusive patch method for skin sensitization in guinea pigs: the Buehler method. Fd. Chem. Toxic. 32:97–101.

14. Robinson, M.K., Nusair, T.L., Fletcher, E.R., Ritz, M.L. (1990). A review of the Buehler guinea pig skin sensitization test and its use in a risk assessment process for human skin sensitization. Toxicology 61:91–107.

15. Buehler, E.V. (1982). Comment on guinea-pig test methods. Food Chem. Toxicol. 20:494–495. Toxicol. Appl. Pharmacol. 84:93. 142/Miles.

16. Bruynzeel, D.P. (1995). Excited Skin Syndrome. In: van der Valk, P.G.M., Maibach, H.I., eds. The Irritant Contact Dermatitis Syndrome. New York, CRC Press, 279–282.

17. Gad, S.C., Dunn, B.J., Dobbs, D.W. Reilly, C., and Walsh, R.D. (1986). Development and validation of an alternative sensitization test: the mouse ear swelling test (MEST).

18. Crowle, A.J. (1959). Delayed hypersensitivity in mice: Its detection by skin test and its passive transfer. Science 130:159.

19. Asherson, G-L. and Ptak, W. (1968). Contact and delayed hypersensitivity in the mouse 1. Active sensitization and passive transfer. Immunology 15:405.

20. Chapman, J.R., Ruben, Z., and Butchko, C.M. (1986). Histology of and quantitative assays for oxozolone-induced allergic contact dermatitis in mice. Am. J. Dermatopathol. 8:130.

21. Gad, S.C., Auletta, C.S., Dunn, B.J., Riles, R.A., Reilly, C., Reagan, B., and Yenser, B. (1986). A double blind intralaboratory validation of the mouse ear swelling test (MEST). Toxicologist 6:242.

22. Kimber, I. and Dearman, R.J. (1991). Investigation of lymph node cell proliferation as a possible immunological correlate of contact sensitizing potential. Fd. Chem. Toxic. 29:125–129.

23. Kimber, I., Hilton, J., and Weisenberger, C. (1989). The murine local lymph node assay for identification of contact allergens: a preliminary evaluation of in situ measurement of lymphocyte proliferation. Contact Derm. 21:215–220.

24. Kimber, I. (1995). The local lymph node assay. In: Burlson, G.R., Dean, J.H., and Munson, A.E., eds. Methods in Immunotoxicology. Vol. 2. New York: Wiley-Liss, 279–290.

25. Kimber, I., Hilton, J., Dearman, R.J., Gerberick, G.F., Ryan, C.A., Basketter, D.A., Scholes, E.W., Ladics, G.S., Loveless, S.E., House, R.V., and Guy, A. (1995). An international evaluation of the murine local lymph node assay and comparison of modified procedures. Toxicology 103:63–73.

26. Cole, C.A., Forbes, P.D., and Davies, R.F. (1984). Different biological effectiveness of blacklight fluorescent ramps available for therapy with psoralens plus ultraviolet A. J. Am. Acad. Dermatol. 11:599.

6

Genetic Toxicology Testing

Ann D. Mitchell
Genesys Research, Inc., Research Triangle Park, North Carolina

I. INTRODUCTION

Genetic toxicology is the branch of toxicology that is concerned with the genetic effects of toxic materials. This specialized field incorporates both theoretical sciences and applied sciences. Selected research approaches have been utilized to examine the effects of chemical and radiation exposures to enhance our understanding of both the structure of genetic material and the mechanisms involved in genetic changes. This understanding has then been applied to develop and utilize relatively rapid and economical tests to assess the potential of chemical agents and radiation to induce adverse genetic effects.

A major impetus for the development and use of genetic toxicology test systems has been a recognition that long-term animal testing resources are insufficient for evaluating the universe of chemicals to which humans and the environment may be exposed. Thus, genetic toxicology tests that assess specific mechanisms observed in the whole animal (including humans) are used as initial tests for regulatory submissions because they have been shown to be useful in predicting the outcome of long-term animal tests. In addition, they are used to conserve resources, reduce animal usage, provide rapid assessments of potential risk, including the risk of exposing human volunteers to drugs under development, and generally to assist in determining whether additional testing would be productive.

When the earlier edition of *Product Safety Evaluation Handbook* was published (1), over 100 genetic toxicology tests were available (see Table 1), and, as described by Barfknecht and Naismith (2) in that edition, a "cafeteria-style" testing approach was often followed in which tests developed to evaluate different theoretical aspects of genetic alterations were selected to address various

Table 1   Representative Genetic Toxicology Assays

Assay type	Organism and/or cell type	Endpoints measured
Bacterial DNA repair	*Escherichia coli polA*[+]/ *polA*[−]	Differential toxicity due to DNA damage not repaired
	Bacillus subtilis Rec[+]/*Rec*[−]	Differential toxicity due to DNA damage not repaired
Bacterial mutation	*Salmonella typhimurium*	Reverse mutation (Ames assay)
	Salmonella typhimurium	Forward mutation
	Escherichia coli (WP2)	Forward and reverse mutations
Fungal/yeast mutation	*Saccharomyces cerevisiae*	Reverse mutation
	Schizosaccharomyces pombe	Forward mutation
	Neurospora crassa	Forward and reverse mutation
Yeast chromosome effects	*Saccharomyces cerevisiae*	Mitotic recombination
	Saccharomyces cerevisiae	Mitotic aneuploidy and meiotic nondisjunction
Mammalian cell DNA damage	Various cells (*in vitro* and *in vivo*)	Adduct formation
	Various cells, e.g., lymphocytes	DNA damage: Comet assay
Mammalian cell DNA repair	Human fibroblasts	Unscheduled DNA synthesis (UDS)
	Rat and mouse hepatocytes	UDS
	Chinese hamster cells and human lymphocytes	Sister chromatid exchange (SCE)
Mammalian cell gene mutation	L5178Y mouse lymphoma cells	Forward mutation
	Chinese hamster cells (CHO/V79/AS52)	Forward mutation
	Human lymphoblasts (TK6)	Forward mutation
Mammalian cell cytogenetic damage	Chinese hamster cells (CHO/V79)	Chromosomal aberrations
	Human lymphocytes	Chromosomal aberrations
	L5178Y mouse lymphoma cells	Small colony formation
Mammalian cell transformation	Mouse or hamster cells	Change in growth characteristics in vitro

Table 1 Continued

Assay type	Organism and/or cell type	Endpoints measured
Insect mutation	*Drosophila melanogaster*	Sex-linked recessive lethal mutations
Insect chromosomal effects	*Drosophila melanogaster*	Translocation and sex chromosome loss
Whole animal DNA repair	Mouse or rat hepatocytes	Unscheduled DNA synthesis
	Mouse bone marrow cells	Sister chromatid exchange
Whole animal mutation	Transgenic mice and rats	Reverse mutation of (bacterial) transgene
	Mouse/specific locus	Forward mutation and deletions
	Mouse/spot test	Forward mutation and deletions
Whole animal cytogenetic damage	Mouse or rat	Bone marrow chromosomal aberrations
	Mouse or rat	Lymphocyte chromosomal aberrations
Whole animal germ cell DNA damage	Mouse or rat	Spermatocyte unscheduled DNA synthesis
Whole animal germ cell cytogenetic damage	Mouse or rat/dominant lethal	Non-viable fetuses
	Mouse/heritable translocation	Sterility and detection of translocations
	Mouse (with heritable translocation)	Spermatocyte chromosomal rearrangements
Host-mediated	Mouse or rat	Gene mutation in bacterial or mammalian cell test system
Body fluids analysis	Urine samples from mouse, rat or man	Various genetic endpoints in bacterial cells or mammalian cell culture

[a]Adapted from Reference 2.

regulatory requirements. Further, because testing requirements had evolved independently within separate governmental agencies and in different geographical regions, numerous tests, and sometimes several modifications of the same tests, were required for companies wishing to market their products internationally. Therefore, in the earlier edition, the authors provided guidance for developing a practical approach for mutagenesis testing.

However, the field of genetic toxicology testing has undergone a dramatic change in the last decade. Because of a recognized need to harmonize testing requirements for national and international regulatory submissions, only a few of the developed tests are routinely used today, with their selection based on considerations such as the mechanistic relevance of the effects that are measured, the extent that the test systems have been defined and evaluated, and the experience, ease, and economy in performance of the tests for laboratories worldwide. Therefore, this chapter will not attempt to provide detailed descriptions of genetic toxicology tests that, although used for prior assessments and important in establishing the relevance of the field, are seldom used for current regulatory submissions.

Instead, to provide a practical guide for professionals responsible for evaluating the safety of current products, this chapter begins with a review of cellular and molecular processes important for understanding currently used genetic toxicology tests and then provides a chronological overview of the development and application of the field of genetic toxicology, including a summary of the current status of regulatory requirements. This is followed by a detailed description of the tests that are most frequently used today to address these regulatory requirements, together with a summary of advantages and limitations of these tests.

Should additional information be required concerning other genetic toxicology tests, e.g., for interpreting previously obtained test results, or for selecting additional tests to augment those that are most frequently used, the reader may wish to consult the 1988 edition of this *Handbook* (1), as well as genetic toxicology texts (3,4), the series *Chemical Mutagens* (5), and a number of established journals in the field, including *Environmental and Molecular Mutagenesis* (Wiley-Liss), *Mutagenesis* (IRL Press), and *Mutation Research* (Elsevier). In the latter may be found the series of U.S. Environmental Protection Agency (EPA) Gene-Tox reviews of specific test systems. Internet resources for additional information include: http://www.fda.gov/ for the FDA homepage; http://www.pharmweb.net/pwmirror/pw9/ifpma/ich5.html for the International Council on Harmonization (ICH) of Technical Requirements of Pharmaceuticals for Human Use guidelines; http://www.epa.gov/epahome/rules.html for EPA environmental regulations; and http://www.oecd.org/ehs/test/testlist.htm for the Organization for Economic Cooperation and Development (OECD) guidelines.

II. BASIC MECHANISMS ASSESSED IN THE GENETIC TOXICOLOGY TESTS MOST-FREQUENTLY USED FOR REGULATORY SUBMISSIONS

Genetic toxicology test systems measure the outcome of damage or alterations in DNA, which is the basic blueprint for transmission of hereditary information to daughter cells. If DNA is damaged, it may: (a) be correctly repaired with no genetic consequences; (b) lead to cell death, again with no genetic consequences; or (c) be replicated with the damage incorrectly repaired. Only the third consequence leads to mutations, DNA alterations that are propagated through subsequent generations of cells or individuals.

Hence, genetic toxicology tests that assess DNA damage and repair, such as sister chromatid exchange tests and tests for unscheduled DNA synthesis (the repair of DNA damage at times other than the scheduled phase of the mitotic cycle, i.e., the S-phase), are less frequently used for regulatory submissions today because they provide only indirect evidence of mutagenesis. Instead, the harmonized testing approaches for regulatory submissions, which will be described, consist of tests for gene and chromosomal mutations.

A. Gene Mutations

Gene mutations can be assessed in bacteria, mammalian cells in culture, and whole organisms. A gene is the simplest functional unit in a DNA molecule. Gene (or point) mutations are changes in the nucleotide sequence at one or a few coding segments. Molecular genetic techniques have now become sufficiently powerful to allow routine identification of the specific DNA sequence changes responsible for mutant phenotypes. About 5,000 diseases in humans are now known to be due to defective genes. These inherited disorders cause 20% of all infant mortalities, half of all miscarriages, and 80% of all cases of mental retardation (6). In addition, considerable research during the last two decades to identify the genes involved in the alteration of normal cellular processes has resulted in the identification of over 100 different cancer genes (7).

1. Gene Mutations in Bacteria

Gene mutations in bacteria can occur in a number of ways. In one of the simplest cases, a *base-pair substitution mutation*, a single nucleotide is changed, which is followed by a subsequent change in the complementary nucleotide on the other strand of the DNA double helix. Such mutations are deleterious when they alter a protein coding sequence to conclude translation prematurely (a *nonsense mutation*) or to incorporate a different amino acid (a *missense mutation*). Similarly, *frameshift mutations* occur following the deletion or insertion of one nucleotide, which then changes the "reading frame" for the remainder of the gene, or even for multiple genes. Both base-pair substitution and frameshift mutations are routinely measured in bacterial cells by the cells' acquisition of the capability of growth in an environment containing a missing amino acid, and for these tests large numbers of bacteria are examined in order to demonstrate significant increases over spontaneous mutation frequencies. A *forward mutation* occurs when there is a change in the native DNA; a *reverse mutation* occurs when a mutated cell is returned to its initial phenotype. The currently used bacterial tests are reverse mutation assays.

2. Gene Mutations in Mammalian Cells

Gene mutations in mammalian cells are generally forward mutations and include base-pair substitution and frameshift mutations. Measurements of gene mutations in mammalian cells reflect the greater complexity of mammalian cells and chromosomes in comparison to those of prokaryotes, and, thus, they more closely approximate the genetic effects of chemicals in rodent species and humans.

In contrast to bacteria, mammalian cells are essentially diploid (2n, with two copies of each chromosome). Mammalian chromosomes are located within the nucleus of the cell and contain nonfunctional and noncoding, as well as functional, coding sequences. In addition, whereas in bacterial cells all genes are usually expressed, in diploid cells there are usually two copies of each gene (one on each chromosome). One (dominant) form of the gene may be expressed while the other (recessive) gene remains unexpressed, unless both copies are recessive. If both copies of the gene are the same, the cell is homozygous for that trait; a heterozygous condition exists if the copies are different, and, if only one chromosome is present to carry the trait, the condition is hemizygous. Hemizygous traits are found on the X chromosome in mammals because males have only one X chromosome and only one X chromosome is expressed in female cells. The first mammalian cell mutation assays that were developed (8,9) utilized a gene found on the X chromosome of Chinese hamster cells, i.e., a hemizygous gene; the mouse lymphoma cell mutation assay (10) utilizes heterozygous cells.

Gene mutations are routinely measured in mammalian cells following the mutant cells' acquisition of the capability of growth in the presence of a selective agent, an otherwise toxic drug that can no longer be utilized by the mutated cell. As for the bacterial assays, large numbers of cells are examined in order to demonstrate significant increases over spontaneous mutation frequencies. However, in mammalian cell gene mutation assays, the chemical exposure step must be followed by an expression period, during which mutant (and nonmutant) cells increase in number and the nonmutant protein (enzyme) present in the mutated cells and the RNA coding for that protein are depleted. Only then can the selective agent be added to permit only the mutated cells to grow and form colonies.

B. Chromosomal Mutations

Chromosomal mutations are large-scale numerical or structural alterations in eukaryotic chromosomes—including small and large deletions (visualized as breaks), translocations (exchanges), nondisjunction (aneuploidy) and mitotic recombination—that may affect the expression of numerous genes with gross effects, or be lethal to affected cells. Chromosomal abnormalities are associated with neoplasia, spontaneous abortion, congenital malformation, and infertility, which occur in approximately 0.6% of live births in humans. It has been estimated that up to 40% of spontaneous abortuses have chromosomal defects (11), and essentially all tumors harbor chromosomal mutations.

1. Chromosomal Mutations in Mammalian Cells

Chromosomal mutations can be measured in several mammalian cell mutation assays, but the L5178Y mouse lymphoma assay is routinely used because it is the most extensively characterized of the several assays. This assay was first developed as a test for gene mutations at the *tk* (thymidine kinase) locus; however, it was subsequently noted that a biphasic curve of colony sizes is obtained, and that the biphasic size distribution is resolved into small (σ) colonies of slowly growing mutant cells and large (λ) colonies of more rapidly growing mutant cells. Banded karyotype and molecular analyses of the σ and λ mouse lymphoma colony mutants have revealed that whereas most λ colony mutants have only gene mutations or small chromosomal deletions, most σ colony mutants represent a full array of possible mutational damage, including gene mutations, small and large deletions, translocations, nondisjunction, and mitotic recombination.

2. Chromosomal Aberrations, In Vitro and In Vivo

In contrast to the assays that have been described which assess gene and chromosomal mutations at only one or a few genes, but in millions of cells per treatment, the in vitro and in vivo assays for chromosomal aberrations assess mutagenic events in multiple genes, but usually for no more than 200 cells per culture, or for up to 100 cells per animal. However, because these cells must be arrested at the appropriate interval after exposure, and because of the need for an experienced cytogeneticist to carefully evaluate each of the cells, the chromosomal aberration assays are generally more time consuming and costly.

Chromosome breakage, which is necessary for chromosomal rearrangements, is the classical end point in chromosomal aberration assays. To visualize chromosomes and chromosomal aberrations with a light microscope following in vitro or in vivo treatment with a chemical, cells are arrested in metaphase, treated with a hypotonic solution to swell the chromosomes, fixed, transferred to microscope slides, and stained. The first metaphase (M) following chemical exposure, M_1, is the time when the greatest number of chromosomally damaged cells may be observed. The extent of damage declines rapidly after M_1 because of the greatly extended cell cycle times of some cytogenetically damaged cells (e.g., while the cells attempt to repair the damage), and because the most severely damaged cells are often incapable of progressing through another cell cycle.

When the chromosomes of diploid somatic cells are replicated, each chromosome then consists of two (sister) chromatids that separate at mitosis to become the chromosomes of the daughter cells. If chromosomal mutations occur before replication (DNA synthesis), both chromatids will be affected. This damage will be visualized as *chromosomal* breaks (deletions) and exchanges (translocations). However, if these mutations occur during replication (the most sensitive stage), or following replication, the damage is visualized as *chromatid* breaks and exchanges. Hence, by enumerating chromatid and chromosome breaks and exchanges an index can be obtained of the time that the damage occurred. Very large deletions are tolerated only if they do not incapacitate essential genes. In diploid cells, this is usually accomplished when a normal gene is retained by the homologous chromosome of paired chromosomes, yielding a heterozygous condition for that trait. Exchanges result when the broken ends of the same or different chromatids or chromosomes rejoin in an aberrant manner.

Although not currently utilized in cytogenetic testing for regulatory submissions, Fluorescence In Situ Hybridization (FISH) staining techniques have been recently developed for human and mouse chromosomes in which each chromosome can be differentially stained, revealing chromosomal rearrangements that are not apparent with conventional staining techniques (12). When FISH staining is translated from a research approach to a testing protocol, it may be possible to reduce the number of chromosomes to be analyzed and, hence, the time for chromosomal aberration tests.

3. Micronuclei

Micronuclei result when nuclear membranes form around broken pieces of chromosomes or around chromosomes that fail to separate at cell division. Therefore, micronucleus tests measure chromosome breakage, the classical end point for chromosomal aberration assays, and aneuploidy, the loss or gain of a chromosome or a chromosome segment. Micronuclei are readily observed microscopically in stained preparations of (otherwise anucleate) polychromatic erythrocytes (PCEs) from the bone marrow of rats or mice or from the peripheral blood of mice; the latter because, in mice, the spleen does not remove micronucleated cells from the blood. With appropriate staining techniques, the PCEs can be differentiated from the more mature normochromatic erythrocytes (NCEs) because the PCEs still contain RNA, which has been lost by the NCEs. For example, with Giemsa staining the PCEs are blue and the NCEs are salmon pink or red.

Peripheral blood erythrocytes can be obtained for micronucleus evaluations without sacrificing the animal, e.g., from animals under treatment for longer-term studies; however, a greater number of cells must be evaluated because the newly formed erythrocytes (PCEs, the cells of interest) are diluted in the population of pre-existing erythrocytes. Hence, bone marrow cells, which give a more informative index of toxicity, are routinely used for the micronucleus test as well as for in vivo chromosomal aberration assays. Because micronuclei can be evaluated more rapidly and economically than chromosomal aberrations, the micronucleus test in rodents is now used more extensively than the rodent bone marrow chromosomal aberration test.

III. DEVELOPMENT AND APPLICATION OF GENETIC TOXICOLOGY TESTS

The origins of genetic toxicology testing date from 1900 and the rediscovery of Mendel's classic paper on the basis of inheritance (13), which was closely followed, in 1901, by the first use of the term "mutation" to signify changes in hereditary material (14). As illustrated in Table 2, which highlights some of the relevant events in the development and application of genetic toxicology testing, the focus of mutagenesis research during the first six decades of the century was directed toward using recently developed techniques to gain an increased understanding of the nature of genetic material. However, the relationship between cancer and an abnormal chromosomal constitution was proposed as early as 1914 (15), and in 1927 it was suggested that mutations could cause cancer (16).

Because of concerns that arose especially in the years following World War II that many chemical products of benefit to industrialized society might adversely affect human health and the environment (17,18), numerous regulations have been promulgated, from 1970 until the present, which include a mandate that industry assess the potential adverse genetic effects of their products. In the 1960s several laboratories developed methods suitable for testing radiation and chemicals for mutagenicity, and by the end of the decade the first in vivo tests—the heritable translocation, specific locus, and dominant lethal tests, the host mediated assay, and in vivo cytogenetics—had been defined (19).

Exponential growth of the field of genetic toxicology testing occurred during the 1970s, shortly after Malling (19) demonstrated, in 1971, that a mammalian liver homogenate could be added to in vitro systems to mimic in vivo metabolism. Then a wide range of in vitro tests, as well as additional in vivo methods, to evaluate the genotoxic effects of chemicals were developed and published. The goal of using such tests to predict carcinogenicity gained momentum in the mid-1970s when McCann, Ames, and associates published test results suggesting that most carcinogens were mutagens in *Salmonella* (20). Support for the role of mutagenesis in carcinogenesis has also included the clonal origin of tumors, the association of specific chromosomal abnormalities with certain cancers, information about genetically determined cancer-prone

Table 2 Development and Application of Genetic Toxicology Testing

1900	Rediscovery of Mendel's classic 1865 paper on the basis of inheritance (18).
1901	de Vries (14) applies the term "mutation" to changes in hereditary material.
1914	Boveri (15) proposes the somatic mutation theory of cancer: that the primary cause of cancer may be abnormal cell division resulting in an abnormal chromosomal constitution.
1927	Muller publishes the first demonstration of the induction of mutations by x-rays, in *Drosophila* (16), and shows that an induced response must be evaluated in relation to background mutations. He also suggests the possibility that mutations may cause cancer.
1938	Federal Food, Drug and Cosmetic Act enacted to provide for the regulation of foods (except meat and poultry products), food and color additives, human and animal drugs, medicated animal feeds, medical devices, and cosmetics.
1938	Sax shows that x-rays can induce chromosomal alterations in plant pollen cells (27).
1941	Auerbach and Robson demonstrate that nitrogen mustards can induce mutations in *Drosophila* similar to the mutations induced by x-rays (28). (Because of censorship, publication was delayed until 1947, after World War II, although nitrogen mustards were not used in World War II.)
1943	Earle establishes continuous cultures of rodent cell lines (29).
1947	Federal Insecticide, Fungicide and Rodenticide Act (FIFRA) enacted.
1951	Russell (30) demonstrates that x-rays can induce genomic mutations in mice.
1952	Gey (31) establishes a continuous cell line (HeLa) from a human tumor.
1953	Watson and Crick elucidate the double-helical structure of DNA (32).
1956	Tjio and Levan (33) utilize colchicine to arrest human cells in metaphase and establish 46 chromosomes as the normal (diploid) compliment of humans.
1959	Lejeune and associates (34) discover that children with Down syndrome have an extra chromosome (number 21).
1960	Nowell and Hungerford (35) discover a consistent chromosome change (the Philadelphia chromosome) associated with a specific type of human tumor (chronic granulocytic leukemia).
1960	In a paper entitled "Chemical Mutagenesis in Animals," Auerbach (36) states that as more and more chemicals are used in therapeutics, food processing, and other industries, the testing of the substances for mutagenic ability will become a necessary protective measure. During the remainder of this decade, numerous similar warnings were issued by the scientific community, and by the end of the 1960s the first *in vivo* tests for mutagenic effects had been established.
1961	Hayflick and Moorehead (37) demonstrate that normal cells have a finite lifespan (~50 generations) before the cells exhibit abnormal growth. It has recently been found that maintenance of normal cell growth is related to telomerase which facilitates DNA replication at the ends of chromosomes.
1962	Publication of *Silent Spring* by Rachel Carson (38) warning of the hazards of radiation and chemicals, especially pesticides, and calling for more regulation of industry.

Table 2 Continued

1968	Two teams of scientists, Kao and Puck (8), and Chu and Malling (9), independently demonstrate the chemical induction of increased mutation frequencies in mammalian (Chinese hamster) cells.
1970	The U.S. Environmental Protection Agency is established to regulate matters concerning air and water pollution, the use of pesticides, and other matters affecting the environment.
1970	Occupational Safety and Health Act (OSHA) enacted.
1971	James and Elizabeth Miller demonstrate that many chemicals become carcinogens only after they are metabolized in animals (39).
1971	Malling (19) demonstrates that chemicals can become mutagenic in vitro by the addition of mammalian liver enzymes to mimic in vivo metabolism. During the remainder of the 1970s numerous research approaches for examining mutations, DNA damage and repair, and chromosome alterations were utilized to define a wide range of in vitro and in vivo genetic toxicology tests.
1971	Knudson (40) explains the origin of retinoblastoma tumors by proposing that two sequential mutations are required. This two-stage genetic model has been found to apply to additional forms of cancer.
1972	Clive and associates (10) define the L5178Y/$tk^{+/-}$ mouse lymphoma cell mutation assay.
1972	Consumer Product Safety Act enacted.
1973	Ames and associates (42) introduce a mammalian liver homogenate into a *Salmonella* reverse mutation test system, test 18 carcinogens and publish the results in a paper entitled "Carcinogens are Mutagens."
1973	The first widely publicized alarm about mutagenicity, an unpublished report of an association between human exposure to aerosols of spray adhesives and the appearance of chromosomal abnormalities and birth defects, led the Consumer Product Safety Commission (CPSC) to remove spray adhesives from the market. However, technically poor cytogenetic preparations rather than chromosomal abnormalities were found in an independent examination of the original slides, and the CPSC rescinded the ban after six months (21).
1973	The National Cancer Institute (NCI) initiates the first contracts to evaluate the utility of in vitro genetic toxicology tests, which eventually included the "Ames" test, unscheduled DNA synthesis, the mouse lymphoma cell mutagenesis assay, and tests for mammalian cell transformation.
1974	Safe Drinking Water Act enacted.
1975	Rodent bone marrow micronucleus testing protocol defined by Schmid (41).
1975	McCann, Ames, and associates (20) publish results for 300 chemicals tested in *Salmonella* and find that the system correctly identifies ~90% of the animal carcinogens while maintaining an equally high specificity for noncarcinogens. Although, the concordance of results has been lower as additional chemicals have been tested, this initial finding became a goal for evaluating additional tests, as justification for genotoxicity tests shifted from predicting effects on the human gene pool to predicting carcinogenicity.

(continued)

Table 2 Continued

1976	The Second Task Force for Research Planning in Environmental Health Science estimates that 50–90% of the total cancer incidence is dependent on known or unknown environmental factors, and, citing a backlog of up to 30,000 agents for the costly long-term testing for carcinogenesis, identifies a requirement of short term [genetic toxicology] tests to screen chemicals for carcinogenic activity (43).
1977	Toxic Substances Control Act enacted to provide the U.S. Environmental Protection Agency with the authority "to regulate commerce and protect human health and the environment by requiring testing and necessary use restrictions on certain chemical substances." This was the first Federal law that identified mutagenicity as an endpoint of toxicological concern.
1978	The EPA proposes guidelines for the mutagenicity testing of pesticides (44).
1978	The National Toxicology Program (NTP) is established, and responsibility for the rodent carcinogenesis bioassay and contracts to evaluate in vitro genetic toxicology tests is transferred from the NCI to the NTP.
1981	Publication of the first in a series of U.S. EPA Gene-Tox Program genetic toxicology test system reviews. Each review consists of an evaluation by an expert work group of a database of published literature for that test system together with recommendations for use of the test system. The Gene-Tox database currently contains mutagenicity information for about 3,000 chemicals from 39 assay systems.
1981	Organization for Economic Cooperation and Development (OECD) Genetic Toxicology Guidelines for the Testing of Chemicals and the OECD Principles of Good Laboratory Practice (GLP) are published. The approximately 30 industrialized member countries of the OECD agree that data generated in the testing of chemicals in an OECD member country in accordance with OECD Test Guidelines and OECD GLP Principles shall be accepted in other member countries for purposes of assessment and other uses relating to the protection of man and the environment.
1984	The National Research Council publishes a report for the NTP entitled *Toxicity Testing. Strategies to Determine Needs and Priorities* (45) which concludes that of the universe of over 5,000,000 chemicals, 65,725 substances are of possible concern because of their potential for human exposure and that, for the vast majority, there is a lack of sufficient data for conducting human health hazard assessment.
1987	Tennant and associates (22) publish an assessment of NTP test results obtained in four short term in vitro genetic toxicology tests—the *Salmonella* and mouse lymphoma mutagenesis assays and tests for chromosomal aberrations and sister chromatid exchanges—which finds their tests to be poorly predictive of rodent carcinogenicity. This finding resounded throughout the scientific community and led to an immediate decline in usage for some of the tests and a reassessment of testing methods for others.
1989	Ames (23) reports that a wide variety of edible plants have high levels of toxins and carcinogens, that these natural toxins may have evolved to protect the

Table 2 Continued

	plants from insects and other predators, and that humans are consuming 10,000 times more natural than man-made pesticides.
1993	Fluorescence in situ hybridization (FISH) techniques are developed (12) for detecting specific chromosomes, chromosomal alterations and specific genes. Currently, each of the human chromosomes and most of the mouse chromosomes can be individually identified.
1997	A multilaboratory comparison of in vitro tests for chromosome aberrations (24) demonstrates that several chemicals including carcinogens that were previously positive in the mouse lymphoma assay but negative for chromosomal aberrations with the NTP protocols were positive for aberrations when a longer treatment time and different sampling times were used.
1997	Publication of Gene-Tox review of data for over 600 chemicals tested in the L5178Y mouse lymphoma cell mutation assay which finds > 90% predictivity of rodent carcinogenicity for adequately tested chemicals (25). In a separate publication (48), the cells used for this assay are shown to harbor mutant $p53$, the tumor suppressor gene found in > 50% of human tumors.
1997	Revised TSCA test guidelines published which include four genetic toxicity testing guidelines adopted from the revised OECD guideline series: the bacterial reverse mutation test, the in vitro mammalian cell gene mutation test, the mammalian bone marrow chromosomal aberration test, and the mammalian erythrocyte micronucleus test.
1997	International Conference of Harmonization of Technical Requirements for Registration of Pharmaceuticals for Human Use (ICH) Guideline entitled "Genotoxicity: A Standard Battery for Genotoxicity Testing of Pharmaceuticals" identifies a standard three test battery: i) a test for gene mutation in bacteria; ii) an in vitro test with cytogenetic evaluation of chromosomal damage with mammalian cells *or* an in vitro mouse lymphoma tk assay; and iii) an in vivo test for chromosomal damage using rodent hematopoietic cells, e.g., a test for chromosomal aberrations *or* a micronucleus test. The ICH also states that the in vitro tests should be completed prior to the first human exposure of candidate pharmaceuticals and the standard three-test battery should be completed prior to the initiation of Phase II clinical trials.
1998	Revised OECD Genetic Toxicology Guidelines for the Testing of Chemicals approved and published.
1998	The EPA's Office of Pollution Prevention and Toxics urges chemical companies to voluntarily provide physical and chemical data and to conduct five types of screening tests (mutagenicity, ecotoxicity, environmental fate, acute toxicity, and subchronic reproductive and developmental toxicology), which comprise the OECD's Screening Information Data Sets (SIDS) Program, for ~3,000 high production volume chemicals that were classified as "existing" chemicals when TSCA became effective in 1977 and, hence, which did not require testing for a PMN (Pre-Manufacture Notice). Concerns have been expressed that resources may be insufficient for completing this testing by the target date of 2005.

conditions, and recent knowledge about the correlation of mutations in onco-
genes and tumor suppressor genes with key steps leading to tumor formation.

Although a number of chemicals are known to be human carcinogens, and
although many of the same mutagenic processes have been shown to be directly
involved in inducing both heritable effects and carcinogenesis in animals, it is
virtually impossible to obtain direct evidence for specific chemicals inducing
inherited defects in humans. Thus, the *Salmonella* results led to a shift from
justifying the genotoxicity testing of chemicals based on potential risk to future
generations to primarily, if not exclusively, justifying the tests as screens for
carcinogenicity. Consequently, to date, positive mutagenicity results in the absence of proven carcinogenicity have been considered insufficient justification
for regulating chemicals already on the market (21).

When positive mutagenicity results are obtained for a new product, however, regulatory agencies may request additional information. The product can
often be marketed if the further testing yields a negative outcome for genomic
mutations or carcinogenicity or, even then, if the product is a drug for a life-
threatening condition with no alternative therapies. In practice, however, because of the time and expense involved in this additional testing, coupled with
the uncertain outcome of the additional test results, the development of new
pharmaceuticals and industrial chemicals is often discontinued if the initial mutagenicity test results are positive (21).

The rapid expansion of the field of genetic toxicology came to an abrupt
halt following the publication, in 1987, of an assessment (22) of National Toxicology Program (NTP) test results for 73 chemicals evaluated in four short term
in vitro genetic toxicology tests in which the NTP found the tests to be only
about 60% accurate in predicting rodent carcinogenicity. In particular, only
about 50% of the carcinogens were found positive in the assays for reverse
mutations in *Salmonella* and chromosomal aberrations in mammalian cells, and,
while positive predictivity (the percentage of chemicals yielding positive genetic
toxicology results that were rodent carcinogens) was 86% in *Salmonella*, positive predictivity was 73% for the aberration assay, 67% for the sister chromatid
exchange (SCE) assay, and only 50% for the mouse lymphoma cell mutation
assay. Thus, the *Salmonella* and chromosomal aberration assays appeared to be
poorly predictive of rodent carcinogenicity, and the SCE assay and particularly
the mouse lymphoma assay appeared to yield an unacceptably high number of
"false positive" results.

Then, less than two years later, Ames tested a wide variety of edible plants
in the *Salmonella* assay and reported that most, if not all, contained mutagens
that were evolved as natural toxins to protect the plants from insects and other
predators and, further, that although even higher levels of some mutagens may
be found in the workplace, humans consume 10,000 times more natural than
manmade pesticides. In addition, Ames noted that the risk of carcinogenesis

may be negligible at the levels of chemicals to which humans are usually exposed, which are far below the maximum tolerated doses used for the rodent carcinogenesis bioassay. He then suggested that basic, instead of applied, research should be emphasized to minimize cancer and other degenerative diseases of aging. Thus, the NTP findings, followed shortly by Ames' assertion that concerns with the risk of exposing humans to mutagens and carcinogens were grossly magnified, resounded throughout the scientific community. This led to a pronounced lack of enthusiasm and subsequent government funding for developing and evaluating additional tests, an immediate decline in use of the mouse lymphoma assay in particular, and essentially a discontinuation of the SCE assay, the latter because direct mechanistic relevance of the SCE test has yet to be established.

Although only one of the four in vitro tests evaluated by the NTP—the measurement of reverse mutations in *Salmonella*—is currently used by the NTP, in the most recent decade independent reassessments of the chromosomal aberration and mouse lymphoma assays have been published (24–26) that clearly illustrate multiple deficiencies in the testing protocols used by the NTP and justify the current recommendation and use of these tests for regulatory submissions. Further, recent dramatic research advances in defining the molecular basis of genetic alterations have led to an enhanced understanding of the theoretical basis of genotoxicity test systems, which will be discussed in the following section. At the same time, as noted above, there have been recent concerted efforts to identify the most reliable genetic toxicology tests and to harmonize testing methodology and agency requirements.

Thus, although the tests used for regulatory submissions through most of the 1980s were often based as much on theoretical considerations as on the actual performance of the tests, with increasing use and evaluation of the test systems only a few have gained universal acceptance and are used today for initial assessments for regulatory agencies, with the selection of protocols usually based on the experience of industry and current regulatory guidance. These few tests, which will be described in greater detail together with the reasons that they are used, include: bacterial reverse mutation, the mouse lymphoma assay, in vitro chromosomal aberrations, and the chromosomal aberration and micronucleus tests in rodent bone marrow cells.

Recent molecular biology advances have led to an expanded awareness of the importance of genotype in susceptibility to cancer, and they promise to yield more reasoned and informed assessments of risk to present and future generations. However, public concerns with the potential hazards of chemicals have not abated, and, from a regulatory perspective, perhaps the most significant recent change at the time of this writing is that the pendulum appears to be again swinging toward an increased volume, if not variety, of genetic toxicology testing. The dramatic growth of the biotechnology industry during the past decade is now yielding numerous potentially useful pharmaceutical products that, under ICH guidelines, must be tested for genotoxicity before they are administered to human volunteers. In addition, there are at least 3,000 high production volume chemical products that were in existence when TSCA became effective in 1977 and, hence, which did not require testing for a PMN (Pre-Manufacture Notice). The OECD and the EPA are now urging that, consistent with industry's product stewardship programs, chemical companies voluntarily test these chemicals for several endpoints, including mutagenicity, in the OECD's Screening Information Data Sets (SIDS) Program. The EPA has also announced plans to issue a "test rule" to be finalized by the end of the century that will require chemical-specific testing of existing chemicals if it has not been done on a voluntary basis and to require testing beyond the SIDS level for almost 500 high production volume chemicals that are used in consumer products (46).

IV. HARMONIZED GUIDANCE FOR REGULATORY SUBMISSIONS

Under the auspices of the OECD, extensive international efforts have been directed toward defining protocols for the genetic toxicology tests that have been used for product registration. Agreement has been reached that the results obtained with an OECD-defined protocol in one country will be accepted internationally. Thus, there is the expectation that testing for the registration of chemical products and pharmaceuticals will be conducted according to the OECD guidelines and that any deviations from these guidelines will be justified.

Until recently, however, the selection of specific protocols for regulatory submissions has been a separate issue, with different groups of test systems used by chemical and pharmaceutical companies, and within different geographical regions. Thus, the harmonization of regulatory requirements has been considered necessary to facilitate more efficient and economical testing strategies for companies that market their products worldwide. To address this need, harmonized testing guidelines have now been published by the OECD for high production volume chemicals, by the EPA for chemicals tested under TSCA, and, for pharmaceuticals, by the International Council for Harmonization. These guidelines, which are summarized in Table 3, are discussed below.

A. OECD/SIDS Guidelines

The OECD Screening Information Data Set (SIDS) voluntary testing program for international high production volume (HPV) chemicals began in 1989 and includes obtaining six types of data: physical/chemical, mutagenicity, ecotoxi-

Table 3 Harmonized Testing Guidelines for Regulatory Submissions

Type of Test	OECD/SIDS	TSCA	ICH
Bacterial reverse mutation test	✔	✔	✔
Nonbacterial in vitro test			
Mammalian cell mutation	✔	✔	✔[a]
	or		or
Chromosomal aberration	✔		✔
In vivo test			
Chromosomal aberration	✔	✔	✔
	or	or	or
Micronucleus	✔	✔	✔

[a]Only the L5178Y mouse lymphoma gene and chromosomal mutation assay is recommended in the ICH guidelines.

city, environmental fate, acute toxicity, and subchronic reproductive and developmental toxicology. The mutagenicity tests identified by OECD/SIDS include: a test for gene mutations in bacteria, a nonbacterial in vitro test (e.g., a mammalian cell gene mutation assay *or* a chromosomal aberration assay), and an assessment of genetic toxicity in vivo (e.g., a micronucleus or chromosomal aberration test). These are tests most frequently identified for testing chemicals in the guidance provided by regulatory bodies in the U.S. and other nations; however, in some countries fewer tests may be identified for chemicals with a lower level of concern, which is based on production volume and use. Then, only one or two of the tests, i.e., a test for gene mutations in bacteria and possibly an in vitro chromosomal aberration assay may be required.

The SIDS program is currently focused on developing base level test information on approximately 600 poorly characterized international HPV chemicals, but only about 80 of the chemicals have been completely evaluated to date. In addition, the U.S. EPA has estimated that there are currently ~3,000 HPV chemicals that were classified as "existing" chemicals when TSCA became effective in 1977 and, hence, which did not require testing for a PMN (Pre-Manufacture Notice), and that are currently produced or imported in amounts of over 1 million pounds per year. At the time of this writing, the U.S. government is preparing to encourage OECD countries to speed up testing by chemical companies, and the EPA is also planning to issue a "test rule" in December 1999 which will require chemical-specific testing. However, the EPA and the Chemical Manufacturers Association (CMA) are currently meeting to address concerns that resources may be insufficient for completing this testing within the first decade of the 21st century (46).

B. TSCA Guidelines

Historically, because of mandates under TSCA and FIFRA that apply to domestically produced and imported chemicals, the U.S. EPA has often taken the lead in providing guidance for the registration of chemicals for companies planning to market their products worldwide. In a series of TSCA test guidelines established in 1985, two TSCA Section 4 mutagenicity testing schemes were followed, one for gene mutations and one for chromosomal mutations, but by the end of the decade it had been proposed that they be combined into one revised mutagenicity testing scheme (47). In 1997, the EPA Office of Pollution Prevention and Toxics (OPPT) published a Final Rule for TSCA Guidelines, including mutagenicity, to harmonize the testing guidelines developed by the Office of Pesticide Programs (OPP), the earlier TSCA guidelines, and the OECD guidelines. The revised guidelines, which incorporate the OECD protocols, establish the following four initial genetic toxicology approaches: a bacterial reverse mutation test; an in vitro mammalian cell mutation test; and either a mammalian bone marrow chromosomal aberration test or a mammalian erythrocyte micronucleus test.

By examination of Table 3 it may be noted that the TSCA guidelines differ from the OECD/SIDS guidelines in that an in vitro chromosomal aberration test is not identified as an alternative for the in vitro mammalian cell mutation test. Although the EPA's harmonized guidelines may be modified at some future date to accept in vitro chromosomal aberration test results as an alternative to the in vitro mammalian cell mutation test, this decision may be delayed until the EPA's Gene-Tox review of in vitro and in vivo chromosomal aberration assays (which is currently in progress) has been completed. It should additionally be noted that although the OECD guidelines, and hence the TSCA guidelines, for the in vitro mammalian cell gene mutation test indicate that L5178Y mouse lymphoma cells, a CHO, AS52 or V79 line of Chinese hamster cells, or TK6 human lymphoblastoid cells may be used, the mouse lymphoma assay is the only one of the identified tests that has been extensively defined and evaluated and shown to be mechanistically relevant, i.e., to detect a full range of chromosomal mutations as well as gene mutations.

C. ICH Guidelines

Historically, in the United States, the FDA has identified tests that might be appropriate for the registration of pharmaceuticals, food additives, biomedical materials, and some veterinary products, e.g., in Red Books I and II. However, it was the responsibility of the pharmaceutical industry to select the tests that were used, then to conduct additional testing if the initial tests were not sufficiently informative. Thus, often based upon the prior experience of specific companies, new products could be evaluated in five or more genotoxicity test systems, including tests for bacterial reverse mutation, mammalian cell mutagenesis, in vitro and/or in vivo cytogenetics, DNA damage and repair, and mammalian cell transformation (a change from normal to abnormal growth characteristics of cultured cells). However, at the same time, initially only a bacterial reverse mutation test, and later a bacterial reverse mutation test plus in vitro cytogenetics, were required for some European submissions, and only a bacterial reverse mutation test plus in vitro cytogenetic testing, but with different protocols, were required in Japan.

This situation presented obvious problems for pharmaceutical companies wishing to market their products internationally. Hence, following a series of formal deliberations by the six-member International Council on Harmonization (ICH), Expert Working Group—consisting of one representative, each, from the appropriate regulatory agency and from the pharmaceutical manufacturers from the U.S., the European Union (E.U.), and Japan—a consensus was reached that pharmaceuticals should be evaluated for genotoxicity in three tests: a test for gene mutations in bacteria; an in vitro test with cytogenetic evaluation of chromosomal damage in mammalian cells, or an in vitro mouse lymphoma *tk* assay; and an in vivo test for chromosomal damage (either chromosomal aberrations or micronuclei) using rodent hematopoietic cells.

The ICH Working Group considered the in vitro cytogenetic evaluation and the mouse lymphoma assay to be interchangeable because of recent evidence that they yield congruent results and because both detect genetic effects that cannot be measured in bacteria. An in vivo test was considered necessary to provide a test model that included factors such as absorption, distribution, metabolism, and excretion that could influence genotoxicity. The ICH Expert Working Group stated that, for compounds giving negative results, the completion of this three-test battery, performed in accordance with current (OECD and ICH) recommendations, will usually provide a sufficient level of safety to demonstrate the absence of genotoxic activity, but compounds giving positive results in the standard battery may, depending on their therapeutic use, need to be tested more extensively. The latter is interpreted as requiring testing in additional genotoxicity test systems to resolve incongruent initial results and/or testing for carcinogenicity in rodents.

As may be noted in Table 3, the first and third of the three approaches identified for testing pharmaceutical products are the same as those defined by OECD/SIDS and TSCA for chemicals; the second approach is the same for the three sets of guidelines only if the L5178Y mouse lymphoma cell mutagenesis assay is used for testing chemical products as well as for pharmaceuticals.

V. GENETIC TOXICOLOGY TESTS FOR CURRENT PRODUCT REGISTRATION

Current OECD/SIDS and ICH regulatory guidance has identified the following five basic genetic toxicology approaches: (a) a test for bacterial reverse gene mutations, (b) the L5178Y mouse lymphoma cell assay for gene and chromosomal mutations, (c) an in vitro chromosomal aberration test, and either (d) an in vivo chromosomal aberration test or (e) an in vivo micronucleus test, both for chromosomal mutations, and TSCA regulatory guidance has identified all but (c) the in vitro chromosomal aberration test. The five identified tests will be described, based on the current OECD guidelines and the author's experience, then the advantages and limitations of these tests will be summarized.

To establish that a chemical is negative, in vitro tests must be conducted in the absence and presence of exogenous metabolic activation, and positive and negative controls must be within historical ranges for the testing laboratory. The latter is also applicable for in vivo tests, and, in addition, the animals must be maintained under conditions that minimize the influence of environmental variables, and bioavailability must be considered when selecting the route of administration. It should also be noted that, although some prior testing guidelines specified that test results should be reproducible in independent experiments, under current guidelines there is no requirement for repeating an appropriately conducted test that yields clearly positive results. Appropriately conducted in vivo tests, e.g., tests in which dosing is by the appropriate route and to a sufficiently high dose level, that yield negative results are seldom, if ever, repeated. However, for in vitro tests, repeat testing with an alternate metabolic activation system or different exposure conditions may be required if negative results are obtained, and ICH guidance for in vitro cytogenetics tests specifies that, in addition, a later harvest time should be used. Repeat testing is clearly required if the initial results are equivocal; although, replication for its own sake (i.e., an exact repeat of the first test) is usually not informative; instead, the repeat test should be designed to correct any deficiencies of the first.

Finally, it is often helpful to evaluate the results in the different test systems for redundancy. For example, chemicals that yield positive results in a bacterial reverse mutation test often yield positive results in the mouse lymphoma assay, and chemicals that yield positive results in an in vivo test for chromosomal mutations usually have yielded positive results in an in vitro test for chromosomal mutations (either an aberration assay or the mouse lymphoma assay).

A. Reverse Gene Mutations in Bacteria

The most extensive testing for gene mutations is in bacteria, particularly using reverse mutation in *Salmonella typhimurium* and *Escherichia coli*. Therefore, bacterial reverse mutation assays are considered by many to be the cornerstone of genetic toxicology testing. Bacterial tests present the advantages of relative ease of performance, economy, efficiency, and the ability to identify specific DNA damage that is induced, e.g., frameshift or base pair substitution mutations. Bacterial tests can also provide information on the mode of action of the test chemical, as the bacterial strains that are used vary in their responsiveness to different chemical classes. Many of the tester strains have features that make them more sensitive for the detection of mutations including responsive DNA sequences at the reversion sites, increased cell permeability to large molecules, and the elimination of DNA repair systems or the enhancement of error-prone DNA repair processes.

The *Salmonella typhimurium* strains that are routinely used were designed for sensitivity in detecting gene mutations that revert the bacteria to histidine independence, and the *Salmonella* strains are histidine auxotrophs by virtue of mutations in the histidine operon. The *E. coli* WP2 *uvrA* strains that are recommended for initial tests are tryptophan auxotrophs by virtue of a base-pair substitution mutation in the tryptophan operon. When these histidine- or tryptophan-dependent cells are grown on minimal medium agar plates containing a trace of histidine or tryptophan, only those cells that revert to histidine or tryptophan independence are able to form colonies. The small amounts of these amino acids allow all the plated bacteria to undergo a few divisions; in many cases, this growth is essential for mutagenesis to occur, and the revertants are easily visible as colonies against a slight lawn of background growth.

In addition to the histidine and tryptophan operons, most of the indicator strains carry a deletion that covers genes involved in the synthesis of the vitamin biotin (*bio*), and all carry the *rfa* mutation that leads to a defective lipopolysaccharide coat and makes the strains more permeable to many large molecules. The strains also carry the *uvrB* mutation, which results in impaired repair of ultraviolet (uv)-induced DNA damage and renders the bacteria unable to use accurate excision repair to remove certain chemically or physically damaged DNA, thereby enhancing the strains' sensitivity to some mutagenic agents. In addition, the more recently developed strains contain the resistance transfer factor, plasmid pKM101, which is believed to cause an additional increase in error-prone DNA repair, leading to even greater sensitivity to most mutagens.

In bacterial reverse mutation testing, usually one strain is used for a preliminary concentration range-finding assay, then mutagenesis assays are conducted with five strains. The strains recommended by the OECD guidelines are:

1. *S. typhimurium* TA1535
2. *S. typhimurium* TA1537 or TA97 or TA97a
3. *S. typhimurium* TA98
4. *S. typhimurium* TA100

5. *E. coli* WP2 *uvr*A or *E. coli* WP2 *uvr*A (pKM101) or *S. typhimurium* TA102

Salmonella strains TA1535 and TA100 are reverted to histidine independence by base pair mutagens; strains TA1537, TA97, TA97a, and TA98 are reverted by frameshift mutagens, and all six have GC base pairs at the primary reversion site. *Salmonella* strain TA102 and the *E. coli* strains have an AT base pair at the primary reversion sites, and they detect a variety of oxidants, cross-linking agents, and hydrazines that are not detected by the other strains.

Basic microbial mutagenesis protocols use the plate incorporation approach or a preincubation modification of this approach. In the standard plate incorporation protocol, the test material, bacteria, and either a metabolic activation mixture (S9) or buffer are added to liquid top agar in a disposable glass tube which is held at 45°C in a heating block while the components are added, then mixed, and the mixture is immediately poured on a plate of bottom agar. After the agar gels, the bacteria are incubated, at 37°C, for 48–72 hours; then the resulting colonies are counted. In a typical mutagenesis assay with and without metabolic activation, each of the five strains of bacteria is exposed to the solvent control (with six cultures per strain and activation condition), and to five concentrations of the test chemical (with three cultures per concentration, strain and activation condition), and to the appropriate positive controls for that strain (with three cultures per activation condition). This yields a total of 240 bacterial plates, and additional plates that are used to check the sterility of the components.

The preincubation modification is used for materials that may be poorly detected in the plate incorporation assay, including short chain aliphatic nitrosamines, divalent metals, aldehydes, azo-dyes and diazo compounds, pyrollizidine alkaloids, alkyl compounds and nitro compounds. In this protocol, the test material, bacteria, and S9 mixture (when used) are incubated for 20–30 min at 37°C before top agar is added, mixed, and the mixture is poured on a plate of bottom agar. Increased activity with preincubation in comparison to plate incorporation is attributed to the fact that the test chemical, bacteria, and S9 are incubated at higher concentrations (without agar present) than in the standard plate incorporation test. Other modifications of the assays provide for exposing the bacteria to measured concentrations of gases in closed containers and/or the use of metabolic activation systems from a variety of species.

For an acceptable assay, the test chemical should be tested to a toxic level, as evidenced by a reduction in colonies or a reduced background lawn, or to a level at which precipitated test material precludes visualization of the colonies, or to 5 mg or 5 µl/plate, whichever is lower. To evaluate a result as positive requires a concentration-related and/or a reproducible increase in the number of revertant colonies per plate for at least one strain with or without activation.

B. The L5178Y/$tk^{+/-}$ Gene and Chromosomal Mutation Assay

The L5178Y mouse lymphoma assay measures gene and chromosomal forward mutations at the thymidine kinase locus, $tk^{+/-} \rightarrow tk^{-/-}$, and, as indicated in the recent EPA Gene-Tox review of published results for over 600 chemicals tested in this assay (25), when used with appropriate protocols and evaluation criteria, the mouse lymphoma assay yields results that are > 90% concordant with the outcome of the rodent carcinogenesis bioassay. The Gene-Tox review, which contains a detailed description of the assay, was published in late 1997, after the most recent OECD guidelines were adopted. Because of the order of publication, the review could not be cited in the guidelines; therefore, for additional information about this assay, the OECD guidelines should be supplemented with information from the Gene-Tox review.

More recently, the L5178Y mouse lymphoma cells were found to harbor gene mutations in *p53* (48) which, in the mouse, is found on the same chromosome as *tk*. The *p53* tumor suppressor gene is considered to be the "guardian of the genome" because its function is to delay the cell cycle progression of cells that have acquired chromosomal mutations until the damage has been repaired. Thus, the presence of mutant *p53* in the mouse lymphoma cells renders the assay more similar to mutation assays in repair-deficient bacteria. In addition, this finding is not only consistent with the sensitivity of this assay for detecting chromosomal mutations, but it enhances the relevance of the assay for predicting carcinogenicity, as mutant *p53* is found in over 50% of human tumors.

L5178Y mouse lymphoma cells, specifically clone 3.7.2C, grow in suspension culture with a relatively short cell generation time, 9–10 hours. A few days before use in an assay, a culture is "cleansed" of pre-existing spontaneous $tk^{-/-}$ mutants by growing the cells for about 24 hours in medium containing methotrexate. After the cells have recovered from cleansing, they are exposed to a series of concentrations of the test chemical, usually for four hours, in the absence and presence of metabolic activation. Testing under nonphysiological conditions must be avoided in this assay and other in vitro mammalian cell assays, as acidic pH shifts, to ≤ 6.5, and high salt concentrations have been shown to produce physiologically irrelevant positive results. Conversely, if the pH of the medium used to culture the cells is ≥ 7.5, cell growth in suspension culture may be depressed, and small colony mutants, in particular, may not be detected (25).

Because chromosomal mutations are usually associated with slower growth rates and because the induction of both gene and chromosomal mutations are associated with cytotoxicity, a chemical cannot be considered to be nongenotoxic in this assay unless testing is performed to concentrations that produce significant cytotoxicity, e.g., 10–20% RTG (relative total growth =

cloning efficiency × relative suspension growth [RSG]). On the other hand, responses observed only at extreme cytoxicity (<10% RTG) are considered to be biologically irrelevant. Therefore, exposure concentrations for each assay are selected, based on the results of a preliminary range-finding experiment, to span a range of anticipated survival from non- or weakly toxic to 10–20% RTG, with the concentrations selected to emphasize the lower RTG values. For relatively noncytotoxic chemicals, the maximum concentration should be 5 μl/ml, 5 mg/ml, or 10 mM, or a concentration that evidences insolubility, whichever is lower. However, scientific judgment should be exercised in evaluating results that appear to be positive only in the presence of a precipitate. In this case, the test chemical may be present in suspension culture during the two-day expression period, thus lengthening the exposure time and leading to erroneous cell counts if cell density values are obtained with a cell counter instead of with a hemacytometer. In addition, erroneous colony counts can be obtained if an automated colony counter is used to enumerate the colonies.

After chemical exposure, the cells are rinsed, then grown in suspension culture for a two-day expression period, with the cells in each culture diluted as necessary to maintain a rapid growth rate; then the cells are cloned to measure mutagenesis and survival. Two methods are currently used for cloning, and for both approaches, the selective agent (TFT) is present in the cloning medium for the mutant colonies. In the original approach (which was used for virtually all test results included in the Gene-Tox review of this assay, and which is used by most, if not all, U.S. laboratories), the cells are cloned in culture dishes in medium containing sufficient soft agar to immobilize the cells. The second approach, cloning the cells without agar in microwell plates (49), was developed in the U.K. by a laboratory that had difficulty in obtaining small colony mutants with the original approach, and it has been used by Japanese laboratories that recently gained experience with the mouse lymphoma assay (50). A number of laboratories that are experienced with both approaches obtain equivalent results with either, and they find the soft agar cloning approach to be less labor-intensive and less subjective.

After cloning, an approximately 10–12 day incubation period is used for the microwell method and a two week incubation period is required for the soft-agar approach before the colonies are counted and sized. With shorter times, the σ mutant colonies may not grow to a sufficient size to be visualized; however, even with only a 10-day incubation period, it is sometimes difficult to determine whether only one or more than one large colony mutant is in a microwell. Because most of the colonies enumerated to obtain cloning efficiency are large colonies, this difficulty can lead to lower cloning efficiency values which, in turn, can lead to an artificially elevated spontaneous mutant frequency or an incorrect conclusion of a positive mutagenic response. Colony counting and sizing are accomplished using colony counters that can discriminate between the size ranges of the objects (colonies) that are counted, and both σ and λ colony mutant frequencies, as well as total mutant frequencies, are reported for positive and negative controls and for treated cultures that yield a positive response. However, many of the older colony counters do not have sufficient resolution to detect all of the small mutant colonies that may be present, a problem that is circumvented by counting the colonies by hand.

For acceptable assays, absolute cloning efficiencies for the solvent controls are expected to be between 80 and 120%; however, lower and higher cloning efficiencies may be acceptable in individual experiments, especially if a test chemical is unambiguously positive. Solvent control mutant frequencies should be consistent with the testing laboratory's historical ranges and generally in a range from $\geq 20 \times 10^{-6}$ to $\leq 120 \times 10^{-6}$. As discussed in the gene-Tox review (25), there is currently *no* statistical method that is considered to be appropriate for this assay. In fact, in a number of published mouse lymphoma assay results, e.g., for the NTP, chemicals were erroneously called positive because of inappropriate reliance on a statistical analysis system (26). Therefore, the Gene-Tox evaluation criteria are recommended for evaluating the results, with the caveat that these criteria were developed for the agar cloning approach and may require modification if results are obtained with the microwell approach. (These criteria are summarized in Table 4.)

C. Chromosomal Aberrations, In Vitro

In vitro chromosomal aberration assays for regulatory submissions are routinely conducted in the absence and presence of exogenous metabolic activation and may use a variety of established cell lines, cell strains, or primary cell cultures, selected on the basis of factors such as growth ability in culture, stability of the karyotype, chromosome number, chromosome diversity, and spontaneous frequency of chromosome aberrations. The most frequently used cells are Chinese hamster fibroblasts (either CHO, Chinese hamster ovary, or CHL, Chinese hamster lung, cells) or human or rat lymphocytes stimulated to divide in vitro. The cell cultures are propagated from stock cultures and seeded in culture medium at a density such that the cultures will not reach confluency before the time of harvest, which should be about 1.5 hours after addition of a mitotic spindle inhibitor (Colcemid® or colchicine). The lymphocytes are usually obtained from whole blood from healthy subjects, treated with heparin (an anticoagulant), and stimulated to divide with a mitogen (e.g., phytohemagglutinin). After a prolonged G_1 stage, the cells enter S-phase, which should be the time of addition of the test chemical to the cells. For a typical protocol, chemical exposure is initiated at 48 hours, a mitotic spindle inhibitor is added at 70.5 hours, and cells in metaphase are harvested at 72 hours.

After the cells are harvested, they are treated with a hypotonic solution to

Table 4   Gene-Tox Evaluation Criteria for the Mouse Lymphoma Assay[a]

++	Definitive positive response with evidence of a dose-response and an induced (treated minus spontaneous) mutant frequency of at least 100×10^{-6} at RTG $\geq 20\%$.
+	Limited positive response with evidence of a dose-response and an induced mutant frequency of at least 70×10^{-6} at a RTG $\geq 10\%$.
−	Negative response for which toxicity is evidenced by a RTG of 10–20%, and the positive control mutant frequency demonstrates that there are no inherent problems with the assay.
−−	Negative response with no toxicity, and the positive control mutant frequency demonstrates that there are no inherent problems with the assay.
I	Inconclusive. Insufficient concentrations tested over the critical range of 10–20% RTG to be able to evaluate the result as clearly positive or negative. The portion(s) of the assay that yield(s) an inconclusive result must be repeated.
E	Equivocal. A negative or inconclusive result is obtained in one mutagenesis assay and a positive result is obtained in another, and there is no apparent reason to give greater weight to either result. In this case, the testing must be repeated a third time. However, some chemicals yield equivocal results regardless of the number of times that an assay is repeated. (Repeat testing is not required if the initial result is clearly positive.)
NT	Not testable. Applied to chemicals that cannot be tested to sufficiently high concentration to obtain a conclusive result in the mouse lymphoma assay because of limited solubility, acidic pH shifts, elevated osmolality, or the test material's physical properties such as dissolving plastic, and this limitation cannot be overcome by use of an alternate solvent or by adjusting the exposure conditions to ensure that they are physiologically relevant.

[a]*Source:* Ref. 25.

swell the chromosomes, fixed, and dropped onto prelabeled slides. Then, the chromosomes are stained and coverslips are attached to permit microscopic analysis with oil immersion ($100 \times$) objectives. At least three concentrations are analyzed that are selected based on a preliminary evaluation of uncoded slides. All slides to be analyzed, including positive and negative controls, should be coded by an individual who will not be involved in the analysis, and, if the slides are to be evaluated by more than one cytogeneticist, the selected concentrations and controls should be divided into equivalent sets before coding. At least 200 well-spread metaphases should be scored per concentration and controls; however, this number can be reduced when high numbers of aberrations are observed.

Among the criteria to be considered when determining the highest concentration to be tested for chromosomal aberrations are cytotoxicity, solubility, and changes in osmolality or pH, to ensure that exposure conditions will be in a physiologically-relevant range (as was described, above, for the mouse lymphoma assay). These criteria are assessed in preliminary concentration range-finding assays, with mitotic index determinations and/or assessments of cell growth (e.g., generation times) in culture used to indicate cytotoxicity and cell cycle delay. As a general rule-of-thumb, to ensure that there will be sufficient numbers of mitotic cells for analyses, mitotic indices need not be depressed more than 50%. For relatively noncytotoxic chemicals, the maximum concentration should be 5 µl/ml, 5 mg/ml, or 10 mM, whichever is lowest. For relatively insoluble chemicals, OECD guidelines advise testing one or more than one concentration in the insoluble range so long as a precipitate does not interfere with the analysis.

OECD guidelines recommend that the cells should be exposed to the test chemical both with and without metabolic activation for 3–6 hours and sampled at a time equivalent to about 1.5 times the normal cell cycle after the beginning of treatment. If the result is unambiguously positive, no further testing is needed. However, if the chemical yields negative results with and without activation, a second experiment without metabolic activation is recommended with continuous treatment until a sampling time equivalent to about 1.5 times the normal cell cycle after the beginning of treatment. The ICH guidelines go one step further and specify that if the second experiment is also negative, a third experiment without metabolic activation is needed, with a continuous 24-hour treatment time, as only with this approach were some carcinogens that had previously been evaluated as negative for aberrations by the NTP detected as positive in this assay (24).

D. Rodent Bone Marrow Chromosomal Effects

In vivo tests for chromosomal effects for regulatory submissions consist of the in vivo chromosomal aberration test and the micronucleus test. They are routinely conducted using bone marrow cells from rodents, e.g., mice or rats, because the bone marrow is highly vascularised and contains a population of rapidly dividing cells that can be readily isolated and processed. However, the micronucleus test can also be conducted with sampling of cells from the peripheral blood that were exposed to the test chemical while in the bone marrow. Because the target cells are exposed to the products of in vivo metabolism under physiological conditions, these tests are particularly useful if positive results have been obtained with an in vitro test for chromosomal effects. However, they are not appropriate tests if there is evidence that the test substance, or a reactive metabolite will not reach the bone marrow. In this case, other tests may be required.

Healthy young adult animals are acclimated before testing and, when weighed before dosing, the weight variation of the animals should be minimal and not exceed ± 20% per sex. The temperature in the room in which the animals are housed should be 22°C (± 3°C), and humidity should be at least 30% and preferably not exceed 70%. Artificial lighting is used with 12 hours light and 12 hours dark. If group housing is used (for each sex), the number of animals per cage should be consistent with the appropriate guidelines, and the animals are identified individually before they are weighed and dosed.

Dosing is routinely accomplished by intraperitoneal injection or gavage, but inhalation exposures are also used, if justified. The maximum dose level required for relatively nontoxic chemicals is 2,000 mg/kg body weight, and the maximum volume that is administered by injection or gavage should not exceed 2 ml/100 g body weight. If available pharmacokinetic or toxicity data demonstrate that there are no substantial differences between sexes, then testing in a single sex, preferably males, is sufficient. However, if human exposure may be sex-specific, the test should be performed in animals of the appropriate sex. Preliminary dose range-finding tests are necessary, sometimes using an evaluation of mitotic indices for the chromosomal aberration test or enumerating polychromatic erythrocyte (PCE) ratios for the micronucleus test, to select a high dose in which there will be at least five analyzable animals per sex with a sufficient number of cells for analysis. Experience has shown that this dose is often significantly lower than the LD_{50} defined in acute toxicology testing, and it is often prudent to use extra animals for toxic chemicals, particularly for the highest dose group.

Concurrent positive and negative (solvent/vehicle) controls are used for each sex and, except for treatment, the positive and negative control animals should be handled in the same way as the treated animals. The positive control may be administered by a different route than the one used for the test chemical, and only one sampling time is required. The negative control is administered by the same route as the test chemical, and negative controls are used for each sampling time, unless it can be demonstrated by the testing laboratory's historical control data that minimal inter-animal variability is obtained for negative control animals irrespective of the sampling time.

1. Chromosomal Aberrations, In Vivo

For the chromosomal aberration test, the highest dose is defined as 2,000 mg/ kg body weight or the dose producing signs of toxicity such that higher dose levels, based on the same dosing regimen, would be expected to produce lethality. The highest dose may also be defined as a dose that produces some indication of toxicity in the bone marrow (e.g., a greater than 50% reduction in the mitotic index). Chemicals are preferably administered as a single treatment, and samples are taken at two separate times following treatment. The first sampling interval is 1.5 times the normal cell cycle length; therefore, the first samples are obtained 12–18 hr after treatment, and a minimum of three dose levels plus the appropriate controls are required. A second sampling time, 24 hr following the first, is recommended to allow for the time required for uptake and metabolism of the test chemical as well as its effect on cell cycle kinetics; however, only the highest dose is used for the second time.

The animals are injected intraperitoneally, approximately 1.5–2 hr before the sampling time, with an appropriate dose of Colcemid® or colchicine. Then the animals are sacrificed, cells are removed from the bone marrow, treated with a hypotonic solution and fixed; then slides are prepared, stained, coverslipped and coded before analysis as described for the in vitro chromosomal aberration test. Mitotic indices are obtained based on at least 1,000 cells per animal, and at least 100 cells per animal should be analyzed for chromosomal aberrations, unless high numbers of aberrations are observed. Criteria for a positive response include a dose-related increase in the number of cells with chromosomal aberrations or a clear increase in the number of cells with aberrations in a single dose group at a single sampling time.

2. Micronucleus Tests

For micronucleus tests, the highest dose is defined as 2,000 mg/kg body weight or the dose producing signs of toxicity such that higher dose levels, based on the same dosing regimen, would be expected to produce lethality. The highest dose may also be defined as a dose that produces some indication of toxicity in the bone marrow (e.g., a reduction in the percentage of PCEs in the bone marrow or the peripheral blood). The test may be performed in two ways. In the first, animals are treated with the test chemical once, and samples of bone marrow cells are obtained at least twice, with the first samples obtained no earlier than 24 hr after treatment and the last samples no later than 48 hr after treatment. Samples of peripheral blood are obtained at least twice, with the first samples obtained no earlier than 36 hr after treatment and the last samples no later than 72 hr after treatment. Three dose levels, plus negative and positive controls are required for the first sampling time, but only the highest dose may be required for the second sampling time. In the second approach, the animals are treated on each of two or more consecutive days to achieve steady state kinetics, and samples are obtained once, between 18 and 24 hr following the final treatment for the bone marrow, or between 36 and 48 hr following treatment for the peripheral blood.

Bone marrow cells are usually obtained from the femurs and/or tibias immediately following sacrifice, e.g., by CO_2 asphyxia followed by cervical dislocation; peripheral blood is routinely obtained from the midventral tail vein, and, unless the animals are to be continued on test, immediately after they are sacrificed, e.g., by cervical dislocation. The proportion of PCEs among total erythrocytes (PCEs plus NCEs), which is a measure of toxicity, is obtained for at least 200 bone marrow erythrocytes, or for at least 2000 erythrocytes from

Table 5 Advantages and Disadvantages of Currently Used Tests

Test System	Advantages	Disadvantages
Bacterial Reverse Mutation	The "cornerstone" of geno-toxicity tests. Economy. The strains are sensitive to specific types of mutations. Several modifications of the test have been sufficiently evaluated for use. A large database of results is available.	Does not detect chemicals that break mammalian chromosomes, i.e., that induce chromosomal mutations. Toxic chemicals often yield a background of small colonies which can be misinterpreted as a positive result.
Mouse Lymphoma Assay	Detects the full range of gene and chromosomal mutations. Highly predictive of carcinogenicity in rodents. An extensively characterized assay. Can be conducted more efficiently and economically than the in vitro chromosomal aberration assay.	Requires careful adherence to a specific protocol. More expensive and time-consuming than the bacterial reverse mutation assay. Chromosomal mutations are assessed indirectly (as small colony mutants).
In vitro Chromosomal Aberrations	Permits direct visualization of chromosomal events and yields information on cell cycle effects. More consistent with the expertise available in some laboratories than the mouse lymphoma assay.	Requires specialized expertise. A more subjective test than the mouse lymphoma assay. A negative result can be obtained if the cells are not sampled at the appropriate time after exposure.
In vivo Chromosomal Aberrations	Permits direct visualization of chromosomal events and yields information on cell cycle effects. Historically, one of the first genetic toxicology tests to be developed. Yields information on the effects of in vivo metabolism.	Requires specialized expertise. A more subjective test than the micronucleus assay. More expensive and time-consuming than the micronucleus test. Sampling times are critical for ensuring valid results.

Table 5 Continued

Test System	Advantages	Disadvantages
Micronucleus Tests	More rapid, less expensive and less subjective than the in vivo chromosomal aberration test. Less specialized expertise required than the in vivo chromosomal aberration test. Yields information on the effects of in vivo metabolism.	Does not permit direct visualization of the full range of chromosomal effects as does the in vitro chromosomal aberration assay, and, as a result, it is less informative of cell cycle effects.

the peripheral blood. Then at least 2,000 PCEs per animal are evaluated to obtain the percentage with micronuclei. Criteria for a positive response include a dose-related increase in the number of PCEs with micronuclei or a clear increase in the number of micronucleated PCEs for a single dose.

VI. ADVANTAGES AND DISADVANTAGES OF THE GENETIC TOXICOLOGY TESTS USED FOR CURRENT PRODUCT REGISTRATION

The objective of this chapter has been to provide practical guidance to professionals responsible for evaluating the safety of current products. Thus, the harmonized testing guidelines have been stressed, and current developments in more theoretically-oriented genetic toxicology research have been largely omitted. Table 5 summarizes some of the advantages and disadvantages of the genetic toxicology tests identified in the harmonized guidelines and, hence, the tests that are currently used for product registration. Other factors to be considered may include previously obtained data for the test chemical, the properties of the test chemical, and the experience of the sponsoring organization and the testing laboratory. The tests most frequently used at the present time in the U.S. are the bacterial reverse mutation assay, the mouse lymphoma assay, and the micronucleus test; these comprise the most economical and rapidly performed set of tests.

Each of the initial genetic toxicology tests that has been described has been shown to be useful to varying degrees in predicting the outcome of the long-term animal tests and, when used together, these tests provide a high degree of confidence that chemicals that yield consistently negative results will be found to be negative in other tests for carcinogenesis and heritable genetic effects. Thus, the basic set of tests identified for current product registration is useful for providing rapid assessments of potential risk, including the risk of exposing human volunteers to drugs under development, and for conserving resources, reducing animal usage, determining whether additional testing would be productive, and reducing the time for obtaining regulatory approval to market new products.

REFERENCES

1. Gad, S.C., ed. (1988). Product Safety Evaluation Handbook, New York, Marcel Dekker.
2. Barfknecht, T.R. and Naismith, R.W. (1988). Practical mutagenicity testing. In: Gad, S.C., ed. (1988) Product Safety Evaluation Handbook, New York, Marcel Dekker, pp. 143–217.
3. Brusick, D. (1987). Principles of Genetic Toxicology. New York, Plenum Press.
4. Li, A.P. and Heflich, R.H. (1991). Genetic Toxicology. Boca Raton, FL: CRC Press.
5. Hollaender, A. and de Serres, F.J. (1971–1983). Chemical Mutagens. Principles and Methods for their Detection, Vols. 1–8, New York: Plenum Press.
6. Anon. (1998). The Promise of Gene Therapy. Newsletter of the Childrens Hospital Los Angeles Research Institute, p. 1.
7. Fox, T.R. and Gonzales, A.J. (1996). Cell cycle controls as potential targets for the development of chemically induced mouse liver cancer. Research Triangle Park, NC: CIIT Activities. 16:1–5.
8. Evans, H.J. (1977). Molecular mechanisms in the induction of chromosome aberrations. In: Scott, D. Bridges, B.A., and Sobels, F.H. eds. Progress in Genetic Toxicology, New York: Elsevier/North-Holland.
9. Trask, B.J., Allen, S., Massa, H., Fetitta, A., Sachs, R., van den Engh, G., and Wu, M. (1993). Studies of metaphase and interphase chromosomes using fluorescence *in situ* hybridization. Cold. Spring Harb. Symp. Quant. Biol. 58:767–775.
10. Mendel, G. (1866). Versuche uber Pflanzenhybriden. Vern des Naturf Vereines in Brunn, 4 (English translation revision published in J.R. Horticulture Soc. 26:1–32, 901).
11. de Vries, H. (1901). The Mutation Theory. Leipzig: Verlag von Veit and Co.
12. Boveri, T. (1914). Zur Frage der Entwicklung maligner Tumoren. Jena, Gustav Fischer.
13. Muller, H.J. (1927). Artificial transmutation of the gene. Science 64:84–87.
14. Efron, E. (1984). The Apocalyptics. How Environmental Politics Controls What We Know About Cancer. New York: Simon & Schuster, Inc.
15. Wassom, J.S. (1989). Origins of genetic toxicology and the Environmental Mutagen Society. Environ. Molec. Mutagen 14(S16):1–6.
16. Malling, H.V. (1971). Dimethylnitrosamine: formation of mutagenic compounds by interaction with mouse liver microsomes. Mutat. Res. 13:425–429.
17. McCann, J., Choi, E., Yamasaki, E., and Ames, B.N. (1975). Detection of carcino-

gens as mutagens in the *Salmonella*/microsome test: Assay of 300 chemicals. Proc. Natl. Acad. Sci. USA 72:5135–5139.

18. Prival, M.J. and Dellarco, V.L. (1989). Evolution of social concerns and environmental policies for chemical mutagens. Environ. Mol. Mutagen. 14(S16):46–50.

19. Tennant, R.W., Margolin, B.H., Shelby, M.D., Zeiger, E., Haseman, J.K., Spalding, J., Caspary, W., Resnick, M., Stasiewicz, S., Anderson, B., and Minor, R. (1987). Prediction of chemical carcinogenicity in rodents from *in vitro* genetic toxicity assays. Science 236:933–941.

20. Ames, B.N. (1989). What are the major carcinogens in the etiology of human cancer? Environmental pollution, natural carcinogens, and the causes of human cancer: Six errors. In: De Vita, V.T., Jr., Hellman, S., and Rosenberg, S.A., eds. Important Advances in Oncology. Philadelphia, J.B. Lippencott Company, pp. 237–247.

21. Galloway, S.M., Sofuni, T., Shelby, M., Thilagar, A., Kumaroo, V., Kaur, P., Gulati, D., Putman, D.L., Murli, H., Marshall, R., Tanaka, N. Anderson, B., Zeiger, E., and Ishidate, M., Jr. (1997). Multilaboratory comparison of *in vitro* tests for chromosome aberrations in CHO and CHL cells tested under the same protocols. Environ. Molec. Mutagen. 29:189–207.

22. Mitchell, A.D., Auletta, A.E., Clive, D., Kirby, P.E., Moore, M.M., and Myhr, B.C. (1997). The L5178Y/$tk^{+/-}$ mouse lymphoma specific gene and chromosomal mutation assay. A phase III report of the U.S. Environmental Protection Agency Gene-Tox Program. Mutat. Res. 394:177–303.

23. Mitchell, A.D., Auletta, A.E., Clive, D., Kirby, P.E., Moore, M.M., and Myhr, B.C. (1998). A comparison of the Gene-Tox and NTP evaluations of the utility of the L5178Y mouse lymphoma cell mutation assay for predicting rodent carcinogenicity. Mutat. Res. (Submitted).

24. Sax, K. (1938). Induction by X-rays of chromosome aberrations in *Tradescantia* microspores. Genetics 23:494–516.

25. Auerbach, C. and Robson, J.M. (1947). The production of mutations by chemical substances. Proc. R. Soc. Edinburgh Section B 62:271–283.

26. Earle, W.R., Schilling, E.L., Stark, T.H., Straus, N.P., Brown, M.F., and Shelton, E. (1943). Production of malignancy *in vitro*. IV. The mouse fibroblast cultures and changes seen in the living cells. J. Nat. Can. Inst. 4:165–212.

27. Russell, W.L. (1951). x-ray-induced mutations in mice. Cold Spring Harbor Symp. Quant. Biol. 16:327–336.

28. Gey, G.O., Coffman, W.D., and Kubicek, M.T. (1952). Tissue culture studies of the proliferative capacity of cervical carcinoma and normal epithelium. Cancer Res. 12:364–365.

29. Watson, J.D., and Crick, F.H.C. (1953). Molecular structure of nucleic acids. Nature. 171:737–738.

30. Tjio, J.H., and Levan, A. (1956). The chromosome number of man. Hereditas 42:1–6.

31. Lejeune, J., Gautier, M., and Turpin, R. (1959). Etude des chromosomes somatiques de neuf enfants mongoliens. Compt. Rend. Acad. Sci. 248:1721–1722.

32. Nowell, P.C., and Hungerford, D.A. (1960). A minute chromosome in human chronic granulocytic leukemia. Science 132:1497.

33. Auerbach, C. (1960). Chemical mutagenesis in animals. Abh Deutsch Akad Wiss Berlin Klin Med 1:1–13.

34. Hayflick, L., and Moorehead, P.S. (1961). The serial cultivation of human diploid cell strains. Exp. Cell Res. 25:585–621.
35. Carson, R. (1962). Silent Spring. Greenwich, CT: Fawcett.
36. Kao, F.-T., and Puck, T.T. (1968). Genetics of somatic mammalian cells. VII. Induction and isolation of nutritional mutants in Chinese hamster cells. Proc. Natl. Acad. Sci. USA 60:1275–1281.
37. Chu, E.H.Y., and Malling, H.V. (1968). Mammalian cell genetics. II. Chemical induction of specific locus mutations in Chinese hamster cells in vitro. Proc. Nat. Acad. Sci. USA 61:77–87.
38. Miller, J.A., and Miller, E.C. (1971). The mutagenicity of chemical carciogens: Correlations, problems, and interpretations, In: Hollaender, A.E., ed. Chemical Mutagens: Principles and Methods for Their Detection, New York: Plennum, Vol. 1, pp. 83–120.
39. Knudson, A.G., Jr. (1971). Mutation and cancer: Statistical study of retinoblastoma. Proc Natl. Acad. Sci., U.S. 68:820–823.
40. Clive, D., Flamm, W.G., Machesko, M.R., and Bernheim, N.J. (1972). A mutational assay system using the thymidine kinase locus in mouse lymphoma cells. Mutat. Res. 16:77–87.
41. Schmid, W. (1975). The micronucleus test. Mutat. Res. 31:9–15.
42. Ames, B.N., Durston, W.E., Yamasaki, E., et al. (1973). Carcinogens are mutagens: A simple test system combining liver homogenates for activation and bacteria for detection. Proc. Natl. Acad. Sci. USA 70:2281–2285.
43. Second Task Force for Research Planning in Environmental Health Science. (1976). Human Health and the Environment—Some Research Needs. Washington, DC, DHEW Publication No. NIH 77-1277, 498 pp.
44. Dearfield, K.L. (1991). Use of mutagenicity data by the U.S. Environmental Protection Agency's Office of Pesticide Programs. In: Genetic Toxicology, Li, A.P., and Heflich, R.H., eds. Boca Raton, FL: CRC Press, pp. 473–484.
45. National Research Council (1984). Toxicity Testing. Strategies to Determine Needs and Priorities. Washington, DC: National Academy Press, 382 pp.
46. Johnson, J. (1998). Administration backs chemical testing. Chem. Eng. News. 76: 7–8.
47. Auletta, A. (1991). Regulatory perspectives: TSCA In: Genetic Toxicology, Li, A.P., and Heflich, R.H., eds. Boca Raton, FL: CRC Press, pp. 435–454.
48. Storer, R.D., Kraynak, A.R., McKelvey, T.W., Elia, M.C., Goodrow, T.L., and DeLuca, J.G. (1996). The mouse lymphoma L5178Y TK$^+$/TK$^-$ cell line is heterozygous for a codon 170 mutation in the p53 tumor suppressor gene. Environ. Molec. Mutagen. 27(S27):66.
49. Cole, J., Arlett, C.F., Green, M.H.L., Lowe, J., and Muriel, W. (1983). A comparison of the agar cloning and microtitration techniques for assaying cell survival and mutation frequency in L5178Y mouse lymphoma cells. Mutat. Res. 111:371–386.
50. Sofuni, T., Honma, M., Hayashi, M., Shimada, H., Tanaka, N., Wakuri, S., Awogi, T., Yamamoto, K.I., Nishi, Y., and Nakadate, M. (1966). Detection of in vitro clastogens and spindle poisons by the mouse lymphoma assay using the microwell method: interim report of an international collaborative study. Mutagenesis. 11: 349–355.

7
Repeated-Dose Toxicity Studies

Vincent J. Piccirillo
NPC, Inc., Sterling, Virginia

I. INTRODUCTION

Many of the standard safety evaluation studies are repeated dose studies designed to characterize the effects of test chemicals upon multidose exposures to experimental animals. These studies include subchronic and chronic toxicity and carcinogenicity studies as well as studies to evaluate developmental and reproductive toxicity. Developmental and reproductive toxicity are extensively discussed elsewhere. This chapter will concentrate on subchronic, chronic, and carcinogenicity studies.

The principal routes of administration in repeated dose studies are oral, dermal, and inhalation. Inhalation exposure is discussed elsewhere. In most cases, the route of exposure is that which most typifies potential human exposure. Physical and chemical properties of the test article must also be considered in selection of the appropriate administration route. For example, instability of the test article in diet may preclude dietary exposure and requiring selection of an alternative oral dosing such as gavage.

Subchronic studies evaluate health hazards that may result from repeated exposure during a limited part of the test animals' lifetime. The standard duration for subchronic toxicity studies is 90-days (13 weeks). Historically, subchronic toxicity studies were designed to provide information that would serve as the basis for dose selection for the chronic toxicity and carcinogenicity studies. Subchronic studies evaluate dose-related effects on survival, body weight, food consumption, hematology, serum chemistry, urinanalysis, and gross and microscopic organ changes. High dose exposure for short durations may be predictive of many of the toxicologic effects that would occur upon low dose, long-term exposure. In recent years, subchronic toxicity study designs have been

expanded to include evaluation for chemical induced neurotoxicity and immunotoxicity. Further, evaluation of mode and/or mechanism of toxicity have become
a critical component of risk characterization. Today, it is not uncommon for
subchronic studies to include procedures to evaluate enzyme induction activity,
changes in hormonal stasis, peroxisomal proliferation, or other physiologic or
histologic changes that may provide relevant data for determining underlying
mechanisms of toxicity.

Chronic toxicity studies assess the potential hazards that may result from
prolonged, repeated exposure over a significant portion of the animals' lifetime.
Oncogenicity is considered a chronic effect. Chronic toxicity and oncogenicity
studies in rats are generally of at least 24 months duration. Chronic exposure in
mice should be for at least 18 months.

In the United States, chemicals, including pesticides, are regulated by the
U.S. Environmental Protection Agency (EPA). In recent years, the EPA Offices
of Prevention, Pesticides and Toxic Substances (OPPTS) developed guidelines
(1) to harmonize the testing requirements of the Office of Pollution, Prevention,
and Toxics (OPPT), the Office of Pesticide Programs (OPP) and the Organization for Economic Cooperation and Development (OECD). The purpose of the
harmonization was to minimize variations among the testing procedures required
to meet the data requirements of the Toxic Substances Control Act (TSCA) and
the Federal Insecticide, Fungicide, and Rodenticide Act (FIFRA) and European
regulatory bodies. Health Effects Test Guidelines are designated as Series 870
and can be downloaded from the Internet (currently found at www.epa.gov/
OPPTS_Harmonized). Specific guidelines for repeated dose toxicity studies are
as follows:

870.3100   90-day oral toxicity (2)
870.3150   Subchronic nonrodent oral toxicity—90 days (3)
870.3200   Repeated dose dermal toxicity—21/28 days (4)
870.3250   Repeated dose dermal toxicity—90 days (5)
870.4100   Chronic toxicity (6)
870.4200   Carcinogenicity (7)
870.4300   Combined chronic toxicity/carcinogenicity (8)
870.6200   Neurotoxicity screening battery (9)
870.7800   Immunotoxicity (10)

The U.S. Food and Drug Administration (FDA) has promulgated separate
guidelines for the toxicological evaluation of food and color additives. Specific
testing requirements are detailed in the "Toxicological Principles: For the Safety
Assessment of Direct Food Additives and Color Additives Used in Food" (11).
This document is commonly referred to as "the redbook" guidelines.

Although some guidance (12,13) has been published regarding study designs for repeated dose studies with pharmaceutical products, the majority of

these studies are specifically prepared based on the intended use of the drug, specific treatment durations, and pharmacologic properties.

In general, the guideline requirements between the OPPTS studies and the "redbook" studies are very similar. Of course, the "redbook" designs are specific for the oral route of administration. The OPPTS guidelines include specific sections and requirements related to oral, dermal, and inhalation exposures. Some important differences in the designs are summarized in Table 1.

II. ORAL TOXICITY

The standard dosing regimens via the oral route are test chemical/diet admixture, test chemical/drinking water admixture, and oral gavage.

Table 1 Differences Between OPPTS and Food Additive Guidelines

Study Type	OPPTS Guidelines	"Redbook" Guidelines
Subchronic toxicity-rodent		
Group size	10 rats/sex/group	20 rats/sex/group
Ophthalmologic exams	All animals	Control and high dose only
Organ weights	Several organs/all animals	Not required
Subchronic toxicity— nonrodent		
Hematology/clinical chemistry	30 days and termination	Termination only
Histopathology	Extensive list of tissues	Limited list of tissues
Oncogenicity		
Maximum required dose	1000 mg/kg/day	5% of the diet
Food consumption	Weekly for 13 weeks, every 4 weeks thereafter	Weekly for 13 weeks, every 3 months thereafter
Organ weights	On animals at interim and terminal sacrifice	None required
Chronic toxicity-rodent		
Ophthalmologic examination	Initiation and termination	Initiation, every 3 months and termination
Urinanalysis	6 months and termination	As indicated by other findings
Chronic toxicity-nonrodent		
Body weight/food consumption	Weekly for 13 weeks, every 4 weeks thereafter	Weekly
Ophthalmologic examination	Initiation and termination	Pretest, every 3 months and termination

A. Dietary Exposure

Dietary exposure is required for all chemicals that may be intentionally or non-intentionally added to the human diet. This route has served as the standard bearer for oral exposure because of its simplicity of presentation to the animals.

1. Diet preparation

The most critical factor to dietary studies is the proper preparation of the test chemical/diet admixture. The range of physical and chemical characteristics of test materials requires that considerations regarding appropriate mixing techniques should be determined on an individual basis. Standard practices generally dictate the preparation of a premix, to which is added appropriate amounts of feed to achieve the proper concentrations. However, direct addition of the test chemical to the untreated feed is often the exception rather than the rule.

a. Liquids. Dietary preparation involving liquid materials frequently results in either wet feed in which the test article does not disperse or formation of "gumballs," feed and test material that form discernible lumps and chemical "hotspots." Drying and grinding of the premix to a free-flowing form prior to mixing the final diets may be required; however, these actions could affect the chemical nature of the test article.

b. Powders, Dusts, Solids. Solid materials require special techniques prior to or during addition to the diets. Materials that are soluble in water may be dissolved and added as described above for liquids. Non–water-soluble materials may require several preparatory steps. The test chemical may be dissolved in corn oil, acetone, or other appropriate vehicles prior to addition to the weighed diet. When an organic solvent such as acetone is used, the mixing time for the premix should be sufficient for the solvent to evaporate. Some solids may require grinding in a mortar and pestle with feed added during the grinding process.

Liquid test chemicals and solvent-test chemical admixtures may "stick"to glassware during the mixing procedure. Analytical measurements of the diet admixtures generally show less than acceptable concentrations at the lower diet levels. Because of this potential problem, it is recommended that the glassware be "rinsed" with small amounts of feed. The feed should be "rubbed" against the surface to physically remove any remaining test chemical.

c. Volatile Liquids and Gases. A new category of chemicals for which dietary evaluation have been required are volatile liquids and gases. These chemicals include fumigants used for both crop protection and vermin control in food storage facilities. The chemical nature of these products does not allow for standard diet preparation. Dog and rodent studies have been performed with fumigants.

Dietary exposure to fumigated feed is a practical approach for dog studies. In these studies, the dogs are "trained" to consume diet during limited feeding periods of 1–2 hr. Fumigation of feed may be accomplished by placing the required amount of feed for a single day into a plastic drum, filling the headspace with known levels of the gas, and tumbling the drum for a period of time to mix and fumigate the feed uniformly. Prestudy trials need to be conducted to determine the appropriate gas headspace concentrations, fumigation times, and the degassing intervals necessary to achieve the study required dietary concentration ranges. Since fumigants will be degassing from the feed, a degassing curve is established by frequent diet analysis. Based on the degassing curve, the appropriate diet preparation and feeding cycle is established. For example, if the intended dietary concentration is 10 ppm, the degassing curve may show that fumigant concentration in the diet declines to 20 ppm after 60 minutes of degassing and 5 ppm after 120 minutes. On this basis, the dogs would be fed beginning 60 min after fumigation for a 1 hr period.

The food consumption patterns of rodents precludes the use of fumigated feed. Since rodents are nocturnal, the majority of feed consumption occurs over the course of the daily animal room darkness cycle. Rodents eat constantly during this period. These factors make limited duration feeding impractical. Dietary exposure of rodents to microencapsulated volatile liquids is a proven option for rodents. The volatile liquid is encapsulated in a material that prevents rapid chemical loss and will not interfere with gastric absorption of the test chemical. The impact of microencapsulation on gastric absorption can be evaluated by conducting comparative acute oral (gavage) studies to determine if the encapsulating material influences toxicity. In cases where the dietary concentrations in the study cover a broad range, it may be necessary to make microcaps containing various concentrations of the volatile liquid. This practice may be necessary to assure homogeneous dispersion of the microcaps in the treated diets. The stability of the microcaps in the diet is the determining factor regarding feeding duration. It should be noted that volatilization from microcaps may require presentation of fresh feed on a daily basis. In these cases, diets are prepared on a weekly basis, separated into 8 aliquots and stored frozen. A single aliquot is used for each day.

2. Homogeneity and Stability Assays

Prior to study initiation, homogeneity and stability of the test chemical in the diet should be determined. The most cost and time effective approach is to conduct homogeneity and stability studies on samples obtained from the same prestudy diet preparation. After diets have been mixed, duplicate or triplicate samples should be taken from the top, middle, and bottom of the mixer for homogeneity determinations. At the same time multiple samples are taken from the middle of the mixer for stability determinations. The number of stability samples depends on the expected test chemical stability and the time period over which the diet admixture will be presented to the animals. In general, diets are mixed weekly and presented to the animals for a seven day period. Room temperature stability for 8 days may be sufficient in this case. If stability is a issue, both room temperature and frozen storage stability are required. Using microencapsulated volatile liquids as an example, room temperature stability should be performed at 16 and 24 hr after removal from frozen storage. The time "0" analysis is derived from the homogeneity samples. At a minimum, frozen storage stability should be performed after 8 days if weekly dietary mixing is expected. Extension of the frozen storage stability interval may allow for less frequent diet mixing.

3. Diet Presentation

A variety of feeders are commercially available for rats and mice. These include various-sized glass jars and stainless steel or galvanized feed cups, which can be equipped with restraining lids and food followers to preclude significant losses of feed due to the animals digging in the feeders. Slotted metal feeders are designed so that animals cannot climb into the feed and also contain mesh food followers to prevent digging.

The frequency of fresh diet presentation depends on the stability of the test chemical in the diet and study design requirements for determination of food consumption.

B. Oral Intubation in Rats and Mice

Oral gavage dosing is an effective alternative to dietary presentation especially in cases where the test material may be unstable in a dietary admixture or when the dietary admixture is unpalatable or unacceptable to the test animal. The accuracy of dosage level is more precise than that of the dietary regimen; however, the toxicological responses of the animal to a single bolus may differ from that seen with ad libitum feeding.

The presence or absence of food in the stomach may influence the response of the animal to the test chemical as well as the acceptability of the gavage technique. Stomach components may interact with the test article, potentially altering both the absorption and toxicological response of the test chemical. Food content in the stomach also limits the volume of dosing solution that can be given to the animal, thereby influencing the maximum achievable dose level that can be presented to the animal. This is an important consideration for materials with low vehicle solubility or those that must be prepared in dilute form for animal acceptability. Test chemicals that cause significant gastrointestinal irritation must be prepared in dilute form or dosed to nonfasted animals to lessen this effect.

Oral intubation in rats and mice is commonly used in acute oral toxicity studies and has been used more frequently in subchronic and chronic toxicity studies over the last several years. Standard dosing needles depend on the size of the animal. A 20-gauge oral dosing needle approximately 1.5 in. (3.8 cm) long with a blunt tip of 1.25 mm diameter is generally used for mice.

Successful gavage dosing requires immobilization of the animal's head such that the esophagus forms a straight line from the mouth to the stomach. The mouse is grasped by the skin behind the neck using the thumb and forefingers. The back of the animal is held against the palm of the hand by the remaining fingers.

Recommended dosing needles for rats are the 16 gauge, 3 in. (7.6 cm) long needle with a blunt tip of 3 mm diameter or a 14 gauge, 3 in. (7.6 cm) long needle with a blunt tip of 4 mm diameter. The rat is held in one hand with the thumb placed under the animal's foreleg pushing the leg upward toward the head. The forefingers hold the animal's body against the palm of the hand.

The tip of the needle is placed in the animal's mouth on either side of the incisors and guided toward the esophagus. With slight pressure and gentle rotation of the needle from side to side, the needle should slide into the esophagus and down toward the stomach. The material is injected into the stomach and the needle is retracted. Forcing the needle may cause esophageal rupture or entry into the trachea and lungs. These trauma injuries may result in infection, clinical symptomatology, and even death of the animal.

C. Exposure to Drinking Water

Industrial, agricultural, and domestic chemical uses may result in the introduction of chemical contaminants into drinking water. For this reason, the OPPTS guidelines include drinking water as a testing regimen.

Physicochemical properties of the test material dictate the acceptability of drinking water as a dosing matrix. Unlike diet preparation or preparation of gavage dose solutions and suspensions where a variety of solvents and physical processes can be utilized to prepare a dosable form, preparation of drinking water solutions are less flexible. Water solubility of the test chemical is the major governing factor and is dependent on factors such as pH, dissolved salts, and temperature. The animal model itself sets limitations for these factors (acceptability and suitability of pH and salt-adjusted water by the animals as well as environmental specifications such as animal room temperature).

Stability of the test chemical in drinking water under study conditions should be determined prior to study initiation. Consideration should be given to conducting stability tests on test chemical/drinking water admixtures presented to some test animals. Besides difficulties of inherent stability, changes in chemical concentrations may result from other influences. Chemicals with low vapor pressure can volatilize from the water into the air space located above the water of an inverted water bottle; thus, a majority of the chemical may be found in the "dead space" not in the water.

Certain test chemicals may be degraded by microorganism contamination. A primary source of these microorganisms is the oral cavity of the rodents. This is especially a concern with guinea pigs. Guinea pigs, and to a lesser extent rats and mice, may "spit back through the sipper tubes into water bottles. Significant bacteria can pass via the sipper tubes and water flow restraints into the water bottles. Sanitation and sterilization procedures for water bottles and sipper tubes must be rigorously maintained to prevent further bacterial growth. A substandard water bottle washer may in fact supply temperature and humidity conditions that may facilitate bacterial growth.

Water bottles should be considered as the least important equipment needed in a drinking water study. Properly fitting rubber stoppers, properly shaped sipper tubes, water restraints, and suitable bottle holders working in conjunction should be considered more important. Worn, poorly fitting, hardened rubber stoppers are the main reason for water spillage. Slight movement of the animal cage racks or activity such as the animal drinking, provide sufficient force to pop these stoppers from the bottle and spill its contents.

Water bottle holders should permit easy accessibility to the animal room staff in changing and replacing the bottles, yet be secure enough to keep the water bottle in place when a rack is moved.

Sipper tubes should be shaped so that access to water is not impaired when the sipper tube is used in conjunction with the bottle, stopper, and holder. Water restrainers are stainless steel ball bearings of sufficient size to preclude water flow and dripping from the bottle and readily movable by the animal to permit it to drink. Water restraints should be checked frequently to assure that water is accessible and that no dripping occurs. Animal saliva and food particles may cause the water restraints to become inoperable so that either water is not accessible to the animal or the water drips continuously from the bottle.

Accurate water consumption data is necessary to calculate meaningful compound intake data. The technical staff involved in the study should be aware of the need for properly fitting equipment and the necessity to prevent water spillage. Whether preparing a few or several hundred bottles, a lack of consistency in the amount of water is generally apparent. The tendency in water bottles filling is to overfill the bottles to assure sufficient water for a specified duration. Technical staff should be aware that an air space above the water in an inverted bottle is essential for the free flow of water. It is frustrating to an investigator to lose study animals to dehydration when an excess of water was available.

III. MOUSE SKIN PAINTING/DERMAL CARCINOGENICITY BIOASSAYS

Skin painting bioassays, generally in mice, have been conducted on a multitude of chemicals. The dermal carcinogenicity of many types of products such as tobacco smoke condensates and oil-based products have demonstrated that continuous application of these classes of materials to the skin of mice produces skin tumors ranging from papillomas to carcinomas. The ability of test chemicals to act as initiators or promoters of dermal tumors can also be demonstrated by proper design of the test protocol. The ability of the mouse skin to respond positively to various test chemicals is thought to be related to the presence of dermal enzymes necessary for producing those intermediates capable of acting as initiators or promoters.

The key point in the design of any skin painting bioassay is to determine the purpose of the study. As discussed above, these studies can be designed to determine the dermal oncogenic potential of the test material itself, as well as the potential of test chemicals to act as initiators and/or promoters. After the purpose of the study has been established, the frequency of test material application must be evaluated. Dosing in skin painting studies can range from daily to weekly applications for study durations ranging from several weeks up to the lifetime of the animal. Unlike standard mouse oncogenicity studies, a single dose level of the test material is generally used rather than multiple dose levels.

The OPPTS guideline for carcinogenicity (7) has expanded the classical design for dermal carcinogenesis studies. The basic designs is that typical of any carcinogenicity study, i.e., at least 3 dose levels should be tested for risk assessment purposes. Animals should be exposed to the tests chemical for at least 6 hr/day and, based on practical considerations, 5 day/week dosing is acceptable.

In dermal carcinogenicity studies, the highest dose should not destroy the integrity of the skin. Acceptance criteria for this high dose include the following:

Gross skin findings:

> Erythema (moderate)
> Scaling
> Edema (mild)
> Alopecia
> Thickening

Histologic skin findings:

> Epidermal hyperplasia
> Epidermal hyperkeratosis
> Epidermal parakeratosis
> Adnexal atrophy/hyperplasia

Fibrosis
Spongiosis (minimal-mild)
Epidermal edema (minimal-mild)
Dermal edema (minimal-moderate)
Inflammation (moderate)

Obvious eschar, fissuring, ulceration or necrosis clearly exceeds the high dose acceptance criteria. The middle dose in a dermal carcinogenicity study should be minimally irritating; the low dose should be the highest nonirritating dose.

A.   Animal Preparation and Test Material Administration

Since these studies are via the dermal route, the hair must be removed from the intended site of application. The test material is generally dosed to the intrascapular area of the mouse in order to prevent potential oral ingestion and to provide a distinct area for observation for the appearance of dermal tumors. An approximate 1 in.^{2} area is shaved free of hair using an electric clipper equipped with a size 40 clipper blade. The predose shaving should be completed a few days prior to the initiation of treatment so that any minor nicks or abrasions have sufficient time for healing. Follow-up shaving should be as needed and once per week is generally sufficient. Care must be taken in the reshaving process so that neither the skin nor any dermal masses are disrupted by the shaving process.

Dosing volumes typically used in the skin painting bioassay are in the microliter range (50–100 μl doses are standard). These small dose volumes can be achieved by using either plastic-tipped calibrated micropipettes or automatic dosing syringe dispensers. Both types of dispensers are commercially available. However, for efficiency in the dosing procedure, the syringe dispenser is preferable. Standard syringe dispensers contain 2500 μl of a test article and precise 50 μl doses can be applied. In this manner a full syringe permits dosing of a group of 50 animals with each receiving a 50 μl dose. These syringes can be cleaned easily; however, it is recommended that one syringe be used for each test article during the course of the study. For both the shaving and dosing procedures, the animal is removed from the cage and allowed to firmly grip the bottom of the wire-mesh cage with its front legs. Gentle pressure is applied to the tail of the animal stretching the animal to a semi-immobile position. In this position, the back can be shaved or the test material can be applied. During the dosing procedure, the tip of the syringe is used to spread the test material evenly in the dosing region.

B.   Tissue Mass Observations

The frequency of observation of the animal for the appearance for dermal tumors depends on the needs of the investigator (skinpainting studies) and the study design. Observation of the animal for dermal tumors on at least a weekly basis is necessary for determination of the time to tumor development. Any skin irregularities that are less than 1 mm and larger masses that do not protrude above the skin surface are generally disregarded. Lesions that measure at least 1 mm but less than 2 mm in diameter are defined as such and are carefully observed since masses of this type have a relatively high incidence of spontaneous regression. A dermal skin lesion is considered to be significant if it reaches or exceeds 2 mm in diameter and protrudes above the surrounding skin. The time previously recorded for a lesion reaching 1 mm in diameter is assumed to be the time of first appearance. Once a lesion has grown to 2 mm the animal is considered to be a lesion bearer even if that lesion regresses or subsequently disappears.

Accurate records of the disposition of each mass are essential. Tissue masses are generally recorded on specifically designed data bearing dorsal and ventral views of the animal. At the time of appearance, the position and size of the mass is drawn onto the diagram. The first mass is numbered 1, and the measurements and location of the mass are recorded in the data record. Additional masses are numbered sequentially and the locations and measurements recorded. In most cases, this procedure is very simple; however, certain procedures must be followed to prevent loss of mass identification under certain circumstances. It is not uncommon for a single animal to bear as many as 6–20 tissue masses in initiation/promotion studies or with positive control substances. Masses may eventually increase in size to the point where two or more masses may merge. In order that the identity of individual masses be maintained, the merged mass should carry the numbers of the individual masses. For example, if masses 1 and 2 merge, the data for the merged mass is recorded as mass 1, 2. If a mass regresses or disappears, these data are also recorded. It is not uncommon for the wartlike lesions noted from 3,4-benzo-(a)-pyrene treatment to disappear. Histological evaluation of the underlying skin shows evidence of a squamous cell carcinoma. The careful maintenance of the tissue mass data through the time of necropsy permits complete accountability so that gross to microscopic determination can be made. In the histopathological evaluation of these tumors, the pathologist should be consulted regarding the necessity of evaluation of all observed masses.

IV. REPEATED PERCUTANEOUS TOXICITY STUDIES

Guidelines for repeated percutaneous toxicity studies are included in the OPPTS Harmonized Test Guidelines (4,5). These studies are commonly conducted in the rat and rabbit and occasionally in the guinea pig. Although the design for these studies is the same, the techniques for shaving and dosing are species specific.

A. Shaving

Approximately 24 hr prior to the first application of the test material, the backs of the test animals are clipped closely of hair using standard small animal clippers. The clipping should be completed so that no abrasions or other disruption of the dermis occurs. It is essential that the clippers be in good condition (not dull) to prevent these types of dermal damage.

The small motor of the clippers tends to overheat and lose efficiency. Therefore several sets of clippers should be available so that they can be alternated, avoiding overheating and eventual breakdown of the clippers. Dull blades also contribute to shaving difficulty. Additional sets of sharpened blades should be available. A stiff brush should be used to remove excess hair and avoid clogging the blades. A clipper lubricant spray used between each animal also assists in the easy removal of hair. Hair should always be clipped in the direction opposite to the hair growth pattern.

For rabbits, clipping is facilitated by using two technicians. One technician removes the rabbit from its cage and places it on a hard flat surface. The rabbit is grasped firmly by the skin at the nape of the neck and at the lower back just above the hind legs. The second person can then clip the hair from the animal. Because of seasonal variations in hair growth for rabbits, a two-step clipping procedure may be necessary. In the first step, an Angra blade is used to shorten the length of the hair. The remaining hair is removed using a size 40 animal clipper blade. The clipped area should approximate 10–15% of the body surface area.

Rats can be held and clipped in the same manner as rabbits. This is particularly required for large rats that have not been placed on study. Clipping of young rats can be completed by one person. Either of two procedures can be utilized. In one procedure, the rat is held by the nape of the neck with the legs hanging. The technician can then remove the hair from the back. In the second procedure, the animal is gently cradled in the palm of the technician's hand. The animal is then clipped. Guinea pigs can be clipped in the same manner as rats.

B. Test Article Application

Liquid test articles are applied directly to the skin and spread evenly over the body surface. If a large volume of liquid is required, the test material can be applied under gauze patches to prevent the test material from flowing to the flanks and abdominal regions of the animal. For test articles in the form of flakes, powders, granules, or other particulates, the appropriate amount of test material can be placed on a gauze pad which has been moistened with a vehicle such as physiological saline and applied to the animal. The design of the study will dictate whether the test sites are occluded or nonoccluded. When occlusion is not required the animal may be fitted with an Elizabethan collar to prevent ingestion of the test chemical. The collars should be used only during the exposure period if possible. Collars should be firm fitting but not so tight that breathing or the animal's ability to eat or drink is impaired. A properly fitting collar for a rat will slide over the animal's head with gentle pressure but be tight enough so that it cannot be easily removed by simple forelimb pressure by the animal. Attachment of the collar is completed by placing it in front of the rat so that the animal explores it with his nose. As the nose pokes through the central hole, the collar is gently pushed over the head and neck with a twisting motion. The collar should be checked for proper fit once it is in place.

In cases where collars are not used, oral ingestion can be precluded by either occlusive or nonocclusive dressings. Nonocclusive dressings include cotton flannel, additional gauze, and elastic bandages. Occlusive dressings include rubber dental dam and impervious plastic sheeting. The entire trunk of the animal is covered with the wrapping material which is secured in place with several long strips of adhesive tape at the anterior and posterior ends. The area of taping should be as distant from the dosing area as possible since tape burns may preclude the appropriate evaluation of the skin for irritation reactions. The tape should not be applied in such a manner to affect the animal's ability to move in its cage or to breathe properly. It is a common mistake for animal technicians to apply the tape so tightly that animals succumb to the dosing and wrapping techniques. At the end of the exposure period the wrappings are cut with scissors and removed. Any test material remaining on the skin may be wiped or washed if required by the study protocol.

C. Dermal Observations

Exposure sites may be graded for appearance of dermal irritation by several different systems. The most frequently used system is that of Draize (14). The design for the study should give consideration as to the frequency of these observations. It is also important to include a provision in the protocol for the early sacrifice of the animals for humane reasons. If excessive irritation, fissuring, or necrosis are observed and these findings are deemed to have an adverse effect on the animal, sacrifice should be considered.

V. CLINICAL ASSESSMENTS

During the course of repeated-dose toxicity studies, the animals are observed on a regular basis for mortality, moribundity, signs of generalized toxicity, and changes in body weight and food consumption. Additional tests may be included in the experimental design to assess potential effects on hematological, biochemical, physiological, neurological, and ophthalmological parameters. The selection of the appropriate tests depends on the use of the chemical, the regulatory body for which the test is conducted, and suspected organ systems that may be affected by ingestion of the chemical.

A. Generalized Toxicity

Every animal is observed at regular intervals for differences in the physical condition and behavior of the animal and for the location and character of specific abnormal findings. Commonly, all animals are observed at least twice daily, once in the morning and once in the late afternoon, for mortality and general physical appearance. These observations should be made on a frequent enough basis to limit the numbers of unobserved animal deaths and tissue loss to autolysis.

Physical examinations include observations for pharmacological and toxicological effects, behavioral abnormalities, and digital palpation for tissue masses. Most laboratories have, as standard operating procedure, defined those clinical findings considered appropriate for each animal specie. Terminology for clinical findings should be standardized by the laboratory. These observations are generally comprised of those obvious signs that can be readily identified by a skilled technician rather than diagnostic evaluations reserved for the study director or other specialists.

Digital palpation of the test animals for suspected tumors is completed on a regular basis and records regarding the time to appearance and disposition of the lesions can be maintained. These records should include the location, size, and any changes that may have occurred since the previous interval. A system for tracking tissue masses has been previously described in the dermal toxicity section. Some laboratories measure tissue masses to include length, width, and height while other laboratories use descriptive terms to serve this purpose (e.g., pea-sized).

B. Clinical Pathology

On a scheduled basis, blood samples are withdrawn to evaluate changes in hematologic and serum chemistry. Urinalysis may be performed based on expected or observed toxicity. Standard hematological evaluations include hemoglobin and hematocrit concentrations, red blood cell count, white blood cell count, differential leukocyte count, platelet count, and a measure of clotting such as prothrombin time or thromboplastin time.

Standard serum chemistry evaluations include assessment of liver and kidney function, carbohydrate metabolism, and electrolyte balance. Serum chemistry evaluation are also expanded to assess chemical specific toxicity (methemoglobin and cholinesterase activity) that may be the basis for risk assessment for a chemical class. In other cases, specific serum chemistry parameters are included to assess potential mechanisms of toxicity (hormonal changes, lipid metabolism, enzyme induction).

C. Ophthalmology

Ophthalmological evaluations are performed to determine changes in the ocular tissues of the animals. The pupils are dilated and evaluations are made by an observer skilled in the use of a slit-lamp biomicroscope, funduscope, or other appropriate equipment.

D. Neurological Assessments

Over the last several years, regulatory agencies have required the evaluation of the potential for drugs and chemicals to elicit neurotoxic responses. It has become a common practice to include at least some additional neurologic evaluations to subchronic toxicity studies or to add satellite groups to these studies to evaluate neurotoxicity. Standard testing protocols to evaluate neurotoxicity include the Functional Observational Battery (FOB) (15,16,17,18,19) Locomotor Activity (20) and Neuropathology (19). In a 13-week study, the FOB and Locomotor Activity assessments are performed prior to study and after 4, 8, and 13 weeks of treatment.

1. Functional Observational Battery

Six observation domains are evaluated in the standard FOB; home cage, handling, open field, sensory neuromuscular and physiological. With the exception of the home cage observations, the FOB should be performed in a soundproof room with minimal disturbance and technician traffic. Some laboratories have custom designed rooms, including some with white noise generators for FOB evaluation. The details of the FOB observation procedures are discussed elsewhere.

Home cage measurements are performed while the animals are in a study cage or a transfer cage. Evaluation of posture, clonic and/or tonic movements, convulsions, tremors, biting, feces consistency, and palpebral (eyelid) closure are generally performed cageside before opening the cage. However, it may be necessary to remove the animal from the cage in order to see the animal's eyes.

Handling observations are made as the animal is removed from the cage and immediately after removal. Some of the observation parameters include ease of removal, reaction to handling, muscle tone, lacrimation/chromodacryorrhea, piloerection, exophthalmus, salivation, fur appearance, respiratory rate and character, and palpebral closure.

Open field evaluation is as the name implies. The animal is placed in the center of an open field testing box and observed for a specified period time, generally 2–5 min. Measurements of open field activity include the number of times that the animal rears, time to first step, number of urine pools and defecations. Scoring of clonic/tonic movements, gait, mobility, backing, arousal, vocalization, respiration, stereotypic behavior, and bizarre behavior is performed in accordance with laboratory scoring systems.

Stimulus reactivity are measured in the sensorimotor assessment. Approach response, touch response, startle (click) reaction, olfactory stimulation, and tail pinch reaction are performed generally in the open field box after the open field evaluation has completed. Pupil response, eyeblink response, righting reflex, temperature (hot plate) response and forelimb/hindlimb extension are performed upon removal of the animal from the open cage activity box.

Forelimb and hindlimb grip strength are determined using strain gauges with wire mesh screens. The animal is allow to grip the screen and the force required to release the grip upon pulling the animal away from the strain gauge is determined. Rotarod performance is measured over a designated time period. Hindlimb splay measurements are performed. Each evaluation should be performed at least 3 times.

Physiological evaluations include body weight, body temperature, and catalepsy.

2. Locomotor Activity

In most laboratories, locomotor activity is performed upon completion of the FOB. Each animal is placed in an individual, computer-controlled Activity Monitor System. This system utilizes a series of infrared photocells surrounding a clear plastic, rectangular cage. The photocells are generally place in a manner to record both horizontal and vertical movements. The number of activity monitoring subsets and durations are generally laboratory specific. The most common subset duration is 10 min, which may be monitored for 4–6 individual subsets.

3. Neuropathology

At the time of necropsy, animals selected for neuropathological evaluation are euthanized and perfused in situ with appropriate fixative (e.g., 3% paraformaldehyde and 3% glutaraldehyde in 0.1M phosphate buffer). Brain weight and brain dimensions (length and width) are recorded and central and peripheral nervous system tissues are collected and preserved for microscopic examination. Central nervous tissues include brain (including cerebrum, cerebellum, pons and medulla oblongata), spinal cord, gasserian ganglion/trigeminal nerves, lumbar and cervical dorsal root ganglion, lumbar and cervical dorsal root fibers, lumbar and cervical ventral root fibers and optic nerves. Peripheral nervous tissue include sciatic nerves, sural nerves, tibial nerves, peroneal nerves. These tissues are appropriate processed and stained and microscopic evaluation performed.

4. Other Procedures

Where appropriate, measurement of plasma, red blood cell, and brain cholinesterase may be included in neurotoxicity studies. Glial fibrillary acid protein (GFAP) immunohistochemistry may also be performed.

E. Immunologic Evaluation

Guidelines (10) have been developed to evaluate the potential for repeated exposure of test substances to induce suppression of immune function. Some information regarding immunotoxicity may be determined from hematology, lymphoid organ weights and histopathology from standard repeated dose toxicity studies. These endpoints alone may not provide sufficient data to predict immunotoxicity (21, 22).

The OPPTS guideline for immunotoxicity requires a minimum of 28 days exposure. Immunotoxicity evaluations may be added to standard subchronic toxicity studies. Immune function as measured by antibody response to antigen are determined by the Antibody Plaque Forming Cell (PFC) Assay (23) or the Enzyme-Linked Immunosorbent (ELISA) Assay (24,25). Immunotoxicity is also assessed by evaluation of Natural Killer (NK) cell activity (26) and by enumeration of splenic or peripheral blood total B-cells, total T-cells, and T-cell subpopulations (27,28).

VI. DATA INTERPRETATION

The primary step in the evaluation of data from repeated dose toxicity studies should include a review of the purpose for which the study was conducted. Since these studies provide the basis upon which regulatory bodies assess the potential risks to humans associated with chemical exposure the most current reporting requirements of that agency should be reviewed. Specific reporting and evaluation requirements can be found in the FIFRA or TSCA test guidelines or in test rules for the specific chemical. The EPA has also prepared data evaluation guidelines for several types of studies.

Data evaluation requires appropriate statistical comparisons of the data from the treated groups to the collateral control groups. Statistically significant differences between the control and treated groups are considered as an indication of chemical-related effect but not as definitive proof.

Because of the limited numbers of animals used in toxicity studies, statistical comparisons of study data to both published and in-house historical control data permits a more valid assessment of potential treatment effects. An organization can provide no better service to their professionals for data evaluation than a properly controlled, statistically compared base of historical laboratory data.

Upon completion of the statistical evaluation of the data, the toxicologist can make an interpretation and evaluation of the study data. This evaluation involves the professional opinion of the study director and other scientists. Therefore, no simple rules or procedures exist or can be provided. Knowledge of dose-response criteria and of "normal" values coupled with the statistical evaluations are most frequently the basis for decision making. In the final analysis, however, it is the experience and intuition of the scientists that arrive at the final conclusions.

VII. COMMON MISTAKES

Some common mistakes and problems associated with the various test procedures have been included in the sections above.

The most basic premise in the conduct of any toxicity study is that the correct animal must receive the correct dose for the duration specified in the protocol. The most serious mistake that can occur in the conduct of a study is the misdosing of the test animals. Errors in observations or procedural errors in dosing (with the exception of animal death or irreversible damage) can generally be corrected without the loss of the entire study. Misdosing of the animals cannot be corrected.

Procedures for the correct identification of the animal and for the test chemical are essential. A simple procedure entails color coding of dosing solution containers and animal cage cards. The labels on the dosing solution containers should include, as a minimum, the study number, the concentration of the test chemical in the solution (diet), the treatment group number, and the mixing date. Animal cage cards should include the permanent animal number, study number, group number, sex, dose level, and study initiation date.

Proper calculations of compound and matrix needs are necessary for proper preparation. These calculations can be made and verified in one step. Two technical personnel (e.g., the study director and the lab supervisor) independently perform the calculations by whatever method each is most familiar with, the results are compared, and any discrepancies resolved. Final calculations should be reverified by each person.

The procedures for the preparation of the dosing solution should be written in recipe form so that anyone could, if the need occurred, be able to properly mix the dosing vehicle. This procedure should be readily accessible also. It serves no purpose to have a detailed procedure that cannot be found when needed. Analytical verification of the dose media should be done prior to initiation of the study to assure the acceptability of the mixing procedures.

An embarrassing situation that occurs more frequently than one would admit is being informed by the laboratory that an insufficient quantity of test chemical is available. This lack of sufficient test article is usually discovered when the most current dosing matrix is being prepared for use the following day or week. Too frequently, calculations of chemical need are performed prior to the study using the appropriate factors (food consumption, dose level, number of animals, weeks of study) without consideration, for example, that the laboratory mixes an excess amount of diet each week to make sure that the animals don't run out of feed. This problem can be avoided by determining the quantity of test material required for the study and multiplying that amount by 2 or 3 fold. The calculated "sufficient" amount of the test article is shipped to the laboratory and the remainder stored as a contingency. This is particularly important for chronic studies where a single lot of test material, if possible, should be used for the entire study or battery of studies. A practical approach to chemical storage is the chemical repository. The repository holds all test chemical and ships the appropriate amount to the test facilities on a prearranged schedule. To assure chemical stability over long term storage, it is a recommended practice to perform purity analysis on the test article prior to shipment.

Selection of the appropriate dose vehicle is essential. The influence of the vehicle on the toxicity of the test chemical is a major consideration since the wrong vehicle may derail the development of a new chemical or affect the risk assessment of an existing chemical. For example, the oral toxicity of the pyrethroids is greater (lower oral LD_{50}) in oil based vehicles as compared to aqueous suspensions. With some pyrethroids, the difference is as great as tenfold (29). A vehicle may also enhance the degradation of the test article to a more toxic moiety. The ethylene bis-dithiocarbamates (EBDCs) degrade to ethylenethiourea (ETU) when dimethylsulfoxide (DMSO) is used as a vehicle.

VIII. SUMMARY

The purpose of this chapter was to discuss some of the methods involved in the conduct of repeated-dose toxicity studies by the oral and dermal routes. The information was not intended as a "how-to" for these types of studies but rather to supply helpful suggestions for conducting these tests and avoiding some of the common problems associated with repeated-dose tests.

REFERENCES

1. U.S. Environmental Protection Agency, 1996. Health Effects Test Guidelines.
2. U.S. Environmental Protection Agency, 1996. Health Effects Test Guidelines. OPPTS 870.3100, 90-Day oral toxicity. EPA Publication number 712-C-96-199.
3. U.S. Environmental Protection Agency, 1996. Health Effects Test Guidelines. OPPTS 870.3150, Subchronic nonrodent oral toxicity-90-day. EPA Publication number 712-C-96-200.
4. U.S. Environmental Protection Agency, 1996. Health Effects Test Guidelines. OPPTS 870.3200, Repeated dose dermal toxicity-21/28 days. EPA Publication number 712-C-96-201.

5. U.S. Environmental Protection Agency, 1996. Health Effects Test Guidelines. OPPTS 870.3250, Subchronic dermal toxicity-90 days. EPA Publication number 712-C-96-202.
6. U.S. Environmental Protection Agency, 1996. Health Effects Test Guidelines. OPPTS 870.4100, Chronic toxicity. EPA Publication number 712-C-96-210.
7. U.S. Environmental Protection Agency, 1996. Health Effects Test Guidelines. OPPTS 870.4200, Carcinogenicity. EPA Publication number 712-C-96-211.
8. U.S. Environmental Protection Agency, 1996. Health Effects Test Guidelines. OPPTS 870.4300, Combined chronic toxicity/carcinogenicity. EPA Publication number 712-C-96-212.
9. U.S. Environmental Protection Agency, 1996. Health Effects Test Guidelines. OPPTS 870.6200, Neurotoxicity screening battery. EPA Publication number 712-C-96-238.
10. U.S. Environmental Protection Agency, 1996. Health Effects Test Guidelines. OPPTS 870.7800, Immunotoxicity. EPA Publication number 712-C-96-351.
11. U.S. Food and Drug Administration, 1982. Toxicological Principles: For the Safety Assessment of Direct Food Additives and Color Additives Used in Food", National Technical Information Service Document PB83170696.
12. United States Pharmaceutical Manufacturers Association. (1977). Guidelines for the Assessment of Drug and Medical Device Safety in Animals.
13. Food and Drug Administration. (1971). Introduction to total drug quality. U.S. Government Printing Office.
14. Draize, J.H. (1959). Dermal toxicity. In *Appraisal of the Safety of Chemicals in Foods, Drugs, and Cosmetics*. Association of Food and Drug Officials of the United States (3rd printing 1975) pp. 46–59.
15. Irwin, S. (1968). Comprehensive observational assessment: Ia. A systematic quantitative procedure for assessing the behavioral and physiological state of a mouse. *Psychopharmacologia* 13: 222–256.
16. Moser, V.C., McCormick, J.P., Creason, J.P., and MacPhail, R.C. (1988). Comparison of chlordimeform and carbaryl using a functional observational battery. Fund. Appl. Toxicol. 11: 189–206.
17. Gad, S. (1982). A neuromuscular screen for use in industrial toxicology. J. Toxicol. Environ. Health 9: 691–704.
18. Haggerty, G.C. (1989). Development of Tier 1 Neurobehavioral Testing Capabilities for Incorporation into Pivotal Rodent Safety Assessment Studies. J. Amer. Coll. Toxicol. 8: 53–69.
19. O'Donoghue, J.L. (1989). Screening for Neurotoxicity Using a Neurologically Based Examination and Neuropathology. J. Amer. Coll. Toxicol. 8: 97–116.
20. Reiter, L.W. and MacPhail, R.C. (1979). Motor activity: A survey of methods with potential use in toxicity testing. *Neurobehav. Toxicol.* (Suppl.) 1: 53–66
21. Luster, M.I., Portier, C., Pait, D.G., White, K.L., Jr., Gennings, C., Munson, A.E., and Rosenthal, G.J. (1992). Risk Assessment in Immunotoxicology. I. Sensitivity and predictability of immune tests. Fundam. Appl. Toxicol. 18: 200–210.

22. Luster, M.I., Portier, C., Pait, D.G., Rosenthal, G.J., Germolec, D.R., Corsini, E., Blaylock, B.L., Pollock, P., Kouchi, Y,. Craig, W., White, D.L., Munson, A.E., and Comment, C.E. (1993). Risk Assessment in Immunotoxicology. II. Relationship Between Immune and Host Resistance Tests. Fundam. Appl. Toxicol. 21: 71–82.

23. Holsapple, M.P. (1995). The plaque-forming cell (PFC) response in: "Immunotoxicology: and approach to monitoring the primary effector function of B lymphocytes". In *Methods in Immunotoxicology* (G.R. Burleson, J.H. Dean, and A.E. Munson, Eds.), Vol. 1, pp. 71–108, Wiley-Liss, Inc., New York.

24. Temple, L., Butterworth, L., Kawabata, T.T., Munson, A.E., and White, K.L. (1995). Elisa to Measure SRBC Specific Serum IgM: Methods and Data Evaluation. In *Methods in Immunotoxicology* (G.R. Burleson, J.H. Dean, and A.E. Munson, Eds.), Vol. 1, pp. 137–157, Wiley-Liss, Inc., New York.

25. Ladics, G.S., Smith, C. Heaps, K. and Loveless, S.E. (1994). Evaluation of the humoral immune response of CD rats following a 2-week exposure to the pesticide carbaryl by the oral, dermal, or inhalation routes. J. Toxicol. Environ. Health 42: 143–156.

26. Djeu, Julie Y. (1995). Natural Killer Activity. In *Methods in Immunotoxicology* (G.R. Burleson, J.H. Dean, and A.E. Munson, Eds.), Vol. 1, pp. 437–449, Wiley-Liss, Inc., New York.

27. Ladics, G.S., and Loveless, S.E. (1994). Cell surface marker analysis of splenic lymphocyte populations of the CD rat for use in immunotoxicological studies. Toxicol. Methods 4: 77–91.

28. Cornacoff, J.B., Graham, C.S., and LaBrie, T.K., (1995). Phenotypic identification of peripheral blood mononuclear leukocytes by flow cytometry as an adjunct to immunotoxicity evaluation. In *Methods in Immunotoxicology* (G.R. Burleson, J.H. Dean, and A.E. Munson, Eds.), Vol. 1, pp. 211–226, Wiley-Liss, Inc., New York.

29. Litchfield, M.H. (1985). Chapter 3. Toxicity to Mammals. In *The Pyrethroid Insecticides* (J.P. Leahey, editor) Taylor and Francis, London and Philadephia.

8

Neuro and Behavioral Toxicology Testing

Shayne Cox Gad
Gad Consulting Services, Raleigh, North Carolina

I. INTRODUCTION

Though nervous system toxicity has been with us since antiquity (in such forms as mercury and lead poisoning), and there were significant incidents associated with specific synthetic chemicals earlier in this century ("ginger jake" paralysis due to cresyl phosphates in 1930 and polyneuritis associated with exposure to carbon disulfide in the 1940s, for example), it is only since 1970 that awareness of the scope and importance of the problem has become generally acknowledged. In the last 25 years this domain, originally restricted to a few researchers, has broadened to a vast field for scientists from such diverse disciplines as biochemistry, physiology, pharmacology, neurology, psychiatry, psychology, occupational health, epidemiology, and internal medicine. The increased interest stems mainly from advances in the field of neuroscience and from enhanced public awareness of the major problems arising from deliberate or unintentional exposure to potentially neurotoxic chemicals. Such exposure might involve substance abuse, neurological and psychiatric disorders caused by drugs, and poorly controlled or unavoidable levels of chemicals present it the work place or in the environment.

Research and test evaluations developed and approaches applied since 1980 (neurophysiology, morphological techniques, neurochemistry, and behavioral measures) have both greatly increased our ability to detect abnormalities and led to confusion over their interpretation.

Our limited understanding of both the mechanisms underlying neurotoxic-induced diseases and of the structure–activity relationships involved with neurotoxicity still complicates (and perhaps precludes) any firm classification of neurotoxicants based on either changes they produce (in structure or function) or on structural similarities between neurotoxic compounds or their active components. Indeed, in most cases, the actions of neurotoxic compounds are arrays of damage or dysfunction in various portions of the nervous system, and not single discrete target actions. Significant progress has been made in understanding effects at the cellular level, however.

One can consider a working classification of neurotoxicants based on their primary or first seen target site. One such classification is:

Sensory
Motor
Peripheral (both sensory and motor)
Central (integrative or behavioral)

The approach to identifying and evaluating potential neurotoxicants that will be presented in this chapter is a tier-type approach. This approach is presented in diagrammatic form in Figure 1. This particular approach is from Gad (1), but others (2,3) have made similar recommendations.

The front end of this tier approach is a screen, the functional observation battery (FOB). This is the tool of choice for initial (and for most of the compounds covered by this volume, the only screen tests for) identification of potentially neurotoxic chemicals. The use of such screens, other behavioral test methods, or what are generally called clinical observations does, however, warrant one major caution or consideration. That is that short-term (within 24 hr of dosing or exposure) observations are insufficient on their own to differentiate between pharmacologic (reversible in the short term) and toxicological (irreversible) effects. To so differentiate, it is necessary to either use additional means of evaluation (such as indicated in Fig. 1, and including morphological evaluations) or to have the period during which observations are made expanded through at least 3–4 days after the cessation of dosing. The use of a brain (specifically, hippocampal) slice screening method has also gained popularity (Chang & Slilelser, 1995).

Table 1 presents a summary of neurotoxic agents identified to date.

II. GENERAL TEST DESIGNS

The most generally useful test of detector for a neurotoxicant is enhanced careful observation of animals during such traditional toxicology studies as acute and subchorionic oral and reproductive and teratology studies. A formal means of ensuring such a set of observations is to use an observational screen as proposed by several researchers (4–6,45). Such a screen, integrated into the normal course of other systemic toxicity studies, is the initial step in evaluating the

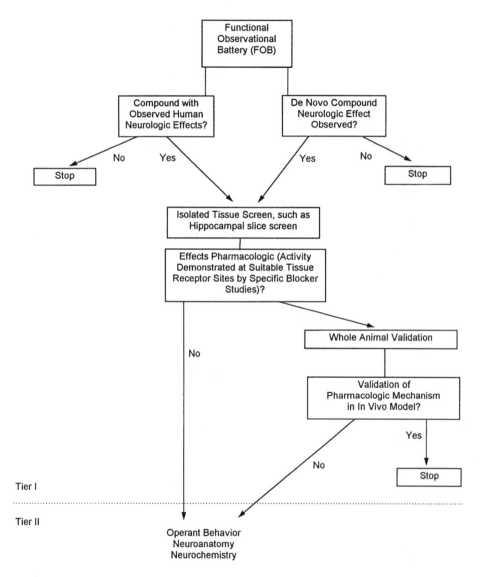

Figure 1 Tiered–decision-tree approach to neurotoxicity screening.

Table 1 Known Neurotoxic Agents

Agents	Effects
Methylmercury	Purkinje cell loss
	Sensory deficits
Lead	Parietal pyramidal cell loss
	Learning deficits
	Motor deficits
X-irradiation	Cortical pyramidal cell loss
	Hyperactivity
Arsenic	Sensory and motor deficits
Organic phosphates	Peripheral neuropathy (sensory and motor deficits)
DDT	Hyperexcitability
Carbon disulfide	Polyneuropathy; central nervous system effects (acute psychosis and motor and sensory effects)
Acrylamide	Sensory and motor deficits
Hexachlorophene	Convulsions; central nervous system effects
Methyl n-butyl ketone (and n-hexane)	Peripheral neuropathy (sensory and motor)
Thallium	Peripheral neuropathy
Triethyitin (Ortganotins)	Hyperexcitability; motor deficit; myclinotoxicity
Kepone (Chlorodecone)	Tremors; central nervous system effects
Styrene	Central nervous system, sensory, and motor effects
Dimethylaminoproprionitrile	Sensory and motor deficits
5, 7, 11-Dodectrilyn-1-01	Sensory and motor deficits; central nervous system effects
Cadmium	Central and peripheral nervous system effects
Carbon monoxide	Sensory and central nervous system effects
Clioquinol	Optic nerve; central nervous system effects; sensory deficits
Soman (and other OP war gases)	Acutely and reversibly—peripheral nervous system Hippocampal effects of longer duration

potential for neurotoxicity of a compound and the one step I believe is essential for all new materials in terms of protecting against possible neurotoxicity.

There are many variations on the design and conduct of such a screen. All have their origin in the work of neurologic and behavioral pharmacologists such as Smith (7), Irwin (8,9), and Campbell and Richter (10). The approach presented here is based on the author's own methodology (6), which has been adopted as the starting point for such a screen by the Environmental Protection Agency (EPA), Food & Drug Administration (FDA), and the Organization for Economic Cooperation and Development (OECD).

The following set of observations/measures are performed on animals (rats and/or mice) that constitute the experimental and control groups in standard acute, subacute, subchronic, reproductive, developmental, and chronic toxicity studies. Technicians can be trained to screen animals after approximately 6 hr with reinforcement conducted over one week. The screen replaces clinical observations performed prior to dosing, and, in the case of an acute study at 1 hr, 24 hr, 4, 7, and 14 days after dosing/exposure (unless a vehicle such as propylene glycol, which masks neurological effects by its transitory character is used, in which case the 1 hr measurement is replaced by a 6 hr measurement). For a repeated dosage study, as appropriate, the screen can be performed at 1 hr, 1, 7, 14, 30 days, and once a month thereafter. A trained technician takes from 3 to 5 min to screen a single animal. Table 2 gives a listing of all the procedures utilized, along with their probably neural correlates and the nature of the data generated by the observation. Each specific test procedure is then briefly described.

In preparation for the screen, a sufficient number of scoring sheets are filled in with the appropriate information. Then the cart employed as a mobile testing station is checked to ensure that all the necessary equipment (empty wire-bottom cage, blunt probe, penlight, 1/2 in. diameter steel rod, force transducer, ink pad, pad of blotting paper, ruler, and electronic probe thermometer) are on the cart and in forking order. Each animal is then evaluated by the following procedures.

Locomotor Activity. The animal's movements (walking, jumping) while on the flat surface of the cart are evaluated quantitatively on a scale of 1 (hypoactive) to 5 (hyperactive), with 3 being the normal state. The data can be upgraded to interval data if one has and utilizes one of the electromagnetic activity-monitoring instruments.

Righting Reflex. For rats and mice, the animal is either grasped by its tail and flipped in the air or held upside down and allowed to drop (2 ft above the cart surface) so that it turns head over heels. The normal animal should land squarely on its feet. If it lands on its side, score 1 point; if on its back; score 2 points. Repeat 4 times and record its total score. For a rabbit, when placed on its side on the cart, does the animal regain its feet without noticeable difficulty?

Grip Strength. For rats and mice, the animal is held by the tail and allowed to grasp the crossbar of a strain gauge designed for the purpose. The tension on the tail is slowly increased until the animal loses its grip, and the resulting value recorded. This procedure is repeated twice for each animal (Meyer, 51).

Body Temperature. The electronic probe thermometer (with a blunt probe) is used to take a rectal temperature, allowing equilibration for 30 sec before the reading is recorded.

Salivation. Discharge of clear fluid from mouth, most frequently seen as beads of moisture on lips in mice and rats or as a fluid flow from the mouth in

Table 2 Observational Screen Components

Observation	Nature of data generated[a]	Correlates to which neutral component
Locomotor activity	S/N	M/C
Righting reflex	S	C/M
Grip strength (fore limb)	N	M
Body temperature	N	C
Salivation	Q	P
Startle response	Q	S/C
Respiration	S	M/P/C
Urination	S	P/M
Mouth breathing	Q	S
Convulsions	S	Reflex
Piloerection	QW	P/C
Diarrhea	S	G.I. tract/PM
Pupil size	S	P/C
Pupil response	Q	P/C
Lacrimation	Q	S/P
Impaired gait	S	M/C
Stereotypy	Q	C
Toe pinch	S	S (surface pain; spinal reflex)
Tail pinch	S	S (deep pain)
Wire maneuver	S	C/M
Positional passivity	S	S/C
Tremors	S	M/C
Extensor thrust	S	C/M
Hind limb splay	N	M/C/P
Positive geotropism	Q	C
Limb rotation	S	M/C

[a]Data quantal (Q), scalar (S), or interval (N). Quantal data is characterized by being of either/or variety, such as dead/alive or present/absent. Scalar data is such that one can rank something as less than, equal to, or greater than over values, but cannot exactly quantitate the difference between such rankings. Interval data is continuous data where one can assign (theoretically) an extremely accurate value to a characteristic that can be precisely related to other values in a quantitative fashion.
Abbreviations: P, peripheral; S, sensory; M, muscular; C, central.

rabbits. Normal state is to see none, in which case the score sheet space should be left blank. If present, a plus sign should be recorded in the blank.

Startle Response. With the animal on the cart, the metal cage is struck with the blunt probe. The normal animal should exhibit a marked but short-duration response, in which case the space on the scoring sheet should be left blank. If present, a plus sign should be entered.

Respiration. While at rest on the cart, the animal's respiration cycle is observed and evaluated on a scale from 1 (reduced) to 5 (increased), with 3 being normal.

Urination. When returning the animal to its case, examine the pan beneath the cage for signs of urination and evaluate on a scale of 1 (lacking) to 5 (polyuria).

Mouth Breathing. Rats and mice are normally obligatory nose breathers. Note whether each animal is breathing through its mouth (if it is, place a check in the appropriate box).

Convulsions. If clonic or tonic convulsions are observed, they should be graded for intensity (1, minor, 5, marked) and the type and intensity recorded.

Pineal Response (Rabbits Only). When a blunt probe is lightly touched to the inside of the ear, the normal animal should react by moving its ear and head reflexively. If this response is present (normal case), the space should be left blank. If absent, a minus sign should be entered in the blank.

Piloerection. Determine whether the fur on the animal's back is raised or elevated. In the normal case (no piloerection), leave the space blank. If piloerection is present, a plus sign should be entered in the blank.

Diarrhea. In examining the pan beneath an animal's cage, note if there are any signs of loose or liquid stools. Normal state is for there to be none, in which case a 1 should be recorded in a scale of 1 (none) to 5 (greatly increased).

Pupil Size. Determine if pupils are constricted or dilated and grade them on a scale of 1–5, respectively.

Pupil Response. The beam of light from the pen light is played across the eyes of the animal, and changes in pupil size are noted. In the normal animal, the pupil should constrict when the beam is on it and then dilate back to normal when the light is removed. Note if there is no response by recording a minus sign in the blank space).

Lacrimation. The animal is observed for the secretion and discharge of tears. In rats and mice the tears contain a reddish pigment. No discharge is normal, and in this case the box should be left blank. If discharge is present, a plus sign should be entered.

Impaired Gait. The occurrence of abnormal gait is evaluated. The most frequent impairments are waddling (W), hunched gait (H), or ataxia (A, the inability of all the muscles to act in unison). Record the extent of any impairment on a scale of 1 (slight) to 5 (marked).

Stereotype.   Each animal is evaluated for stereotypic behavior (isolated motor acts or partial sequences of more complex behavioral patterns from the repertoire of a species, occurring out of context and with an abnormally high frequency). These are graded on a scale of 0–5 (as per Sturgeon et al. (11) if such signs are present.

Toe pinch (rats and mice only).   The blunt probe is used to bring pressure to bear on one of the digits of the hind limb. This should evoke a response from the normal animal, graded on a scale from 1 (absent) to 5 (exaggerated).

Tail Pinch.   The procedure detailed above is utilized with the animal's tail instead of its hind limb, and is graded on the same scale.

Wire Maneuver (rats and mice).   The animal is placed on the metal or wooden rod suspended parallel to the card 2 feet above it. Its ability to move along the rod is evaluated. If impaired, a score of from 1 (slightly impaired) to 5 (unable to stay on the rod) is recorded. The diameter of the rod relative to the animal is critical. Larger animals need thicker rods.

Hind Leg Splay.   After the method of Edwards and Parker (52), the rat or mouse is then held 30 cm above a sand table placed on the cart, and dropped, and the distance between the prints of the two hind paws is measured.

Positional Passivity.   When placed in an awkward position (such as on the edge of the top of the wire-bottom cage) on the cart surface, does the animal immediately move into a more normal position? If not, a score should be recorded on a scale of 1 (slightly impaired) to 5 (cataleptic).

Tremors.   These are periods of continued fine movements, usually starting in the limbs (and perhaps limited to them). Absence of tremors is normal, in which case no score is recorded. If present, they are graded on a scale of 1 (slight and infrequent) to 5 (continuous and marked).

Extensor Thrust.   The sole of either hind foot is pressed with a blunt object. A normal animal will push back against the blunt object. If reduced or absent, this response should be graded on a scale of 1 (reduced) to 5 (absent).

Positive Geotropism.   The animal is placed on the inclined (at an angle of $-30°$) top surface of the wire cage with its head facing downward. It should turn 180° and face "uphill," in which case the space on the form should be left blank. If this occurs, a negative sign should be recorded in the blank.

Limb Rotation.   Take hold of a animal's hind limbs and move them through their normal place of rotation. In the normal state, they should rotate readily but there should be some resistance. The variations from normal are no resistance (1) to markedly increased resistance or rigidity (5), with 3 being normal.

There are a number of other tests which may be added to a behavioral screen to enhance its sensitivity. These methods tend to require more equipment and effort, so if several compounds are to be screened, their inclusion in a screen must be carefully considered. An example of such methods is the "narrowing bridge" technique. All these methods require some degree of training of animals prior to their actual use in test systems. This approach has served the author well in the case of a number of varied industrial chemicals (48–50).

The narrowing bridge test measures the ability of a rat to perform a task requiring neuromuscular control and coordination. Any factor that renders the neuromuscular system of the rat less effective will be expected to result in the rat obtaining a higher score in this test. Therefore, the test cannot by itself discriminate between injuries to the brain (e.g., degenerative changes or tumors), spinal cord, muscle, or peripheral nerve. In addition, compounds that exert a pharmacological action on the central or peripheral nervous systems will be expected to alter the performance of rats on this test. However, a study of the manner in which the performance of the rat alters with time plus clinical examination will enable, in many cases, a distinction to be made between these different possibilities.

The main use of the test is in the study of peripheral neuropathy. It has been demonstrated that this test will detect acrylamide neuropathy 1 week before any clinical signs of neuropathy are apparent. It also claimed that this test is the most sensitive method for detecting hexane neuropathy.

The narrowing bridge consists of three 1.5 m wooden bridges, 23 cm above the ground arranged at right angles. The widths of the three bridges are 2.5, 2.0, and 1.8 cm, respectively. The rat is placed at the end of the 2.5 cm wide bridge and must traverse the three bridges to get to the home cage. The number of times the rat slips is counted. The score on each section of the bridge is calculated as follows:

Bridge width	Score
2.5 cm	number of slips × 3
2.0 cm	number of slips × 2
1.8 cm	number of slips × 1

The total is calculated by adding the scores from the three sections of the bridge. The test is repeated 3 times and the measure of the performance of the rat in the test is the mean of the three total scores. Animals are trained to navigate the bridge system for 5 consecutive days prior to receiving any test compound.

A. Isolated Tissue Assays

The second phase in the tier I screen is a series of isolated tissue preparation bioassays, conducted with appropriate standards, to determine if the material acts pharmacologically directly on neural receptor sites or transmission properties. Though these bioassays are normally performed by a classical pharmacologist, a good technician can be trained to conduct them. The required equipment consists of a Magnus (or similar style) tissue bath (12,13,46), a physiograph or kymography, force transducer, glassware, a stimulator, and bench spectrophotometer. The assays utilized in the screening battery are listed in Table 3, along with the original reference describing each preparation and assay. The assays are performed as per the original author's descriptions with only minor modifications, except that control standards (as listed in Table 3) are always used. Only those assays that are appropriate for the neurological/muscular alterations

Table 3 Isolated Tissue Pharmacologic Assays

Assay system	Endpoint	Standards (agonist/antagonist)	References
Rat ileum	General activity	None (side-spectrum assay for intrinsic activity)	15
Guinea pig van deferens	Muscarinic nicotinic	Methacholine/atropine Methacholine/ hexamethonium	16
Rat serosal strip	Nicotinic	Methacholine/ hexamethonium	17
Rat vas deferens	Alpha adrenergic	Norepinephrine/ phenoxybenzamine	18
Rat uterus	Beta adrenergic	Epinephrine/propanol	19
Rat uterus	Kinin receptors	Bradykinin/none	20
Guinea pig tracheal chain	Dopaminergic	Dopamine/none	15
Rat serosal strips	Tryptaminergic	5-Hydroxytryptamine (serotonin)/dibenzyline or lysergic acid dibromide	21
Guinea pig tracheal chain	Histaminergic	Histamine/benadryl	22,23
Guinea pig ileum (electrically stimulated)	Endorphin receptors	Metenkephalin/none	24
Red blood cell hemolysis	Membrane stabilization	Chlorpromazine (not a receptor-mediated activity)	25
Frog rectus abdominis	Membrane depolarization	Decamethonium iodide (not a receptor-mediated activity)	26

observed in the screen are utilized. Note that all these are intact organ preparations, not minced tissue preparations as others (14) have recommended for biochemical assays.

The first modification in each assay is that, where available, both positive and negative standard controls (pharmacological agonists and antagonists, respectively) are employed. Before the preparation is utilized to assay the test material, the issue preparation is exposed to the agonist to ensure that the preparation is functional and to provide a baseline dose–response curve against which the activity of the test material can be quantitatively compared. After the test material has been assayed (if a dose-response curve has been generated), one can determine whether the antagonist will selectively block the activity of the test material. If so, specific activity at that receptor can be considered as established. In this assay sequence, it must be kept in mind that a test material may act to either stimulate or depress activity, and therefore the roles of the standard agonists and antagonists may be reversed.

Commonly overlooked when performing these assays is the possibility of metabolism to an active form that can be assessed in this in vitro model. The test material should be tested in both original and "metabolized" forms. The metabolized form is prepared by incubating a 5% solution (in aerated Tyrodes) or other appropriate physiological salt solution with strips of suitably prepared test species liver for 30 min. A filtered supernatant is then collected from this incubation and tested for activity. Suitable metabolic blanks should also be tested.

B. Electrophysiology Methods

There are a number of electrophysiological techniques available that can be used to detect and/or assess neurotoxicity. These techniques can be divided into two broad general categories; those focused on central nervous system (CNS) function and those focused on peripheral nervous system function (47).

First, however, the function of the individual components of the nervous system, how they are connected together, and how they operate as a complete system should be very briefly overviewed.

Data collection and communication in the nervous system occurs by means of graded potentials, action potentials, and synaptic coupling of neurons. These electrical potentials may be recorded and analyzed at two different levels depending on the electrical coupling arrangements: individual cell (that is, intracellular and extracellular) or multiple cell (e.g., EEG, evoked potentials (Eps), slow potentials). These potentials may be recorded in specific central or peripheral nervous system areas (e.g., visual cortex, hippocampus, sensory and motor nerves, muscle spindles) during various behavioral states or in in vitro preparations (e.g., nerve-muscle, retinal photoreceptor, brain slice).

C.   CNS Function: Electroencephalography

The electroencephalogram (EEG) is a dynamic measure reflecting the instantaneous integrated synaptic activity of the CNS, which most probably represents, in coded form, all ongoing processes under higher nervous control. Changes in frequency, amplitude, variability, and pattern of the EEG are thought to be directly related to defined aspects of behavior. Therefore, changes in the EEG should be reflected by alterations in behavior and vice versa.

The human EEG is easily recorded and readily quantified, is obtained noninvasively (scalp recording), samples several regions of the brain simultaneously, requires minimal cooperation from the subject, and is minimally influenced by prior testing. Therefore, it is a very useful and recommended clinical test in cases in which accidental exposure to chemicals produces symptoms of CNS involvement and in which long-term exposures to high concentrations are suspected of causing CS toxicity.

Since the EEG recorded using scalp electrodes is an average of the multiple activity of many small areas of cortical surface beneath the electrodes, it is possible that in situations involving noncortical lesions, the following acute or long-term low-level exposures to toxicants are well documented in neurotoxicology (27). The drawback mentioned earlier can be partially overcome by utilizing activation or evocative techniques, such as hyperventilation, photic stimulation, or sleep, which can increase the amount of information gleaned from a standard EEG.

As a research tool, the utility of the EEG lies in the fact that it reflects instantaneous changes in the state of the CNS. The pattern can thus be used to monitor the sleep–wakefulness cycle activation or deactivation of the brainstem, and the state of anesthesia during an acute electrophysiological procedure. Another advantage of the EEG, which is shared by all CNS electrophysiological techniques, is that it can assess the differential effects of toxicants (or drugs) on various brain areas or structures. Finally, specific CNS regions (e.g., the hippocampus) have particular patterns of after-discharge following chemical or electrical stimulation, which can be quantitatively examined and utilized as a tool in neurotoxicology.

The EEG does have some disadvantages, or, more correctly, some limitations. It cannot provide information about the effects of toxicants on the integrity of sensory receptors or of sensory or motor pathways. As a corollary, it cannot provide an assessment of the effects of toxicants on sensory system capacities. Finally, the EEG does not provide specific information at the cellular level and therefore lacks the rigor to provide detailed mechanisms of action.

Rats represent an excellent model of this as they are cheap, resist infection during chronic electrode and annual implantation, and are relatively easy to train so that behavioral assessments can be made concurrently.

Depending on the time of toxicants exposure, the type of scientific information desired, and the necessity of behavioral correlations, a researcher can perform acute and/or chronic EEG activity and thus can complicate subtle effects of toxicants. However, this limitation can be partially avoided if the effect is robust enough. For sleep–wakefulness studies, it is also essential to monitor and record the electromyogram (EMG).

Excellent reviews of these electrophysiology approaches can be found in Fox et al. (28) and Takeuchi and Koike (29).

D. Neurochemical and Biochemical Assays

Though some very elegant methods are now available to study the biochemistry of the brains and nervous system, no one has yet discovered any generalized marker chemicals to serve as reliable indicators or early warnings of neurotoxic actions or potential actions. There are, however, some useful methods. Before looking at these, however, one should understand the basic problems involved.

Normal biochemical events surrounding the maintenance and functions of the nervous system center around energy metabolism, biosynthesis of macro-molecules, and neurotransmitter synthesis, storage, release, uptake, and degradation. Measurement of these events is complicated by the sequestered nature of the components of the nervous system and the transient and liable nature of the moieties involved. Use of measurements of alterations in these functions as indicators of neurotoxicity is further complicated by our lack of a complete understanding of the normal operation of these systems and by the multitude of day-to-day occurrences (such as diurnal cycle, diet, temperature, age, sex, and endocrine status) that are constantly modulating the baseline system. For detailed discussions of these difficulties, the reader is advised to see Damstra and Bond (30,31).

There are two specific markers that may be measured to evaluate the occurrence of specific neurotoxic events. These are neurotoxic esterase (NTE; the inhibition of which is a marker for organo-phosphate–induced delayed neuropathy) (44) and β-galactosidase (which is a marker for Wallerian degeneration of nerves). Johnson and Lotti (32–34) have established that inhibition of 70–90% of normal levels of NTE in hens 36 hours after being dosed with test compound is correlated with the development some 15 days later of ataxia and other classic physiologic signs of delayed neuropathy. Johnson's 1977 article (33) clearly describes the actual assay procedure.

β-galactosidase is associated not with a single class of compounds but rather with a particular expression of neurotoxicity—degeneration following nerve section, the activity of β-galactosidase increases by over a thousand percent. There is also evidence that this enzyme is elevated in the peripheral nerves and ganglia of rats suffering from certain toxic neuropathies. This assay, therefore, can be used as a biochemical method for detecting neurotoxic effects of compounds (35).

β-galactosidase is a constituent of lysosomes whose function is to split β-galactosidase; for example, it will convert lactose into galactose and glucose. The assay method below utilizes an artificial substrate, 4-methylumbelliferyl β-D-galactopyranoside (MUG). At an acid pH, β-galactosidase will split galactose from this compound to leave a product that fluoresces in alkaline solution.

In summary, animals exposed to or dosed with the chemical are necropsied and peripheral nervous tissue is collected. The β-galactosides activity of peripheral nervous tissue homogenates is determined by incubating 0.3 ml of 1% w/v homogenates with 1×10^{-3} methylumbelliferyl β-galactoside in 0.1M glycine buffer, pH 3.0 for 1 hr at 37°C. The enzyme releases methylumbelliferone, which can be measured fluorometrically in alkaline solution (excitation wavelength 325–380 nm, emission wavelength 450 nm) (36).

Progress in the more generalized methodologies of evaluating alterations in neurotransmitter levels has not been as conclusive and is reviewed by Bondy (37,38) and specific methodologies are presented by Ho and Hoskins (39). That such methodologies can be useful is demonstrated by the compendium of results presented by Damstra and Bondy (31), that many neurotoxicants have been shown to be associated with alterations in nervous tissue metabolism in in vivo levels of neurotransmitters or neurotransmitter binding.

E. Pathology

Just as there are special biochemical measurements associated with the study of neurotoxicity, the methodology used in evaluating morphological alterations is also specific. The newly introduced techniques of tissue preparation and examination have been adopted slowly by neuropathologists and, to this day, conventional histological methods are overwhelmingly utilized for the routine examination of human nervous tissue. Toxicologists have been slow to exploit the potential of these new techniques to detail pathological changes and to illuminate the mechanisms by which toxic damage is effected. Modern techniques of tissue preparation and examination will be utilized more heavily for experimental neurotoxicology, and may even become accepted as the method of choice for routine pathological examination of all organs.

Many of these new techniques are presented or reviewed in detail by Spencer et al. (40) and Spencer and Bischoff (41). Three additional generalized methodologies for collection and staining of nervous tissue will be presented in brief below.

Sciatic Nerve Dissection

1. Terminate animal by appropriate rapid and humane means.
2. Remove fur from the hind limb and lower dorsal surface.

3. Make incisions at perpendicular angles in the region of the new joint to expose the sciatic nerve from the spinal cord to the foot.
4. Raise the limb away from the abdomen to reveal a small white section of sciatic nerve.
5. Make two cuts to either side of the nerve mare to produce a plug for well of tissue.
6. Carefully remove the resulting circular area of nerve and muscle and fix in appropriate preservative or process for biochemical analysis.

Rat Trigeminal Ganglion Dissection

1. Terminate animal by appropriate rapid and humane means.
2. Remove the scalp from the top of the skull.
3. Using bone scissors, puncture the skull along the edges of the region from which the scalp has been removed, and carefully remove the top of the skull, exposing the brain.
4. Using a blunt probe, carefully tease the brain from the skull.
5. Identify the trigeminal nerves on either side of the bottom of the brain. These are two cream-colored triangles of tissue.
6. Hold each ganglion with forceps and detach any connective tissue.
7. Remove the ganglia and process them as appropriate.

Rat Dorsal Root Ganglion Dissection

1. Terminate the animal by appropriate rapid and humane means.
2. Remove the fur and skin from the dorsal surface.
3. Remove the muscle layers from above the spinal cord to reveal the terminal vertebra.
4. Remove all connective tissue so that the bone is exposed.
5. Remove the upper section of the neural arch by cutting through the bone on either side of the neural spine. Then cut through the vertebrae so that the bone can be lifted away.
6. Remove the sympathetic nerve processes and clear all connective tissue from the central canal. Separate the connective tissue to expose each dorsal root ganglion.
7. Remove as many ganglia as needed to cold (below 10°C) saline, then process further as needed.

F. Nerve Cell and Tissue Slice Culture

Since 1975, numerous cultured cell and tissue slice models have been developed for screening for study of specific target organ toxicities. Nervous system toxicity has been no exception: there are a number of very active groups in this area. Some of these studies focus on single forms of neurotoxicity (such as that of Fedalei and Nardone (44) on cultured cells to screen for organophosphate neuropathy via NTE inhibition), while most are designed or intended as generalized screens for particular mechanistic forms of neurotoxicity (see Chang and Slipper (53) and Blum and Manzo (54), and Salem and Katz (55)).

Culture of nervous system components was pioneered in the early 1960s. Various methodologies, each with specific advantages and drawbacks, were developed by different laboratories. The major difficulty has been that neurons, as soon as they are sufficiently differentiated to be recognizable as such, probably are not capable of significant additional multiplication in the culture milieu. This purification and cloning of neurons is difficult and very tedious at best. The more complex the culture system, and thus the closer to normality the surrounding nervous system cells, the less likely are the neurons to be capable of multiplication. Although the use of several nervous system tumors in culture and the appearance of cultures of purified cell types have reduced dependence on primary cultures, the disadvantages of isolating any nervous system cell type out of an organ, in which the intercellular interdependencies of function are so great, is frightening. The mystique of the culture of nervous system components has been reduced to the degree that, although all of the details have not been explained, any well-equipped laboratory should be able to reproduce most of the culture systems that have been reported.

The original promised project for the culture techniques, that of rapid and complete dissection of complex nervous system functions within a few years, has not yet been realized. In fact, it seems as if the capacity to produce useful experimental systems has outstripped the capacity of the investigators to ask meaningful questions with those systems. Are the brain and its functions may be so complex that our minds cannot be stretched sufficiently to make meaningful or reasonable hypotheses and test them out? One hopes that these culture systems are simply poised for the time when they will be employed to raise and answer fundamental questions about the nervous system, its functions, and its development. Such breakthroughs will only come after more investigation to find the weakest point.

Neurotoxicology has provided this effort with some essential tools in developing this mode, as agents with known neurotoxic effect on the intact organism can be used as probes in cultured cell systems to correlate organism level effects with cellular mechanisms.

Cultured screening systems used in neurotoxicology include whole embryos, intact organs, explants (i.e., portions of organs, primary cells, and cell lines, that is, tumor cells). Each of these in turn has strengths and weaknesses. Interested readers should see Schrier (42) or Vernadakis et al. (43) for in-depth presentations in this area.

G. Old Hen Test for Organophosphate-Induced Delayed Neuropathy

The most established (and until recently, the only regulatorily recognized) test method in neurotoxicology is the "old hen test," or delayed neurotoxicity test in hens following acute (single) exposure to a test compound.

A basic design for this test may be summarized as:

Three groups of adult hens are selected and treated as follows:

Experimental group	Dosed orally with the test compound
Positive control group	Dosed orally with tri-o-tolyl phosphate
Negative control group	Not dosed

If the hens are to be dosed with a compound possessing a pronounced cholinergic effect, they are given an intramuscular injection of stropine sulfate and pralidoxime chloride prior to dosing. This helps ensure a sufficient number of survivors.

The birds are observed daily for signs of locomotor ataxia, and birds showing persistent signs of ataxia are sent for pathology. If no persistent ataxia is observed in the experimental group after 21 days, the dosing regime is repeated and the hens observed for a further 21 days, after which they are sent for pathological investigation.

REFERENCES

1. Gad, S.C. (1981). A sensory/neuro screen for use in industrial toxicology. Toxicologist 1:150.
2. Weiss, B. (1975). Behavioral methods for investigating environmental health effects. In Proc. Intl. Symp. Recent Adv. Assessment Health Effects. Environ. Pollution, Paris, 1974, Lumembourg; Community of European Committees, pp. 2415–33.
3. Evans, H.L. and Weiss, B. (1978). Behavioral toxicology. In: Contemporary Research in Behavioral Pharmacology. Edited by D.E. Blackman and D.J. Sanger. New York; Plenum, pp. 449–487.
4. Zbinden, G. (1981). Experimental methods in behavioral teratology. Arch. Toxicol. 48:69–88.
5. Mitchell, C.L. and Tilson, H.A. (1982). Behavioral toxicology in risk assessment: Problems and research needs. Crit. Rev. Toxicol. 10:265–274.
6. Gad, S.C. (1982). An neuromuscular screen for use in industrial toxicology. J. Toxicol. Environ. Hlth. 9:691–704.
7. Smith, W.G. (1961). Pharmacological screening tests. In: Progress in Medicinal

Chemistry, vol. 1. Edited by G. Ellis and G. West, Washington, D.C.; Butterworth, pp. 1–33.

8. Irwin, S. (1962). Drug screening and evaluation procedures. Science 136:123–128.

9. Irwin, S. (1964). Drug screening and evaluation of new compounds in animals. Animal and clinical pharmacologic techniques. In Drug Evaluation. Edited by J. Nodine and P. Siegler. Chicago, Year Book Medical Publishers, Inc., pp. 36–54.

10. Campbell, D. and Richter, W. (1967). Whole animal screening studies. Act. Pharmacol. 25:345–363.

11. Sturgeon, R.D. Fessler, R.G., and Meltzer, H.Y. (1979). Behavioral rating scales for assessing phencyclidine induced locomotor activity, stereotyped behavior and ataxia in rats. Eur. J. Pharmacol. 59:169–179.

12. Turner, R.A. (1965). Screening Methods in Pharmacology, vols. I and II. New York, Academic, pp. 42–27, 60–68, 27–128.

13. Offermier, J. and Ariens, E.G. (1966). Serotonin I. Receptors involved in its action. Arch. Int. Pharmacodyn. Ther. 164:92–215.

14. Bondy, S.C. (1979). Rapid screening of neurotoxic agents by in vivo means. In: Effects of Food and Drugs on the Development and Function of the Nervous System: Methods for Predicting Toxicity. Edited by R.M. Gryder and V.H. Frankos. Washington, D.C., Office of Health Affairs, FDA, pp. 133–143.

15. Domer, F.R. (1971). Animal Experiments in Pharmacological Analysis. Springfield, IL; Charles C. Thomas, pp. 98, 115, 155, 164, 220.

16. Leach, G.D.H. (1956). Estimation of drug antagonisms in the isolated gui pig was deferens. J. Pharm. Pharmacol. 8:501.

17. Khayyal, M.T., Tolba, N.M., El-Hawary, M.B., and El-Wahed, S.A. (1974). A Sensitive Method for the Bioassay of acetylcholine. Eur. J. Pharmacol. 25:287–290.

18. van Rossum, M. (1965). Different types of sympathomimetic β-receptors. J. Pharm. Pharmacol. 17:202.

19. Levy, B. and Tozzi, S. (1963). The adrenergic receptive mechanism of the rat uterus. J. Pharmacol. Exp. Ther. 142:178.

20. Gecse, A., Zsilinsky, E., and Szekeres, L. (1976). Bradykinin antagonism. In: Kinins; Pharmacodynamics and Biological Roles. Edited by F. Sicuteri, N. Back, and G. Haberland. New York, Plenum Press, pp. 5–13.

21. Lin, R.C.Y. and Yeoh, T.S. (1965). An improvement of Vane's stomach strip preparation for the assay of 5-hydroxytryptamine. J. Pharm. Pharmacol. 17:524–525.

22. Castillo, J.C. and De Beer, E.J. (1947). The guinea pig tracheal chain as an assay for histamine agonists. Fed. Proc. 6:315.

23. Castillo, J.C. and De Beer, E.J. (1947b). The tracheal chain. J. Pharmacol. Exp. Ther. 90:104.

24. Cox, B.M., Opheim, K.E., Teschemach, H., and Goldstein, A. (1975). A peptide-like substance from pituitary that acts like morphine 2. Purification and properties. Life Sci. 16:1777–1782.

25. Seeman, P. and Weinstein, J. (1966). Erythrocyte membrane stabilization by tranquilizers and antihistamines. Biochem. Pharmacol. 15:1737–1752.

26. Burns, B.D. and Paton, W.D.M. (1951). Depolarization of the motor end-plate by decamethonium and acetylcholine. J. Physiol. (London) 115:41–73.

27. Norton, S. (1980). Toxic responses of the central nervous system. In: Toxicology:

The Basic Science of Poisons, 2nd edition. Edited by J. Doull, C.D. Klaassen, and M.O. Amdur. New York, Macmillan, Inc.

28. Fox, D.A., Lowndes, H.E., and Bierkamper, G.G. (1982). Electrophysiological techniques in neurotoxicology. In: Nervous System Toxicology. Edited by C.L. Mitchell. New York, Raven Press, pp. 299–336.

29. Takeuchi, Y. and Koike, Y. (1985). Electrophysiological methods for the in vivo assessment of neurotoxicology. In: Neurotoxicology. Edited by K. Blum and L. Manzo. New York, Marcel Dekker, Inc., pp. 613–629.

30. Damstra, T. and Bondy, S.C. (1980). The current status and future of biochemical assays for neurotoxicity. In: Experimental and Clinical Neurotoxicology. Edited by P.S. Spencer and H.H. Schaumburg. Baltimore, Williams and Wilkins, pp. 820–833.

31. Damstra, T. and Bondy, S.C. (1982). Neurochemical approaches to the detection of neurotoxicity. In: Nervous System Toxicology. Edited by C.L. Mitchell. New York, Raven Press, pp. 349–373.

32. Johnson, M.K. (1975). The delayed neuropathy caused by some organophosphorus esters: Mechanism & challenge. Crit. Rev. Toxicol. 3:289–316.

33. Johnson, M.K. (1977). Improved assay of neurotoxic esterase for screening. Organophosphates for delayed neurotoxicity potential. Arch. Toxic. 37:113–115.

34. Johnson, M.K. and Lotti, M. (1980). Delayed neurotoxicity caused by chronic feeding of organophosphates requires a high-point of inhibition of neurotoxic esterase. Toxicol. Letts. 5:99–102.

35. Dewar, A.J. and Moffett, B.J. (1979). Biochemical methods for detecting neurotoxicity: a short review. Pharmacol. Ther. 5:545–562.

36. Dewar, A.J. (1981). Neurotoxicity testing with particular references to biochemical methods. In: Testing for Toxicity. Edited by W. Gorrod. London, Taylor & Francis, Ltd., pp. 199–217.

37. Bondy, S.C. (1982). Neurotransmitter binding interactions as a screen for neurotoxicity. In: Mechanisms of Actions of Neurotoxic Substances. Edited by K.N. Prasad and A. Vernadakis. New York, Raven Press, pp. 25–50.

38. Bondy, S.C. (1984). Especial consideration for neurotoxicological research. Crit. Rev. Toxicol. 14(4):381–402.

39. Ho, I.K. and Hoskins, B. (1982). Biochemical methods for neurotoxicological analyses of neuroregulators and cyclic nucleotides. In: Principles and Methods of Toxicology. Edited by A.W. Hayes. New York, Raven Press, pp. 375–406.

40. Spencer, P.S., Bischoff, M.C., and Schaumburg, H.H. (1980). Neuropathological methods for the detection of neurotoxic disease. In: Experimental and Clinical Neurotoxicology. Edited by P.S. Spencer and H.H. Schaumburg. Baltimore, Williams and Wilkins, pp. 743–757.

41. Spencer, P.S. and Bischoff, M.C. (1982). Contemporary neuropathological methods in toxicology. In: Nervous System Toxicology. Edited by C.L. Mitchell. New York, Raven Press, pp. 259–276.

42. Schrier, B.K. (1982). Nervous system cultures as toxicological test systems. In: Nervous System Toxicology. Edited by C.L. Mitchell. New York, Raven Press, pp. 337–349.

43. Vernadakis, A., Davies, D.L., and Gremo, F. (1985). Neural culture: A tool to study

cellular neurotoxicity. In: Neurotoxicity. Edited by K. Blum and L. Manzo. New York, Marcel Dekker. Inc., pp. 559–583.

44. Fedalei, A. and Nardone, R.M. (1983). An in vitro alternative for testing the effect of organo-phosphates on neurotoxic esterase activity. In: Product Safety Evaluation. Edited by A.M. Goldberg. New York, Mary Ann Liebert, Inc., pp. 253–269.

45. Mitchell, C.L., Tilson, H.A., and Cabe, P.A. Screening for neurobehavioral toxicity: Factors to consider. In: Nervous System Toxicology. Edited by C.L. Mitchell. New York, Raven Press, pp. 237–245.

46. Nodine, J.J. and Siegler, P.E. (eds.) (1964). Animal and Clinical Techniques in Drug Evaluation. Chicago, Year Book Medical Publishers, Inc.

47. Seppalainen, A.M. (1975). Applications of neurophysiological methods in occupational medicine: A review. Scand. J. Work Envirn. Health 1:1–14.

48. Gad, S.C., McKelvey, J.A., and Turney, R.A. (1979). NIAX catalyst ESN-subchronic neuropharmacology and neurotoxicology. Drug and Chem. Toxicol. 3(3): 223–236.

49. Gad. S.C., Conroy, W.J., McKelvey, J.A., and Turney, R.A. (1978). Behavioral and neuropharmacological toxicology of the macrocyclic ether 18-Crown 6. Drug Chem. Toxicol. 1:339–354.

50. Gad, S.C., Dunn, B.J., Gavigan, F.A., Reilly, C., and Peckham, J.C. (1987). Acute and Neurotoxicity of 5, 7, 11-dodecatriyn-1-ol and 4, 7, 11, 13-octadecatetrayne-1, 18-Diol. J. Appl. Toxicol. (In press).

51. Meyer, O.A., Tilson, H.A., Byrd, W.C., and Riley, M.T. (1979). A method for the routine assessment of fore- and hind-limb grip strength of rats and mice. Neurobehav. Toxicol. 1:233–236.

52. Edwards, P.M. and Parker, V.H. (1977). A simple, sensitive and objective method for early assessment of acrylamide neuropathy in rats. Toxicol. Appl. Pharmacol. 40:589–591.

53. Chang, L.W. and Slikker, W. (1995). Neurotoxicology: Approaches and Methods. Academic Press, San Diego.

54. Blum, K. and Manzo, L. (1985). Neurotoxicology. Marcel Dekker, Inc., New York.

55. Salem, H. and Katz, G.A. (1988). Advances in Animal Alternatives for Safety and Efficacy Testing, Taylor & Francis, Washington, D.C.

9

Techniques for Evaluating Hazards of Inhaled Products

Paul E. Newton
MPI Research, Inc., Mattawan, Michigan

I. INTRODUCTION

The potential for exposure to toxic materials is greater via inhalation than any other route of exposure. Whereas adult humans consume 1–2 l of water and 1–2 l of food per day, they inhale 10,000–20,000 l of air per day. In addition, the surface area for potential absorption of a test article in the lung far exceeds the surface area of the skin or the gastrointestinal tract. Inhalation exposures in the workplace environment can come from solid or liquid aerosols, fumes, vapors, or gases. Inhalation exposures in the home environment can come from combustion by-products from the furnace, stove, or cigarettes, from solvents degassing from adhesives or synthetic products such as carpets, from aerosolized consumer products, or from radon. Inhalation exposures to a myriad of air pollutants occur in the ambient environment.

The respiratory tract may be the target organ, such as with pulmonary function changes after exposure to ozone or sulfur dioxide, fibrosis after exposure to silica, or with lung cancer after exposure to beryllium, cadmium, or benzo(a)pyrene. The toxicant need not even be absorbed into the body to produce a toxic effect as exemplified by fibrous materials that produce pulmonary fibrosis and cancer. Or the respiratory tract may just serve as the route of exposure with systemic toxic effects such as bladder cancer seen after exposure to benzidine, liver cancer after exposure to vinyl chloride, and hematopoietic effects after exposure to benzene.

As with all routes of exposure, toxic effects may occur directly from exposure to the toxin or they may occur indirectly after metabolic activation. There is significant cytochrome P450 metabolic activity in the respiratory tract in both the olfactory region in the nose as well as in the lungs.

The respiratory tract is composed of a complex cell population with over 40 cell types and it performs many vital functions in the body. In addition to gas exchange, the respiratory tract is involved in the sense of smell and taste, temperature and humidity adjustment, gas and particle collection, inactivation and clearance, metabolism, and other functions. The lung removes, metabolizes, or excretes vasoactive hormones. It regulates angiotension and prostaglandin concentrations in the circulation.

The lung is a unique organ in that it receives all of the cardiac output. The lungs therefore offer rapid access of inhaled and absorbed toxins to all tissues throughout the body. The lungs can also serve as an excretory organ as volatile solvents can be excreted through the lung and expired air. Consequently, evaluation of inhalation toxicity is very important, whether it be from occupational exposures in the industrial setting or environmental exposures in the home and ambient air.

Inhalation toxicology studies involve all of the standard types of toxicity studies conducted with other routes of exposure and their various endpoints. These include acute lethality and sensitization, subchronic and chronic toxicity, oncogenicity, developmental, reproductive, neurotoxicity, immunotoxicity, and both in vivo and in vitro genetic studies. In addition to the expertise needed to conduct the appropriate in-life evaluations, engineering expertise is also needed. In many inhalation toxicity studies the actual study is the easy part. Being able to create the exposure atmosphere at the desired concentration accurately and precisely can be the most difficult part of the study.

A lot of care must be given to the generation, monitoring, and exposure systems before any animal exposures occur. The inhalation exposures are dynamic. Every day is a new day. Exposure parameters are monitored frequently during the exposures and any necessary adjustments are made. Whereas the monitoring and control of a gaseous exposure level is usually the easiest to conduct, if the test article is reactive, such as ozone, loss of the test article on chamber surfaces can dramatically affect the exposure level.

Inhalation exposures to vapors of pure liquids are probably the next easiest to conduct. But if the test article is a mixture, such as gasoline, then the composition of the test article must be shown to be the same in the exposure atmosphere as it is in the neat material. The composition must also be the same at each exposure level and it must be constant during the exposure day.

Inhalation aerosol studies are the hardest to conduct whether it be for a liquid aerosol, or droplets, or for a solid aerosol, or dust. In addition to controlling the exposure level accurately and precisely, the size of the aerosol particles must also be measured and shown to be the same among all exposure groups and a size respirable to the test animal.

In inhalation studies, the actual dose is not always clearly known. Unlike oral studies where the amount of test article gavaged or consumed in the diet can be measured, in inhalation the exposure concentration is measured. To calculate a dose, the exposure duration, ventilation rate, and percent absorption or deposition must be also be measured or assumed. This then adds another dimension of difficulty when extrapolating from animals to man because assumptions about the human ventilation rate and absorption or deposition fractions must also be made.

II. INHALATION DOSE

Estimates of the actual dose of a test article into a test animal are accurate for a study where the test article may be injected intravenously or intraperitoneally. The volume and concentration of a test article administered by oral gavage may also be known accurately. But how much is actually absorbed from the gastrointestinal tract? The same problem exists with dermal studies where the amount of test article applied is known, but the amount absorbed, or the dose, is unknown. Estimating the dose for inhalation studies is even more complex.

While the concentration of the test article being inspired may be accurately measured, what is the test animal's ventilation rate? How much of the inspired test article is being retained in the body and how much is being exhaled? Where is the test article being retained? In the case of gases and vapors, retention depends on the gas or vapor solubility and reactivity. In the case of inhaled particles, the site of deposition is a function of the particle size. The site of deposition significantly influences retention and whether the test article is absorbed into the body or, in the case of particulate matter depositing on the ciliated airways, the particles are removed from the lung up the mucociliary ladder and swallowed.

A. Gases and Vapors

The exchange of oxygen and carbon dioxide occurs in the alveolar region of the lung across the alveolar membrane, while the uptake of toxic vapors and gases can occur throughout the respiratory tract, starting in the nasopharynx or nose. Highly soluble and reactive gases or vapors may never even make it past the nose.

The airways are lined with protective and functional layers of mucus or liquids through which the gas or vapor must penetrate. The thickness of these lining layers varies from the thick mucus layer in the upper airways to the thin surfactant layer in the alveoli. The dominant factors for penetration of a gas or vapor through these layers into the body are diffusion and solubility. The mass transfer is directly proportional to the concentration of the gas or vapor in the air and inversely proportional to water solubility.

When test articles permeate the linings, highly reactive test articles may react directly with those cells and produce locally toxic effects. Less reactive test articles may diffuse across the cells lining the airways and cause toxic effects in endothelial cells. Or even less reactive test articles are absorbed into the blood and transported throughout the body.

Gas and vapor exposure levels are usually reported in parts per million (v/v) of the test article in air. At high concentration alternatively, the concentration can be expressed in percent (10,000 ppm = 1%). The concentration is sometimes expressed in terms of mass per unit volume of air. These units are necessary in calculating the amount of test article that will be required to conduct exposures at the designated ppm levels and exposure duration. At room temperature (25°C) and standard pressure (760 mmHg), a molar volume of gas occupies 24.5 l. A vapor concentration in ppm for a liquid with a molecular weight MW can be converted to mg per cubic meter using

$$C_{ppm} \; MW/24.5 = C_{mg/m3}$$

B. Aerosols

Many airborne materials can be considered under the generic term of "aerosols." An aerosol is suspension of solid particles or liquid droplets in a gaseous medium. Several terms have been used to describe aerosols. Solid particle aerosols, or dusts, arise from processes such as milling, grinding, or mechanical breakage of the test article and are therefore identical in chemical composition to the parent test article. Depending on the method of generation, they can vary in size from 0.5 to 100 μm in diameter.

Fumes are small solid particles that result from condensed vapors usually arising from combustion. Usually the formation of fumes is associated with a change in chemical composition. Fumes tend to be less than 0.1 μm in diameter but tend to flocculate and form larger particles as the aerosol ages. Metal oxide fumes are good examples of fumes of toxicological importance.

Mists are liquid particle or droplet aerosols typically formed by physical shearing of liquids such as in spraying, nebulizing, or bubbling. Fogs are also liquid particle aerosols but typically formed by the condensation of supersaturated vapors. The term smog is applied to the complex mixture of particles and gases formed in the atmosphere by irradiation of automobile exhaust and other combustion products.

The concentration of aerosols is usually reported in terms of mass per unit volume of air. Acute studies, which are conducted at very high exposure levels, are reported typically in mg/l. Longer term studies at much lower concentrations are typically reported in mg/m^3 where 1 m^3 = 1000 l.

Inhaled particles deposit in the lungs via four mechanisms: impaction, sedimentation, diffusion, and interception. Impaction is the primary mechanism for aerosol deposition for large particles. Owing to inertia, particles suspended in air tend to continue along their original path. Therefore, if there is a bend in the airway, the larger particles do not make the bend but impact into the airway wall. Smaller particles are able to make it through the same bend but as the air flow rate decreases in the outer parts of the lung, gravity takes over and the particles settle out in the smaller airways. The smallest particles make it all the way into the alveoli where there they move around or diffuse by Brownian movement and randomly impact the alveolar wall. Interception is involved with the deposition of fibers where the end of a fiber may make a bend but the fiber is so long the trailing end impacts on the side.

The inhaled dose for aerosols is calculated as the product of the exposure level times the duration of the exposure times the ventilation rate of the test animal. However, 100 percent of the inhaled dose is not deposited within the lungs. Some of the small particles are exhaled. In addition, even for those particles that are retained in the body, the size of the particles greatly affects their pattern of deposition. The pattern of deposition greatly affects the particles' toxicity. Larger materials may be removed by the cleaning mechanism of the nose. Smaller particles may escape or pass through the filtering mechanism of the nose but deposit on the mucus lined upper airways. The particles deposited on the airways are removed or cleared from the lung by the mechanism known as the "mucociliary ladder." The mucociliary ladder is composed of the mucus lining of the airways lying on top of rhythmically beating ciliated cells. This rhythmic beat propels the particle-laden mucus upwards to the pharynx where the particles are swallowed. Only the smallest particles, 1–3 μm in the case of the rat, are deposited in the alveolar region. Therefore, the particle size and the pattern of deposition must be taken into consideration when estimating dose.

Percent deposition for various aerosol sizes varies in different species (1). Whereas some 6 micron particles may reach the alveolar region in human lungs, essentially none reach the alveolar region in rodent lungs. Therefore differences in the percent and pattern of particulate deposition becomes critical in risk assessment and extrapolation from animal data to humans.

III. EXPOSURE SYSTEMS

There are four basic types of inhalation exposure systems: whole-body chambers (in which the test animal is completely immersed in the exposure atmosphere), head-only systems (where only the head is placed into the exposure atmosphere), flow-past nose-only chambers (in which only the nose protrudes into the exposure atmosphere flowing past the nose), and directed flow-past nose-only chambers (where the exposure atmosphere is delivered or directed as a separate flow to each animal's nose and then exhausted). In addition to the above systems, test articles can also be delivered to the lung via intratracheal instillation or insufflation. Each of these systems has its own advantages and disadvantages.

A. Whole-Body Exposure Chambers

Whole body stainless-steel and glass chambers are used to provide whole-body inhalation exposures to a variety of test animals. Advantages of the whole body exposure chambers are their large size, which can accommodate many animals and allow easy animal care. The animals are unrestrained providing less stress. In many cases the animals are housed in the same cages both during and after the exposure. One disadvantage of whole-body exposure chambers is, because of their large size, a high consumption rate of the test article. A 2-yr inhalation oncogenicity study with a high exposure level of 10,000 ppm consumed 230 gal of the test article (2).

Whole-body exposures are usually conducted for gases and vapors unless skin absorption of the test article is significant and a problem. Whole-body exposures are usually not conducted for aerosols. During whole-body exposures aerosols deposit on the fur and then get preened after the exposure. This can lead to a significant oral dose. As seen in Table 1, the exposure level necessary to produce a lethal effect in 50% of the animals exposed was considerably less in whole-body exposures than in head-only exposures (3). Since 1992 when the U.S. EPA recommended that aerosol studies be conducted via nose-only exposures, there has been a significant switch from whole-body to nose-only exposures.

The size of the whole-body chamber used in a study is usually the smallest chamber which can be efficiently used for the required number of animals. Three basic guidelines are usually followed. First, the animals are individually housed in open mesh cages to prevent animals from huddling in the corner of their cage, burying their noses, and filtering out the test article. Second, the animal volume should be less than 5% of the chamber volume. And third, the total chamber air flow should provide at least 10 air changes per hr. These latter

Table 1 Effect of Inhalation Exposure Route on Toxicity of Anilines

| Compound | LC_{50} in ppm | | Ratio of whole-body to nose-only |
	Whole-body	Head-only	
Aniline	478	839	0.57
N-ethylaniline	263	424	0.62
N,N-diethylaniline	315	679	0.46

two guidelines provide for good mixing of the chamber air flow and minimal buildup of heat, and waste products or by-products such as CO_2 and ammonia. If the test animals are also being housed within the same cages during the nonexposure periods, then the cage size must also meet the AAALAC requirements for cage sizes (4). This can significantly affect how many cages can be housed within a chamber.

Exposure of only a few animals on a single level, such as in acute studies, are often conducted in rectangular boxes. Studies with larger number of animals, or larger sized animals are usually conducted in chambers equipped with a pyramidal or conical top, which allows for mixing and even distribution of the test article throughout the chamber (5). The chamber air flow enters tangentially at the top to aide in mixing of the test article within the chamber atmosphere. Some chambers however have been also designed with horizontal air flow. Whole-body chambers have ranged in size from as small as 1 l to as large as 25,000 l (6). These large Thomas Dome chambers located at Wright-Patterson Air Force Base in Dayton, OH, were equipped with airlocks, to permit entry by technical personnel in positive pressure ventilation suits and continuous exposure to test articles.

Smaller whole-body chambers may be operated under positive pressure with the only air being supplied through the generator. Larger whole-body chambers are usually operated under a push–pull system where conditioned air is supplied, or pushed, into the chamber inlet port and exhausted, or pulled, from the chamber exhaust port. The exhaust flow is maintained slightly greater than the supply to keep the chamber pressure slightly negative to the room in case of any chamber leaks.

Leak testing should be conducted prior to the start of the actual study and any time the integrity of the chamber seal is questioned. To check for chamber leaks, with the chamber under a negative pressure, a smoke generating tube is place near any potential leak locations. Doors are notorious for leaks. Leaks are identified as smoke being pulled into the chamber. These locations are marked and repaired as required. Alternatively, with the chamber under positive pressure, leaks may be detected using a bubble forming fluid on the outside of the chamber or a smoke bomb inside the chamber.

The homogeneity of the test article distribution in each exposure chamber is determined by sampling the chamber concentration at representative points in the front and back, left and right, and if more than one level of animals is used, from the top and bottom of the chamber. The sampling system should be the one to be used for the study. The various sample location results are compared to the standard monitoring location and they should be within ±5% for gases and vapors and ±20% for aerosols. Variations outside these ranges could indicate chamber leaks. Or, a premixing chamber may need to be added or total chamber air flow may need to be increased to help better disperse the test article. Test article homogeneity should be checked prior to the start of the actual study and periodically thereafter in longer term studies.

Air exchange or air flow through a chamber is characterized by two basic parameters: chamber volume V(l), and air flow rate Q(l/min) (see Figure 1). Regulatory guidelines specify the inhalation chambers should be operated with a minimum of 10–12 air changes per hour. This minimum number of air changes are specified to provide adequate oxygen for the test animals and to prevent heat and CO_2 buildup within the chamber. By definition, 1 air change per hour is provided if the total volume of air flowing through the chamber in an hour equals the volume of the chamber. Thus, for 1 air change per hour in a 1,000 l chamber, a total of 1,000 l must pass through the chamber in an hour. For 12 air changes per hour, 12 times the volume of the chamber, or 12,000 l must pass through the chamber. This equates to a mean chamber air flow rate of 200 l/min.

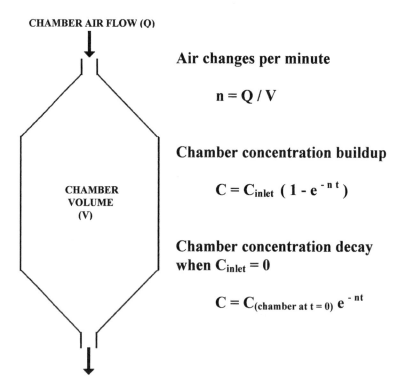

CHAMBER AIR FLOW (Q)

CHAMBER VOLUME (V)

Air changes per minute

$$n = Q / V$$

Chamber concentration buildup

$$C = C_{inlet} (1 - e^{-nt})$$

Chamber concentration decay when $C_{inlet} = 0$

$$C = C_{(chamber\ at\ t = 0)}\ e^{-nt}$$

Figure 1   Air exchange and test article concentration buildup and decay in whole-body inhalation exposure chambers.

The rate at which the concentration of a test article may build up in a chamber is equal to the concentration of the test article in the air flow entering the chamber times the quantity $1 - e^{-nt}$, where n is the air change rate, or air flow Q divided by chamber volume V (7). At the end of an exposure period when the inlet air concentration is set to zero, the concentration at any subsequent time is $C_0 e^{-nt}$ where C_0 is the chamber concentration at the end of the exposure period. For both the buildup and decay of the test article concentration in the chamber, the time it takes to move from a starting concentration to 50% of the equilibrium concentration (i.e., the target concentration for buildup and zero for decay) is referred to as the half time, $t_{1/2}$, and is equal to $\ln 2/n$ or $0.693/n$ or $0.693\ V/Q$. The time it takes to reach 50% of that level, or 75% of the equilibrium level, is $2\ t_{1/2}$, or $1.386\ V/Q$. The time for it takes to reach 99% of the equilibrium, which is the most frequently cited time and referred to as t_{99}, is $4.61\ V/Q$. In our example above with 200 l/min air flow in a 1,000 l chamber, the t_{99} would be 23 min. The t_{99} must be considered when making adjustments to a generation system. It must be kept in mind that it take 23 minutes in our example case for the full effect of any adjustment made to the generation system to take effect.

B. Nose-Only Exposure Chambers

As stated above, whole-body exposures deposit test article onto the fur of the test animals. Preening then results in an additional oral test article dose, which can lead to increased toxicity. In 1992 the U.S. Environmental Protection Agency (EPA) recommended that all aerosol studies be conducted using nose-only exposures. In nose-only exposures the test animals are restrained in acrylic tubes with a conical end. An adjustable tailgate keeps the animal in position in the tube with only its nose or snout sticking out into the exposure atmosphere.

Nose-only exposures can eliminate the majority of the oral dose obtained from preening. The animals still receive an oral dose from inhaled particles deposited in the upper respiratory tract and those cleared through mucociliary action from the airways into the gastrointestinal tract. Immediately after a brief 20 min exposure of rats to a radiolabeled particle, only 23% of the labeled particles were within the trachea-lungs, 10% of the particles were within the nose, 30% of the particles were on the external snout, and 37% of the particles were already in the gastrointestinal tract (8). This effect is influenced by the test animal species. After a 10 min nose-only exposure 20% of inhaled dye particles were in the lungs of rats but 57% were in the lungs of guinea pigs (9).

In addition to minimizing the oral dose from preening, nose-only exposures are also very useful when there is a very limited amount of the test article available and it is very expensive to produce. Nose-only exposures are also the preferred method of exposure to radiolabeled test articles in adsorption, deposition, metabolism, and excretion studies where radiolabeling may be expensive and containment of the radiolabeled test article is essential.

Nose-only exposure systems also have their own potential problems. Handling and/or restraint in the nose-only exposure tubes may cause stress (10,11). This stress could be seen in increased epinephrine and norepinephrine levels (12), increased body temperature (13), alteration in pulmonary function (14), suppression of pulmonary defenses (15), increased toxicity (16,17). Testicular lesions seen in a nose-only study but not in a whole-body study to the same test article at the same exposure level and for the same duration imply a nose-only procedural effect (18). In rats the testes are sensitive to hyperthermia-induced degeneration and atrophy (19). This testicular effect seen in only some nose-only studies however may be due to, or confounded with, the age of the test animals when the study started. The younger or less mature animal may be more sensitive.

Rats maintain their body temperature by regulating heat exchange via their tail. Therefore, the older bottle type nose-only tube design that enclosed their tail can lead to heat stress. The newer tube design, which allows the tails to extend beyond the tail gate and which also have air slits in the top, allows for much better heat exchange. The slit in the bottom of the tubes also allows for urine to drain away, keeping the rats drier. Keeping the room temperature cool also helps keep the animals cooler. After a few days of acclimation to nose-only exposure tubes, if a rat is placed on the table next to the tube he will run into it and stick his nose out the end. The rats seem to like being in that environment and are not stressed. Exposure tube acclimation however is important.

1. Flow-Past

The older nose-only system consists of a cylindrical tube or rectangular box with animal ports around all sides (20). The test animals are restrained in tapered acrylic restraint tubes that orient the animals' noses into the chamber for exposure (see Figure 2). The test animals are therefore breathing from the same volume of air. Cross contamination from one animal to another is therefore possible. In addition, if more than one level of test animals is used and the levels are in-line with respect to the flow of the exposure atmosphere, the animals on the second level, or downstream, receive less test article than those upstream. This is due to the exhaled air of the animals on the first level upstream. If the chamber's inlet flow is twice the minute ventilation of the test animals, and assuming the exhaled breath contains no test article, the downstream level animals will receive 20% less exposure than the upstream level animals (21). Addition of a third or fourth level would reduce the inlet concentration 27 and 30%, respectively (21).

2. Directed Flow-Past

The directed flow-past nose-only system was designed to avoid the above problem of a decrease in concentration going down the chamber (see Figure 2). The

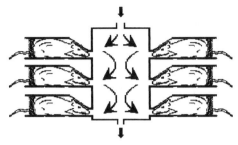

FLOW-PAST NOSE-ONLY CHAMBER

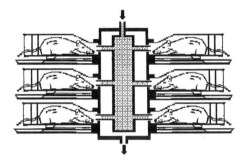

DIRECTED FLOW-PAST NOSE-ONLY CHAMBER

Figure 2   Flow-past and directed flow-past nose-only exposure chambers.

directed flow-past nose-only exposure system consists of two vertical concentric cylindrical chambers (22). Animal ports are arranged in a radial pattern at various levels on the outer chamber. The system operates as a push–pull system. Test atmosphere supplied by a generation system enters the inner chamber and is pushed out via delivery tubes directed at each individual animal's nose. The atmosphere is then pulled by the exhaust flow through the outer chamber.

Because of the individual delivery and exhaust of the test article laden atmosphere to the test animals, there is no cross contamination among the animals. If at least 3 to 4 times the minute ventilation is delivered, approximately 0.6 l/min/animal for rats, there is minimal, or no, rebreathing of the animal's own exhaled air (21,23).

C.   Head-Only Exposures

With the use of a soft rubbery material to seal around the neck, head-only exposures may be conducted. A hole in the material allows the head to protrude into the exposure atmosphere. With the proper hole size, a tight seal is maintained to eliminate leaks around the neck and yet the material is loose enough or flexible enough not to restrict respiration. The head-only exposure system also takes less acclimation time than mask exposures.

Head-only exposures may be conducted in rodents restrained in exposure tubes, dogs restrained in a sling, or primates restrained in a chair (24). The head-only exposure is also used for mice when evaluating respiratory irritation (RD_{50}) as discussed elsewhere in this chapter.

D. Intratracheal Instillation

Alternatively, test articles may be intratracheally instilled into the lungs of animals. In the case of microbial pest agents, it is the preferable route of exposure and specified by the EPA (25). The instilled volume is suggested to be less than 0.2 ml/100 g body weight.

After anesthesia with a volatile anesthesia such as methoxyflurane the animals are suspended from their incisors on a lighted laryngoscope to facilitate correct placement of the dosing needle. The calculated amount of dosing solution is instilled into the trachea using a ball tipped or rounded end needle and a 1 ml sterile disposable syringe. Only 1 dose is drawn into the syringe at a time. After dosing, the animals are removed from the laryngoscope and returned to their home cage. With the use of a volatile anesthetic, the animals can be anesthetized and dosed and then will return to normal activity in a manner of only a few minutes.

Advantages to intratracheal or IT dosing include: 1) Being able to deliver exact doses in terms of mg/kg into the tracheobronchial regions of the lung (26) to generate a dose-response curve; 2) An IT dose can be delivered without regard to particle size and ventilation rate; 3) The IT dose eliminates any interference from particles being deposited in the oro- and nasopharyngeal regions of the respiratory tract; 4) The IT dose can be many times higher if necessary than the maximum dose attainable via conventional inhalation; 5) An IT dose uses far less test article to deliver the dose. Repeated, daily IT dosing is also possible (27).

The disadvantages of IT dosing include: first, the test article is delivered as a bolus and the pattern of deposition within the respiratory tract is different than during normal respiration (28). The vehicle used to instill the test article may affect the response of the lung. Both the normal physiologic responses to particle deposition and pathologic effects may therefore be different in IT dosed animals than from those occurring during conventional inhalation exposures. With IT dosing it is also possible that the test animal can be exposed to an exaggerated and unrealistic dose relative to anything that might occur in a real world setting.

In chrysotile asbestos studies, upper airway granulomas were found in IT dosed rats rather than diffuse interstitial fibrosis as seen in rats that inhaled this fiber (29). However, similar effects of bronchoalveolitis and granulomatous lesions in bronchial associated lymphoid tissue have been produced from exposure to dusts after either IT dosed or inhalation exposure (30). Therefore the use of IT dosing should be used carefully.

The IT technique has proved to be very useful when the IT dosed animals have shown the same responses in the lungs as those produced from acute inhalation exposure. The effects on the lung can be evaluated using bronchoalveolar lavage as discussed elsewhere in this chapter. Subsequent comparison studies among similar test articles, such as in slightly varied formulations, can then be effectively conducted using the IT procedure.

E. PBPK Models and Closed Recirculating Chambers

Physiologically based pharmacokinetic models (PBPK) have been developed to account for the ultimate disposition of inhaled chemicals (31). The models are based on dividing the mammalian system into a series of anatomical compartments such as the lung, fat tissue, muscle tissue, a richly perfused tissue group, and the liver or metabolizing tissue group in the system. A series of mass balance equations are used to describe the movement and disposition of the test article through the system. Additional components can be added to the model system if necessary to account for other potential components in the system, e.g., metabolizing tissues in the nose.

The equations incorporate estimates of real-life values for the various parameters in the test animal. These could include alveolar ventilation, cardiac output, blood flow rates to the various tissue groups, and tissue volumes. These values can be measured, obtained from the literature, or estimated by animal scaling techniques, which use allometric relationships that relate these parameters to body mass. The model also requires estimates of the tissue solubilities or partition coefficients of the test article between blood/air, liver/blood, muscle/blood, and fat/blood. Several in vitro methods are used to calculate these coefficients.

The model also incorporates biochemical constants for the metabolism of the test article. One approach for determining these parameters such as V_{max} (maximum enzymatic reaction rate), K_m (Michaelis constant for enzymatic reaction), and k_f (first order rate constant) uses a closed chamber recirculation technique (32). In the closed chamber studies, animals are placed within the chamber at a designated concentration. The air is continuously recirculated and the animals are exposed for several hours. Carbon dioxide and water are scrubbed from the recirculating air and oxygen is added to maintain the oxygen level at 19–21%. The concentration of the test article is measured in the chamber over time and the drop in concentration is produced by the uptake of the test article by the test animals. The uptake is dependent on the rate of metabolism and the solubilities of the test article in the various tissues. A series of exposures and uptake curves over a wide range of concentrations is obtained. Using an optimization technique, the metabolic parameters are adjusted to achieve calculated uptake curves that best fit the experimental data. Once the parameters have been determined, this model can be use to predict the effect of various changes in one parameter or another, e.g., ventilation rate or tissue volumes. Furthermore, the model will then allow extrapolation to other species or humans by replacing the model values with appropriate human values. This then becomes a very useful tool in risk assessment.

IV. TEST ATMOSPHERE GENERATION SYSTEMS

A. Gases

Gaseous exposure atmospheres are certainly the easiest to generate. Using mass flowmeter-controllers, the test gas may be metered very accurately and precisely into the chamber air supply prior to entry into the chamber. Calibrated mass flowmeter-controllers may be purchased for specific gases but typically a mass flowmeter-controller calibrated for air is recalibrated for the test gas using a primary standard such as an electronic bubble-meter.

Safety should always be a concern when working with any test article, and gases are no exception. In addition to following safe handling procedures for compressed gas cylinders, care must be taken in testing the delivery system for leaks. In the case of highly toxic gases, a small leak could be fatal. In addition, if the gas is pyrophoric such as phosphine, until the gas is diluted down below its lower explosive limit with an inert gas such as nitrogen, any contact with oxygen could produce an immediate explosion.

If the gas is reactive, such as ozone, the test gas may need to be generated in situ to minimize loss of the gas in delivery lines. The interior surface of the chambers may also need to be covered with a nonreactive material.

B. Vapors

Vapor test atmospheres of a test article can be generated by flowing air over the liquid test article. For very volatile liquids this can be done by simply pumping or metering the test article into one neck of a 3-neck flask. Air or nitrogen is pumped into the second neck of the flask and vapor laden air exits from the remaining neck of the flask. If insufficient vapor is being generated, a heating mantle may be placed under the flask to provide additional heat for evaporation. In addition, the supply air may also be heated.

Other generation devices also use a similar principle. The "J" tube generator (Figure 3) is a vertical glass column filled with glass beads (33). The test article is metered in at the top of the column and flows down over the beads. The increased surface area provided by the beads facilitates evaporation. Heat may also be applied to this generator by wrapping and heating the column with a heating tape and heating the supply air.

Another vapor generator uses two concentric glass columns with a glass coil inside the outer column rotating down around the inner column. The test article again is metered in at the top and spirals down around the coil. A heating element inside the inner coil can provide additional heat if necessary.

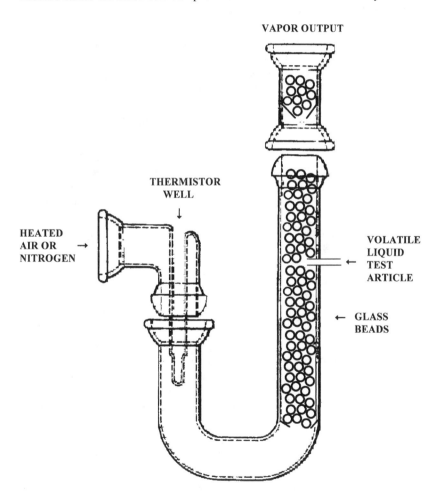

Figure 3 "J" Tube used to evaporate volatile liquids to produce vapor exposure atmospheres.

Vapor atmospheres may also be generated from solids. This poses special problems however, in that it is more difficult to sublimate the test article in the solid state than evaporate it from the liquid state and the test article condenses more easily. A stable vapor exposure level can be achieved by using the 3-neck flask system described above but with the entire flask inside a constant temperature furnace. Alternatively, the test article can be melted and used to coat glass beads. The dried test article coated beads can then be placed within a column. This achieves a greater surface area for generation than just a solid chunk of test article.

Generation of vapors poses a safety problem in that as the test article evaporates and is diluted down to the target level in air it passes through its explosive limits. If air is used as the gas flowing through the generator and heat is being applied to help evaporate the test article the potential for a disaster is increased. The risk can be minimized. If any heat that is needed for evaporation can be supplied through the inlet air, then the situation of a heating mantle or heating tape in contact with the test article through a layer of glass can be avoided. In addition, if nitrogen is used as the gas flowing through the generator instead of air, then no oxygen is present where the evaporation is occurring. At some point the vapor laden nitrogen must be mixed with air prior to entry into the exposure chamber but that can be done in a grounded mixing chamber with no heat present.

A final comment may be made about generating a vapor by atomizing a liquid as a fine mist which then evaporates. This certainly may be done and can possibly avoid the safety problems associated with heating a flammable liquid. However, the generation of any aerosol, including liquid aerosols, can produce a static charge buildup on the particles. Therefore this technique is not without its own safety concerns.

C. Liquid Aerosols or Mists

The atomization of solutions and suspensions with compressed air is one of the simplest ways to generate a liquid aerosol. An atomizer is a device used to produce liquid particulate or droplets by mechanical disruption of a bulk liquid. The nozzle on the end of a garden hose is a good example. A nebulizer is a special type of atomizer. In a nebulizer, an added impaction plate or surface only allows the smallest liquid particles to escape. The larger particles impact against the plate and are removed from the atmsophere. Several types of nebulizers are available for generating liquid aerosols for inhalation toxicity studies (34–36).

The DeVilbiss nebulizer, shown in Figure 4, is a classic example of how a nebulizer works. Compressed air enters the nebulizer and expands as it passes through an orifice and past a liquid inlet tube. Due to a venturi effect, a lower

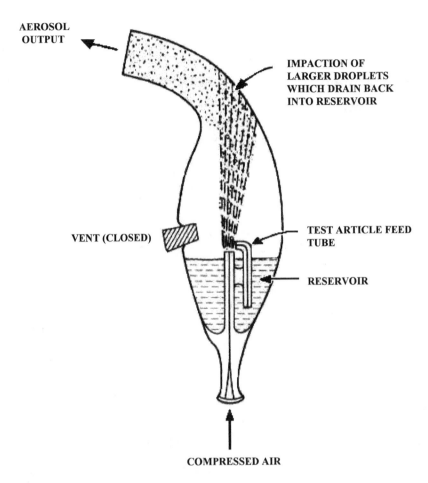

AEROSOL
OUTPUT

IMPACTION OF
LARGER DROPLETS
WHICH DRAIN BACK
INTO RESERVOIR

VENT (CLOSED)

TEST ARTICLE FEED
TUBE

RESERVOIR

COMPRESSED AIR

Figure 4 DeVilbiss liquid aerosol generator.

pressure draws a stream of liquid into the airstream where it breaks into droplets. The droplet spray is directed toward a curved wall or baffle where larger droplets are removed by impaction. Small droplets are able to follow the airstream around the baffle and out of the nebulizer.

Because the largest droplets do not leave the nebulizer whereas the solvent is constantly evaporating, the solution in the nebulizer becomes more concentrated with time. This can produce increased particle size over time and even plug the nebulizer fill tube. Presaturating the compressed air and cooling the reservoir can reduce, but not eliminate, the problem. For long term generation periods the nebulizer can be modified with the addition of a supply line to constantly replenish the reservoir.

D. Solid Aerosols or Dusts

1. Generators

Several different types of solid aerosol or dust generators may be used including the Wright Dust Feeder, fluidized bed, venturi, and others. The Wright Dust Feeder (Figure 5) involves prepacking the test article particles into a cake within a cylindrical holder. This can be done either manually or with a hydraulic press (37). The packed cylinder is then inverted and attached to a threaded spindle. As a motor causes the cylinder to travel slowly down the spindle a scraper blade advances up into the cylinder and test article cake. In this way, with each revolution of the cylinder, a very thin layer of test article is scraped off the cake into a groove in the scraper blade. The loose particles are dispersed by a stream of high velocity compressed air flowing through the groove.

If the test article has the right physical properties and the proper packing pressure can be empirically determined to produce the proper test article consistency within the feed cylinder cake, the Wright dust feeder can be a reliable generator. The generator does not work well for coarse or nonpackable particles. Generator output can be adjusted by the size of the feed cylinder and the rotation speed of the blade. Older models required changing gears and motors to change the blade rotation speed. Newer models now do this electronically, which makes changing generator output a lot easier.

Another dust generator based on a similar type process (Figure 6) involves prepacking the test article in the bottom of a glass cylinder (38). A few small beads are then dropped onto the top of the test article cake. A suction tube is place down the center of the cylinder to within close proximity of the test article surface and beads. A finer tube delivers a tangential air stream that sets the beads spinning around the surface. The spinning beads pick up and aerosolize the test article particles.

Another generator used in inhalation toxicity studies (Figure 7) is the fluidized bed generator (39). In this generator the test article is fed at a constant rate via a chain conveyor from a reservoir into a cylinder containing a bed of metal beads. The beads are supported on a nylon screen above an inlet compressed air plenum. If the compressed air flow rate is sufficient, the metal beads "boil" or become fluidized within the column. In this process test article particles are deagglomerated and aerosolized. Smaller particles are entrained into the airstream and carried out the top. Larger particles may initially be carried upwards but due to the gravitational pull, settle back down. The fluidized bed generator works well with free flowing test articles. However, unless the test

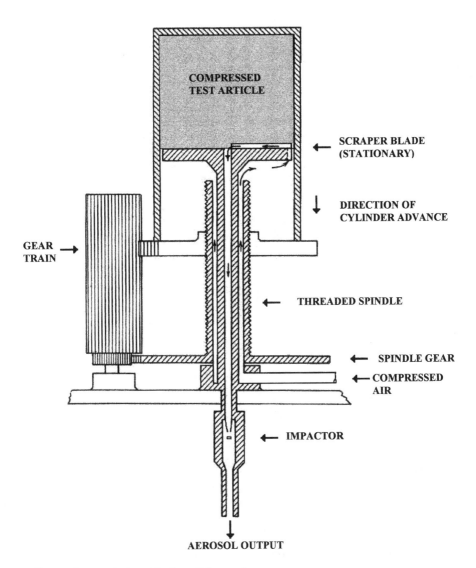

COMPRESSED
TEST ARTICLE

SCRAPER BLADE
(STATIONARY)

DIRECTION OF
CYLINDER ADVANCE

GEAR
TRAIN

THREADED SPINDLE

SPINDLE GEAR

COMPRESSED
AIR

IMPACTOR

AEROSOL OUTPUT

Figure 5   Wright Dust Feeder solid aerosol generator.

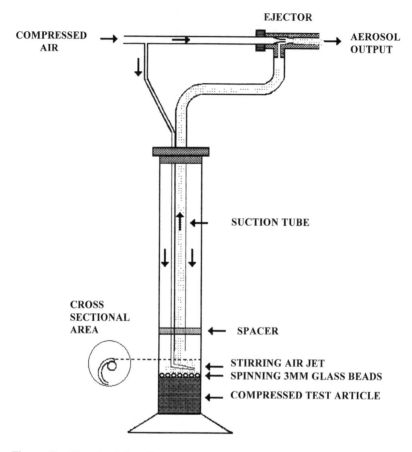

Figure 6 Glass bead dust dispenser.

article is initially mixed with the metal beads it can take considerable time before the generator output becomes stable.

The venturi principle can also be used to generate solid aerosol exposures. Using this technique test article particles are placed within a circular track on a platter. A motor rotates the platter such that the circular track is moved continuously under a feeder tube. Compressed air flowing through the main delivery tube creates a negative pressure and flow within the feeder tube, which sucks the test article particles into the main delivery tube air stream. This process will work well for free flowing test article and provides a reliable means for introducing test article into a delivery system at a constant rate.

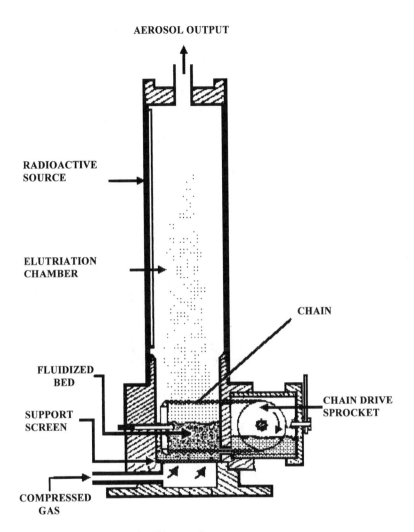

AEROSOL OUTPUT

RADIOACTIVE
SOURCE

ELUTRIATION
CHAMBER

CHAIN

FLUIDIZED
BED

CHAIN DRIVE
SPROCKET

SUPPORT
SCREEN

COMPRESSED
GAS

Figure 7 Fluidized bed solid aerosol generator.

2.   Dust Generator Maximization

During chamber trials prior to any animal exposures the operating conditions of
the dust generators are determined for each exposure level. Maximization of
generator output occurs in acute inhalation studies where target exposure levels
of 2–5 mg/l are required, and frequently difficult if not impossible to achieve.
Maximization of generator output may also be necessary for studies requiring
large generator flow rates such as for whole-body chamber studies or nose-only

studies with large number of animals. In the case of the fluidized bed generator, where the mass output is increased by increasing the test article feed rate and by increasing air flow through the generator, the effect on particle size must also be measured. Higher flow rates up through the generator entrained larger particles. Therefore the desired concentration may be achieved but the increase in concentration may be due to larger particles that have a different deposition pattern. As an example, consider the data in Table 2 for a rat inhalation study. The exposure level is increased by increasing the generator flow rate and entrainment of larger particles. Therefore, the percent of the test article mass or exposure level contained in particles less than 5 microns decreases. From deposition curves for a rat, the percent of particles depositing in the alveolar region is 5 percent. Therefore, the calculated alveolar exposure level data shows that the tenfold increase in exposure level produced no increase in the alveolar level. Any toxic effect due to alveolar deposition would consequently not show any dose related effect as expected from the tenfold increase in concentration.

One way to eliminate the above problem is to use fluidized bed generators of different diameters. Instead of using commercially available fluidized bed generators made of metal, relatively inexpensive generators may be produced from glass columns fitted with a fritted glass bottom. Because they are inexpensive, they can easily be replaced if broken or contaminated with a test article. In addition, they can be purchased with different internal diameters. Therefore, in the above example where the increased air flow entrained larger particles, if the diameter of the generator increased proportionately, then whereas the volume of air flow increased with the increased diameter, the velocity of the air flowing up through the generator stays the same. Consequently higher output with the same size particles can be achieved.

3. Static Charge

Static charge buildup can be a problem with aerosols. As the particles impact against each other a charge can develop on the particles. This can result in loss

Table 2   Rat Inhalation Study

Exposure group	Exposure level (mg/l)	Percent of particles less than 5 microns	Alveolar exposure level (mg/l)
Low	0.1	100	0.1
Mid	0.3	33	0.1
High	1	10	0.1

While the test article exposure concentration can be set at appropriate intervals, if the particle size in each is not also maintained constant, the alveolar exposure level will not be appropriately spaced.

of the test article particles to surfaces within the generation and chamber expo- sure systems and the charge buildup produces a safety concern. The generation system and chamber exposure system should be electrically grounded.

Charge neutralizers may also be used. The aerosol laden airstream is deliv- ered through a tube containing, for example, Kr-65 or Ni-63. The result is a neutralization of the total charge within the aerosol particles. This does not mean that all particles have a charge of zero but that all of the charges are distributed equally around zero.

This problem is not limited to solid aerosols. Charge can also develop on liquid aerosols droplets as well. Therefore it is safer to evaporate a liquid test article to produce a vapor exposure than it is to generate a fine mist, which would then evaporate, from the liquid.

4. Large Particles

As discussed previously, differences in generation parameters can increase the particle size being generated. One method to counter the production of the larger particles is to use elutriation chambers or cyclonic devices. Elutriation chambers are simply large chambers through which the particle laden air stream flows, allowing gravitational forces to remove the heavier particles. The column of air at the top of the fluidized bed in a fluidized bed generator serves as an elutria- tion chamber. Long horizontal delivery tubes from the generator to the chamber can also provide the same functionality.

A cyclonic device uses the principle of inertia to remove larger particles. By varying the physical dimensions of the cyclone and the flow rate through it, larger particles with greater inertia impact internal surfaces and are removed from the air stream. Only small particles are able to traverse through the cy- clone.

In some cases, its not a function of the generator but the neat test article may just be primarily large particles. In this situation, cyclonic devices may be used to separate the smaller particles from the neat material.

E. Fibers

The brush generator was developed as a result of the need for nondestructive aerosolization of fibers. The Wright Dust Feeder would not work because the scraping blade would cut the fibers. In the brush generator (see Figure 8) a column is packed with the fibrous material and a plunger pushes the packed material upward toward the spinning brush. The brush is spinning at a slow enough rate so that the fibers are picked up by the brush but not broken. A jet stream then blows the fibers off the top of the spinning brush into the delivery port of the chamber exposure system.

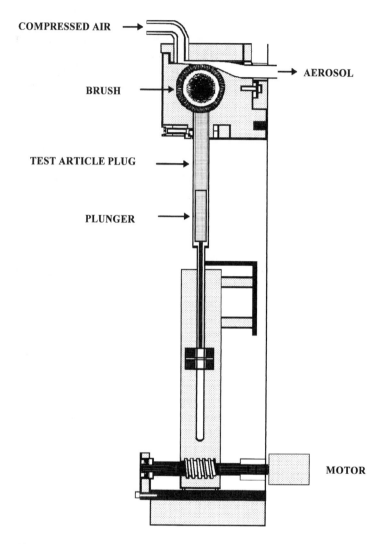

COMPRESSED AIR →

AEROSOL

BRUSH →

TEST ARTICLE PLUG →

PLUNGER →

MOTOR

Figure 8 Brush generator for generation of solid aerosols and in particular for fibers.

V. CHAMBER MONITORING SYSTEM

Chamber exposure levels are frequently reported both as nominal and analytical exposure levels. The nominal exposure level is calculated from the amount of test article consumed during the generation period divided by the volume of air passing through the chamber. The air volume is calculated as the chamber flow rate times the generation time. The analytical exposure level is calculated using a variety of monitoring techniques to obtain samples from the breathing zone of the test animal.

For nonreactive gases and vapors from liquids with high vapor pressures, the nominal and analytical exposure levels should be in very good agreement. Due to the formation or agglomeration of large droplets and impaction or settling on chamber surfaces, the nominal to analytical ratio for liquid aerosols can be 5 or 10 to 1. For solid aerosols with inherently large particle size, and where loss due to static charge buildup can be significant, nominal to analytical rations can be much higher.

A. Breathing Zone Samples

Because an inhalation chamber is a dynamic operation and there can be differences in test article concentration within a chamber over time or from one area to another area within the chamber, the actual exposure level should be measured in the breathing zone of the animals. That is, samples should be taken as close as practical to the test animals. During chamber trials, samples may be collected from within the animal exposure cages. If these samples reflect the same concentration and particle size as a sampling point exterior to the cage, then the exterior sampling point may be used.

The goal of any sampling technique is that the technique itself will not affect the system by its presence. This holds for measuring chamber concentration. The sample flow rate should not be significant relative to the overall chamber air flow rate. For example, take the case of a small whole-body chamber being operated at 20 l/min air flow by a downstream pump. If a sampling system were turned on also pulling 20 l/min, then the total air flow through the chamber doubled. The concentration of any test article being generated would drop to one half its original value. Sampling air flow rates should be small relative to chamber air flow rates.

In the case of a directed flow-past nose-only chambers where the test article laden air is being delivered at approximately 1 l/min per rat, the sampling system should be set up at an animal port and the sample drawn at 1 l/min. Sampling at this flow rate would therefore not affect chamber operation.

B. Gases and Vapors

The infrared spectrophotometer (IR) is a very useful device for monitoring gases or vapors in inhalation exposure chambers. After comparing a scan of a test article to background air, specific wavelengths where the test article absorbs energy can be determined. The best wavelength for monitoring exposure levels is determined by selecting the sharpest defined peak in a relatively flat region of the spectra and away from such confounding peaks as water and carbon dioxide.

The IR can be calibrated in one of two ways. The first method involves a closed loop. A pump circulates air through the loop of known volume and a calculated amount of test article is injected through a septum into the loop. If a liquid test article is injected and it has a low vapor pressure the response of the IR may be sluggish. Heat may have to be added to the IR cell and loop in order to completely vaporize the test article. Conversely, injection of test articles with high vapor pressures can also be problematic. Chilling syringes and the test article as well as the use of gloves may be necessary to keep the test article from vaporizing in the syringe prior to injection.

A second way to calibrate the IR is with the use of standard gas bags. A known volume of air is pumped into a standard bag. The air is pumped through a glass bulb equipped with a septum through which a calculated amount of test article is injected. The air flowing through the bulb evaporates the test article. Use of the glass bulb allows the visual confirmation that all of the test article has been evaporated.

Gas standard bags can be composed of many materials, e.g., Teflon®, Tedlar®, Mylar®, aluminum coated Mylar®, Saran®, and 5-layer bags. There is no perfect bag for all test articles (40). Losses of test article in these bags can occur from permeation, sorption, reactions, and simple leaks. Factors that can affect these losses include the chemical nature of the bag and test article, temperature (permeation is temperature dependent), the concentration of the test article (permeation is also concentration dependent), relative humidity, and time. If gas bag standards are being made to monitor a test article in humidified air, then the standards should be prepared in humidified air. Standards in new bags may have to be discarded until the inside is "conditioned." Gas standard stability must be evaluated to determine the length of time a prepared standard remains accurate.

The IR may not be the best monitoring device for mixtures. By setting on the carbon–hydrogen bond absorption wavelength the IR can be used as a total hydrocarbon analyzer. But the composition of the test article could be changing. Analysis of the exposure atmosphere with a gas chromatograph (GC) allows for analysis and quantification of individual peaks. With very complex mixtures, such as gasoline, the elution time may be so long to separate the peaks for the individual components that the technique cannot be used to monitor the test article exposure level.

This problem can be solved using a combination of the two techniques. The IR could be used as a total hydrocarbon monitoring device to give real time results, which would allow for the control of the exposure level. One or two GC samples per day could then also be run to verify that the composition of the mixture in the exposure atmosphere is the same as the neat material and that this composition doesn't change during the day.

If there were concern over intra-day stability, the elution time could be shortened to allow for chamber monitoring. However, this shortened elution time would merge the individual components into several major peaks. By monitoring the ratio of these peaks to the largest peak, test article stability throughout the day can be demonstrated. To monitor each of four or five exposure chambers hourly means a maximum elution time of about 12–15 minutes. A single long elution could be done on another GC to document composition. In the case of multiple component mixtures such as gasoline, the logarithmic Kovats Retention Index is a very useful GC tool in the qualitative identification of chromatographic peaks (41).

Impingers provide another monitoring technique for reactive gases and semivolatile organic compounds. Impingers work by causing the test article laden air to be broken into bubbles as it passes through a liquid. There are basically two types of impingers. In the first, the air is simply blown into the liquid where it dissolves or reacts with the liquid. In the second, the air is pumped through fritted glass, which is fused glass with porous openings, into the liquid.

Initial evaluations of the impinger must include analysis for breakthrough of the test article into a second in tandem impinger (42). Both the direct delivery and fritted glass impingers can work equally well and may be test article dependent. In the case of formaldehyde, the fritted impinger performed better. In the case of ammonia, the direct impinger performed better. Use of relatively nonvolatile liquids or chilling the impinger may be necessary to prevent liquid loss from the impinger. Analytical techniques for many compounds or classes of compounds have been published by NIOSH (National Institute of Occupational Safety and Health).

Absorbent tubes can also be used similar to impingers. In this case the absorbing liquid is replaced by a solid absorbent. Coconut-shell activated carbon is the sorbent of choice in sample tubes for collecting organic compounds present in workplace atmospheres. The characteristics of coconut carbon are not well suited for sampling polar or reactive compounds and other sorbents such as a carbon molecular sieve may be used. Analysis of the exposure level then involves the extraction of the test article off the absorbent material.

A good rule to follow when calibrating any monitoring system is to calibrate the entire sampling system exactly as it is going to be used. That is, don't calibrate by direct injections onto a GC column or into an impinger or absorbent tube when an exposure chamber is going to be monitored via sampling lines. Prepare gas bag standards and attach them to the end of the sampling lines for calibration. Differences in pressure in the GC sample loop, leaks, test article loss in the sampling lines, or other unknown problems could significantly affect the results.

C. Liquid and Solid Aerosols

1. Concentration

Filtration is the most commonly used method for analysis of aerosol concentration within inhalation exposure chambers because of its simplicity, flexibility, and economy. The collection sampling scheme collects a representative sample from the exposure atmosphere onto a porous filter by pulling a measured volume of air through the filter. If the exposure level is to be measured gravimetrically, the filter weight gain divided by the volume of air sampled provides the aerosol exposure level. Alternatively, the analytically determined mass of the test article on the filter can be used to calculate the exposure level. A critical aspect of the sampling scheme is that the volume of air sampled is known accurately and that there are no leaks in the sampling line or around the filter itself.

In order to get a representative sample of what is being inhaled, the sample should be collected from within the breathing zone of the test animals. The collection filter should be on the end of the sample probe to eliminate sample loss within any sampling lines. Open-faced as opposed to in-line filters are used to provide assurance of uniform particle deposition onto the filter and to eliminate sample loss in the inlet. In cases where in-line filters are used, the filter holders use a gradual expansion from the inlet to the filter as well as from the filter to the outlet. This allows uniform deposition over the filter, which may be critical if subsequent analysis utilizes only a fraction of the filter. However, sample loss in the inlet due to electrostatic or diffusional loss can be significant.

A wide selection of fibrous and membrane filters are available for use. Glass fiber filters are commonly used for exposure level measurements because they are not affected by moisture as are cellulose or paper filters. Teflon coated glass fiber filters are even less moisture-sensitive and are more inert than glass fiber filters to catalyzing chemical transformations. If analytical procedures are to be used, consideration must be given in the selection of the filter as to extraction efficiency of the test article from the filter, as well as contamination of the subsequent analysis with trace components from the filter itself.

Filter analysis may work very well for solid or nonvolatile aerosols. But care must be taken that the test article is not sublimating or evaporating from the filter (43). To test this, filters should be spiked with a known amount of test article and the intended air sampling volume pulled through the filter. Filter weight loss will demonstrate any potential problem.

Filter analysis however can be used even for semivolatile test articles. The technique involves empirically determining the percent volatility of the test article. This is accomplished by spiking a filter with a known amount of test article, pulling the intended air sampling volume through the filter, and then desiccating. The change from the postspiking weight to the postdesiccating weight will give the percent volatility. Chamber samples can then be collected, desiccated in a similar manner, and the original formulation concentration calculated based on the dry sample weight and the test article volatility.

Alternatively, samples can be collected using devices such as impingers or granular bed filters. These devices collect both the volatile and nonvolatile components of the test article atmosphere.

2. Particle Size Distribution

Evaluation of particle size is critical in evaluating the potential dose and pattern of particle deposition of any inhaled aerosol. Particle size distribution can be measured using microscopy, the cascade impactor, or other techniques such as light scattering or time of flight devices.

Collected solid aerosol particles can be measured using a microscope. While nonvolatile liquid aerosol particles can be collected, a liquid droplet on a solid surface may no longer be a sphere but flattened. A slide of the test material is made and by use of a reticle in the eyepiece the diameter of the particle may be measured. Optical microscopy is limited to the detection of particles larger than about 0.3 microns. Scanning electron microscopy or transmission electron microscopy allow the measurement of smaller particles. In addition, electron microscopy allows elemental analysis on a particle by particle basis.

When the diameter is irregular in shape, several dimensions may be chosen as particle "diameters." The investigator could estimate the diameter of a circle with the same area as that of the particle, or measure the maximum dimension of the particle (Feret's diameter), or measure the length of a line bisecting the particle into two equal areas (Martin's diameter). Measuring the size of a particle from a 2-dimensional projection of the particle can be difficult and misleading, especially if the particle is not spherical but a rod, flake, or fiber.

The microscopic technique can be useful in characterizing the particle size distribution of the bulk test article prior to and after milling, or to get an indication of how much of a bulk test article may be respirable, or to differentiate fibers from other particles. The data obtained is the number of particles of a certain diameter. The distribution is described by the count median diameter (CMD) and the geometric standard deviation σ. The distribution is frequently log normal as shown in Figure 9.

If the particle size distribution is log normal, then the count, surface area, and volume distributions are all log normal. Therefore, the MMD can be calculated from the CMD data as follows (44).

$$MMD = CMD \exp(3 \ln^2 \sigma)$$

If the CMD = 0.3 microns, and $\sigma = 1.7$, then the MMD would be 0.7 microns. If σ were only 20% larger the MMD would be 1.38 microns, or nearly double the original estimate. This illustrates how sensitive to error these calculations are when converting from count data.

The most common and meaningful diameter however is the aerodynamic diameter. The aerodynamic diameter is defined as the diameter of a sphere of unit density (1 g/cm^3) having the same terminal settling velocity as that of the particle in question. Because the larger particles are deposited in the respiratory tract by impaction or gravitation the aerodynamic diameter is preferred to any

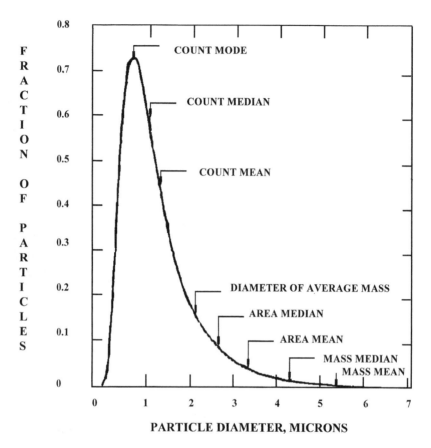

Figure 9 Typical log-normal aerosol particle size distribution.

geometric diameter found by 2-dimensional analysis. The aerodynamic diameter is frequently determined by an inertial impaction device such as the cascade impactor described below. This device separates particles based upon mass. The cascade impactor gives results indicating that irrespective of being a solid or liquid aerosol, or irrespective of shape, the particle is behaving aerodynamically and will deposit in the respiratory tract as if it were a spherical particle with the measured mass median aerodynamic diameter (MMAD).

The MMAD is more relevant in inhalation toxicology because toxicity is related to the dose or mass of the test article particles, not the number of particles per se. Because the volume of a particle, and hence its mass, goes up by the cube of the radius, the mass of a 3-micron spherical particle is 27 times that of a 1-micron particle.

A cascade impactor is a multistage, multi-orifice sampler designed to measure size distribution and mass concentration levels of liquid and solid aerosols (see Figure 10). The impactor is calibrated with unit density (1 g/cm^3) spherical particles so that the particles collected are sized aerodynamically equivalent to the particles regardless of their physical size, shape, or density.

The cascade impactor is made of classification stages consisting of a series of nozzles, or jets, and impaction surfaces, or collection plates. At each stage the aerosol stream passes through the jet and impinges upon the surface. Particles in the aerosol stream with a large enough inertia will impact upon the collection plate, smaller particles pass as aerosols onto the next stage. By designing stages with higher aerosol velocities in the jet, smaller diameter particles are collected at each stage. Particles too small to be collected on the first stage are collected on an after filter.

The cascade impactor is calibrated to operate at a specific flow rate. When operated at this flow rate each stage has a specific cutoff diameter. Each stage

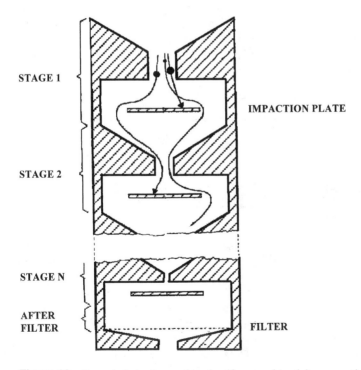

Figure 10   Cascade impactor used to classify aerosol particles as per their aerodynamic diameter.

is assumed to collect all particles of an aerodynamic diameter larger than its cutoff size.

Particles may bounce off the collection surface. These particle may bounce and be reentrained by the same collection surface, succeeding collection surfaces, or other surfaces within the impactor. Coating the impaction surface with a sticky substance, such as silicone, may improve particle collection.

3. Fibers

The term fiber is applied to aerosol particles having a length greater than or equal to 5 microns and a diameter less than or equal to 3 microns. The National Institute for Occupational Safety and Health (45) and the World Health Organization (46) have analytical methods for assessing the levels of airborne fibers. Samples are collected on a 25-mm cellulose ester filter, pore size 0.8–1.2 microns, with a backup pad. The filter is held within a 25-mm cassette fitted with a 50-mm electrically conductive extension cowel. Sampling is conducted with the filter in an open faced position. A section of the filter is then evaluated by positive phase-contrast microscopy. Specific counting rules regarding required aspect ratios and fiber length are followed and measurements are made using a calibrated graticule in the eyepiece of the microscope. Bivariate length and diameter fiber dimensions may be determined by scanning electron microscopy.

Other fiber characterization is also essential in evaluating fiber toxicity. Because the fibers tend to align with the air flow streams, the aerodynamic diameter of a fiber is about 3 times its actual diameter. Therefore very long fibers may deposit in the deep lung. But what are their physiochemical properties? Will the fibers dissolve or persist? Will they be cytotoxic to recruited macrophages? Will they be mutagenic? Thus nondimensional characteristics are also important in evaluating fiber toxicity.

VI. STUDY TYPES

A. Acute Toxicity

Determination of acute toxicity is usually an initial step in the assessment of the toxic characteristics of a test article. It provides information on health hazards arising from short-term exposures. Acute inhalation studies are single uninterrupted inhalation exposures. The exposure period is usually 4 hours but the stipulated duration can range from 1 hour for the Department of Transportation (47), the International Maritime Dangerous Goods Code (48), the International Air Transport Association Dangerous Goods Regulations (49), the Occupational Safety and Health Act (50), and the Federal Hazardous Substance Act (51) to 7 hours for OECD (52), or 8 hours for the new EPA guideline (53) (see Table 3). The animals (5 per sex) are singly housed in open-mesh cages within a whole-

Table 3 Acute Inhalation Testing Guidelines

	EPA			Europe OECD(52)	Japan JMAFF(61)
	FIFRA(111)	TSCA(112)	TSCA(53)		
Study Design					
Species	Rat	Rat	Rat	Rat	Rat
Sex and Number	5 males 5 females	5 males 5 females	5 males 5 females	5 males 5 females	5 males 5 females
Weight Range	125–250 g	Group mean ± 20%	Group mean ± 20%	Group mean ± 20%	Group mean ± 20%
Exposure Time	4 hours	4 hours	1,4,8 hours	4,7 hours	4 hours
Pathology	Gross necropsy	Gross necropsy	Gross necropsy	Discretionary	Gross necropsy
Limit Test	5 mg/l	2 mg/l	2 mg/l aerosols; 50,000 ppm gases and vapors	5 mg/l	5 mg/l
Exposure Conditions					
Temperature	22 ± 2°C	22 ± 2°C	22 ± 2°C	22 ± 2°C	Unspecified
Relative Humidity	40–60%	40–60%	40–60%	30–70%	Unspecified
Oxygen	≥19%	≥19%	≥19%	≥19%	Unspecified
Particle Size Distribution	"Respirable"	MMAD 1–4 µm	MMAD 1–4 µm	Unspecified	"Respirable"
Frequency of Measures					
Concentration	≥2 times	>3 times	≥3 times	Discretion	Unspecified
Air flow	every 30 minutes	every 30 minutes	every 30 minutes	Discretion	Unspecified
Particle Size	Discretion	Discretion	Discretion	Discretion	Unspecified
Temperature and Humidity	every 30 minutes	every 30 minutes .	every 30 minutes	Discretion	Unspecified

body chamber, or in nose-only exposure tubes for a nose-only study. Feed and water are removed during the exposure.

Whole-body exposures are usually used for gas or vapor studies. To minimize deposition of aerosols on the fur and the subsequent oral exposure due to animal preening, aerosol studies are usually conducted via nose-only exposures.

Lethality is the primary endpoint although possible mode of toxic action, behavioral or clinical abnormalities, body weight changes, gross lesions, and other endpoints are also evaluated. The first exposure is to 2 mg/l of the test article or the maximum attainable concentration, a limit test. For several years and for various regulatory agencies the limit test was 5 mg/l but this high a level of concentration with the also required particle distribution to have 25% of the particles less than 1 micron is not possible (54). Newer and harmonized regulations now have 2 mg/l as the limit test exposure level.

For aerosol studies the particle size is critical for penetration into the lung. The mass median aerodynamic diameter should be less than 4 microns to permit deposition throughout the entire respiratory tract of the rat. After the exposure the animals are held for 14 days before they are euthanized and evaluated macroscopically. During the 14-day period, the animals are frequently observed for clinical signs of toxicity and body weights are recorded. If toxic signs are reversing but not yet complete, the 14-day observation period may be extended.

If no lethality occurs, the exposure is considered to be a limit test and no further exposures are required. If the exposure level was not over 2 mg/L or the aerosol MMAD was not less than 4 microns, then the final report must detail all efforts made to meet those requirements in order for the study to be accepted by a regulatory agency.

If lethality occurred, then at least 2 additional exposures are conducted. The incidence of mortality from these 3 or more exposure levels will then allow for the calculation of the median lethal dose or the LC_{50} (55). The LC_{50}, which is analogous to the oral or dermal LD_{50}, is the exposure concentration that will kill 50% of the animals. The results should be given with the exposure length, such as a 4-hour LC_{50}. Data from these studies are used for classification and labeling.

The EPA, under the Toxic Substance Control Act (TSCA) issued new or revised health effect guidelines in 1997. These guidelines now include a 3 group, 4-hour duration, acute inhalation toxicity study with histopathology (56). There should be minimal lethality in the high dose group. Test animals are sacrificed 24 hr postexposure and in addition to microscopic examination of the respiratory tract, liver, and kidney, effects on the lung are also evaluated using bronchoalveolar lavage (BAL). If the test article is toxic, then those endpoints must also be evaluated after 8-hour exposures as well as 1-hour (optional). In addition, this guideline also requires a test of respiratory sensory irritation, the RD_{50}. Both the BAL and RD_{50} are discussed elsewhere in this chapter.

An alternative method has been recently proposed for adoption by OECD. The method is a stepwise method utilizing only 3 animals per sex per group. Utilization of this method is projected to allow accurate classification by all regulatory agencies around the world and use 50–80% fewer animals (57).

B. Subchronic Toxicity

The acute study is traditionally a step in establishing exposure levels for sub-chronic and other studies. The high dose for a 28-day subchronic inhalation study may be set at approximately 1/2 the calculated LC_{10} or less, depending on the steepness of the lethality curve.

Subchronic inhalation toxicity describes the adverse effects occurring as a result of repeated daily exposures for a part (up to approximately 10 percent) of a life span (see Table 4). The exposures are usually carried out 6 hr per day, 5 days per week, mimicking the industrial exposure. For studies relevant to ambient air quality, exposures may be carried out up to 23 hr per day, 7 days per week, allowing 1 hr per day for exposure chamber cleaning. Food and water are not provided during the exposures to preclude contamination of the food or water by the test article.

Endpoints evaluated during subchronic inhalation exposures are the same as for studies using other routes of exposure such as in the diet or gavage. Body weights are recorded weekly. The animals are removed from their cages weekly and given a detailed clinical examination. Observations of the animals during the exposure are also usually conducted at least once daily from outside the chamber to the extent possible and to how well and how many of the test animals can be seen.

After completion of the subchronic exposure period, hematology and clinical chemistries are evaluated. The animals are then euthanized. They receive a complete necropsy and macroscopic examination and organ weights are obtained. The absolute organ weights are evaluated as well as the relative organ weights, that is the organ to body weight or the organ to brain weight ratios. The organ to brain weight ratio can be useful when there is a significant test article effect on body weight. The brain weight is resilient to effects of weight loss. Therefore the organ to brain weight ratios are not confounded by changes in body weight and test article effects on organ weights are more easily discerned. Tissues from the control and high exposure group animals are evaluated microscopically. In the lower exposure groups the lungs are evaluated for any signs of disease as well as any target organs.

C. Chronic Toxicity

Chronic inhalation toxicity describes the adverse effects occurring as a result of repeated exposures for usually at least 12 months (58–61). The exposures are

Table 4 90-Day Subchronic Inhalation Testing Guidelines

	EPA			Europe OECD(116)	Japan JMAFF(61)
	FIFRA(113)	TSCA(114)	TSCA(115)		
Study Design					
Species	Rat	Rat	Rat	Rat	Rat
Sex and Number	10 males 10 females	10 males 10 females	10 males 10 females	10 males 10 females	10 males 10 females
Weight Range	Intergroup Variation <20%	Intergroup Variation <20%	Intergroup Variation <20%	Intergroup Variation <20%	Intergroup Variation <20%
Exposure Time	6 hrs/day, 5 days/ week; 90 days	6 hrs/day, 5 days/ week; 90 days	6 hrs/day, 5 days/ week; 90 days	6 hrs/day (after equilibrium) 5 days/ week; 90 days	6 hrs/day, 5 days/ week; 90 days
Exposure Levels	3 + control; optional 28 day recovery groups	3 + control; optional 28 day recovery groups	3 + control; optional 28 day recovery groups	3 + control; optional 28 day recovery groups	3 + control; optional 28 day recovery groups
Exposure Conditions					
Temperature	22 ± 2°C	22 ± 2°C	22 ± 2°C	22 ± 3°C	
Relative Humidity	40–60%	40–60%	40–60%	30–70%	
Oxygen	≥19%	≥19%	≥19%	≥19%	≥19%
Particle Size Distribution	"respirable"	MMAD 1–3 μm	MMAD 1–3 μm	unspecified	unspecified
Frequency of Measures					
Concentration	≥1	≥3	≥2	discretionary	unspecified
Air flow	60 minutes	30 minutes	≥2	discretionary	unspecified
Particle Size	≥1	discretionary	1–3	discretionary	unspecified
Temperature and Humidity	60 minutes	30 minutes	≥3	discretionary	unspecified

typically 6 hr per day, 5 days per week. The study should generate data from which to identify the majority of chronic effects and to define long-term dose-response relationships. The design of the study is similar to the subchronic study as far as endpoints of evaluation. Usually more animals are exposed per group and interim evaluation of such endpoints as hematology and clinical chemistries may occur. The chronic study may also be combined with an oncogenicity study. The test animals designated for the chronic study are treated as satellite animals to the main oncogenicity study and sacrificed at the appropriate intervals.

D. Oncogenicity

The objective of a long-term inhalation carcinogenicity study is to observe test animals for a major portion of their life span for development of neoplastic lesions during or after exposure to various doses of a test article (61,62). The study is usually performed from 18–24 months in mice, hamsters, and rats. In some studies, the actual chamber exposures are halted after 24 months and the animals are held until approximately 50% survival.

The high exposure level in oncogenicity studies is to set at the highest exposure concentration that would elicit signs of minimal toxicity without significantly decreasing the animal's life span. This is referred to as the maximum tolerated dose (MTD) (63). It is difficult however to set high exposure levels in chronic inhalation toxicity or oncogenicity studies of particulate test articles when many of the signs of toxicity usually signifying the MTD are not present. In point, lung tumors have occurred in studies of high concentrations of insoluble dusts that are considered to be benign, e.g., carbon black and titanium dioxide (64).

These tumors are believed to be secondary to excessive lung burdens, i.e., particle overload (65). That is, any poorly soluble particulate when inhaled at concentrations that will overwhelm the lungs ability to clean itself will induce lung tumors. Therefore evaluation of pulmonary clearance of a test article should be made in any subchronic study to be used to set exposure levels for a chronic study (66). This information will then allow appropriate exposure levels to be set for the chronic studies.

E. Other Study Types

Inhalation is just the route of exposure. Other types of toxicity studies commonly run such as neurotoxicity, developmental and reproductive toxicity, and genetic toxicity can also be run via the inhalation route of exposure. In the case of neurotoxicity studies, a unique problem associated with inhalation is the dose isn't given at one brief time point but during an exposure which frequently lasts up to 6 hr per day. Because of the time involved in conducting evaluations such as a functional observational battery and motor activity, in subchronic studies evaluations are staggered over several days and the animals aren't exposed on their respective days of evaluation. In developmental and reproduction inhalation studies, effects of stress from the exposure may show up as low pup weights and reduced weight gain, which can confound interpretation of test article-related effects. In vitro genetic toxicity studies pose an interesting problem on how to expose the cells bathed in a media to a vapor or gas. One approach to this is to place the cells on a rotating round flask. As the flask rolls, the cells alternately pass through the media and the test atmosphere.

VII. SPECIALIZED TECHNIQUES

A. Bronchoalveolar Lavage

Bronchoalveolar lavage (BAL) is a saline wash of the bronchoalveolar region of the respiratory tract. Changes in the enzyme and cellular components of the wash, or bronchoalveolar lavage fluid (BALF), can provide information on test article induced pulmonary injury. Use of the BALF results as biomarkers of pulmonary injury has become popular in recent years (67,68). BAL is now included in the E.P.A. guidelines for evaluating acute inhalation toxicity (56).

While acute inhalation exposures can be conducted, intratracheal instillation is also used to expose animals. Intratracheal instillation is less expensive than inhalation studies, can provide an exact dose, and can be used when there is little test article to use or inhalation exposure atmospheres are too difficult to generate. Intratracheal instillation has been criticized because it is not physiologic and the test article is given in a nonuniform bolus, which could produce an inflammatory response that would not be observed if the test article were accumulated gradually. In a recent study however, Henderson et al. (69) showed that the relative potentials for two materials to produce bronchoalveolitis and granulomatous lesions in bronchial-associated lymphoid tissues could be appropriately evaluated using either intratracheal or inhalation exposure.

At various times after acute exposure to a test article, test animals are sacrificed to perform the BAL. The heart and lungs can be removed en bloc to perform the BAL, or it can be done in situ. Usually both lobes of the lung are washed together but alternatively, to conserve animal use, one lobe can be tied off. The BAL is then performed in one lobe while the other lobe is fixed for histopathologic evaluation. The lungs are lavaged using physiologic saline at a volume of about 80% of the total lung or lobe capacity.

Enzymes frequently measured in the BALF include lactate dehydrogenase, beta glucuronidase, n-acetylglucosaminidase, and total protein. Cell viability as well as a total and differential count are measured. An inflammatory response can be detected by the appearance of polymorphonuclear leukocytes. Release of cytoplasmic enzymes such as lactate dehydrogenase can indicate cellular death or damage. An index of macrophage phagocytosis can also be measured (70).

Sustained or increasing levels over time can be indicative of long term pulmonary effects such as fibrosis (68). BAL can be used as an effective screening tool. If lung injury is the primary toxic effect of a test article, then BAL results after a single exposure can be used to evaluate toxicities among various potential formulations of the test article.

B. RD_{50}

Alarie has described an animal bioassay for use in detecting the sensory-irritating response of airborne chemicals (71). A dose related decrease in the respiration rate of mice is in proportion to the concentration of the exposure. The concentration that decreases the respiration rate by 50% is known as the RD_{50}. Using the RD_{50} the relative potency of chemicals as sensory irritants can be estimated. Of greater importance is the use of the RD_{50} to estimate what exposure level humans would find irritating.

Threshold Limit Values (TLVs) have been developed by the American Conference of Governmental Industrial Hygienists as guidelines for worker exposure (72). Based on industrial experience human and animal studies, it is believed that workers may be repeatedly exposed to the TLV without adverse health effects. The TLV frequently is based upon irritation unless further studies have shown other hazardous effects from exposure, such as the test article is a teratogen or carcinogen, which would necessitate the TLV to be lower. A plot of TLVs versus 0.03 * RD_{50} in Figure 11 from Schaper (73) shows an excellent

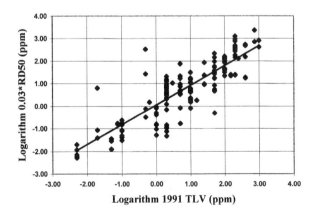

Figure 11   Plot of the logarithm of the 1991 TLV and the logarithm of 0.03* RD_{50} values showing agreement between respiratory depression in mice and subjective irritation in humans. Adapted from Schaper (73).

correlation between the decrease in respiration rate in mice and subjective irritation in humans.

The American Society for Testing and Materials (ASTM) has published a standard method for determining the RD_{50} (74). Four mice are simultaneously exposed to the airborne chemical via head-only exposure. The exposure tubes, or plethysmographs, are equipped with pressure transducers, which sense the change in pressure within the tube caused by the animal's respiration. The amplified signals are recorded on a recorder or by a computer. The respiration rate is recorded during a 10 min baseline or acclimation period and then during a 30 min exposure. A sufficient number of animal groups are exposed to generate a concentration response curve between the exposure concentration and the percent decrease in respiration rate from the baseline period.

The decrease in respiration rate is produced by a characteristic pause during exhalation (71). Recently, further analysis of the breathing pattern has been used to detect 3 different types of reactions along the respiratory tract: sensory irritation in the upper airways, airway limitation along the conducting airways, and pulmonary irritation at the alveolar level (75).

C. Pulmonary Sensitization

There is increasing interest in the potential for industrial chemicals to produce allergic reactions in the respiratory tract. The interest has developed because of the association between allergies and the development of asthma, and because the incidence of asthma has been increasing for unclear reasons. In 1992 the EPA convened a workshop to determine the availability, applicability, and status of test methods that might be applied to chemicals to evaluate their potential to produce respiratory hypersensitivity (76). There was a general consensus that the currently available test methods are not ideal and more validation needs to be conducted.

The evaluation of the test article could use a tiered approach (77). If initial evaluation of the structure activity of the test article, or its class of compounds, indicates potential for pulmonary hypersensitivity, further testing could be performed. The presence of chemical-specific cytophilic antibody in either the guinea pig or mouse, or an increase in total immunoglobulin E in the mouse are useful markers in a screen for this effect (76). Chemicals testing positive in this screen could then be evaluated using an animal model of allergic bronchoconstriction.

The most established test method for detection of potential pulmonary allergy is the Karol guinea pig procedure (78). In this procedure, guinea pigs are exposed via whole-body inhalation exposure to a test article for 60 min per day on Study Days 1–5. These animals are then challenged with the test article on Study Days 19 and 33. In the challenge exposures the guinea pigs are exposed using whole body plethysmographs attached to the primary chamber. Respiration rate is recorded preexposure, during the 60 min exposure and for 10 hr post each challenge exposure. Immunologically sensitized animals will typically respond to the challenge with an increase in respiratory rate and a decrease in tidal volume. During severe reactions with severe bronchoconstriction, the response is a slow gasping pattern. A positive control chemical, such as trimellitic anhydride, is usually used in each study.

D. Cardiac Sensitization

The use of aerosol products is ubiquitous in our society primarily because of the convenience of pressurized containers to the consuming public. Aerosolized products necessarily contain one or more propellants, chiefly chlorinated and/or fluorinated methane or ethane derivatives. Two problems are associated with the use of these propellants. The first is the depleting effect of these propellants on the ozone layer in the stratosphere. The second involves the cardiotoxicity of the halogenated hydrocarbons. In an attempt to get "high," some users have inhaled these products. Sudden deaths associated with these episodes without any known cause of death have suggested the fatalities were due to cardiac arrhythmias which culminated in ventricular fibrillation and cardiac arrest.

Cardiac sensitization is not a new phenomenon. It has been known since 1911 that sudden death in cats under chloroform anesthesia was the result of its sensitization of the myocardium to epinephrine induced arrhythmia (79). By 1971 over 40 compounds had been identified which sensitize the heart to epinephrine, resulting in the production of arrhythmias (80). Many more have been identified since then.

The test method to evaluate cardiac sensitization uses dogs (81). Six healthy male dogs are trained to maintain a standing position in a sling while wearing an inhalation mask over their snout and mouth. Because dogs can vary markedly in their cardiac response to epinephrine injected intravenously, each dog is evaluated to determine the appropriate dose which would induce some but not too many ectopic beats.

The actual test is completed in 17 min. The dog to be tested is positioned in the sling breathing fresh air through the mask. Electrocardiogram leads are applied and an ECG recording is initiated. At 2 min, the selected dose of epinephrine is administered. At 7 min the article exposure commences. At 12 min a challenge dose of epinephrine is injected. At 17 min the vapor exposure is halted.

The dogs are exposed to a 2.5% concentration the first time. If necessary, the dogs are successively exposed to 5, 10, 15, and 20%. As soon as ventricular tachycardia is evident, the testing is stopped for that dog. A dose response curve may be constructed by plotting the percent of dogs responding versus the inhaled concentration.

This test is primarily a screening tool to permit a rank order of the cardiac sensitization potential of the test article tested. If no arrhythmias occur at the highest concentration, then no cardiac sensitization has occurred.

E. Pulmonary Function

Because the lung is potentially a target organ in any inhalation toxicity study, measurement of changes in lung function are of particular interest. Tests of pulmonary function have been developed in both large and small laboratory animals. These tests were developed on the basis of similar tests used in humans to diagnose and manage patients with lung disease. In some cases pulmonary function tests have been found to show evidence of test article-related damage before it is possible to detect it histologically.

The battery of tests developed allow assessment of pulmonary mechanics (lung volumes, quasistatic pressure-volume curves), pulmonary dynamics (resistance, compliance, partial and full forced maneuvers), gas distribution (nitrogen washout and closing volume), and gas transfer (carbon monoxide diffusion) (82–84). Because of the small lung volumes and rapidity of such maneuvers as forced vital capacities in rodents, the frequency response of the measuring equipment, pressure transducers, flowmeters, etc. must be carefully evaluated (85). Failure to do so can produce significant errors in measuring the amplitude and phase of measure signals and calculated endpoints.

F. Pathology

In order to perform microscopic evaluation of respiratory tract tissues, the tissues must be properly collected, prepared, and examined. In the case of the respiratory tract however, certain tissues require special techniques (86).

1. Lung Infusion

To ensure that the lung tissue is fixed, the fixative should be infused via the trachea. To standardize the amount of lung inflation, the lung should be fixed at a constant pressure of about 20 cm H_2O. This pressure will inflate the lungs to near total lung capacity without overinflation. This technique will also minimize or eliminate the overinflated or conversely underinflated lobes or regions of the lungs frequently seen when the fixative is infused once using a syringe.

A simple device for maintaining a constant fixation pressure in the lungs is presented in Figure 12. The sealed container is set up as shown with the fixative level well above the bottom of the vent tube. The bottom of the vent tube is placed even with the outlet. When the outlet is opened, fixative will drain out the outlet and air will come down the vent tube. Eventually air will fill the tube and start to bubble up through the fixative. Once the air starts to bubble, the vent tube is full of air and the pressure of the air at the bottom of

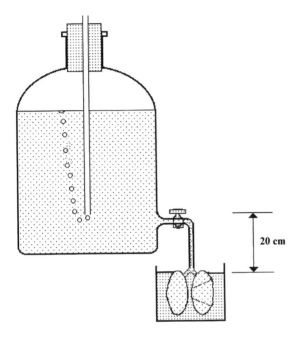

Figure 12 Lung infusion apparatus to provide uniform inflation and fixation of lung tissue for microscopic examination at 20 cm of water pressure.

the vent tube, and correspondingly the pressure of the fixative at that level, is atmospheric. As the fixative has drained out it has created a vacuum in the top of the sealed container. This vacuum or negative pressure now equals the head or positive pressure of the fixative above the bottom of the vent tube. As more fixative drains out, more air will bubble in. The bottom of the vent tube is therefore at atmospheric pressure irrespective of the fixative level until the fixative level is below the vent tube. If the outlet is connected to a manifold with attached lungs 20 cm below the outlet, when each lung's respective valve is opened the lung will be inflated and maintained at a constant 20 cm H_2O pressure. The pressure will be maintained even as other lungs are added to a system or even if there are small nicks and leaks in the lungs themselves. The lungs are usually maintained in a container of fixative during this period with a fixative saturated gauze pad lying over the top.

2. Lung Volume

When a potential toxic effect in the lung includes edema, a measurement of lung density can be a useful endpoint. The lung density can be calculated as the lung weight divided by the volume of the lungs. The volume of the lungs can be measured based upon the principle that the volume of water displaced by an object submerged within a container of water will equal the weight gain in grams of the container containing the water.

More specifically, to determine the volume of a lung, place an appropriately sized beaker, partially filled with saline, onto a balance. Insert a piece of coiled wire to be used to submerge the lung into the saline to a line marked on the wire. Tare the balance. Submerge the lungs under the coil of wire to the same mark on the wire. Do not allow the wire or lungs to touch the sides or bottom of the beaker. Assuming 1 g/ml, the weight gain in grams equals the lung volume in milliliters.

3. Nose

The nose provides several functions for the body including olfaction, filtering of airborne particulates, and heating and humidifying inspired air. The filtering or scrubbing of inhaled test article places the nose at risk to injury. The extent of this injury is a consequence of the regional deposition of the test article and the local tissue susceptibility. The amount of test article deposited or absorbed is a function of the exposure concentration, duration of exposure, and chemical properties of the test article, such as reactivity and water solubility. Nasal toxicity and carcinogenicity of inhaled compounds has been demonstrated for such compounds as formaldehyde (87), acetaldehyde (88), hexamethylphosphoramide (89), and 1,2 dibromoethane (90).

Less appreciated however, is the fact that the nose is also a site for xenobiotic metabolism. The distribution of enzymatic activity, like the distribution of air flow discussed before, is not uniform. But unlike air flow, enzymatic activity is predominantly in the olfactory mucosa (91). The potential roles for this metabolic activity include degradation of test articles to terminate olfactory stimulation, metabolic deactivation of inhaled toxicants, and protection of the lower respiratory tract (92). But this metabolism can also produce toxic metabolites. Therefore test article-related effects which require metabolic activation are seen in the olfactory region of the nose and metabolic activation may be relevant in the toxic effects produced by test articles administered orally such as certain nitrosamines (93), 1,4-dioxane (94), and phenacetin (95).

Nasal toxicity can occur by venue of this first contact with deposited test article, which is affected by the regional flow of the inspired air through the nose. The nasal cavity is not uniformly ventilated (96). Inspiratory air flow follows a distinctly asymmetrical pattern with the majority of the air flow being apportioned to the respiratory mucosa. Therefore test article-related effects from direct contact with the test article are seen in this epithelium. If effects are not seen in the respiratory epithelium but are seen in the olfactory region, an area of relatively reduced air flow, these effects are probably associated with metabolic activation.

The issue of nasal toxicity is even more complex than the difference between air flow and enzyme distributions. Whereas the olfactory mucosa may only receive a small part of the inspiratory flow during normal inspiration, this is not true with higher inspiratory flow rates such as during sniffing or exercise. At low flows, olfactory metabolism is limited by gas or vapor delivery to the mucosa; at high flow rates it is not. Even within the olfactory region itself, asymmetrical distribution of specific enzymes can lead to asymmetrical toxic effects (97). Nasal mucosa blood flow and its distribution throughout the nose is also important in removing deposited test article. Analysis of nasal uptake of test article and related effects must take all of these factors into account (98).

Knowledge of the pattern of lesions within the nose can therefore provide insight into the relative roles of air flow and metabolic activation. Localization also permits subsequent studies of site specific responses to a test article. Sectioning of the nose is a critical issue in determining the pattern of distribution of any test article-related lesions. The first description of a systematic approach to sectioning of the nose included 4 standard sections (99). The use of these 4 sections allowed for the evaluation of the 4 major epithelial types in the nose including squamous, transitional, respiratory, and olfactory regions. This evaluation has been taken a step further with the use of nasal mapping (100).

In nasal mapping, multiple cross-sectional diagrams of the noses of Fischer-344 rats and B6C3F1 mice have been prepared. Each diagram indicates the various epithelia present. After selecting the appropriate diagram for the cross section being evaluated, the investigator can record the distribution of the lesion on the diagram. This information is not readily available from routine tabulation of incidence data. Location of the lesion on these diagrams can then be transferred to a sagittal diagram to show the location of the lesion along the long axis of the nose as well. Use of these diagrams allows visualization of where the lesion is occurring and to what extent within a certain epithelial type it is occurring. These diagrams can help visualize the location and distribution of a test article on the nose (see Figure 13). Site specificity of a lesion can provide important clues about the underlying mechanism responsible for the lesion. Understanding the principle factors that produced the observed lesion is then very useful in extrapolating from this animal data to estimate potential human risks (101).

If a test article has selectively induced lesions in only part of the olfactory region, how much olfactory epithelia must be lost to produce a loss in olfaction? An olfactometer has been developed to answer that question (102). The device uses a commercially available rat shuttle box which has been modified to create 2 separate exposure chambers into either of which an odorant can be added. A central air curtain serves as a physical barrier for odor movement and washes odorant from the fur of the animal as it passes through the air curtain from one chamber to the other. The test animal is trained to move to the other chamber

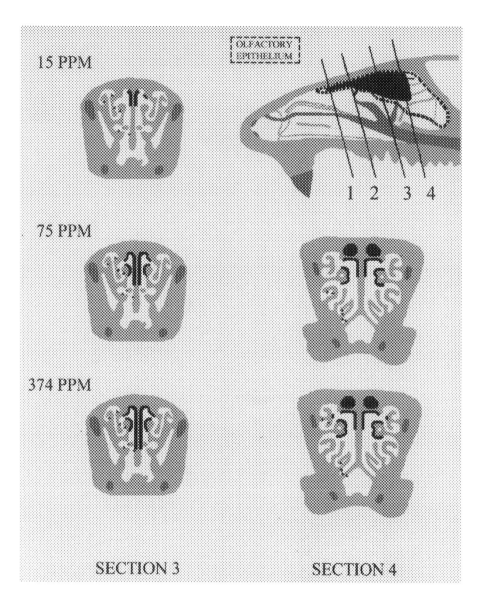

Figure 13 Map of test article-related lesion sites within the nose after exposure to methylethylketoxime (117).

and avoid a mild electric shock by providing an odor as a warning signal. A decrease in the rat's performance suggests that the animal is losing its sense of smell. Nasal histopathology is the more sensitive indicator of olfactory damage. Severe olfactory degeneration must be present before a loss of olfaction can be seen.

4. Larynx

The larynx is an organ which has gotten a lot of recent interest in inhalation toxicity studies. Where a simple section through the larynx may miss test article-related effects, there are regions which are highly responsive to inhaled materials. These regions include the base of the epiglottis, ventral pouch, and the medial surfaces of the vocal processes of the arytenoid cartilages. The specific anatomical sites can be difficult to find and consistent histological sampling must be employed (103). These sites seem to be particularly sensitive to test article-related changes (104). Therefore, careful evaluation of these sites should be conducted in all inhalation toxicity studies.

The effect in the larynx is frequently seen as a thickening of the epithelial layers or squamous metaplasia. The squamous metaplasia is also seen in control animals and appears to increase with age (105). An increased incidence and severity of squamous metaplasia response is usually seen in aerosol exposures. This may be resulting from the impaction of test article particles produced by air flow turbulence through this region. This generic type effect may be an adaptive or protective response much as the buildup of a callus on the hand. If true, then the differences in anatomy, air flow, and tissue susceptibility must be considered when trying to extrapolate the findings to man (106).

5. Cell Proliferation

Molecular toxicological endpoints are increasingly important. Altered cell proliferation can be a sensitive indicator of toxicity. Cell proliferation studies combined with histopathology can provide valuable information on both neoplastic and nonneoplastic responses to toxic materials. Measuring cell proliferation in target tissues can help in understanding the mechanism of action, in risk assessment, and in dose selection for chronic inhalation toxicity studies.

In vivo cell proliferation can be measured by the incorporation of radioactively labeled thymidine (^{3}H-thymidine) or the synthetic thymidine analog 5-bromo-2′-deoxyuridine (BrdU) into DNA during replication. The relative advantages and disadvantages of these labeling methods in toxicological studies has been discussed (107). BrdU incorporation is nonradioactive which avoids radiation contamination and hazards, produces results in hours, but uses immunohistochemistry techniques for visualization, which can be costly. Visualization of ^{3}H-thymidine incorporation is simple but the autoradiography may require several weeks of film exposure. Cellular details may also be lost due to overlabeling with ^{3}H-thymidine.

Both labels are rapidly eliminated from the body. Therefore, injection of either of these labels results in a brief "pulse" of label at the target tissue. This pulse may then miss or underestimate an acute burst of cell proliferation. Consequently, unless the timing of the effect is known, continuous infusion of the label using an osmotic pump maximizes the potential for measuring a proliferative response. Both pulse (108) and continuous infusion (109) have been successfully used to evaluate cell proliferation in the respiratory tract.

Cell proliferation can be evaluated using a mitotic index (MI), a labeling index (LI), or a unit length labeling index (ULLI). The MI measures the percent of cells undergoing mitosis. MI may be a more precise measure of DNA replication than LI but since mitosis is a transitory event in the cell cycle very small numbers are seen in respiratory and nasal epithelia with relatively long generation times. The LI measures the percentage of cells in the S phase that have incorporated the label. LI can be a very sensitive measure of DNA synthesis.

The ULLI, which is expressed as the number of labeled cells per mm of basement membrane, may be more appropriate than the LI when evaluating cell proliferation in tissues such as the nose where a single slide may contain several different types of epithelia (110). If the total number of cells counted or the denominator in the LI were from the same epithelia cell population there would be no problem. But if the total number of cells included cells from other perhaps nonaffected cell populations, then supposed test article-related changes may only be due to this change in cell population. The number of labeled cells per mm of basement membrane provides a practical alternative.

VIII. CONCLUDING REMARKS

Inhalation is just another route of exposure to test articles but the potential for exposure is greater via inhalation than any other route of exposure. The techniques involved in the evaluation of inhalation toxicity are greater and more problematic than any other route of exposure. Each test article presents its own unique set of challenges dealing with the generation of stable exposure atmospheres, developing appropriate monitoring techniques, and avoiding the confounding effects of animal handling and stress on the evaluation of endpoints of interest. Because of the labor and equipment involved inhalation studies typically cost 2–3 times what the same study via the oral route would cost. Despite all of the challenges and increased cost, inhalation toxicology can be and should be done. Inhalation toxicology is doable.

REFERENCES

1. Schlesinger, R.B. Deposition and clearance of inhaled particles. In: McClellan, R.O. and Henderson R.F., eds. Concepts in Inhalation Toxicology. New York: Hemisphere Publishing, 1989, chapter 6.

2. Kelly, D.W., Duffy, J.S., Haddock, L.S., Daughtrey, W.D., Keenan, T.H., Newton, P.E., and Rhoden, R.A. Chronic Inhalation Study of commercial hexane in rats. The Toxicologist, 1994; 14:1233.

3. Kennedy, G.L. Evaluating Hazards of Inhaled Products. In: Product Safety Evaluation Handbook, Gad, S., ed. New York: Marcel Dekker, 1988: 261.

4. Guide for the Care and Use of Laboratory Animals, Institute of Laboratory Animal Resources, National Academy Press, Washington, D.C., 1996.

5. Hinners, R.G., Burkart, J.K., and Punte, C.L. Animal inhalation exposure chambers. Arch. Environ. Health 1968; 16:194–206.

6. Mattie, D.R., Alden, C.L., Newell, T.K., Gaworski, C.L., and Fleming, C.D. A 90-day continuous vapor inhalation study of JP-8 jet fuel followed by 20 or 21 months of recovery in Fischer 344 rats and C57BL/6 mice. Toxicol. Path. 1991; 19:77–87.

7. Silver, S.D. Constant flow gassing chambers: Principles influencing design and operation. J. Lab. Clin. Med. 1946; 31:1153–1161.

8. Newton, P.E. and Pfledderer, C. Measurement of the deposition and clearance of inhaled radiolabeled particles from rat lungs. J. Appl. Toxicol. 1986; 6:113–119.

9. Dahlback, M., Eirefelt, S., Karlberg, I.-B., and Nerbrink, O. Total deposition of evans blue in aerosol exposed rats and guinea pigs. J. Aerosol Sci. 1989; 20: 1325–1327.

10. Phalen, R.F., Mannix, R.C., and Drew, R.T. Inhalation exposure methodology. Environ. Health Perspect 1984; 56:23–34.

11. Pare, W.P. Restraint stress in biomedical research. Neurosci. Biobehav. Rev. 1986; 10:339–370.

12. Svendsen, P. Environmental impact on animal experiments. In: Svendsen, P. and Hau, J., eds. Handbook of Laboratory Animal Science, Vol. 1 Selection and Handling of Animals in Biomedical Research. Boca Raton: CRC Press, 1994: 191–202.

13. Mauderly, J. Respiration of F344 rats in nose-only inhalation exposure tubes. J. Appl. Toxicol. 1986; 6:25–30.

14. Landry, T.D., Ramsey, J.C., and McKenna, M.J. Pulmonary physiology and inhalation dosimetry in rats: development of a method and two examples. Toxicol. Appl. Pharm. 1983; 71:72–83.

15. Jakab, G.J. and Hemenway, D.R. Restraint of animals required for nose-only inhalation toxicologic studies suppresses pulmonary antibacterial defenses. Inhalation Toxicol. 1989; 1:289–300.

16. Drew, R.T. Acute carbon monoxide toxicity in restrained vs. unrestrained rats. The Toxicologist 1982; 2:46.

17. Damon, E.G., Eidson, A.F., Hobbs, C.H., and Hahn, F.F. Effect of acclimation to caging on nephrotoxic response of rats to uranium. Lab. An. Sci. 1986; 36:24–27.

18. Frame, S.R., Kelly, D.P., Carakostas, M.C., and Warheit, D.B. Two four-week inhalation toxicity studies with HFC-134a in rats. The Toxicologist 1992; 12:355.

19. Capen, C.C., DeLellis, R.A., and Yarrington, J.T. Endocrine systems. In: Haschek, W.M. and Rousseaux, C.G., eds. Handbook of Toxicologic Pathology. San Diego: Academic Press, 1994:717–736.

20. Green, J.D., Helke, W.F., Scott, J.B., Yau, E.T., Traina, V.M., and Diener, R.M. Effect of equilibration zones on stability, uniformity, and homogeneity profiles of

vapors and aerosols in the ADG nose-only inhalation exposure system. Fundam. Appl. Toxicol. 1984; 4:768–777.

21. Moss, O.R. and Asgharian, B. Precise inhalation dosimetry with minimum consumption of product: the challenge of operating inhalation exposure systems at their design limits. In: Byron, P.R., Dalby, R.N., and Farr, S.J., eds. Respiratory Drug Delivery IV. Buffalo Grove: Interpharm Press, 1994:197–201.

22. Cannon, W.C., Blanton, E.F., and McDonald, K.E. The flow-past chamber: an improved nose-only exposure system for rodents. Am. Ind. Hyg. Assoc. J. 1983; 44:923–928.

23. Pauluhn, J. Validation of an improved nose-only exposure system for rats. J. Appl. Toxicol. 1994; 14:55–62.

24. Allen, D.L., Pollard, K.R., Hughes, B.L., Dorato, M.A., and Wolff, R.K. Use of a head dome system to compare i.v. methacholine-induced bronchoconstriction in conscious vs anesthetized rhesus monkeys. J. Appl. Toxicol. 1995; 15:13–17.

25. U.S. EPA, Pesticide Assessment Guidelines, Microbial Pest Control Agents and Biochemical Pest Control Agents, Subdivision M 152A-12, Acute pulmonary toxicity/pathogenicity study with microbial pest control agents (MPCA)s.

26. Leong, B.K.J., Coombs, J.K., Imlay, M.M., and Sabaitis, C.P. Morphometric analyses of the pulmonary distribution of inhaled particles. The Toxicologist 1986; 6: 35.

27. Sabaitis, C.P., Coombs, J.K., and Leong, B.K.J. Repeated oropharyngeal nebulization of drugs to rats and dogs. The Toxicologist 1989; 9:184.

28. Phalen, R.F. Inhalation Studies: Foundation and Techniques. Boca Raton: CRC Press, 1994.

29. Pritchard, J.N., Holmes, A., Evans, J.C., Evans, N., Evans, R.J., and Morgan, A. The distribution of dust in the rat lung following administration by inhalation and by single intratracheal instillation. Environ. Res. 1985; 36:268–297.

30. Henderson, R.F., Driscoll, K.E., Harkema, J.R., Lindenschmidt, R.C., Chang, I.Y., Marples, K.R., and Barr, E.B. A comparison of the inflammatory response of the lung to inhaled versus instilled particles in F344 rats. Fundam. Appl. Toxicol. 1995; 24:183–197.

31. Gargas, M.L. and Anderson, M.E. Physiologically based approaches for examining the pharmacokinetics of inhaled vapors. In: Gardner, D.E., Crapo, J.D., and Massaro, E.J., eds. Toxicology of the Lung. New York: Raven Press, 1988:449–476.

32. Gargas, M.L., Anderson, M.E., and Clewell, H.J., III. A physiologically based simulation approach for determining metabolic constants from uptake data. Toxicol. Appl. Pharm. 1986; 86:341–352.

33. Miller, R.R., Letts, R.L., Potts, W.J., and McKenna, M.J. Improved methodology for generating controlled test atmospheres. Am. Ind. Hyg. J. 1980; 41:844–846.

34. Miller, J.I., Stuart, B.O., Deford, H.S., and Moss, O.R. Liquid aerosol generation for inhalation toxicity studies. In: Leong, B.K.J., ed. Inhalation Toxicology and Technology. Ann Arbor: Ann Arbor Science, 1980:121–138.

35. Mercer, T.T., Tillery, M.I., and Chow, H.Y. Operating characteristics of some compressed air nebulizers. Am. Ind. Hyg. Assoc. J. 1968; 20:66–78.

36. Gussman, R.A. Note on the particle size output of collison nebulizers. Am. Ind. Hyg. Assoc. J. 1984; 45:B9–B12.

37. Wright, B.M. A new dust-feed mechanism. J. Sci. Inst. 1950; 27:12–15.
38. Rendall, R.E.G. and Coetze, F.S.J. A simple reliable dust disperser. Ann. Occup. Hyg. 1983; 27:189–198.
39. Marple, V.A., Liu, B.Y.H., and Rubow, K.L. A dust generator for laboratory use. Am. Ind. Hyg. Assoc. J. 1978; 39:26–32.
40. Posner, J.C. and Woodfin, W.J. Sampling with gas bags I: Losses of analyte with time. Appl. Ind. Hyg. 1986; 1:163–168.
41. American Society for Testing and Materials, Standard test method for detailed analysis of petroleum naphthas through n-nonane by capillary gas chromatography, ASTM D 5134-92, Philadelphia, 1992.
42. Lin, X., Willeke, K., Ulevicius, V., and Grinshpun, S.A. Effect of sampling time on the collection efficiency of all-glass impingers. Am. Ind. Hyg. Assoc. J. 1997; 58:480–488.
43. McAneny, J.J., Leith, D., and Boundy, M.G. Volatilization of mineral oil mist collected on sampling filters. Appl. Occup. Environ. Hyg. 1995; 10:783–787.
44. Marple, V.A. and Rubow, K.L. Aerosol generation concepts and parameters. In: Willeke, ed. Generation of Aerosols and Facilities for Exposure Experiments. Ann Arbor: Ann Arbor Science Publishers, 1980:3–30.
45. National Institute for Occupational Safety and Health, 1984. Manual of Analytical Methods, Third edition, Volume I (DHHS/NIOSH Pub. No. 84-100). Cincinnati, Ohio; Method 7400 revised, May 15, 1989, pp. 7400–01—7400–14.
46. World Health Organization, Reference methods for measuring airborne man-made mineral fibres (MMMF), WHO/EURO MMMF Reference Scheme, Copenhagen, Denmark, 1985.
47. U.S. Department of Transportation, Fed. Reg. Vol. 55, No.246, December 21, 1990.
48. International Maritime Dangerous Goods Code, Class 6.2-Poisons, Amendment 24-86, January 1, 1991.
49. International Air Transport Association Dangerous Goods Regulations, Division 6.1, 32nd Edition, January 1, 1991.
50. Occupational Safety and Health Administration, 29 CFR 1920.1200, July 1, 1988.
51. Federal Hazardous Substance Act, 16 CFR Part 1500.3, January 1, 1987.
52. Organization for Economic Cooperation and Development (OECD), Guideline 403.
53. U.S. EPA, Toxic Substances Control Act (TSCA), Guideline 799.1350.
54. Commentary—Recommendation for the conduct of acute inhalation limit tests (Prepared by the technical committee of the Inhalation Specialty Section, Society of Toxicology), Fundam. Appl. Toxicol. 1992; 18:321–327.
55. Litchfield, J.T., Jr. and Wilcoxon, F. A simplified method of evaluating dose-effect experiments. J. Pharmacol. Expt. Ther. 1949; 96:99–115.
56. U.S. EPA, Toxic Substances Control Act Test Guidelines, 40 CFR 798.1150.
57. Diener, W., Kayser, D., and Schlede, E. The inhalation acute toxic class method: test procedures and biometric evaluations. Arch. Toxicol. 1997; 71:537–549.
58. U.S. EPA, Toxic Substance Control Act Test Guidelines, 40 CFR 798.3300.
59. U.S. EPA, Federal Insecticide, Fungicide and Rodenticide Act, Series 83-2, 40 CFR Part 158.

60. Organization for Economic Cooperation and Development (OECD), Guideline 452.

61. Japanese Ministry of Agriculture, Forestry and Fisheries Guidance on Toxicology Study Data for Application of Agricultural Chemical Registration, 59 NohSan 4200, January 28, 1985.

62. Organization for Economic Cooperation and Development (OECD), Guideline 451.

63. Sontag, J.M., Page. N.P., and Saffiotti, U. Guidelines for carcinogenicity bioassay in small rodents. DHHS Publication (NIH) 76-801, Washington, D.C., 1976.

64. Morrow, P.E., Haseman, J.K., Hobbs, C.H., Driscoll, K.E., Vu, V., and Oberdoerster, G. Workshop overview, the maximum tolerated dose for inhalation bioassays: toxicity versus overload. Fundam. Appl. Toxicol. 1996; 29:155–167.

65. Oberdorster, G. Lung clearance of inhaled insoluble and soluble particles. J. Aerosol Medicine 1988; 1:289–330.

66. Morrow, P.E. and Mermelstein, R. Chronic inhalation toxicity studies: protocols and pitfalls. In: Mohr, U., ed. Inhalation Toxicology: The Design and Interpretation of Inhalation Studies and Their Use in Risk Assessment. Berlin: Springer Verlag, 1988:103–117.

67. Henderson, R.F. Use of bronchoalveolar lavage to detect lung damage. Environ. Health Perspect 1984; 56:115–129.

68. Lindenschmidt, R.C., Driscoll, K.E., Perkins, M.A., Higgins, J.M., Maurer, J.K., and Belfiore, K.A. The comparison of fibrogenic and two nonfibrogenic dusts by bronchoalveolar lavage. Toxicol. Appl. Pharm. 1990; 102:268–281.

69. Henderson, R.F., Driscoll, K.E., Harkema, J.R., Lindenschmidt, R.C., Chang, I.Y., Maples, K.R., and Barr, E.B. A comparison of the inflammatory response of the lung to inhaled versus instilled particles in F344 rats. Fundam. Appl. Toxicol. 1995; 24:183–197.

70. Burleson, G.R., Fuller, L.B., Menache, M.G., and Graham, J.A. Poly(1):poly©-enhanced alveolar and peritoneal macrophage phagocytosis: quantification by a new method utilizing fluorescent beads. Proc. Soc Exp. Biol. Med. 1987; 184: 468–476.

71. Alarie, Y. Irritating properties of airborne materials to the upper respiratory tract. Arch. Environ. Health 1966; 13:433–449.

72. American Conference of Governmental Industrial Hygienists: Threshold Limit Values for Chemical and Physical Agents and Biological Exposure Indices, Cincinnati, OH.

73. Schaper, M. Development of a database for sensory irritants and its use in establishing occupational exposure limits. Am. Ind. Hyg. Assn. J. 1993; 54:488–544.

74. American Society for Testing and Materials, Standard test method for estimating sensory irritation of airborne chemicals, ASTM E 981-84, Philadelphia, 1984.

75. Boylstein, L.A., Luo, J., Stock, M., and Alarie, Y. An attempt to define a just detectable effect for airborne chemicals in the respiratory tract. Arch. Toxicol. 1996; 70:567–578.

76. Selgrade, M.K., Zeiss, C.R., Karol, M.H., Sarlo, K., Kimber, I., Tepper, J.S., and Henry, M.C. Workshop on status of test methods for assessing potential of chemicals to induce respiratory allergic reactions. Inhalation Toxicol. 1994; 6:303–319.

77. Sarlo, K. and Clark, E.D. A tier approach for evaluating the respiratory allergenicity of low molecular weight chemicals. Fundam. Appl. Toxicol. 1992; 18:107–114.

78. Karol, M.H., Stadler, J., and Margreni, C.M. Immunotoxicologic evaluation of the respiratory system: animal models for immediate- and delayed-onset pulmonary hypersensitivity. Fundam. Appl. Toxicol. 1985; 5:459–472.

79. Levy, A.G. and Lewis, T. Heart irregularities resulting from the inhalation of low percentage of chloroform vapor, and their relationship to ventricular fibrillation. Heart 1911/12; 3:99–111.

80. Reinhardt, C.F., Azar, A., Maxfield, M.E., Smith, Jr., P.E., and Mullin, L.S. Cardiac arrhythmias and aerosol "sniffing." Arch. Environ. Health 1971; 22:265–279.

81. American Society for Testing and Materials Standard E 1674-95, Philadelphia.

82. O'Neil, J.J. and Raub, J.A. Pulmonary function testing in small laboratory animals. Environ. Health Perspec. 1984; 56:11–22.

83. Mauderly, J.L. Respiratory function responses of animals and man to oxidant gases and to pulmonary emphysema. In: Miller, F.J. and Menzel, D.B., eds. Fundamentals of Extrapolation Modeling of Inhalaed Toxicants. New York: Hemisphere, 1984:165–181.

84. Newton, P.E., Becker, S.V., and Hixon, C.J. Pulmonary function and particle deposition and clearance in rats after a 90-day exposure to shale-oil-derived jet fuel JP4. Inhalation Toxicol. 1991; 3:195–210.

85. Jackson, A.C. and Vinegar, A. A technique for measuring frequency response of pressure, volume and flow transducers. J. Appl. Phsio.: Respir. Environ. Exercise Physiol. 1979; 47:462–467.

86. Rasmussen, R. Tissue acquisition and processing. In: Phalen, R.F., ed. Methods in Inhalation Toxicology. New York: CRC Press, 1996:101–122.

87. Swenberg, J.A., Kerns, W.D., Mitchell, R.I., Gralla, E.J., and Parkov, K.L. Induction of squamous cell carcinomas of the rat nasal cavity by inhalation exposure to formaldehyde vapor. Cancer Res. 1980; 40:3398–3402.

88. Woutersen, R.A., Appelman, L.M., VanGarderen-Hoetmer, A., and Feron, V.J. Inhalation toxicity of acetaldehyde in rats III. Carcinogenicity Study, Toxicology 1986; 41:213–231.

89. Lee, K.P. and Trochimowicz, H.J. Induction of nasal tumors in rats exposed to hexamethylphosphoramide by inhalation. J. Natl. Cancer Inst. 1982; 68:157–171.

90. Stinson, S.F., Reznik, G., and Ward, J.M. Characteristics of proliferative lesions in the nasal cavities of mice following chronic inhalation of 1,2-dibromoethane. Cancer Lett. 1981; 12:121–129.

91. Dahl, A.R. and Hadley, W.M. Nasal cavity enzymes involved in xenobiotic metabolism: effects on the toxicity of inhalants. CRC Crit. Rev. Toxicol. 1991; 21:345–372.

92. Dahl, A.R. The effect of cytochrome p-450 dependent metabolism and other enzyme activities in olfaction. In: Margolis, F.L., and Getchell, T.V., eds. Molecular Neurobiology of the Olfactory System. New York: Plenum Press, 1990:51–70.

93. Reznik-Schuller, H.M. Nitrosamine-induced nasal cavity carcinogenesis. In: Reznik, G. and Stinson, S.F., eds. Nasal Tumors in Animals and Man, Vol. III. Boca Raton: CRC Press, 1983:47–77.

94. Kociba, R.J., McCollister, S.B., Park, C., Torkelso, T.R., and Gerhing, P.J. 1,4-Dioxane. I. Results of a 2-year ingestion study in rats, Toxicol. Appl. Pharm. 1974; 30:275–286.

95. Isaka, H., Yashii, H., Otsuji, A., Nagai, Y., Koura, M., Sugiyasu, J., and Kanabayashi, T. Tumors of Sprague-Dawley rats induced by long term feeding of phenacetin. Gann. 1979; 70:29–36.

96. Morgan, K.T., Kimbell, J.S., Monticello, T.M., Patra, A.L., and Fleishman, A. Studies of inspiratory air flow patters in the passages of the F344 rat and rhesus monkey using nasal molds: relevance to formaldehyde toxicity. Toxicol. Appl. Pharmacol. 1991; 110:223–240.

97. Genter, M.B., Owens, D.M., and Deamer, N.J. Distribution of microsomal epoxide hydrolase and glutathione s-transferase in the rat olfactory mucosa: relevance to distribution of lesions caused by systemically-administered olfactory toxicants. Chem. Senses 1995; 20:385–392.

98. Morris, J.B., Hassett, D.N., and Blanchard, K.T. A physiologically based pharmacokinetic model for nasal uptake and metabolism of nonreactive vapors. Toxicol. Appl. Toxicol. 1993; 123:120–129.

99. Young, J.T. Histopathologic examination of the rat nasal cavity. Fundam. Appl. Toxicol. 1981; 1:309–312.

100. Mery, S., Gross, E.A., Joyner, D.R., Godo, M., and Morgan, K.T. Nasal diagrams: a tool for recording the distribution of nasal lesions in rats and mice. Toxicol. Path. 1994; 22:353–372.

101. Morgan, K.T. and Monticello, T.M. Air flow, gas deposition, and lesion distribution in the nasal passages. Environ. Hlth. Perspec. 1990; 88:209–218.

102. Owens, J.G., James, R.A., Moss, O.R., Morgan, K.T., Struve, M.F., and Dorman, D.C. Design and evaluation of an olfactometer for the assessment of 3-methylindole-induced hyposmia. Funda. Appl. Toxicol. 1996; 33:60–70.

103. Sagartz, J.W., Madarasz, A.J., Forsell, M.A., Burger, G.T., Ayres, P.H., and Coggins, C.R.E. Histological sectioning of the rodent larynx for inhalation toxicity testing. Toxicol. Path. 1992; 20:118–121.

104. Gopinath, C., Prentice, D.E., and Lewis, D.J. Atlas of Experimental Toxicological Pathology. Lancaster, England: MTP Press, 1987:24–42.

105. Burger, G.T., Renne, R.A., Sagartz, J.W., Ayres, P.H., Coggins, C.R.E., Mosberg, A.T., and Hayes, A.W. Histologic changes in the respiratory tract induced by inhalation of xenobiotics: physiologic adaptation or toxicity? Toxicol. Appl. Pharm. 1989; 101:521–542.

106. Renne, R.A., Sagartz, J.A., and Burger, G.T. Interspecies variations in the histology of toxicologically important areas in the larynges of CRL:CD rats and Syrian Golden Hamsters. Toxicol. Path. 1993; 21:542–546.

107. Doolittle, D.J., McKarns, S.C., Ayres, P.H., and Bombick, D.W. Molecular approaches for quantifying DNA synthesis and cell proliferation during rodent bioassay. Toxicol. Methods 1992; 1:215–230.

108. Roemer, E., Anton, H.J., and Kindt, R. Cell proliferation in the respiratory tract of the rat after acute inhalation of formaldehyde or acrolein. J. Appl. Toxicol. 1993; 13:103–107.

109. Ayres, P.H., McKarns, S.C., Coggins, C.R.E., Doolittle, D.J., Sagartz, J.E., Payne,

V.M., and Mosberg, A.T. Replicative DNA synthesis in tissues of the rat exposed to aged and diluted sidestream smoke. Inhalation Toxicol. 1995; 7:1225–1246.

110. Monteicello, T.M., Morgan, K.T., and Hurtt, M.E. Unit length as the denominator for quantitation of cell proliferation in nasal epithelia. Toxicol. Path. 1990; 18: 24–31.

111. U.S. EPA, Federal Insecticide, Fungicide and Rodenticide Act, Series 81-3, 40 CFR Part 158.

112. U.S. EPA, Toxic Substances Control Act Test Guidelines, 40 CFR 798.1150.

113. U.S. EPA, Federal Insecticide, Fungicide and Rodenticide Act, Series 82-4, 40 CFR Part 158.

114. U.S. EPA, Toxic Substance Control Act Test Guidelines, 40 CFR 798.2450.

115. U.S. EPA, Toxic Substance Control Act Test Guidelines, 40 CFR 799.9346.

116. Organization for Economic Cooperation and Development (OECD), Guideline 413.

117. Newton, P.E., Bolte, H.F., Lake, B.G., Derelanko, M.J., and Rinehart, W.E. Olfactory epithelium and liver peroxisome proliferation evaluations after inhalation exposure to methylethylketoxime. The Toxicologist 1996; 30:96.

10
Reproductive Hazards

James L. Schardein
WIL Research Laboratories, Inc., Ashland, Ohio

I. INTRODUCTION

The toxic effects of chemicals on the human reproductive system have become a major health concern to scientists and the populace alike, due to several factors. First, the number of reproductive hazards to which we are being exposed in the environment is increasing. Best estimates indicate about 100,000 chemicals in common enough use to be of interest, 500–1,000 chemicals of which are added new each year into our environmental milieu intentionally (1). The near global use of pesticides and accounts of incidents such as Love Canal, Three Mile Island, Minamata Bay, Times Beach, Seveso, Hopewell, Bhopal, and countless other industrial chemical spills, leaks, and other accidents, both real and exaggerated, fortify the perception of potential hazards in the environment. Unfortunately, only scant data exist on the reproductive effects of the large array of existing chemicals. The information that is available usually relates to accidental overexposures, whereas most real-life exposures are low level (which may impart greater significance as hazards to reproductive health).

Second, a relatively large number of individuals are exposed more directly because of occupational exposure in the workplace, through manufacture, packaging, or handling of manmade chemicals, than through the environment. In this regard, 50% of pregnant American women are employed during at least part of their gestation (2); thus, while emphasis has been directed toward protection of the *pregnant woman and conceptus* when potential industrial risks have been suspected, exposure of either males or nonpregnant females may cause abnormalities that result in reproductive failure. Disorders of reproduction, infertility, abortion, and teratogenesis are in fact, the sixth leading cause of work-related disease according to OSHA (1982).

Finally, it is generally perceived that sensitive biological indicators of such toxic exposures (i.e., impotency, infertility, stillbirths, abortions, malformations and cancers) are on the increase. In addition, it is generally recognized that human reproductive processes may be reactive to a wide variety of other conditions, including climate, altitude, social class, parity, age, diet, infections, stress, and social habits. Thus, there is heightened concern over environmental hazards being added to an already overburdened number of potentially detrimental factors.

It is very likely that environmental toxins have taken their toll on reproductive capacity in the human species. For instance, approximately 10–12% of couples who desire children fail to achieve pregnancy (3); this number rises to 20–25% of those who conceive but who do not have live offspring and those that fail to conceive a second time are included (4). Then, only ¼ to ⅓ of all embryos conceived develop to become liveborn infants (5). From a different clinical perspective, it has been speculated that "normal" sperm counts in American men may have been decreasing in the recent past: In 1950, 44% of men sampled had sperm counts in excess of 100 million, while in 1977, only 22% of men assayed had sperm counts of this magnitude (6). To the extent that reduction in sperm counts affects reproduction, these data may reflect a serious decline in reproductive potential. An associated problem here is that basic physiologic parameters of normalcy have not yet been established with respect to human male reproduction (4).

Consider for a moment the critical prerequisites for successful reproduction: It requires the completion, in both sexes, of a series of complex interdependent cellular, molecular, and physiological events, involving the capacity of a male to produce and release viable sperm in adequate numbers, a female to produce and release viable ova, and the union to produce a conceptus, through gametic interaction, which will flourish and develop (7). Is it any wonder that every sexual union does not result in a perfect outcome?

II. TARGET ORGANS AND SPECTRUM OF REPRODUCTIVE OUTCOMES

For our purposes, reproductive toxicity shall be defined simply as adverse effects of chemicals that interfere with the ability of males or females to reproduce. It is important in this context to realize that effects to either sex may result in the same endpoint of reproductive failure. Because miscarriage/abortion, stillbirth, intrauterine growth retardation (IUGR)/low body weights at birth and congenital malformations are important reproductive outcomes and at the same time represent developmental toxicity, there can be no clear-cut separation of these events from strictly reproductive toxicity. However, this presentation shall be directed toward reproductive hazards as defined above, rather than developmental ones. The discussion thus will be largely confined to preconception and pregnancy reproductive outcomes (Table 1).

A. Characteristics of Gonadotoxins and Their Outcomes

The range of reproductive outcomes possible is depicted in Table 1. The background frequencies for these events in the human are given in Table 2.

In general, damage to gonads and their function by chemicals can result from any of several mechanisms including direct actions on germ cells, actions affecting the accessory sex organs, or inhibition of hormonal-controlling mechanisms at either the gonadal or the hypothalamic-pituitary level. It should be kept in mind that a reproductive toxin in one species may not be toxic in another, because of differences in reproductive or toxicological mechanisms. In this respect, gender differences in toxicity are crucial: As a result of the accessibility of gametes and gonads, more compounds have been demonstrated to be toxic in males than in females (8).

Evidence to date indicates that the most likely outcome of exposure to environmental toxicants is *infertility* in the male and *spontaneous abortion* in the female (9). In laboratory animals as well as in humans, fertility rates are commonly used as reproductive endpoints, but these are hampered by a large number of variables influencing reproductive potential, especially in the human. This is because of psychological and physiological factors in the latter, and in addition, personal habits (i.e., smoking, alcohol, and caffeine use) may affect reproductive outcome (10). Additionally, infertility appears not to be gender

Table 1 Range of Reproductive Outcomes

Prior to conception	During pregnancy	After delivery
Altered libido	Maternal toxicity	Low birth weight (IUGR)
Abnormal sperm production/transport	Miscarriage	Congenital malformation
Impotence (males)	Spontaneous abortion	Congenital malformation
Ejaculatory disorders (males)	Premature labor	Congenital malformation
Ovulatory disorders (females)	Altered/prolonged gestation	Developmental disability
Abnormal menses (females) (dys-, oligo-, amenorrhea, dysfunctional uterine bleeding)	Dystocia	Death (late fetal, neonatal, childhood) Behavioral disorders
Effect on fertility (reduced, infertility/sterility)		Altered reproductive capacity

Table 2   Background Frequency of Reproductive
Outcomes (Human)

Parameter	Reported normal (approximate) rate (U.S.)	Reference
Maternal mortality	0.7/10,000	14
Infertility[a]	15%	15
Spontaneous abortion[b]	15%	15
karyotypical abnormal	60%	16,17
Livebirths[k]	86.7%	18
Prematurity	6.4–9.2%	14
Prolonged labor	2.4%	14
Low birthweight[d]	7%	15
Birth defects		
minor[e]	140/1000	19
major[e]	4%	15
minor mental retardation[e]	3–4/1000	19
severe mental retardation[e,j]	0.4%	15
among deaths after		
gestation of: 2–8 wks	3.4%	19
9–15 wks	8%	19
14–18 wks	5.7%	19
at birth[e]	20–30/1000	19
at 1 year	60–70/1000	19
Death		
early embryonic/fetal[h]	11–25%	19
late fetal[c]	9.8/1000	19
stillbirth[c]	2%	15
neonatal[g]	9.9/1000	19
infant[e,f]	14.1/1000	19
childhood, 1–4 years	0.95/1000	20
Chromosomal abnormalities[e]	5–6/1000	19
among early fetal deaths[i]	50%	19
among stillbirths	6%	16,19
among nonmalformed	1.7%	21
among lethally malformed	13–33%	16
Physically handicapped, age 2	16.7%	20

[a]Impaired fecundity. Defined as failure to achieve pregnancy after 1
year without contraceptive use.
[b]<20 weeks gestation.   [g]28 days.
[c]21+ weeks gestation.   [h]End of the 4th week on.
[d]<2500 g.   [i]8–20 weeks.
[e]Of livebirths.   [j]IQ < 50.
[f]<1 year old.   [k]As % of total pregnancies.

specific: Male factors have been identified in approximately 40% of the cases, and female dysfunction in 35–50%; unknown causes account for 10–20% of the cases of infertility in human populations (11).

Abortion has been suggested as one of the most useful outcomes for the evaluation of occupational reproductive hazards (12). Because of the frequency of their occurrence, the power of studies to detect an effect of an exposure is much greater than for other adverse pregnancy outcomes (13).

Reproductive failure in the form of abortion, stillbirth, or birth defects alone is not an adequate measure of the extent of reproductive hazards from toxic agents among humans (9). Reproductive toxins can manifest themselves in a variety of ways, including adversely affecting the male or female reproductive cycle, possibly leading to infertility; causing the production of insufficient or defective sperm; preventing the successful implantation of fertilized ova; or inducing functional defects not readily observed at birth and hence, not associated with reproductive failure. Thus, reproductive toxins may have subtle as well as overt effects on reproduction.

1. Male

Specifically in the male, dysfunction can be reflected in altered hypothalamo-pituitary-gonadal interactions, spermatogenesis, Sertoli cell function, hormone synthesis and action, accessory sex organ function, gene integrity, libido, potency, and ejaculation (22,23).

It is vital to know the mechanism by which chemicals interfere with gonadal function, because the severity of, and in some cases the reversibility of, the toxicity depends on the process being disrupted. Some of these have been reviewed specifically in the male (24,25). For instance, a number of toxicants, in particular hormones, inhibit gonadal function through negative feedback, based on the androgen dependency of the testis. A number of others may interfere with gonadotropin secretion. Some inhibit enzymes involved in androgen biosynthesis, while still others, like the heavy metals, destroy the blood-testis barrier. Antimetabolites cause irreversible nutritional disturbances that affect testicular function. The antimitotic and anticancer chemicals act directly on the germ cells, especially those cells most active in nucleic acid synthesis (i.e., the spermatocytes).

A large number of chemicals have been reported to affect male reproduction. More than 100 chemicals have shown this potential in male laboratory animals, while fewer than 15 of this number have been shown conclusively to have this effect in the human (26). A list of metals and trace elements, pesticides, food contaminants, industrial chemicals, investigational antispermatogenic drugs, and miscellaneous chemicals have been tabulated as inferred reproductive toxicants in males in several publications (5,22,24–31).

Physicochemical characteristics of reproductive toxins in the male have been reviewed elsewhere (32). In general, the stereotypic gonadotoxin is usually lipophilic, of diverse chemical structure, and has avidity for androgen receptors and a propensity for rapidly dividing cells. Its molecular weight is frequently less than 400, thus it can permeate the testes-blood barrier.

2. Female

In the female as well as in the male, the ways in which reproductive dysfunction can be expressed are multitudinous. Female reproductive dysfunction can appear as altered hypothalamo-pituitary-gonadal interactions; oogenesis, steroidogenesis, and ovulation; and accessory sex organ function (22). Some 30 reproductive processes have been identified as potentially susceptible to toxicants in nonpregnant subjects and at least half that number in pregnant women (33).

In the larger dimension, the reproductive hazards to which the female is exposed may precede fertilization, occur between fertilization and implantation, or placentation and parturition, at parturition, postnatally, or through accelerated reproductive senescence. Each of these events is vulnerable to adverse toxicity.

Damage to primary oocytes usually occurs through cell death, but sublethal injury may result in oocytes capable of fertilization but culminate in early abortion (34). Some gonadotoxins, polycyclic aromatic hydrocarbons for instance, may not be so directly, but become metabolized by the ovary to reactive intermediates that are cytotoxic (35). Exposure of ova to chemicals near meiosis may result in death of the ova or affect fertilizability. However, ovarian toxicity which produces periods of infertility or subfertility may be difficult to identify (36). Tabulations of chemicals affecting reproductive function in the female have been summarized elsewhere (5,8,22,28,29,36–39).

B. Origin and Differentiation of Gonads And Gametes

It is important that fundamentals of germ cell development in both males and females be well understood if we are to devise methods and evaluate meaningfully reproductive events and gonadal toxicity in laboratory animals in order to extrapolate these into realistic assessments of human hazard. The development of reproductive capacity occurs during a critical period in time, and while undergoing development, the reproductive system is a highly vulnerable target for toxic injury (40).

1. Male

In mammals, gonadal origins occur early in embryonic development, prior to sexual differentiation (41). Thus the initial stages described here are equally pertinent to male and female alike. Descriptions of development and differentiation of the duct system and external genitalia in either gender will not be discussed in this presentation, since an understanding of their embryology is not critical to considerations of gonadal toxicity.

Derivation. The gonads appear initially as a pair of longitudinal genital ridges formed by proliferation of the coelomic epithelium and a condensation of the underlying mesenchyme of the mesonephros renal system. The *primordial germ cells* appear at an early stage of development among the endoderm cells in the wall of the yolk sac close to the allantois, migrate along the dorsal mesentery of the hindgut, and invade the genital ridges. This occurs in the sixth week of development in the human or days $10\frac{1}{2}$–12 in the rat.

Shortly before and during the arrival of the primordial germ cells, the coelomic epithelium of the genital ridge proliferates and epithelial cells penetrate the underlying mesenchyme, forming a number of irregularly shaped elements, the primitive sex cords. At this time, it is impossible to differentiate between the male and female gonad: It is thus known (at about 8 weeks in the human or day 12.5 in the rat) as the *indifferent gonad.* It should be emphasized that it is the Y chromosome in the male and the XX chromosome configuration in the female that cause the development of the respective gonadal structures.

In genetically male embryos (carrying an XY sex chromosome complex), the primitive sex cords of the indifferent gonad continue to proliferate and penetrate deep into the medulla to form the medullary cords or *testis.* The secondary cortical cords typical of the female constitution regress at this time. Toward the hilus of the gland, the testis cords break up into a network of strands which later give rise to the tubules of the rete testis; during further development, the testis cords become separated from the surface epithelium by the tunica albuginea.

Later on, the extremities of the testis cords are continuous with those of the rete testis. They are now composed of primitive germ cells (spermatogonia) and Sertoli cells, derived from the surface of the gland. The interstitial cells (Leydig cells) develop from the mesenchyme located between the testis cords: They are particularly abundant at months 4–6 of development in man (day 15 in the rat). The male gonad is now able to influence the sexual differentiation of the genital ducts and external genitalia. The cords remain solid until puberty, when they acquire lumens, thus forming the seminiferous tubules.

Spermatogenesis. Spermatogenesis is a two-phase process comprised of spermatocytogenesis and spermiogenesis (42). The spermatogenesis process is the sum of transformations that result in formation of spermatozoa from spermatogonia while maintaining spermatogonial numbers. The process begins at puberty and continues almost throughout life. Spermatogonia are dormant following birth until puberty when proliferative activity begins again. In simplistic terms, the process evolves as follows: The *spermatocytogenesis* phase is the spermatogenic tissue growth phase of the testis; in it, proliferation occurs through mitotic division of germ cells to form spermatids.

In the testis there exist a number of germ cells recognized as cellular associations: Depending on the species and the observer, 8 or 14 different cellular associations have been discerned (75). Each contains 4 or 5 types of germ cells organized in a specific layered pattern within the seminiferous tubules of the testis, with each layer representing one cell generation. The entire series of cellular associations is termed the cycle of the seminiferous epithelium. Progression through the series of cellular associations occurs in a predictable, sequential fashion and continues repeatedly over and over. The interval required for one complete series of cellular associations to appear at a fixed point within a tubule is termed the duration of the cycle of the seminiferous epithelium. This duration is uniform for each species and ranges from 8.6 days in the mouse to 16 days in man (Table 3).

The process of spermatogenesis is initiated when type A stem spermatogonia become committed to produce a cohort of spermatids. The onset accompanies functional maturation of the testes; the germ cells proliferate in a protected environment created in part by the blood-testis barrier (43). Type A spermatogo-

Table 3 Endpoints in Animal Models for Studying Male Reproductive Function[a]

	Species					
	Mouse	Rat	Rabbit	Beagle dog	Rhesus monkey	Human
Age at sexual maturity (days)	28–35	45–75	150–210	180–240	800	15.1 (yr)
Age at breeding (days)	50	100	180	270–365	2190	—
Cycle seminiferous epithelium (days)	8.6	12.9	10.7	13.6	9.5	16.0
Cycle spermatogenesis (days)	35.0	51.6	48.0	54.4	70.0	64.0
Testes weight (g)	0.2	3.7	6.4	12.0	49	34
Ejaculate volume (ml)	?	?	1.0	0.8–3.1	1.1	3.4
Sperm:						
Count (10^6/ml)	—	50–60	50–250	60–600	100–600	80–110
Abnormal (%)	1.1–2.0	<3	—	10	—	12–27
Motile (%)	—	32–50	—	80	58	58–65
Velocity (μm/sec)	—	65–69	—	—	—	30–68
Daily sperm production (10^6)	5	86	160	300	1100	125
Sperm reserves cauda (10^6)	49	440	1600	?	5700	420
Sperm transit time through cauda (days)	5.6	5.1	9.7	?	5.6	3.7
Breeding life (yr)	1–1.5	1	1–3	5–14	12–15	60

Compiled from numerous sources.

nia germ cells periodically differentiate at a given point within the seminiferous tubule and divide to give rise to more differentiated spermatogonia and ultimately, primary spermatocytes. The spermatogonial stem cell population in its developmental stages is far more vulnerable to chemical injury than differentiated spermatogonia (44). The duration of spermatogenesis is the interval from this point until release of the resulting spermatozoa at spermiation. The interval between commitment of a stem A spermatogonium to differentiation and formation of the resulting primary spermatocytes is not known with certainty, but probably requires between 1.3 and 1.7 cycles of seminiferous epithelium, and the interval between formation of primary spermatocytes and spermiation is close to 3.0 cycles in the common mammalian species. Thus, the duration of spermatogenesis is 4.3–4.7 cycles of the seminiferous epithelium, or about 35–70 days in the common species (Table 3).

As this transformation is in progress, reduction occurs through meiotic division, to ensure that the haploid number of chromosomes in each gamete is maintained (Figure 1a). Because of the complexity of the process, meiosis is one of the most susceptible stages of the entire process for chemical toxicity to occur.

In the *spermiogenesis* phase, the spermatids complete their development into spermatozoa by undergoing reorganization: The nucleus condenses and becomes the sperm head; the two centrioles form the axial filament (flagellum); the Golgi in part becomes the acrosome; and the mitochondria concentrate into the sheath. It is not until the sperm reach the lower corpus or cauda epididymis, a process lasting 10–15 days in most species, that they finally achieve the potential to fertilize the mature oocyte. The immature, immotile spermatozoa transformed by this process depend on follicle-stimulating hormone (FSH) secreted by the pituitary and subtle biochemical and morphological changes acquired during epididymal transit for final maturation into fertile spermatozoa. In the case of the human male's reproductive lifespan of more than 60 years, approximately one quadrillion spermatozoa are produced in this manner (27). This is a superlatively efficient process, even in biologic terms, to say the least!

Sperm storage is within the caudal segment of the epididymis, and upon ejaculation, only sperm present in this region of the duct are discharged (43). Surplus unejaculated sperm are discharged during spontaneous emissions, voided in the urine, and in rodents, emerge in the form of seminal plugs in the urethra; others may also disintegrate in the cauda and vas deferens.

2. Female

Derivation. In embryos predetermined to be female (XX sex chromosome complement), the primitive sex cords comprising the indifferent gonad described above, break up into irregular cell clusters. These contain groups of primitive germ cells, and are located primarily in the medullary part of the

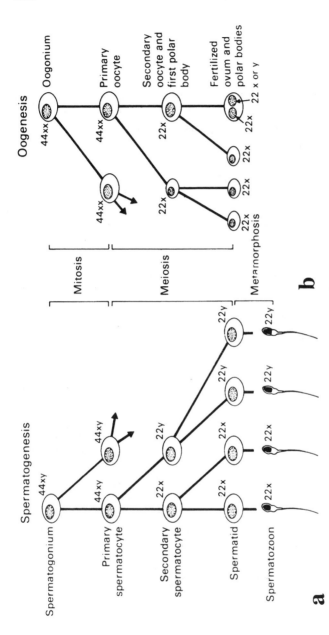

Figure 1 The processes of spermatogenesis (a) and oogenesis (b) (from Ref. 27).

designated ovary. Later they disappear and are replaced by a vascular stroma which forms the ovarian medulla.

Unlike that of the male, the surface epithelium of the female gonad continues to proliferate, giving rise to a second generation, the cortical cords. These penetrate the underlying mesenchyme and in the 4th month in the human (day 13.5 in the rat), these cords are also split into isolated cell clusters, each surrounding one or more primitive germ cells. The germ cells subsequently develop into the oogonia, while the surrounding epithelial cells, descendents of the surface epithelium, form the follicular cells.

Oogenesis/Folliculogenesis. In contrast to the process of spermatogenesis in the male, oogenesis in the female is a discontinuous process. The process is outlined below (27,39).

As previously mentioned, the oogonia proliferate during the fetal period within the cortex of the ovary and become surrounded by epithelial cells to form the primary follicle. Shortly after birth, oogonia cease to proliferate and become oocytes, folliculogenesis begins, with formation of the follicle complex.

The follicle complex is the smallest functional unit of the ovary, and consists of oocyte, granulosa cells, basement membrane, and thecal cells. Oocytes require the follicular complex for support. Those oocytes which are not a part of a follicular complex following completion of folliculogenesis are lost through extrusion from the surface of the ovary or by cell death within the ovary. After sexual maturation, three types of follicular complexes are found in the ovary: Resting or primordial follicles, growing follicles, and preovulatory follicles, and are distinguished on the basis of size of oocyte and zona pellucida, and number of granulosa cells. This classification is important because follicle complexes of different size having varying susceptibility to reproductive toxins.

In mammals, germ cells in the ovary are arrested at the primary oocyte stage (diplotene), where they remain until just before they are ovulated. During the 30 yr or more that constitute the human reproductive period (or in the 1-yr breeding interval in the rat), follicles in various stages of growth can always be found. Following this (menopause in the human), follicles are no longer present in the ovary.

Follicular growth requires recruitment of follicles from a resting pool into a growing pool, the mechanisms of which are poorly understood. Further growth and ultimate ovulation of the oocyte from the follicle complex requires the presence of gonadotropins and steroid hormones produced by dynamic interactions between the ovary, hypothalamus, and pituitary. Ovulation occurs predictably in the various species (Table 4); in the human it is 28–32 hours after the onset of the luteinizing hormone (LH) surge (45). The final event of this process, follicle rupture, is probably the result of the action of prostaglandins. Following ovulation, the follicle complex differentiates into the corpus luteum, and those follicle complexes recruited into the growing pool which do not ovulate undergo atresia.

Table 4 Endpoints in Animal Models for Studying Female Reproductive Function[a]

	Species					
	Mouse	Rat	Rabbit	Beagle dog	Rhesus monkey	Human
Age at sexual maturity (days)	28	46–53	120–240	270–425	1,642	15.2 (yr)
Age at breeding (days)	35–60	100	150–180	270–365	1,825	—
Duration estrous/ menstrual cycle (days)	4–5	5	N/A	120–240	28	28
Duration estrus (hr)	10	13–15	continuous	168–216	N/A	N/A
Conventional fertility rates (%)	~90	~90	>80	—	—	85
Duration gestation (days)	19	21	31	63	165	260
Ovulation (hr from estrus onset)	2–3	8–12.5	10–12[b]	24–72	264–336[c]	336[c]
Number oocytes ovulated	10–12	12–14	8–10	6–12	1	1
Fertilization (hr after ovulation)	5	4	immed.	~48	<48	<36
Implantation (days after coitus)	4–5	5–6	7–8	18	9–11[d]	7[d]
Litter size	8–11	10–12	7–9	4–8	1	1
Breeding life (yr)	<1 (6–10 litters)	1	1–3	5–10	10–15	30

[a]Compiled from numerous sources.
[b]After coitus.
[c]Of menstrual cycle.
[d]After ovulation.

While in the ovary, the primary oocyte undergoes two specialized meiotic divisions: In the first stage, the primary oocyte is in preparation for entering prophase. Each prophase chromosome doubles and each doubled chromosome is attracted to its homologous mate to form tetrads; chromosomes of the same parental origin are connected to one another by their centromeres. The members of the tetrads synapse, but before separation, the chromosomes exchange genetic material by a "crossing-over" process, which accounts for most of the qualitative differences between the resulting gametes. The subsequent meiotic stages distribute the members of the tetrads to the daughter cells so that each cell receives haploid chromosomes. At telophase, one secondary oocyte and polar body have been formed which are no longer genetically identical, and the mature ovum is released from the ovary at this stage.

The second meiotic division in the oocyte is triggered in the oviduct by the entry of the sperm. The stimulus of sperm penetration into the mature ovum and decondensation of the sperm chromatin initiates the resumption of meiosis and extrusion of the second polar body. Meanwhile, the first polar body attempts division shortly before degenerating. The early product of ovulation and fertilization is thus one large ovum with maternal and fraternal haploid chromosome complements and three rudimentary ova known as polar bodies each with haploid chromosomes (Figure 1b).

In humans, between 300,000 and 400,000 follicles are present at birth in each ovary. Under normal conditions, there is a continual reduction in the number of viable ovarian follicles: About half the number of oocytes present at birth remain at puberty; the number is reduced to about 25,000 by age 30, and further loss occurs to menopause at about age 50. Thus, on an average during the reproductive life of a woman, only about 400 primary follicles will yield mature ova, and only a very few of these are likely to be fertilized. This disparity in female and male gametogenesis is depicted in Figure 2.

With respect to ovarian toxicity induced by various chemicals, it is clear from the description of the oogenesis and folliculogenesis processes, that several stages in the process are particularly vulnerable to toxins. Obviously any chemical agent that blocks the process in toto will decrease the number of oocytes and thus may affect fertility. Likewise, any agent that damages the follicles or oocytes proper will accelerate the depletion of the follicle pool and lead to reduced fertility. Further, in both experimental animals and humans, follicle complexes have differing sensitivity to ovarian toxins, depending on the strain, species, agent, and dosage used. Effects on dominant follicles are immediate, while resumption in fertility occurs following repopulation of the preovulatory pool and selection of another dominant follicle (36). Toxicity to growing gonadotropin-independent follicles will cause a delay in onset of infertility proportionate to the time necessary for follicles to progress through the gonadotropin-dependent pool. Finally, toxicity to resting follicle complexes is most delayed with respect to effects on reproductive function. Hypothetical effects on fertility based on the type of oocyte destruction in the female are shown in Figure 3.

C. The Processes of Fertilization and Implantation

The formation, maturation, and intersection of gametes produced by the male and female are all preliminary to their actual union into a zygote by the process of fertilization. Fertilization can be arbitrarily divided into three phases: Penetration of the egg by the sperm; activation of the egg; and union of egg and sperm nuclei (27). The process is short-lived, ranging from about 0.25–12 hours in duration, depending on the species (47).

A proper state of maturity of both male and female germ cells must exist

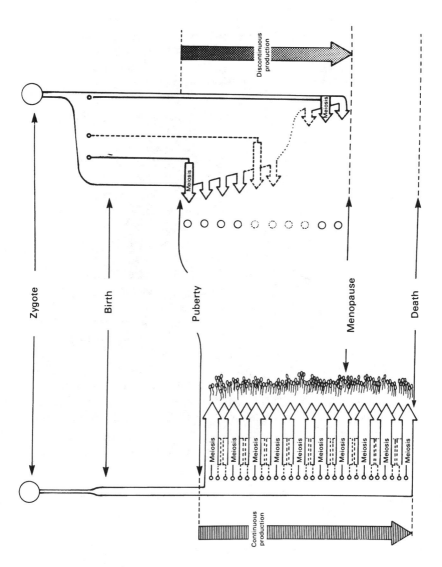

Figure 2 The contrast of the gametogenesis process between males (left) and females (right) (from Ref. 46).

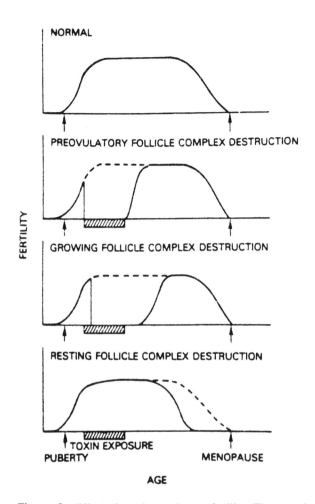

Figure 3 Effect of ovarian toxins on fertility. The cross hatched area represents the period of ovotoxin exposure: (–) the expected fertility; (—) the normal fertility in absence of toxin exposure (from Ref. 39).

for union of sperm and egg. In almost all mammals, the first polar body must be extruded and the second polar body must be in a state of arrest before penetration of the sperm can take place. As mentioned above, the second meiotic division is completed only during the preliminary events of fertilization. The sperm, to be successful, must possess high motility and also must be in a functionally potent phase. The actual site of fertilization is in the ampulla of the oviduct within one day of ovulation.

Preparation of the sperm for fertilization requires the initiation of complex events termed capacitation and involves labilization of the sperm plasma membrane, requiring about 5 hours. Subsequent to this, sperm membrane changes allow breakdown of the acrosome and release of enzymes instrumental in passage of sperm through the follicular cells prior to penetration of the sperm cell through the zona pellucida into the egg cytoplasm. This process, the acrosomal reaction, is thought to be prerequisite for fertilization in mammals (45). The sperm pass through the cumulus, then the zona pellucida, and enter the eperivite-line space. In the great majority of animals, only one sperm finds its way into the egg. Upon attachment of the fertilizing spermatozoan to the egg, rapid changes take place in the membrane composition of the egg which reduce the possibility of penetration by a second sperm. Finally, the sperm penetrates the plasma membrane of the oocyte, and intense nuclear activity ensues, with eventual formation of a male pronucleus. At the same time, a female pronucleus forms and the two join (syngamy), restoring the diploid state and establishing the sex of the individual. This is followed almost immediately by the first cleavage division, signaling the end of fertilization. As with a number of reproductive processes already described, any of the sequences of steps in the process of fertilization may be a target for insult by chemically hazardous agents (48).

In the mammal following fertilization, the cleaving ova pass through the oviducts into the uterus, and after a variable period in its lumen, adhere to the endometrium. Tubal passage is relatively constant, generally lasting about 3–4 days. Adherence is followed by firm attachment, or implantation, and formation of a placental connection from the fusion of maternal and fetal tissues. During this phase the developing conceptus is nourished, first by its own yolk substance and the tubal fluids, then by the secretions of the uterine glands. Once formed, the placenta becomes chiefly responsible for maintenance and growth of the embryo.

On arriving in the uterus, in polytocous species, the eggs distribute through the two horns: Attachment of the blastocyst is a relatively rapid process (see Table 4), and results from precise synchronous interactions between the embryo and the uterus. The preimplantation stage is critical in this scheme, because injuries to the embryo at this time are likely to result either in death of the conceptus or in repair and recovery.

Based on morphological criteria, implantation can be divided into five phases: hatching, apposition, attachment/adhesion, invasion, and peri-implantation development. Physiological correlates to these events ascribe these changes to interactions between progesterone and estrogen (49). Chemicals interfering with the timing of the entry of embryos into the uterus, the development of embryos, and the differentiation of the uterus will have a bearing on the occurrence or absence of implantation; a number have been described (50). From here on, the very early implanted embryo undergoes a complicated series of morphogenic events leading to an embryo with recognizable organ systems capable of insult by developmental toxins, the whole of which is outside the scope of this presentation. A very high rate of embryonic loss is a normal phenomenon in mammals, especially in the very early stages of pregnancy: Upon exposure to sperm, the probability of fertilization of a human ovum is estimated to be 84%, but by the time pregnancy is recognizable, one-half of all embryos have been lost (5). During the remainder of pregnancy, another 25% perish and are aborted, thus the entire process, from fertilization until birth, results in an estimated probability of a livebirth of only 31 out of 100.

III. SOURCES OF REPRODUCTIVE HAZARDS

As alluded to earlier, there are a number of sources of environmental toxins that present a potential hazard to reproduction as shown in the following:

Developmental and Reproductive Toxicants in Perspective*		
	Animals	Humans
Known teratogens	~1,500	21
Known reproductive toxicants	Hundreds	~45
Number of agents tested	>4,700	?

*Personal data, 1998.

Chief among these are chemicals or groups of chemicals and/or physical factors to which individuals are exposed in the workplace or in the environment at large. There are also exposures to needed medications and usage of social chemicals and workplace situations in which the specific hazards are yet to be even identified, yet alone proven. These two situations are beyond the intended scope of this work. Finally, there are accidental hazards in which chemical contaminants through spills, leaks, or other industrial accidents may provide significant exposures. We will consider these in turn.

A. Environmental and Occupational Exposures

The largest source of reproductive hazards has been identified through occupational or environmental exposures of specific chemicals, chemical groups, or physical factors. Forty-three of these have been characterized to date, of which 22 have been identified as affecting only females (Table 5). Nine have been identified as affecting only males, and 12 agents in this group affect both sexes and thus would appear to constitute even greater hazard. These include cadmium, carbon disulfide, chloroprene, estrogens, gossypol, elevated temperature,

Table 5 Environmental/Occupational Exposures: Adverse Reproductive Outcomes

| Chemical/group | Occupation/situation | Effects on Exposed | | Comments |
		Males	Females	
Androgens	In manufacturing employees		Altered menses (51)	
Aniline	Occupational exposures		Increased spontaneous abortion and infertility (cited, 22)	
Antimony	Occupational exposure to dust		Spontaneous abortion, premature births, gynecological problems (52)	Evidence weak
Arsenic	Among women living close to or working in smelters emitting pollutants		Increased spontaneous abortion (55), low birth weight (53)	
Benzene	With heavy occupational exposures		Menstrual disorders (54), increased spontaneous abortions, premature births (55)	Females more sensitive than males, Benzene exposures impossible to separate from petroleum and chlorinated hydrocarbon exposures
Boric acid	In manufacturing employees and high boron level in drinking water (Russia)	Reduced sexual function (56,57)		

Agent	Exposed population	Male effects	Female effects	Comments
Butiphos	Agricultural workers occupationally (Russia)		Aggravated parturition, stillbirths, birth defects (58)	
Cadmium	In manufacturing plant workers	Testicular damage (59)	Low birth weight (60)	Female effects refuted Food is also a major source of exposure
Caprolactam	Textile spinners		Menstrual and childbearing disturbances (61)	
Carbaryl	Workers exposed during manufacture and application	Sperm abnormalities (62)		
Carbon disulfide	Textile workers	Decreased libido, impotence, sperm abnormalities (63)	Menstrual irregularities (64), decreased fertility (65), increased spontaneous abortion (65,66), birth defects (67)	Declared reproductive hazard by NIOSH in 1985
Carbon monoxide	Environmental exposure to gas		Increased fetal death and neuropathy (cited, 68)	
Chlordecone (kepone)	Among manufacturing workers	Loss of libido (cited, 69), reduced sperm count and motility, abnormal sperm morphology (70), infertility (71)		76 Exposures in 1975; use banned in 1977
Chloroprene	Factory workers and among wives of exposed male workers (Russia)	Sperm abnormalities (72)	Menstrual disorders (cited, 73), increased sterility and abortion (72)	Most claims anecdotal
Chromium	In manufacturing employees		Menstrual disorders (74)	

(continued)

Table 5 Continued

| Chemical/group | Occupation/situation | Effects on Exposed | | Comments |
		Males	Females	
DDT	Agricultural workers (Russia)		Pregnancy complications (72), miscarriages, toxemia, and low birth weight (77)	Use halted in U.S. in 1972
Dibromochloropropane (DBCP)	Agricultural workers and manufacturing employees	Testicular atrophy (78); infertility (79)		Most potent testicular toxin yet found. No recovery in severely affected cases No adverse effects in families of exposed men (80) Production partially banned in 1977
Dimethylformamide	Environmental exposure		Increased abortion (81)	
Dinitro-dipropyl-sulfanilamide	Hospital exposure		Stillbirths (82)	Report unconfirmed
	Manufacturing plant spouses exposed		Miscarriage and birth defects (83)	
Estrogens	In manufacturing employees	Impotence (cited, 69), decreased libido, infertility (84)	Abnormal menses (84)	
Ethylene oxide	Production plant workers		Increased gynecological disorders and abortions (85,86)	Data inadequate A major industrial chemical
	Hospital workers		Increased spontaneous abortion (87)	

Agent	Exposure	Effect	Comments
Formaldehyde	Occupational exposures	Menstrual disorders, increased spontaneous abortion, increased infertility and low birth weight (88); weak association to miscarriages (89)	Limited study, inadequate for analysis Male study negative: further studies needed
Gasoline	Environmental, occupational contact	Birth defects (90), altered menses and impaired fertility (cited, 36)	
Gossypol	Exposure through cooking	Antispermatogenic effects (91) Menstrual disturbances (cited, 22)	
High altitude	Environmental exposure	Decreased sperm, reduced motility, abnormal sperm (92)	Data limited
High temperature	Occupational, environmental	Inhibition spermatogenesis, testicular pathology at 30–37°C (93) Birth defects at >40°C (94)	
Insecticides (general)	Environmental exposures	Fetal death and birth defects (95,96)	
Irradiation	Occupational exposure	Spermatogenesis alterations, reduced hormone levels (97)	Testicular function altered at >15 rads
Lead	Pottery glazers Male workers in auto and storage battery plants	Sterility (98), abnormal sperm (98,99) hypogonadism (100) Increased prematurity and spontaneous abortion, neurological defects in children (cited, 101), menstrual disorders (102)	
	Female refinery workers	Increased abortion (103)	Work restrictions on women in some countries

(continued)

Table 5 Continued

Chemical/group	Occupation/situation	Effects on Exposed		Comments
		Males	Females	
Manganese	Mineworkers	Decreased libido (104), impotence (105)		
Mercury (inorganic)	Industrial poisoning (male) Occupational exposures (female)	Reduced libido & potency, disturbed spermatogenesis (105,106)	Menstrual disturbances and increased spontaneous abortion (106–108), abnormal ovarian function (109)	Association unconfirmed
Methyl parathion	Environmental exposure		Fetal death and birth defects (110)	
Microwaves	Long-term occupational exposure	Decreased libido, sperm reduced motility, abnormal sperm (111)		Evidence in males incomplete, female studies indicated
Nonionizing radiation	Physiotherapists		Perinatal death and birth defects (112)	Association weak
Pesticides (general)	In women producing organochlorine/ phosphorus chemicals Environmental exposure in men spraying chemicals	Impotence (113)	Abnormal menses (114–117), ovarian malfunction (118), decreased fertility (119), gynecological disorders (120)	Adverse effects not confirmed in spouses of males (121)
Phthalate plasticizers	Among those manufacturing chemicals		Abnormal menses and increased spontaneous abortion (122)	

Agent	Exposure	Male effects	Female effects	Comments
Selenium	Laboratory workers		Increased spontaneous abortion and birth defects (123)	Report unconfirmed
"Stress"	Environmental	Decreased sperm (cited, 5)		Anecdotal reports of amenorrhea
Styrene	Plastics processing plant		Menstrual disturbances (124,125)	Human effects not corroborated (126)
Tetraethyl lead	Exposure to fuel fumes	Reduced libido and potency with reduced semen volume, sperm count and motility, abnormal morphology (127,128)		
Thallium	Poisoning		Low birth weight (129)	
Toluene chemicals	Exposure in manufacturing industries, abuse	Sperm abnormalities (130)	Menstrual disorders (131), low birth weight (132), birth defects (133–135), spontaneous abortion (130)	Exposure to other solvents as well clouds effect of toluene
Vinyl chloride	Among manufacturing plant workers	Loss of libido and impotence (136)	Increased miscarriage, stillbirth (137,138), irregular menses (139)	Effects in females need validation

lead, psychological stress, inorganic mercury, toluene, vinyl chloride, and pesticides.

Additionally, a number of substances affect more than single endpoints in both sexes, and thus would also appear to constitute higher priority factors for control. For example, carbon disulfide among textile workers affects libido, induces sperm abnormalities, and causes impotence in males, and produces menstrual irregularities, and results in decreased fertility and increased spontaneous abortion in females. Metals industries (lead and mercury) are other good workplace examples of sources of reproductive toxins affecting multiple endpoints.

The data generated thus far for agents in this group are admittedly weak in a number of cases: chloroprene, DDT, dinitrodipropyl-sulfanilamide, ethylene oxide, formaldehyde, methylparathion, nonionizing radiation, selenium, "stress," and styrene are examples where evidence of reproductive toxicity is inadequate and additional confirmatory data are needed.

Unfortunately, identification of a number of potent reproductive toxins among agents in this group has evoked little change in industrial practice. In a few cases, there are restrictions on workers, in the lead industry in Europe for instance. Some pesticides have been banned from production and use, and extensive suits have been litigated by affected DBCP workers, but precious little else has ensued either for protection of the worker or the individual exposed through a natural course in the environment.

B. Occupational Exposure (Agent Unidentified)

There is a small group of occupations or industries that has been associated with adverse reproductive outcomes in females, but in which the specific agents inducing the effects have not been clearly identified. A representative group of these have been tabulated in Table 6.

Little comment can be made of these sources of potential hazard except to indicate that in most cases the available data demonstrate these may represent likely sources of reproductive toxins. Additional epidemiological data are needed to isolate the agents responsible for this hazard.

C. Drug Exposures

Another major source of reproductive hazards is therapeutic use of drugs. At least 27 drugs or drug groups have been documented as having adverse reproductive effects in either males or females, but this subject is outside the intended scope of this work.

D. Social Uses/Abuses

Chemical exposures resulting from social habits constitute a significant source of hazard to reproductive health in the human.

Table 6 Occupational Reproductive Hazards—Exposure Unidentified

Occupation/Industry	Reproductive effects	Reference	Comments
Chemical	Increased spontaneous abortion	141	
	Abnormal menses	142	Chlorine responsible?
Electrical	Adverse reproductive effects	143	
Factory workers	Decreased viability and body weight at birth	144	
	Malformations	145	
Laboratory technicians	Increased spontaneous abortion	146	Effect not confirmed (147)
	Increased perinatal death rate	147	
	Malformations	149–151	Negative reports (146,151)
Leatherworkers	Increased stillbirths and perinatal death	153	
Metals	Increased spontaneous abortion	154	
Plastics	Abnormal menses	155–157	
	Malformations	158	
	Increased spontaneous abortion	141,159	
Pulp and paper industry	Pregnancy complications	160	
Rubber	Altered menses	161	Hydrocarbons responsible?
Video display terminal operators	Abnormal pregnancy outcomes	162	Results not confirmed (161)
Wastewater treatment	Increased fetal loss	164	From paternal exposures
Workers, laborers (generalized)	Increased spontaneous abortion	165	

Alcohol use, tobacco smoking, abuse of "recreational drugs" and coffee (caffeine) consumption in females are examples, but discussion is outside the scope of this work.

E. Accidental Contamination

There are a number of potential sources of reproductive hazards due to strictly accidental exposure. These have been recorded for wartime bombing, accidental contamination of food or water supplies, or contact with the toxin through industrial or hazardous waste (Table 7).

Table 7 Exposures Due to Accidental Contamination; Reproductive Outcomes

Location (date)	Chemical(s) identified	Source	Reproductive outcomes	Comments
Hiroshima/ Nagasaki (1945)	Atomic radiation	Wartime bombing	Birth defects (164)	
Minamata, Japan (1952)	Methylmercury salts	Entry into food chain	Death, birth defects (165)	Subsequently occurred in Sweden, Japan, U.S.S.R., U.S., Iraq 1 of only 3 putative chemical teratogens in humans
Kyusho, Japan (1968)	PCBs	Entry into food chain	Menstrual dysfunction (166), low birth weight (167), "Cola" babies (168)	Poisoning termed "Yusho" Also in Taiwan in 1979 1 of only 3 putative chemical teratogens in humans
Vietnam (1970–)	2,4,5-T/Agent Orange (TCDD?)	Spraying/contaminated drinking water	Abortion, stillbirths, birth defects (169–171)	Allegations refuted (172, 173)
		Direct contact	Birth defects from father's exposure (174)	Negative study published (175)
New Zealand, U.S. Gulf Islands (1972–)	2,4,5-T (TCDD?)	Spraying/contaminated drinking water	Increased miscarriages and/ or birth defects (176–181)	Negative studies on this issue have been published (182–188)
Michigan (1974)	PBBs	Entry into food chain	Reproductive problems, birth defects (189)	Fetal mortality not affected (190)

Location	Chemical(s)	Event	Outcome	Notes
Michigan (up to 1975)	TCDDs	Contact through manufacture	No adverse pregnancy outcomes from father's exposure (191)	
Seveso, Italy (1976)	TCDD	Plant explosion	Abortion (192), birth defects (193–195)	Effects not proven (196)
Love Canal, NY (1978)	Benzene Dichloroethylene Lindane Chloroform Toluene (of some 82 chemicals isolated)	Hazardous waste site	Increased miscarriages and birth defects (197)	Effects not corroborated (198)
Drake Waste Site, PA (1978)	Numerous chemicals	Hazardous wastes	No related birth defects could be ascertained (199)	
Three-Mile Island, PA (1979)	Radiation	Nuclear power plant accident	No increased spontaneous abortions (200)	
Bhopal, India (1984)	Methylisocyanate	Plant exploded	Increased spontaneous abortion and neonatal deaths (385)	

There are both well-documented and uncorroborated exposure effects from agents in this list. Several of the agents are recognized developmental toxins in the human, including methyl mercury and PCBs. Others, like 2, 4, 5-T and its incorporated contaminant TCDD (dioxin) and PBBs have not been confirmed as reproductive toxins, and their reported effects must be regarded as dubious. Several other incidents, widely publicized in the press in recent years, such as hazardous waste sites at Love Canal and situations such as Times Beach and Three-Mile Island, also have not been shown to have any detrimental effects on reproduction. Perhaps future research will prove differently.

IV. LABORATORY METHODS AND ANIMAL MODELS FOR DETERMINING REPRODUCTIVE EFFECTS

A. Male

The choice of a laboratory animal model to predict reproductive hazards to the human male is conditioned in part by two factors, the higher prevalence of infertility in humans than in laboratory animals or in signal species, and the numbers of progressively motile and morphologically normal sperm in human semen typically are inferior to values characteristic of males of other species (42). Human testes may function at the threshold of pathology, and may be particularly sensitive to toxins compared with the testes of animals used to study testicular function (33). Thus, it appears that men are more vulnerable than animals (male) to potential reproductive toxins and raises the issue of whether animal models are really sensitive in detecting reproductive hazards in humans. Furthermore, the very nature of the reproductive process in males (in contrast to females), in which spermatogenesis is a continuous process and therefore usually fully restorative following chemical injury, necessitates an entirely different strategy in assessing reproductive parameters in the laboratory.

Despite these factors, and as in other toxicity assessments, evaluation of potential reproductive toxins requires evaluation of one or more laboratory species. Let it be stated at the onset that no animal model has reproductive characteristics similar to those of humans, but in general, rodents and rabbits offer several advantages in comparison to the dog and subhuman primate (33,42). Early age at sexual maturity, short gestational and lactational periods, ease of handling, large litters, and cost are considerations in their favor (201). Of these species, the rat is probably preferable to the mouse or hamster for reasons of size, well-characterized reproductive processes, and widespread use in other toxicological studies. The major disadvantage of the rat in this context is that ejaculates cannot be collected; thus semen or spermatozoa cannot be evaluated by longitudinal protocol. The rabbit is an ideal second species because it is the smallest common species from which semen can be quantitatively and conveniently collected in longitudinal studies, and as in the rat, a wealth of background information exists for this species. Both species can be subjected to fertility testing, probably the most important criterion in selecting male laboratory models, although multigenerational use in the rabbit is not practical due to the length of its reproductive cycle.

Among other laboratory species considered for use as models, the dog is suitable for semen collection but impractical for use in fertility testing, and subhuman primates are sufficiently rare and too costly for routine use (42). Monkeys are also considered unsuitable for investigation of semen parameters (25). Other species recommended include the chicken (202), hamster, tree shrew, guinea pig, and gerbil (203). Only the latter species of this group is considered acceptable by one investigator (203), but recent utility has not been explored.

Useful endpoints for studying reproduction in male animal models compared to those of the human are tabulated in Table 3. Methods for studying effects on reproduction include whole animal testing, routine methods of analyses of target organs (testes, semen), and other nonroutine and largely unvalidated methods, some of which may have potential for use in the future.

1. Whole Animal Model Testing

Reproduction/Fertility Study. The most commonly applied animal test for detecting effects on reproductive function is the reproduction or fertility (generation) study, usually carried out in the rodent.

The sterotypic testing design for product testing in the United States was promulgated initially by the Environmental Protection Agency (EPA) to regulate pesticides, agrochemicals, and residues under FIFRA Series 83 Guidelines (204), and published in somewhat revised form by a different branch (TSCA) Part 798 Guidelines within the agency (205) to regulate chemicals in general. The guidelines were mandatory prior to registration of a new chemical entity or re-registrating old entities if their databases were inadequate. They were modeled in part on the first segment phase of the guideline authored for the U.S. Food and Drug Administration (FDA) in 1966 to regulate pharmaceuticals prior to entering in the marketplace (206). Similar but not identical guidelines for chemicals other than pharmaceutical products by other countries, including Japan (207,208) and the countries of the European Union (209) also appeared. The multigeneration study evolved over the years, the current model being the one proposed in 1968 by Fitzhugh (210). The design is an elaboration of the older "2-litter" test originally intended for evaluating food additives and pesticides by the FDA.

The basic test is typically termed a Segment I test or reproduction/fertility study. Several versions of the test are used in industry (Figure 4). The test provides for treatment of the male (usually about 6 weeks of age) over the cycle of spermatogenesis prior to cohabitation with a female treated over several estrous cycles prior to mating and usually through gestation and weaning (Figure 4a). The British add behavioral and reproduction phases as well. In this manner, the effects of a test chemical over a broad spectrum of gonadal functions, estrous cycles, mating behavior, conception, parturition, lactation, weaning, and growth and development of the resultant offspring can be assessed. Specifically, this is the sole test suggested by various regulatory agencies to determine male reproductive function. Alternatively, either males or females treated alone and bred to untreated mates in a similar manner can be employed to isolate gender-specific effects. However, this is seldom necessary in actual practice.

A widely used variation of this test design and one used for potential food additives (211), pesticides (204), and regulated chemicals (205) is one that selects F_1 offspring at weaning to become parents of a second generation, with treatment continuing through the process, to weaning F_2 offspring. This is the so-called 2-generation 1-litter study (Figure 4b). The protocol for chemicals, including pesticides, has been recently modified (212). A further variation, stemming from the perception that the quality of litters varies between matings of the same parents, allows for two litters each ("a" and "b") being produced by F_0 and F_1 parents over two generations, the 2-generation 2-litter study. A third generation could be produced in a similar manner and a teratology phase added to the second or third generation if so desired (Figure 4c). The primary objectives of multigeneration protocols are twofold: To detect injury to the developing gonads and to fertility from the progressive accumulation of body burdens, and to determine the potential adverse consequences of metabolic transformation (213). This type of study is the testing method of choice when there is need for an overall view of reproductive function that cannot be achieved by discrete, shorter tests. In terms of specific information obtained, the parental animals provide data on fertility and pregnancy. The first generation provides information on the uterine environment, lactation, and growth and maturation of offspring, and the second (or third) generation assess the effect of chemical accumulation and gene alteration (203). It should be noted that an Advisory Panel has questioned the value of multigeneration reproduction studies beyond the second filial generation (214). Reproduction/fertility tests carried out according to these different protocols vary in duration from about 3 to 13 months (Table 8).

Strictly speaking, since spermatogenesis requires over 4 cycles (about 52 days) of the seminiferous epithelium in the rat, a test to evaluate effects of an agent on spermatogenesis should extend over 6 cycles (77 days) for this species (33,42). The same concept for length of treatment applies to other species as well (i.e., rabbit, 65 days; dog, 82 days; rhesus monkey, 57 days). This interval is based on the time required to attain steady-state concentrations of the agent in the target organs, the concept that an agent acting on the germinal epithelium

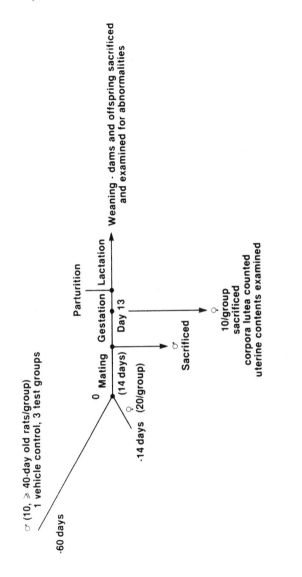

Figure 4 Reproduction/fertility study schemes: (a) Segment I, (b) 2G 1-litter, (c) 3G 2-litter, with teratology phase (modified from Ref. 217).

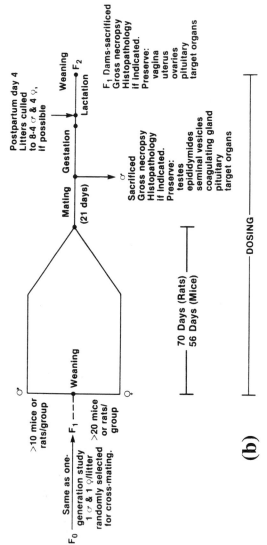

Figure 4 Continued.

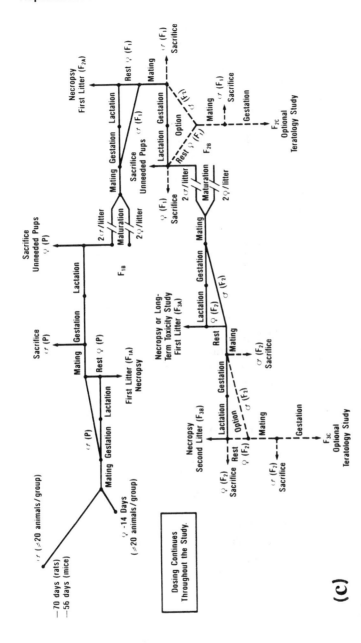

(c)

Figure 4 Continued.

Table 8 Characteristics of Evolving Reproduction/Fertility Studies

Agency (year)	Parental treatment (days premating)			Study duration (months)
	F_0	F_1	F_2	
FDA (drugs) (1966)	60 M, 14 F			3.5
United Kingdom (1974)	60 M, 14 F ⟶			7
Canada (pesticides) (1981)	~80 ⟶ (2 litters)			13
FDA (additives) (1982)	70 M, 14 F ⟶ w/wo teratology			11–12 or 20
OECD (1996)	70 M, 70 F	70 M, 70 F		10
EPA OPPTS (1998)	70 M, 70 F	70 M, 70 F		10
Japan MAFF (1985)	56 ⟶			8
Harmonized (drugs) (1994)	14–28 M, 14 F			3

may require some time prior to degeneration of the affected cells, the fact that damage to the germinal epithelium is most evident by absence of more mature germ cells, and finally, by the knowledge that qualitative changes in germ cells may not be readily discernable until abnormal sperm pass into the cauda epididymis or ejaculated semen. For monitoring recovery, 12–18 complete cycles of the seminiferous epithelium are necessary (25,33).

Criticisms regarding all aspects of the various designs for reproduction studies have been published (203,213,215–227). These center mainly on the limited group sizes, lack of testing F_1 progeny reproductive ability, excessively long premating periods, no provision for behavioral testing, undue complexity in study design, requirement of spermatogenesis testing of male animals, histopathology, and time and cost required for testing. Additional criticism of conventional fertility tests has also been made on the grounds that such tests are simply insensitive (42). In this context, it has been pointed out that since male rats produce and ejaculate 10 to 100 times more sperm than are necessary for normal fertility and litter size, the number of sperm available can be reduced by 90% before the decrease in ejaculate is sufficient to cause sterility. Thus, there may be difficulties identifying reproductive toxicity even if the agent reduces sperm counts significantly. Also, the quality of measurements of conventional reproductive parameters from tests as currently performed are really not very good (222). The latest study designs address most of these concerns, and generation reproduction studies of the types just described remain the primary method for reproductive toxicity testing. The methods of performing fertility and generational tests are crucial in obtaining the proper information for assessing reproductive hazards in the animal model, and the reader would do well to study closely the details in the publications cited above. Pitfalls and discussion pertinent to conducting fertility/reproduction studies is found in Section IV.B.1.

Parameters obtainable in males from reproduction/fertility studies include only endpoints relating to mating (e.g., libido and fertility). The ultimate index of male fertility is, of course, induction of successful pregnancy in the receptive female (25). Conventional indices are as follows, given as % ($\times 100$):

$$\text{Copulatory index} = \frac{\text{no. males mating}}{\text{no. males paired}}$$

Copulatory interval = day (mean) animals paired until mating

$$\text{Fertility index} = \frac{\text{no. males shown to be fertile}}{\text{no. males paired}}$$

$$\text{Conception rate} = \frac{\text{no. males shown to be fertile}}{\text{no. males mating}}$$

Continuous Breeding. In order to satisfy some criticisms of reproduction-type studies in cost-effective yet scientifically acceptable ways, another type of comprehensive reproductive toxicology protocol has been designed which tests both male and female reproductive function, with the mouse the animal model (228).

The design of the protocol maximizes the number of litters that can be measured by continuous breeding of paired mice over a 98-day period following a 7-day treatment period (Figure 5). Through discarding the offspring as they are produced, several litters can result and at the end of 98 days, the last litter is followed through weaning. If effects are observed, crossover matings can be performed with control mice to assess sex-specific effects, and target organ toxicity can be determined through histopathology, if necessary. Should there be no effect, the weanlings can be treated, reared, and bred to test their reproductive capacity after prenatal, lactational, and developmental exposure.

Limited testing has shown the protocol to be predictive and sensitive in discriminating effects of several developmental toxicants (218,229–231), but further validation is needed to determine if the pattern of reproductive toxicity of a number of different test chemicals can be shown. To date, over 40 chemicals from the glycol ether, polyglycol, phthalate ester, methylxanthine and other classes have been studied, but full results are not available at present (232). Of particular interest is the fact that the continuous breeding protocol has been accepted by U.S. agencies in lieu of the fertility or generational-type reproduction studies (233).

Serial Mating. Serial mating in rodents, such as used in so-called dominant lethal assay, is another type of test used, but it assesses male reproductive effects only.

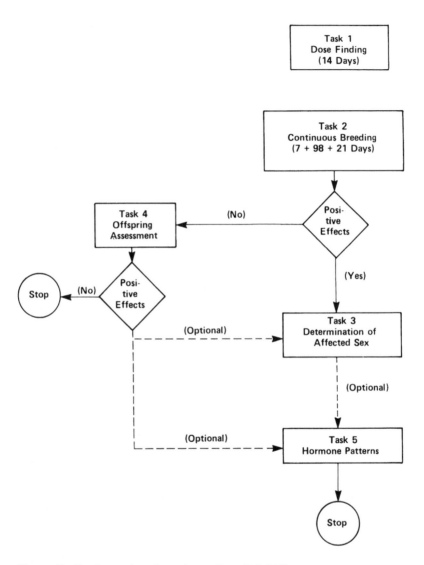

Figure 5 Continuous breeding scheme (from Ref. 220).

The protocol for such tests consists of a short, 5–7 day treatment regimen at acute or subacute dosages to male mice or rats, followed by serial matings, usually to two untreated females each over short (usually 7 day) cohabitation periods over the total spermatogenesis cycle of 8–10 weeks. About two weeks after evidence of copulation, the females are sacrificed and evidence of dominant lethal mutations (decreased embryo viability) is assessed. The time that treatment affected viability indicates when the spermatogenesis process was interfered with. For example, decreased viability of implant sites in the first week of treatment in the mouse indicates an effect on epididymal sperm, whereas in the sixth week or earlier would point to effects on spermatogonia; intermediate intervals would affect spermatids and spermatocytes (234). It appears that few, if any, compounds tested exert their effect in one week only (235). Treatment-related decreases in sperm-positive matings might indicate effects on libido or semen quality. Thus, the serial mating protocol has proven to be a valuable tool in assessing the effects of chemicals on male reproductive function. Among the alternatives that can be used to serial mating as described above is to continue the treatment exposure over all stages of spermatogenesis and then conduct a single-mating trial. This procedure was successfully used to test one potential developmental toxicant, dimethyl methyl phosphonate in rats (cited, 218).

A number of criticisms of serial mating procedures, such as the propensity of the assay for showing preimplantation loss which is not correlated with dead implants, aberrancies in statistical analysis, dose-response problems, and the inordinate time to conduct the test have resulted in modifications leading to adoption of better protocols (236).

Limited/Competitive Fertilization. To compensate for the insensitivity of conventional reproduction/fertility tests due to excessive sperm production in rodents, several other approaches have been suggested.

The first is the use of artificial insemination, allowing introduction of a controlled and limited number of sperm into the reproductive tract of the female (42). In this way, insemination with only a number of sperm that is marginally adequate for normal fertility, a functional alteration in the number of sperm brought about by an agent could be detectable by a decrease in fertility.

Another approach that has been used is one termed "competitive fertilization." In this technique, sperm from a control and a treated male are placed in direct competition by simultaneously inseminating equal numbers of sperm from the two males into a single female (237). The parentage can be determined by any of several phenotypic marker systems. Such a technique was successfully employed to detect toxic levels of caffeine in semen in avian species (202).

Copulatory Behavior. One of the most logical endpoints for reproductive assessment is whether the animals are mating. In the most commonly used species, the rodent, mating is traditionally confirmed by inspection of the females for the presence of a vaginal or copulatory plug, or smearing of vaginal contents for the presence of sperm. Coitus usually occurs at night, thus examination is done the following morning. Presence of a vaginal plug is more predictive of pregnancy outcome than is presence of sperm in the vagina (238). In male rodents, multiple intromissions are the rule: Four or more penile intromissions are necessary to achieve successful pregnancy (239).

It is very important to correlate copulation with the actual results at termination of pregnancy of the female in order to detect sterile matings. This obviously is different from the situation where males do not mate, indicating potential behavioral and/or neuromuscular effects.

A simple method of assessing libido and fertility in the male was first detailed many years ago (210). A male is cohabitated with a female for two estrous cycles; if no copulation occurs, it is replaced by another male. The number of copulations divided by the number of pregnancies provides a mating index.

As part of the development of other models that could provide information on the overall function of the male reproductive system, another simple scheme for assessing copulatory behavior in rodents has been devised (240). In this model, male and female rats are placed together at 100 days of age (maximum sperm production in the male) and mating behavior observed following exposure to the chemical under test. Either subacute (5 days) or subchronic exposures (70–80 days) are used. The mount latency (interval between introduction of male to female and the first mount), the number of mounts, the number of intromissions, and ejaculation latency (interval between first mount and ejaculation) are scored. The animals are then euthanized and additional reproductive assays conducted if desired. Although not validated at present, this model has detected two chemicals that alter copulatory behavior, trichloroethylene and carbon disulfide (240). Similar methods are underway in other laboratories to assess adverse effects on the nervous system through disturbances of behavior, libido, erection, and ejaculation in rats (241).

2. Target Organ Analysis

Semen Assessment.   Semen analysis is considered to be very useful in studies on the possible effects of drugs, chemicals and environmental hazards on testicular and epididymal function and on male fertility (242). In fact, the single most sensitive and important parameter for human fertility is the total number of motile sperm in an ejaculate (33). Three lines of indirect evidence suggest that monitoring sperm can indicate reproductive impairment (15): Male exposures affect fetal loss independently of female factors; there is a general association between fertility and sperm counts, proportion of abnormally shaped sperm and proportion of abnormally shaped sperm and proportion of motile sperm; sperm quality is a sensitive indicator of testicular function, and impaired quality is correlated with increased incidence of spontaneous abortion. Sperm has additional advantages of being readily obtainable, is subject to objective evaluation, is regarded as a sensitive indicator of recent exposures, is free from consideration of female factors, and requires modest sample size to demonstrate presence or absence of hazard (15).

Semen is a composite solution formed by the testes and accessory male reproductive organs whose function is to provide a nutritive medium of proper osmolality and volume for conveying sperm to the endocervical mucus. Semen is assessed according to three main parameters: Sperm concentration or density (counts), motility, and morphology. Semen characteristics (volume, color, consistency, pH) themselves are of little value in assessing reproductive detriment.

Paradoxically, infertile human males tend to have increased semen volume (243), while postcoital studies suggest that greatly decreased semen values in men may result in poor penetration of cervical mucus by the sperm (244). Much of the data related to semen analysis in laboratory animals has come from the work of Amann and his associates, and the reader desiring more detailed information is referred to those and other publications (3,42,245–249).

Sperm Counts. Measurements of sperm numbers are the most feasible component of semen evaluation (250). It is possible that reproductive toxicants can affect daily sperm production; thus this endpoint may be an important one in reproductive toxicology. However, only an accurate determination of the total number of sperm in an ejaculate can provide this information, and this is not feasible in many laboratory species (33,42). Nonetheless, sperm production can be assessed indirectly in any one of several ways.

Semen for quantitation in laboratory animals is typically taken from the cauda epididymides following euthanization of the animal; counts of spermatozoa are performed in a hemacytometer. For larger laboratory animals like rabbits, and in humans, sperm counts may be made directly from ejaculates. In animal studies, a uniform interval of 1 or 2 days, or less ideally 3 or 4 days between semen collection is essential, and the series of ejaculates should extend over 20 days if semen is not collected continuously throughout the experiment (42,245,246). The methods for counting sperm are simple and well established, and techniques and instrumentation exist for accurate quantitation. Background data on sperm production is provided for the common laboratory species in Table 6.

A low sperm count is in itself not a reason for infertility (242). In fact, sperm concentration is considered the least informative of all semen tests (249). Dysfunctional sperm, rather than a deficient number of sperm, is the probable cause of reduced fertility (251). Although 10 to 40 million spermatozoa/ml semen has been a dividing line between infertile and fertile (249), the only valid data concerning sperm count and its relationship to fertility has been the observation that men with sperm counts less than 20 million/ml were encountered more frequently in an infertile group than in a fertile group in an older, classic study (252). In reality, more than 80% of apparently infertile men have sperm counts which meet or exceed the normal standards (250). In fact, pregnancies have been achieved by men who had sperm counts below 2 million/ml upon semen analysis (253). A similar situation exists in animals. For instance, in one experiment in rats, the only disturbance of reproduction following a 80% reduction of morphologically normal, motile sperm by chemical administration was a small reduction in the number of implants per pregnant female (254).

The use of sperm counts for reproductive risk assessment is confounded by several other factors as well: Normal day-to-day variations in sperm count and the fact that sperm counts may reflect relatively late signs of testicular toxicity (250) are two such factors. Further, while there are a number of chemicals that can induce severe damage to spermatogenesis, much less is known about agents with weak or moderate inhibitory effects on spermatogenesis or sperm maturation.

Sperm Motility.   Motility of spermatozoa is a functional parameter, because successful fertilization depends on the sperm being actively motile (48). It has been said that fertility potential is related to the total number of motile sperm (255); motility has been found to be a sensitive indicator of male fertility (252). Essentially, two aspects of motility can be distinguished: percent progressive motile sperm and velocity of sperm.

Percent progressive motile sperm can be quantitated from the same diluted semen sample collected from the cauda epididymides of the animal following euthanization as was the sperm count, or ejaculated samples can be used. Though visual estimation of sperm motility is not ideal, it can be very useful provided the estimations are made in a careful manner, especially controlling for time and temperature after collection and dilution to allow proper visualization (42,246,256). Acceptable techniques and discrete criteria for categorizing motility have been published (246,257,258). While no rigid standardization exists for motility, it is felt by many investigators that semen should be considered abnormal if fewer than 60% of spermatozoa show progressive motion in specimens examined within three hours of collection (243).

Scientifically, rapidly declining motility seems compatible with fertility, while a low motility soon after ejaculation can be regarded a sign of decreased fertility, at least in the human (242). In rats, the presence of a high percentage of immotile sperm is clear evidence for abnormal testicular or epididymal function (42). A number of chemical agents are known to inhibit motility, enhance it, or immobilize sperm altogether (48).

The other motility factor important in assessment is velocity, or the swimming speed of sperm.According to one investigator, the velocity of spermatozoa may be the most important factor in predicting fertility in men (259). Freshly ejaculated sperm from fertile subjects in one study averaged 75 μm/second but in men with impaired fertility, a high proportion of the sperm moved <40 μm/second

(260). Spermatozoal velocity is assessed visually or by a number of techniques including photomicrography and turbidimetric methods. How sperm velocity is applicable in animal models is unclear at present, but experimentation continues.

Sperm Morphology. The morphological characteristics of sperm have long been regarded as a parameter closely related to fertility as a measure of testicular toxicity. However, it remains difficult to define specific criteria for the shape and percentage of "normal" sperm necessary to establish fertility (5). Sperm morphology is regarded as the most stable and predictive semen parameter of fertility potential in animals by some (261). The mouse sperm morphology test has, in fact, been the predominant test conducted on sperm used as an indicator of germ cell mutation and it has been used in testing over 150 chemicals in the mouse (262–264). The test is based on the premise that an agent that induces abnormal forms of sperm is one that clearly interferes with the normal differentiation of germ cells, and about 27% of chemicals tested have had this propensity (264). Its full utility in assessing reproductive toxins is unconfirmed however, as is its applicability in other species (240); however, the test is feasible in rats (265).

There is no commonly accepted method of morphological assessment. One way of course, is to examine cells microscopically in a diluted sample of semen from that already procured from the cauda epididymides and that from which sperm counts and motility have been evaluated as described above. Sperm from ejaculates can also be utilized. Properly prepared stained smears should be used, and evaluation based on an appropriate classification scheme. Several techniques have been published (262–264,266).

Both head and tail of spermatozoa should be evaluated. Changes in sperm head shape have been associated with effects on fertility in humans and animals (42,268). In rats, the presence of sperm containing a proximal cytoplasmic droplet is clear evidence of abnormal testicular or epididymal function (42). In humans, excessive numbers of sperm with coiled tails have been correlated with infertility (242).

Testicular Morphology. Morphology of the testes can be evaluated subjectively or quantitatively, the latter being more sensitive (42). An understanding of spermatogenesis is essential for evaluation of testicular histology and function; the process has been described in detail (269–271).

Examination of suitably fixed testes can establish whether all cellular associations and types of germ cells are present in the tubules; however, subtle changes in spermatogenesis are not detectable. The various cell types, which can be identified by relatively simple histological examination of the seminiferous tubules of the testis, include spermatogonia, primary and secondary spermatocytes, spermatids, and spermatozoa. It is imperative that testes be properly prepared for these evaluations: Helly's, Bouin's, Zenker's, and formalin in descending order of preference, have been established by one major laboratory as fixatives for morphological studies with tissue embedding in methacrylate preferred (218).

For quantitative evaluations, different types of germ cells can be counted (e.g., leptotene spermatocytes, Sertoli cells). Counting spermatid nuclei in testicular homogenates is probably the most sensitive and simplest approach for detecting degeneration or death of primary spermatocytes or spermatids according to one investigator (42). Enumeration of germ cells per Sertoli cell or per tubule cross section was the most sensitive measure of testicular response in a recent study in the rabbit with the testicular toxin, dibromochloropropane (272). Quantitation can also be applied by scoring tubule cross sections with respect to mature spermatid luminal alignment and evidence of active spermatogenesis. Significant deviations in these values between control and treated male rats would be clear evidence of treatment effect. It is also important to identify which cells are the first to be visibly affected by treatment with the compound under study. Appreciation of biological variability and spontaneous pathology of aging of the testis has been stressed in toxicity testing in the various species (25).

Sex Organ Weights. This parameter is useful because testicular size largely determines daily sperm production (245), and because testicular degeneration induced by toxins will result in reduction in testis size (42). However, it is not as sensitive as other tests for detecting testicular damage. For instance, a 50–60% weight reduction of the testes is correlative to an atrophic gland that has lost all or most of its germ cells (218).

One testis freed of the epididymis and spermatic cord of each male on test should be weighed as an indication of testicular toxicity (42). Since testes weight and body weight in adult males are independent variables, absolute testis weights are the appropriate parameter for assessment.

Weighing the distal half of the epididymis may also be an informative measurement (42). The weight of accessory male sex glands is an objective indicator of whether or not the androgen status of the animal has been significantly compromised (218); it is thought to be a crude bioassay of testosterone production by the testes and normalcy of the number of available steroid receptors (42).

A product of the sex organs, the postmating seminal plug may be weighed, its size serving as a marker of hormone status since it is a product of androgen-dependent glands (240), but the method appears to have little practical significance.

Endocrine Function. Historically, the male endocrine system has been an infrequent target of reproductive toxicants. In some cases however, routine endocrine analyses may be desired. In fact, it is clearly established in all mammalian species investigated that an endocrine defect in the brain, pituitary, or testis may inhibit spermatogenesis and normal sexual behavior (33).

Luteinizing hormone (LH) controls testosterone secretion by the testes which in turn, is responsible for the maintenance of accessory glands and spermatogenesis. Prolactin synergizes with LH in the regulation of testosterone synthesis, secretion, and inhibition (25). Follicle-stimulating hormone (FSH) on the other hand, controls Sertoli cell function and spermatogenesis, testosterone playing a pivotal role in the latter process. Thus, one infamous reproductive toxicant, dibromochloropropane (DBCP), through destruction of germ cells, induced a measurable increase in FSH without any concurrent changes in either testosterone or LH (273). In contrast, an experimental drug, PMHI, caused severe testicular weight depression and affected Sertoli cells without altering hormone levels (274).

Direct toxic effects on the testes can lead to abnormally high levels of gonadotropins because of the feedback relationship existing between the pituitary gland and the gonads (250). In such cases, radioimmunoassays for gonadotropins may provide useful information. However, laboratory assays of circulating hormones are likely to provide only late signs of reproductive effects.

3. Others

The need to assess multiple endpoints of reproductive function is clearly evident. Assessment has obviously not developed to the point where a single animal endpoint is indicative of reproductive risk in the human male (275–277). As a consequence, a number of qualitative and quantitative reproductive toxicity tests have been described (33). A very useful manual providing methods that help identify toxicant-induced changes at all levels in the male animal have been published by Chapin and Heindel (298). The following represent some of the assays currently being explored or already in limited use.

Sperm Penetration Tests.   Since cervical mucus is a well-defined fluid accessible for laboratory study and sperm travel to the site of fertilization, passing first through it, important functions of the sperm cell can be assessed by examination of sperm interaction with the cervical mucus (278). Thus, sperm penetration of cervical mucus is one type of examination that may be useful in reproductive toxicology. The ability of sperm to penetrate cervical mucus has been correlated with fertility in humans (279,314). Several different in vitro methods are available to assess the ability of sperm cells to enter into the mucus and to characterize and/or quantify their swimming behavior (280,281).

Another sperm penetration test that may be useful utilizes hamster ova. Hamster ova treated enzymatically to digest the zona pellucida membrane can be fertilized by sperm from other species, including the human (282). Thus, the percentage of capacitated sperm observed to penetrate the zona pellucida-freed hamster egg and fuse can be determined. Clinically, there are a number of reports associating male fertility and the success of sperm fusion (283,284), but the test at present remains controversial, based largely on the fact that sperm unable to fuse hamster ova may not represent infertile sperm (250,251). This subject has been reviewed in detail recently (285).

Double Y Bodies. This test is based on staining of fluorescent spots in sperm by a quinacrine dye (286). The spots are thought to be Y chromosomes. Thus sperm containing two Y bodies are thought to represent abnormal sperm due to meiotic nondisjunction (287). Unlike other tests on males discussed thus far, the double Y-body test has no direct counterpart in common laboratory species; it appears to be of unique applicability to humans and certain other primates (256).

Acrosomal Proteolytic Activity. Proteolytic activity in the sperm acrosome is essential for penetrating the zona pellucida of the ovum. Therefore, loss of this activity may reflect decreased fertility. A method has been developed to demonstrate proteolytic activity in sperm acrosomes based on staining of sperm suspensions with toluidine blue (288). The method has been used by one group of investigators in mice to successfully identify two reproductive toxicants, cyclophosphamide and mitomycin C (289). Further application of the method is in order.

Serum Chemistry. A number of tests have been used in the past in humans to evaluate different chemical entities in semen which may be markers of infertility. These include tests for seminal fructose (290), zinc (291), polyamines (292), fumarase (293), cyclic nucleotides (294,324), various cations (295), and adenine triphosphate (ATP) (296). Only ATP content of semen has been shown to be correlated with sperm count, motility and the ability of sperm to penetrate zona-free hamster ova (285). Application of these and other chemical analyses to animals warrants attention.

Pubertal Development. A testing protocol has been developed recently to screen chemicals for reproductive effects in male hamsters in order to identify potential reproductive toxicants for more thorough testing (297). A series of pubertal alterations are measured following chemical administration including preputial separation, flank gland development, sexual behavior, development of gonads, sperm motility, caudal sperm reserves, and pituitary hormone levels. The reproductive toxicant methoxychlor induced a number of changes in pubertal development, and indicates the screen may have future utility.

B. Female

In contrast to the male, animal model selection and study design for assessing reproductive hazards in the female require a somewhat different strategy. This is due primarily to the fact that in the female, a *finite* number of germ cells (oocytes) is formed during the fetal period. Additional germ cells cannot be produced; thus chemical injury may be irreversible. Another important factor in these considerations is the cyclicity of reproductive functions characterizing the female (i.e., estrus or menses at fixed intervals) that have no true counterpart in the male. One additional factor influencing choice of animal models for determining reproductive effects in females is that laboratory animals, with the exception of primates, are polytocous. Thus, even more important than in males, no animal model has reproductive characteristics similar to those of human females.

Nonetheless, current viewpoints favor the use of one or more laboratory animal species to assess potential reproductive hazards to the female of different chemical agents. The choice of species rests largely on the negative aspects of most all species, leaving the *rat* and *rabbit*, as in male studies, as first and second species preferential in the study of effects on female reproductive processes. Fertility testing can be carried out, timed ovulation is possible, and evaluation of oocytes, embryos, uterine morphology, hormone receptors, and longitudinal hormonal analyses can be conducted in both species (42). These species have the further advantage of having the potential of producing multiple numbers of large litters (10–12 in the rat, 7–9 in the rabbit) during their reproductive lives. Of several other species, the long anestrus, the inability to predict the onset of proestrus or to induce estrus or ovulation, together with the impossibility of conducting fertility testing in the bitch, severely limit the use of the dog (42). Inbred mice may represent the most sensitive species for oocyte and follicle toxicity assay (33). And while subhuman primates offer several advantages related primarily to having menstrual cycles and bearing single young, widespread use in reproductive toxicology is unlikely for a variety of reasons. The guinea pig is more satisfactory than other species for assessing the effects of toxicants on gonadotropic function or luteinization (33). Pigs and cows are desirable large species for steroidgenesis toxicity assays (33).

Useful endpoints for studying reproduction in female animal models compared to those of the human are tabulated in Table 4. Methods and techniques for assessing reproductive effects in female animal models include fertility-type studies (whole animal testing), a number of target organ (ovary) analyses, and nonroutine methods perhaps having potential utility in the future.

1.　Whole Animal Model Testing

Reproduction/Fertility Study.　As in assessing male reproductive function, the standard reproduction/fertility study in rodents remains the most sensitive indicator of chemical effects on reproduction in use at present as it relates to the female gender.

Reproduction/fertilities studies in females provide a wide range of parameters that may reflect reproductive effects. One of these is evaluation of the estrous cycle. This is typically done prior to administration of a test chemical, prior to mating concurrent with chemical administration, and/or following chemical treatment during mating. One of the ways to assess estrus is to simply score the cycle in relation to normal duration of the stages, for example, in the rat, a diestrus greater than three consecutive days or shorter than two consecutive days, or proestrus, estrus or metestrus longer than 1 day. In this manner, adverse effects on normal reproductive cycling can be discerned. It is important to stress that changes observed with treatment are in fact different than they were in the untreated period, since there is some variation in cycle periodicity from animal to animal.

As already indicated, females in reproduction/fertility studies are usually administered the test chemical for periods ranging from 2 weeks to 10 weeks prior to mating (minimum 3 estrous cycles). The females are paired with males in 1 : 1 ratios, usually to treated animals, over 2- or 3-week mating intervals. Appropriate subtests may also be performed to establish cause of sex-induced infertility or offspring mortality due to maternal toxicity. Several useful endpoints can be determined from these pairings to include effects on libido and ability to copulate. These are given as % ($\times 100$):

$$\text{Copulatory index (sometimes termed "mating index")} = \frac{\text{no. females mating}}{\text{no. females paired}}$$

$$\text{Mating index} = \frac{\text{no. females mating}}{\text{no. estrous cycles}}$$

The copulatory interval or precoital time (days animals paired before mating) is also of interest here, but refers more to the male than to the female. At termination of gestation, the dams are either euthanized and the offspring taken by Cesarean section, or more commonly, are allowed to deliver. At this time, pregnancy status is determined by any of several endpoints:

$$\text{Fertility index} = \frac{\text{no. pregnant}}{\text{no. females paired}}$$

$$\text{Pregnancy index ("fecundity index" = conception rate)} = \frac{\text{no. pregnant}}{\text{no. females mating}}$$

$$\text{Gestation index} = \frac{\text{no. live litters born}}{\text{no. pregnant}}$$

$$\text{Parturition index} = \frac{\text{no. deliveries}}{\text{no. females mated}}$$

Careful observations are made of delivery, since protracted or difficult labor (dystocia) may be chemically induced. An endpoint of significance at this point in the reproductive process is concerned with viability of offspring at birth, assessed in the following manner:

$$\text{Gestation survival index} \atop \text{("live birth index")} = \frac{\text{no. live pups at birth}}{\text{no. pups born}}$$

Another parameter evaluated at this time is data reflective of litter size (live + dead term fetuses), since reductions may reflect adverse chemical effects on early embryonic or fetal viability.

Growth and survival of the pups during lactation are then evaluated and are important on two counts. This is because reduced growth as measured by body weights and pup viability, quantitated by survival indices (see below), may be due to chemical toxicity. In the first instance, the dams, through inherent toxicity and/or behavioral alteration, or both, may affect nursing and/or care of their litters; as one might expect, maternal neglect can have profound effects on neonates. If there is chemical toxicity to the pups directly through in utero and/or nursing chemical exposure, failure to thrive and death may ensue. Pups are usually culled to 8 or 10 per litter on day 4 (or 5) of lactation in order to minimize intralitter competition during nursing. Traditional survival indices are as follows:

$$\text{Reproduction index} = \frac{\text{no. pups surviving 4 days}}{\text{no. pregnant animals}}$$

$$\text{4- (or 5-) day survival index} \atop \text{("viability index")} = \frac{\text{no. pups surviving 4 days}}{\text{no. live pups at birth}}$$

$$\text{7-day survival index} = \frac{\text{no. pups surviving 7 days}}{\text{no. live pups at 4 days}}$$

$$\text{14-day survival index} = \frac{\text{no. pups surviving 14 days}}{\text{no. live pups at 4 days}}$$

$$\text{21-day survival index} = \frac{\text{no. pups surviving 21 days}}{\text{no. live pups at 14 days}}$$

$$\text{Lactation index} = \frac{\text{no. pups surviving 21 days (weaned)}}{\text{no. pups retained day 4 (or 5)}}$$

There are a number of important considerations to be taken into account in order to avoid pitfalls in conducting reproduction/fertility studies, whether they be done to assess reproductive effects in males or in females.

For the prototype fertility study of the Food and Drug Administration (206), separate protocols exist for treatment of males and females. In the author's opinion this is unwarranted as a general rule, and combined treatment of both sexes in a single study is appropriate. Actually, from practical experience, the necessity for conducting them separately would occur in less than 1% of cases according to one experienced investigator (220). Gender-specific effects can be determined in a combined study by adding additional groups of each sex to high dose and control groups and mated to each other as has been suggested by others (299) or simply repeating the study using treated animals of both sexes mated to untreated mates in the rare case where such effects are suspected or realized.

Virtually all regulatory guidelines recommend a minimum of 20 animals per group for parental and litter observations. For all practical purposes, this requires placing 24, 26, or preferably 30 animals per group on study to ensure adequate numbers for evaluation. Otherwise, toxic, seasonal, or other factors may result in too few litters for adequate analysis. The advantages of group sizes even larger than 30 each in detecting reproductive effects have been described (222).

Another almost universal requirement of the various protocols is the criteria for dose selection. The highest dose should elicit toxicity of undefined quantity, but little or no mortality. Seldom are doses in reproduction studies the same as those for determining developmental toxicity; the higher doses used in the latter are deliberately set to induce maternal toxicity. At the lower levels the recommendation is minimal toxicity (again of undefined severity or nature) at the mid-dose level, while the low dose should be a "no observable effect level" (NOEL). This ideal set of dosage criteria is difficult to achieve as a general condition.

The age at which the females are mated is a critical factor: Rats should be approximately 9–10 weeks of age at first mating (220); guidelines and regulations specify ages ranging from immediately after weaning (PND 21) to 9 weeks. Toxicants, particularly those that possess steroidal activity, will diminish the success of pregnancy and number of offspring of older but not those of younger females; thus while testing at earlier ages is more economical, it might yield false-negative results (33). Further, declining fertility as a normal phenomenon of advancing age can occur within the range of ages specified by some protocols for matings intended to produce litters from which a further generation will be derived, pointing further to the critical nature of this factor (203,300). Presently, treatment regimens range from 2–10 weeks; thus duration impacts directly on breeding age. It should be recognized too, that body weight is a more critical factor than age in the determination of reproductive capacity in rodents (220). The wide variability experienced in fertility rates among control animals is in itself a real concern in studies of this type (222).

Several reproduction/fertility protocols specify that postnatal evaluation be conducted on F_1 issue. They state that late effects of the chemical on the progeny in terms of auditory, visual, and behavioral function should be assessed.

What specific evaluation this statement is meant to convey is not known, but the reproductive toxicologist would be wise to include assessments concerned with postnatal maturation (e.g., eye opening, pinna detachment), reflexes (e.g., negative geotaxis, Preyer's reflex), and learning (e.g., maze, shuttle box) from representatives of both sexes from each litter in order to provide sufficient data to satisfy the intent of these regulations when given. Neurotoxicity screening is an increasing topic under consideration for universal testing in some protocols as well. With recent emphasis on endocrine dysruption, assessment of sexual maturation (e.g., vaginal opening in females, preputial separation in males) in the postnatal period is mandatory.

The disposition of offspring as described in the various protocols is variable. Certainly the 13-day midterm embryo examination as defined in the FDA Fertility and General Reproductive Performance Study (206) can, in my judgement, be better replaced with euthanization one day prior to term, primarily because direct and indirect fetal effects can be discriminated, and intrauterine growth can be more fully assessed. Detailed examination of offspring for malformations from reproduction studies as suggested in U.K. (301) and Japanese guidelines (211) would appear to be a meaningless exercise since treatment is chronic in both designs and ends prior to organogenesis in the latter as well. Neither regimen could be expected to elicit teratogenicity under any but the most unusual circumstances, and fortunately have been superceded by ICH Guidelines (303).

Requirements for reproductive phases of the offspring also vary widely: Most protocols recommend production of one litter per generation, but the practice in Canada with pesticides (386) and the trend in the United States with additives (304) toward evaluation of two litters per generation is, in my opinion unfounded; the evidence provided to date (305) indicating that additional information gained from the second litter in such studies is less than convincing. In fact, it is my experience and that of others (220) that first matings are as successful as second matings in most litter parameters, and analysis of 20 multiple generation studies reported in the literature indicated that *one generation* was sufficient for evaluation of reproductive effects (219).

Notwithstanding the large number of perhaps less significant variations (e.g., mating schemes, culling practices) in protocol design among the various international protocols, undoubtedly the most important consideration is the apparent lack of universal acceptability from country to country and agency to agency at the present time. Do sufficient scientific reasons exist to disallow in any country a fertility study in which adequate numbers of 1 : 1 mated rats are euthanized at term for fetal morphological examination, suitable numbers allowed to deliver and wean for postnatal testing and selection for producing a second generation, the treatment period encompassing all reproductive events? Global study designs typified by this oversimplified example would go a long way in standardizing testing requirements to the benefit of all, and without sacrificing scientific principles. It is anticipated that the EPA/OECD guidelines currently under discussion for revision will be constructed along similar lines and eventually merged with MAFF Guidelines and eventually with the recently harmonized drug guidelines in the three major venues.

As pointed out by others (220), the chief concern with reproduction studies is with the interpretation of differences around the limits of normal variation, not with clear-cut dose-related toxicity. The validity of such studies can be seriously compromised by the coincidental or treatment-related death or infertility of an occasional male or more often, less than absolute mating performance and pregnancy rate. So it is that protocol design in these types of studies assumes great importance, and the inexperienced investigator would do well to take great care in planning reproduction studies for specific objectives.

Reproductive Capacity. The total reproductive efficiency assessment is very suitable for determining reproductive toxicity in rodents. It is particularly powerful for identification of chronic, low dose exposures. The test is based on the irreplaceable nature of oocytes; thus, animals are intentionally depleted of the ovarian complement of oocytes through repetitive matings. Single treated females are paired with single fertile males and as litters are born, the young are removed and the females bred repeatedly. The cumulative number of live young per dam over an extended period of time (usually 35 weeks) is a measure of reproductive capacity. Failed fertilization, preimplantation loss and dominant lethality are some of the reproductive parameters that can be assessed in this test. It has been used successfully to determine the reproductive capacity of mice following gestational exposure to a well-known reproductive toxicant, DES (306).

Reproductive Behavior. Sexual behavior is another important observation to make in the female. These are mainly indicators of hypothalamic function or dysfunction (33). In the mammalian female, a recurring estrous cycle ("heat") induced by gonadal hormones produces the two measurable behaviors proceptivity and receptivity (213). Proceptivity is a display of a variety of patterns including darting, hopping and ear vibration, obviously representing solicitation of the male. Receptivity then follows, with the female assuming the lordosis posture for mounting by the male. Methods for assessing sexual behavior and quantifying it have appeared (307–310). Since mating occurs in the dark hours in rodents, this assessment is inconvenient, if not difficult.

A notable example of alteration of female receptivity has been provided in a study reported in rats, in which females rejected males and practiced pseudocopulation with each other following treatment with a potential new CNS agent (311).

2. Target Organ Analysis

Endpoints for quantitation of reproductive injury in the female take advantage of the fact that normal fertility is the result of the integration of normally differentiated, developed and maintained central nervous system, ovarian, and reproductive tract functioning (213). The endpoints specifically would include sexual differentiation and maturity, estrual cyclicity and stability, oocyte quantitation, corpora lutea function, follicle atresia, and reproductive senescence. Several other endpoints such as reproductive capacity and reproductive behavior, which might be included here, are included more appropriately in Section IV.B.1.

Sexual Differentiation and Maturity. There are several ways to assess the level of sexual differentiation and maturation as might be influenced by reproductive toxicants. These assessments are particularly useful for toxicants having hormonal activity (33,213). The first externally visible effect with the reproductive hormones is androgenization of the vulva; with such masculinization, the anogenital distance is increased. This effect was reported in female pups of rats injected with androgens during gestation (312). A similar effect is the uterotrophic response, assessed either by alterations in uterine weight or in histology of the uterus following treatment. Still another method is through assay of estrogen receptor binding in target tissues. Another method with utility in assessing sexual development and maturity is examination of the female offspring to determine the time of appearance of the vaginal opening (after postnatal day 30 in the rat). Reproductive toxicants, especially those with hormonal activity, can advance or delay this process.

A testing protocol has been developed recently to screen chemicals for reproductive effects in female hamsters in order to identify potential reproductive toxicants requiring further testing (313). A number of pubertal alterations are measured following chemical administration including age at first behavioral estrus, estrus cyclicity, fertility, litter size, viability, and the number of implant sites. Methoxychlor induced a number of alterations, and the screen may be suitable for screening of other potential toxicants.

Estrous Alterations. Initiation of regular estrous cycles at the time of sexual maturity occurs shortly after vaginal opening and is dependent on hormone coordination that is reflected in mating behavior. Although the human does not have an estrous cycle, alterations found in a model species estrous cycle may signal possibly important though subtle changes in the menstrual cycle as well. Several characteristics can be evaluated, including simple cyclicity, senescence, and postpartum stability. It is important to remember that proper lighting is critical to estrous cycling in rodents (314).

The estrous cycle in the rat consists of a proestrus stage (12 hours), estrus or "heat" (12 hours), metestrus (21 hours), and diestrus (57 hours), the different stages characterized microscopically by vaginal cellular contents over a 4–5 day interval. The endpoint in mature animals is the cyclic appearance of leucocytes and noncornified squamous cells in the vagina during the latter two stages. Alterations in either the timeliness of the stages of estrous or inability to cycle altogether is indicative of a disruption of a sensitive pituitary-ovarian balance, possibly reflecting reproductive toxicity. Successful pregnancies in the presence of such changes however, may indicate minor, reversible or insignificant alterations. In this regard it has been shown that the copulatory response in the rat represents a better index of heat than does vaginal cornification, the marker for estrus (315).

Reproductive senescence may be determined in a similar manner by examining vaginal smears prior to and subsequent to resting intervals of 2–3 months duration. The lack of estrous cycling (anestrous) is indicative of senescence and may have possible relevance for humans. The method has been shown to be more predictive for chronic anovulation than is gonadotrophin assay (316).

A "stress test" of sorts has been devised to determine any cause for reduction in reproductive potential, predicated on the observation that within 8–10 hours after delivery in the rodent, the first postpartum estrus occurs in the majority of dams (213). On this basis, the test is conducted during four consecutive cycles by mating the postpartum females beginning 8 hours after delivery; the number of vaginal plugs and the number and weight of the offspring determined, with cumulative reproductive performances compared to controls.

Quantitation of Oogenesis and Ovulation.   There are several quantitative measures that may demonstrate reproductive toxicity in the female animal. While the only direct method of assessing ovulation in laboratory animals depends on collecting free oocytes, there are several indirect methods that may be used to quantitate these processes based on morphological features of the ovary and reproductive outcome (317).

The first of these is determination of the number of oocytes in the ovary through histologic examination; the number observed represents a direct measure of oocyte toxicity. Determination of the precise developmental stage of oogenesis or folliculogenesis is indicative of when exposure to a reproductive toxicant occurred.

Another of these methods is serial counting of oocytes and/or ovarian follicles for detecting and measuring follicle atresia or destruction. Alteration of counts, especially those indicating accelerated loss of either oocytes or follicles might be reflective of reproductive toxicity. Another method of assessing follicular function is the simple but very subjective evaluation of secondary sex characteristics at the time of sexual maturation. Several other ways of assessing folliculogenesis have been described, but are indirect, and not feasible in many laboratories.

3. Others

A number of qualitative and quantitative reproductive toxicity tests have been described in addition to the ones just outlined (33) and some may hold promise for the future. A very useful manual providing methods that help identify toxicant-induced changes at all levels in females has been published (318).

V. USE AND PREDICTABILITY OF ANIMAL MODELS IN IDENTIFYING REPRODUCTIVE HAZARDS

The main source of relevant information relating to reproductive hazards in the human comes largely from animal studies. It is therefore pertinent to determine whether animal models have predictive value in identifying potential reproductive hazards. Several sources have inferred from review of comparative data that the predictive value of animal models in determination of potential reproductive chemical hazards is high in both males and females (319,320). To be sure, humans are certainly not less sensitive than animals with respect to reproductive effects; thus it appears reasonable to assume that where animal data do exist showing reproductive effects, it is also reasonable to conclude that there may be reproductive effects in humans as well. Let us see what the actual data show (Table 9).

Of the approximately 75–80 individual agents or groups of agents thus far identified as potential reproductive hazards in the human (Tables 5–7,9), about half have also demonstrated concordant reproductive effects in laboratory animal models. Thus, as a generality, identifiable reproductive hazards in humans at present have also been associated with reproductive effects in animals about half of the time. Of these, effects in males were mimicked in 74% and effects in females were observed in 81%. Moreover, many other agents have been identified as inducing adverse reproductive effects in animals, but have not yet been confirmed as hazards in human reproduction. As far as the ability to successfully predict whether a given agent will be a reproductive hazard in humans because it produces reproductive effects in animals, it appears that this propensity is not very great.

Some reproductive effects, such as menstrual/estrous cycles and fertility appear to show good correlation in animals and humans because such effects are modulated much the same in the various species. Others, like specific effects on pregnancy, appear not to correlate closely, presumably because of basic biochemical and physiologic differences among species (e.g., pituitary and ovarian

Table 9 Predictability of Animal Models in Identifying Reproductive Hazards

Chemical/group	Effects in				Comments
	Males		Females		
	Human[a]	Animal	Human[a]	Animal	
Alcohol	+	Reproductive dysfunction in rat (321)	+	"FAS" in mouse, dog, rat, and sheep (cited, 322)	Putative human teratogen
Antimony	○		+	Abortion in rabbit (323)	
Antineoplastic drugs	+	Infertility in rat (324)	+	○	Putative human teratogens
Arsenic	○		+	Fetal body weight reduced in mouse (325) and rat (326) with salts	
Benzene	○		+	Estrous cycle changes In rat (327)	
Boric acid	+	Testicular atrophy In rat (328) and dog (329)	○		
Cadmium	+	Testicular damage and reduced fertility in mouse, rat, hamster, rabbit, guinea pig, dog, and squirrel (cited, 320)	+	Reduced fetal body weight in rats (330)	
Carbon disulfide	+	Male sterility (331) and decreased sperm counts in rat (332)	+	○	
Carbon monoxide	○		+	Reduced fetal survival in mouse, rat, rabbit, sheep, and pig (cited, 320)	

Agent				
Chlordecone	+	Testicular atrophy in rat (333) and rabbit (334)	o	Female effects reported in animals: persistent estrus and anovulation in rat (335) and mouse (336)
Chloroprene	+	Testicular degeneration In rat and cat (337)		Reproductive effects in rat and mouse (338)
Cimetidine	+	Antiandrogenic effects In rat (339)	o	
Clomiphene	+	Testicular lesions in rat (340)	+	
DDT	o		+	Increased embryonic death and reduced fetal body weight in rabbit (341), anovulation and persistent estrus in rat (342)
Diamines	+	Decreased fertility and sperm abnormalities in mouse, rat, dog, and monkey (343)	o	
Dibromochloropropane	+	Testicular atrophy and infertility in rat, rabbit, and guinea pig (344,345)	o	Animals less sensitive than humans
Diethylstilbestrol	+	Gonadal lesions in mouse (346), rat (347), and primate (348)	+	Gonadal lesions in mouse (349), rat (347), ferret (350), hamster (351), and primate (352)
Ethylene dibromide	+	Suppression of reproduction in rat (353)	+	
Gossypol	+	Antifertility effects in rat, hamster, rabbit (354), mouse (355), and primate (356)	+	

(continued)

Table 9 Continued

| | Effects in | | | | |
| | Males | | Females | | |
Chemical/group	Human[a]	Animal	Human[a]	Animal	Comments
High temperature	+	Testis lesions, lowered testosterone levels and abnormal sperm in rat (cited, 261)	+	Malformations readily induced in many species	
Insecticides (general)	o		+	Developmental toxicity induced in multiple species by many (cited, 322)	
^{131}I	+	o	+	Fetal goiter in mouse, rabbit and guinea pig (cited, 322)	
Irradiation	+	Spermatogenesis alterations in mouse (357)	+		
Lead	+	Sperm abnormalities and infertility in rat and mouse (cited, 358)	+	o	
Manganese	+	Testicular damage and infertility in mouse (359), rat (360), and rabbit (361)	o		
Mercury (inorganic)	+	Reduced fertility in mouse (362)	+	Estrous effects in mouse (363), rat (364), and hamster (365)	
Methyl mercury	o		+	Developmental toxicity In variety of species (cited, 322)	

Substance		Male effect		Female/developmental effect
Methyl parathion	o		+	Increased fetal mortality in rat (366)
Narcotics	+		+	Increased neonatal mortality (367) and disrupted estrus in rat (368)
Nitrofurantoin	+	Reversible arrest of spermatogenesis in rat (369)	o	
PCBs	o		+	Prolonged estrus in mouse (370), primate (371), and rat (372)
Phthalate plasticizers	o		+	Increased fetal mortality in rodents (122)
Salicylates				Reproductive effects produced in multiple species by many (cited, 322)
Styrene	o		+	Estrous cycle effects in rat (373)
Thallium	o		+	Reduced fetal body weight in rat (374)
Tobacco smoking	+		+	Reduced fetal body weight in rat (375) and rabbit (376)
Toluene chemicals	+		+	Reduced fetal body weight in mouse and rat (377)
Vinyl chloride	+		+	Increased embryonic lethality in mouse and rat (378)

°, no effect; +, effect.

function is essential in rodent but not in human). Because of these differences, complete understanding of both site and mechanism of action of reproductive toxins will be necessary to extrapolate from experimental animal studies to evaluation of human risk (39).

VI. SAFETY EVALUATION AND RISK MANAGEMENT

As the preceding discussion has demonstrated, there are thousands of potential reproductive hazards to which we are exposed. The 80 or so chemicals that have been identified as possible toxicants constitute risks from occupational, or other exposure patterns in addition to therapeutic agents. It would appear that altered reproductive function is definitely a major health endpoint of substantial proportions.

As pointed out by Schull (7), within the broad context of the workplace and environment, every individual is involved, but some by virtue of their occupations will have even greater risks; thus it is the working males and females of reproductive age in this group that are of special concern. A subset of these persons, whose risks may differ substantially, are *pregnant* women. They warrant special consideration for at least two reasons: Their physiology is altered as a consequence of pregnancy, and this factor may affect their own risks; and their exposure is inextricably confounded with that of the fetuses they carry. Moreover, they constitute a "visible susceptible" group, whereas most other high-risk groups are less readily identifiable.

As might be expected, reproductive hazards constitute multiple risk factors (379), primarily because of differing pregnancy outcomes, but for other reasons as well, including confounding factors leading to problems with data interpretation, synergistic effects, documentation of human exposures, and adequate sample sizes, among others.

A number of factors must be identified if assessment of risk to reproduction is to be made more precise (7). First, there is a need to understand more fully the relationships between the measurable endpoints and reproductive outcomes. As has already been discussed, sperm production in animal models must be reduced to critical levels before reproductive effects can even be ascertained, while in the human, we are not certain what levels, if any, of sperm density are associated with impaired fertility. We need to define more precisely just what endpoints are of greatest predictability in reproduction for both animals and humans.

Since observations on humans are limited and experimental results in animals will be the basis of human risk assessment, the choice of animal surrogates is critical. As we have already pointed out, while the rat and rabbit appear to be the most suitable models at present, they clearly are less desirable than some others with respect to certain endpoints, and additional species and other possible endpoints must be investigated. Very few comparisons of methods for assessing reproductive effects from the same chemical in the same animal species have been made. One recent study conducted on the testicular toxin dibromo-chloropropane (DBCP) in the rabbit demonstrated the most sensitive indicators of effect to be sperm morphology and elevation of FSH in contrast to sperm motility, ejaculate volume, sperm concentration, fertility rate, libido, and LH and testosterone levels (380). Similar studies on a variety of real and potential reproductive toxicants are in order to define appropriate methods for assessing reproductive hazards. Reproduction in its broadest sense is a very sensitive tool in toxicity testing (381), but methods are not sensitive enough and as we have shown, animal models have identified reproductive hazards only about half the time. Hardly convincing evidence for their use as models!

The current Segment I type fertility-reproduction and the multigeneration protocol for certain chemicals are likely for several reasons to remain the standard in vivo testing procedures to assess the potential of chemicals to disrupt reproduction. But the continuous breeding protocol being subjected to further validation may prove to be a valuable tool in this regard as well. A testing strategy based on the biological activity of the compound under study would be meaningful (25). Toxicokinetics should be part of reproductive assessments (319), and characterization of the relationship between dose level and response in animals is crucial to this assessment (382). Ultimately, risk-benefit analysis relies heavily on judgement based on an understanding of both the relevance and limitations of experimental data obtained from animals. At present, extrapolation from no-effect levels in animals to presumably safe levels of human exposure should incorporate a safety margin sufficiently wide to take account of possible species differences in susceptibility. The present 10-to 100-fold NOEL doses should be sufficient in this regard for all but the most unique and ubiquitous hazards.

Also, information routinely collected on potential reproductive hazards must be better utilized to make more valid predictions. Proper evaluation of existing information is critically important in this regard. For instance, it has been said that the infertility due to DBCP exposure at one manufacturing plant could have been identified within 4 years just from monitoring the numbers of births to their spouses, instead of the 20-year period that passed following notice by the workers (383). As already pointed out, reproduction data on individual toxicants and epidemiologic information on workers exposed to a chemical in production, let alone adverse reaction reports, are available only for a small number of chemicals. In fact, a large study conducted in 1981 of reproductive hazards could only identify two agents—smoking and alcohol, as having substantial effects in the general population and only two-anesthetic gases (not considered here) and lead, as risk factors to workers exposed in the workplace; data on others were considered fragmentary and incomplete (319).

Part of the formidable task of identifying reproductive hazards could be expedited if the mechanism of a chemical agent's action could be inferred from knowledge of its structure and physicochemical properties. Studies on these aspects need to be greatly expanded. Even in those instances where exposure to known reproductive toxins is believed to have occurred, it is not yet possible to assess the effects of low levels of exposure. Since in many instances it may be economically impractical to remove completely a particular hazard, permissible levels of exposure will presumably have to be set for a number of toxicants, much as they have already been set for exposure to radiation for instance.

Lastly, we must utilize more fully the information now available to minimize untoward occurrences in the workplace. Of the three major informational sources: alert observations by clinicians, systematic toxicological testing in non-human systems, and epidemiological studies and surveillance among humans, the observational report has been the most productive to date (304,384). Probably the best example is the effort by workers in a DBCP manufacturing plant to gain an explanation for their infertility.

One of the main problems in estimating risk from potential reproductive toxins is the number of chemicals, knowledge of exposure, and numbers of potential victims of exposure. Benefits and economics are radically different between drug and industrial chemical testing, and affect both the philosophy of testing and the acceptable risk.

ACKNOWLEDGMENT

The author is grateful to Mrs. Carmen Walthour for aiding in the preparation of this manuscript.

REFERENCES

1. Huff, J., Haseman, J., and Rall, D. (1991). Scientific concepts, value, and significance of chemical carcinogenesis concepts. Ann. Rev. Pharmacol. Toxicol., 21: 621.
2. Chamberlain, G. (ed.). (1984). Pregnant Women at Work, London: Macmillan.
3. Alexander, N.J. (1982). Male evaluation and semen analysis. Clin. Obstet. Gynecol. 25:463.
4. Steinberger, E. (1981).Current status of studies concerned with evaluation of toxic effects of chemicals on the testes. Environ. Health Perspect. 38:29.
5. Reproductive Health Hazards in the Workplace. (1985). Washington, D.C.: OTA.
6. Lee, I.P. and Dixon, R.L. (1978). Factors influencing reproduction and genetic toxic effects on male gonads. Environ. Health Perspect. 24:117.
7. Schull, W.J. (1984). Reproductive problems: fertility, teratogenesis and mutagenesis. Arch. Environ. Health 39:207.

8. Mattison, D.R. (1981). Effects of biologically foreign compounds on reproduction. In: Drugs During Pregnancy, Clinical Perspectives. Philadelphia: George F. Stickley Co., pp. 101–125.

9. Stellman, J.M. (1979). The effects of toxic agents on reproduction. Occup. Health Saf. 48:36.

10. Hogue, C.J. (1981). Coffee in pregnancy. Lancet 1:554.

11. Coulam, C.B. (1982). The diagnosis and management of infertility. In: Gynecology and Obstetrics. Edited by J.J. Sciarra. New York: Harper & Row, pp. 1–18.

12. Kline, J., Stein, Z.A., Susser, M., and Warburton, D. (1977). Smoking: A risk factor for spontaneous abortion. N. Engl. J. Med. 297:793.

13. Sever, L.E. and Hessol, N.A. (1984). Overall design considerations in male and female occupational reproductive studies. In: Reproduction: The New Frontier in Occupational and Environmental Health Research. Edited by J.E. Lockey, G.K. Lemasters, and W.R. Keye. New York: Alan R. Liss, pp. 15–47.

14. Chez, R.A., Haire, D., Quilligan, E.J., and Wingate, M.B. (1976). High risk pregnancies: Obstetrical and perinatal factors. In: Prevention of Embryonic, Fetal, and Perinatal Disease. Edited by R.L. Brent and M.I. Harris. DHEW Publ. No. (NIH) 76–853, pp. 67–95.

15. Rosenberg, M.J. (1984). Practical aspects of reproductive surveillance. In: Reproduction: The New Frontier in Occupational and Environmental Health Research. Edited by J.E. Lockey, G.K. Lemasters, and W.R. Keye. New York: Alan R. Liss, pp. 147–156.

16. Boue, J., Boue, A., and Lazar, P. (1975). Retrospective and prospective epidemiological studies of 1500 karyotyped spontaneous human abortions. Teratology 12:11.

17. Shepard, T.H. and Fantel, A.G. (1979). Embryonic and early fetal loss. Clin. Perinatol. 6:219.

18. Slater, B.C.S. (1965). The investigation of drug embryopathies in man. In: Embryopathic Activity of Drugs. Edited by J.M. Robson, F.M. Sullivan, and R.L. Smith. Boston, Little, Brown & Co., pp. 241–260.

19. Hook, E.B. (1981). Human teratogenic and mutagenic markers in monitoring about point sources of pollution. Environ. Res. 25:178.

20. Sholtz, R., Goldstein, H., and Wallace, H.M. (1976). Incidence and impact of fetal and perinatal disease. In: Prevention of Embryonic, Fetal and Perinatal Disease. Edited by R.L. Brent and M.I. Harris. DHEW Publ. No. (NIH) 76-853, pp. 1–18.

21. Byrne, J., Warburton, D., Kline, J., Blanc, W., and Stein, Z. (1985). Morphology of early fetal deaths and their chromosomal characteristics. Teratology 32:297.

22. Schrag, S.D. and Dixon, R.L. (1985). Reproductive effects of chemical agents. In: Reproductive Toxicology. Edited by R.L. Dixon. New York: Raven Press, pp. 301–319.

23. Phillips, J.C., Foster, P.M.D., and Gangolli, S.D. (1985). Chemically-induced injury to the male reproductive tract. In: Endocrine Toxicology. Edited by J.A. Thomas, K.S. Korach, and J.A. McLachlan. New York: Raven Press, pp. 117–134.

24. Neumann, F. (1984). Effects of drugs and chemicals on spermatogenesis. Arch. Toxicol. 7(Suppl.):109.

25. Heywood, R. and James, R.W. (1985). Current laboratory approaches for assessing male reproductive toxicity: Testicular toxicity in laboratory animals. In: Re-

productive Toxicology. Edited by R.L. Dixon. New York: Raven Press, pp. 147–160.

26. Dixon, R.L. (1984). Assessment of chemicals affecting the male reproductive system. Arch. Toxicol. 7(Suppl.):118.

27. Dixon, R.L. and Hall, J.L. (1982). Reproductive toxicology. In: Principles and Methods of Toxicology. Edited by A.W. Hayes. New York: Raven Press, pp. 107–140.

28. Mattison, D.R. (1983). The mechanisms of action of reproductive toxins. Am. J. Indust. Med. 4:65.

29. Bergin, E.J. and Grandon, R.E. (1984). How to Survive in Your Toxic Environment, The American Survival Guide. New York: Avon.

30. Zenick, H. (1984). Mechanisms of environmental agents by class associated with adverse reproductive outcomes. In: Reproduction: The New Frontier in Occupational and Environmental Health Research. Edited by J.E. Lockey, G.K. Lemasters, and W.R. Keye. New York: Alan R. Liss, pp. 335–361.

31. Wyrobek, A.J., Watchmaker, C., and Gordon, L. (1984). An evaluation of sperm tests as indicators of germ-cell damage in men exposed to chemical or physical agents. In: Reproduction: The New Frontier in Occupational and Environmental Health Research. Edited by J.E. Lockey, G.K. Lemasters, and W.R. Keye. New York: Alan R. Liss, pp. 385–405.

32. Thomas, J.A. (1981). Reproductive hazards and environmental chemicals: A review. Toxic Subst. J. 2:318.

33. Anon. (1982). Assessment of Risks to Human Reproduction and to Development of the Human Conceptus from Exposure to Environmental Substances. Proc. U.S. EPA Conferences, Atlanta, 1980 and St. Louis, 1980 (EPA-600/9-82-001), NTIS.

34. Chapman, R.M. (1983). Gonadal injury resulting from chemotherapy. Am. J. Ind. Med. 4:149.

35. Mattison, D.R. and Thorgeirsson, S.S. (1978). Smoking and industrial pollution, and their effects on menopause and ovarian cancer. Lancet I:187.

36. Mattison, D.R. (1985). Clinical manifestations of ovarian toxicity. In: Reproductive Toxicology. Edited by R.L. Dixon. New York: Raven Press, pp. 109–130.

37. Mattison, D.R. (1981). Drugs, xenobiotics and the adolescent: Implications for reproduction. In: Drug Metabolism in the Immature Human. Edited by L.F. Soyka and G.P. Redmond. New York: Raven Press, pp. 129–143.

38. Hemminki, K., Axelson, O., Niemi, M.-L., and Ahlborg, G. (1983). Assessment of methods and results of reproductive occupational epidemiology: Spontaneous abortions and malformations in the offspring of working women. Am. J. Ind. Med. 4:293.

39. Mattison, D.R., Nightingale, M.S., and Shiromizu, K. (1983). Effects of toxic substances on female reproduction. Environ. Health Perspect. 48:43.

40. Steinberger, E. and Lloyd, J.A. (1985). Chemicals affecting the development of reproductive capacity. In: Reproductive Toxicology. Edited by R.L. Dixon. New York: Raven Press, pp. 1–20.

41. Langman, J. (1981). Medical Embryology, 4th Ed. Baltimore, Williams & Wilkins.

42. Amann, R.P. (1982). Use of animal models for detecting specific alterations in reproduction. Fund. Appl. Toxicol. 2:13.

43. Desjardins, C. (1985). Morphological, physiological, and biochemical aspects of male reproduction. In: Reproductive Toxicology. Edited by R.L. Dixon. New York: Raven Press, pp. 131–146.

44. Erickson, B.H. (1985). Effects of ionizing radiation on mammalian spermatogenesis: A model for chemical effects. In: Reproductive Toxicology. Edited by R.L. Dixon. New York: Raven Press, pp. 35–46.

45. Keye, W.R. (1984). An overview of female reproduction: Sexual differentiation, puberty, menstrual function, fertilization. In: Reproduction: The New Frontier in Occupational and Environmental Health Research. Edited by J.E. Lockey, G.K. Lemasters, and W.R. Keye. New York: Alan R. Liss, pp. 189–200.

46. Tuchmann-Duplessis, H., David, G., and Haegel, P. (Eds.) (1972). Illustrated Human Embryology. Embryogenesis. Vol. 1. New York: Springer-Verlag.

47. Longo, F.J. (1985). Biological processes of fertilization. In: Reproductive Toxicology. Edited by R.L. Dixon. New York: Raven Press, pp. 173–190.

48. Gwatkin, R.B.L. (1985). Effects of chemicals on fertilization. In: Reproductive Toxicology. Edited by R.L. Dixon. New York: Raven Press, pp. 209–218.

49. Sherman, M.I. and Wudl, L.W. (1976). The implanting mouse blastocyst. In: The Cell Surface in Animal Embryogenesis and Development. Edited by G. Poste and G.L. Nicolson. Amsterdam: Elsevier/North Holland, pp. 81–125.

50. Wu, J.T. (1985). Chemicals affecting implantation. In: Reproductive Toxicology. Edited by R.L. Dixon, New York: Raven Press, pp. 239–249.

51. Agaponova, E.D., Markov, V.A., Shashkina, L.F., Tsarichenko, G.V., and Lyubchenko, P.N. (1973). Effects of androgens on the bodies of women engaged in industrial work. Gig. Truda. Prof. Zabol. 17:24.

52. Belyayeva, A.P. (1967). The effect of antimony on reproductive function. Gig. Truda. Prof. Zabol. 11:32.

53. Nordstrom, S., Beckman, L., and Nordenson, I. (1978). Occupational and environmental risks in and around a smelter in northern Sweden. I. Variations in birth weight. Hereditas 88:43.

54. Mikhailova, L.M., Kobyets, G.P., Lyubomudrov, V.E., and Braga, G.F. (1971). The influence of occupational factors on diseases of the female reproductive organs. Pediatr. Akush. Ginekol. 33:56.

55. Mukhametova, I.M. and Vozovaya, M.A. (1972). Reproductive power and the incidence of gynecological affections in female workers exposed to the combined effect of benzine and chlorinated hydrocarbons. Gig. Truda. Prof. Zabol. 16:6.

56. Tarasenko, N.Y., Kasparov, A.A., and Strongina, O.M. (1972). The effect of boric acid on the generative function in male. Gig. Truda. Prof. Zabol. 16:13.

57. Krasovskii, G.N., Varshavskaya, S.P., and Borisov, A.I. (1976). Toxic and gonadotropic effects of cadmium and boron relative to standards for these substances in drinking water. Environ. Health Perspect. 13:69.

58. Kasymova, R.A. (1976). Experimental and clinical data on the embryotoxic effect of butiphos. Probl. Gig. Organ. Zdravookhr. Uzb. 5:101.

59. Smith, J.P., Smith, J.C., and McCall, A.J. (1960). Chronic poisoning from cadmium fume. J. Pathol. Bact. 80:287.

60. Tsvetkova, R.P. (1970). Influence of cadmium compounds on the generative function. Gig. Truda. Prof. Zabol. 14:31.

61. Martynova, A.P., Lotis, V.M., Khadzieva, E.D., and Gaidova, E.S. (1972). Occupational hygiene of women engaged in the production of capron (6-handecanone) fiber. Gig. Truda. Prof. Zabol. 16:9.

62. Wyrobek, A.J., Watchmaker, G., Gordon, L., Wong, K., Moore, D., and Whorton, D. (1981). Sperm shape abnormalities in carbaryl-exposed employees. Environ. Health Perspect. 40:255.

63. Lancranjan, I. (1972). Alterations of spermatic liquid in patients chemically poisoned by carbon disulphide. Medna Lav. 63:29.

64. Wiley, F.H., Hueper, W.C., and VonOettingen, W.F. (1936). On toxic effects of low concentrations of carbon disulfide. J. Ind. Hyg. Toxicol. 18:733.

65. Ehrhardt, W. (1967). Experience with the employment of women exposed to carbon disulphide. In: International Symposium on Toxicology of Carbon Disulphide. Amsterdam: Excerpta Medica. p. 240.

66. Bezvershenko, A.S. (1967). Environmental Health Criteria 10. Carbon Disulfide, cited by WHO, 1979.

67. Bao, Y.-S., Cai, S., Zhao, S.F., Xhang, X.C., Huang, M.Y., Zheng, O., and Jiang, H. (1991). Birth defects in the offspring of female workers exposed to carbon disulfide in China. Teratology 43:451.

68. Longo, L.D. (1970). Carbon monoxide in the pregnant mother and fetus and its exchange across the placenta. Ann. N.Y. Acad. Sci. 174:313.

69. Sullivan, F.M. and Barlow, S.M. (1979). Congenital malformations and other reproductive hazards from environmental chemicals. Proc. R. Soc. Lond. 205:91.

70. Cohn, W.J., Boylan, J.J., Blanke, R.B., Fariss, M.W., Howell, J.R., and Guzelian, P.S. (1978). Treatment of chlordecone (Kepone) toxicity with cholestyramine (Results of a controlled clinical trial). N. Engl. J. Med. 298:243.

71. Cannon, S.B., Veazey, J.M., Jackson, R.S., Burse, V.W., Hayes, C., Straub, W.E., Landrigan, P.J., and Liddle, J.A. (1978). Epidemic kepone poisoning in chemical workers. Am. J. Epidemiol. 107:529.

72. Sanotskii, I.V. (1976). Aspects of the toxicology of chloroprene: Immediate and longterm effects. Environ. Health Perspect. 17:85.

73. U.S. Department of Health, Education and Welfare. (1977). Criteria document for a recommended standard: Occupational exposure to chloroprene. DHEW (NIOSH) Publication No. 77-210.

74. Makarov, Y.V. and Shmitova, L.A. (1974). Occupational conditions and gynecological illnesses in workers engaged in the production of chromium compounds. In: Gigiena Truda Sostoyanie Spetsificheskikh Funkts. Rabot. Neftekhim. Khim. Prom-sti. Edited by R.A. Malysheva. Sverdlovsk, USSR, Sverdl Nauchno-Issled Inst. Okhr Materum Mladenchestva Minzdrava, pp. 18–186.

75. Russell, L.D., Ettlin, R.A., Sinhahikim, A.P., and Clegg, E.D. (1990). Histological and Histopathological Evaluation of the Testis. Clearwater: Cache River.

76. Kagan, Yu.S., Fudel-Ossipova, S.I., Khaikina, B.J., Kuzminskaya, U.A., and Kou-

ton, S.D. (1969). On the problem of the harmful effect of DDT and its mechanism of action. Residue Rev. 27:43.

77. Nikitina, Y.I. 1974). Course of labor and puerperium in the vineyard workers and milkmaids in Crimea. Gig. Truda. Prof. Zabol. 18:17.

78. Biava, C.G., Smuckler, E.A., and Whorton, D. (1978). The testicular morphology of individuals exposed to dibromochloropropane. Exp. Mol. Pathol. 29:448.

79. Whorton, D., Krauss, M.M., Marshal, S., and Milby, T.H. (1977). Infertility in male pesticide workers. Lancet 1:1259.

80. Goldsmith, J.R., Patasknic, G., and Israeli, R. (1984). Reproductive outcomes in families of DBCP-exposed men. Arch. Environ. Health 39:85.

81. Schottek, W. (1972). Chemicals (Dimethylformamide) having embryotoxic activity. In: Vop. Gig. Normirovaniya Izuch. Otdalennykh Posledstivil Vozdeistviya Prom. Veshchestv. pp. 119–123.

82. Farguharson, R.G., Hall, M.H., and Fullerton, W.T. (1983). Poor obstetric outcome in three quality control laboratory workers. Lancet 1:983.

83. Dickson, D. (1979). Herbicide claimed responsible for birth defects. Nature 282: 220.

84. Harrington, J.M., Rivera, R.O., and Lowry, L.K. (1978). Occupational exposure to synthetic estrogens-the need to establish safety standards. Am. Ind. Hyg. Assoc. J. 39:139.

85. Yakubova, Z.N., Shamova, N.A., Miftakhova, F.A., and Shilova, L.F. (1976). Gynecological disorders in workers engaged in ethylene oxide production. Kazanskii Meditsinskii Zhurnal 57:558.

86. Spasovski, M. Khristeva, V., Pervov, K., Kirkov, V., Dryanovska, T., Panova, Z., Bobev, G., Gincheva, D., and Ivanova, S. (1980). Healthstate of the workers in the production of ethylene and ethylene oxide. Khig. Zdrav. 23:41.

87. Hemminki, K., Mutanen, P., Saloniemi, I., Niemi, M.-L., and Vainio, H. (1982). Spontaneous abortions in hospital staff engaged in sterilising instruments with chemical agents. Br. Med. J. 285:1461.

88. Shumilina, A.V. (1975). Menstrual and child-bearing functions of female workers occupationally exposed to the effects of formaldehyde. Gig. Truda. Prof. Zabol. 19:18.

89. John, E.M. (1991). Spontaneous abortions among cosmetologists. NTIS Rep./PB 91-222703.

90. Hunter, A.G. W., Thompson, D., and Evans, J.A. (1979). Is there a fetal gasoline syndrome? Teratology 20:75.

91. National Coordinating Group on Male Antifertility Agents. (1978). Gossypol, a new antifertility agent for males. Chinese Med. J. 4:417.

92. Donayre, J., Guerra-Garcia, R., Moncloa, F., and Sobervilla, L.A. (1968). Endocrine studies at high altitude. IV. Changes in the semen of men. J. Reprod. Fertil. 16:55.

93. Hueper, W.C. (1942). Testes and occupation. Urol. Cutaneous Rev. 46:140.

94. Smith, D.W., Clarren, J.K., and Harvey, M.A. (1978). Hyperthermia as a possible teratogenic agent. J. Pediatr. 92:878.

95. Nora, J.J., Nora, A.H., Sommerville, R.J., Hill, R.M., and McNamara, D.G. (1967). Maternal exposure to potential teratogens. JAMA 202:1065.

96. Hall, J.G., Pallister, P.D., Clarren, S.K., Beckwith, J.B., Wiglesworth, F.W., Fraser, F.C., Cho, S., Benke, P.J., and Reed, S.D. (1980). Congenital hypothalamic hamartoblastoma, hypopituitarism, imperforate anus, and postaxial polydactyly-a new syndrome? Part 1. Clinical, causal and pathogenetic considerations. Am. J. Med. Genet. 7:47.

97. Popescu, H.I., Klepsch, L., and Lancranjan, I. (1975). Elimination of pituitary gonadotropic hormones in men with protracted irradiation during occupational exposure. Health Phys. 29:385.

98. Hamilton, A. and Hardy, H.L. (1974). Industrial Toxicology, 3rd revised ed. New York: Publishing Science.

99. Lancranjan, I., Popescu, H.I., Gavanescu, O., Klepsch, I., and Serbanescu, M. (1975). Reproductive ability of workmen occupationally exposed to lead. Arch. Environ. Health 30:396.

100. Braunstein, G.P., Dahlgren, J., and Loriaux, D.L. (1978). Hypogonadism in chronically lead-poisoned men. Infertility 1:33.

101. Rom, W.N. (1976). Effects of lead on the female and reproduction: A review. Mt. Sinai J. Med. NY 43:542.

102. Panova, Z. (1973). Cytomorphological characteristics of menstrual cycles in women in occupational contact with inorganic lead. Khig. Zdrav. 16:549.

103. Nogaki, K. (1957). On action of lead on body of lead refinery workers: Particularly conception, pregnancy and parturition in case of females and on vitality of their newborn. Igaku Kenkyu 27:1314.

104. Schuler, P., Oyanguren, H., Maturana, V., Valenzuela, A., Cruz, E., Plaza, V., Schmidt, E., and Haddad, R. (1957). Manganese poisoning, environmental and medical study at a Chilean mine. Industr. Med. Surg. 26:167.

105. Mena, I., Marin, O., Fuenzalida, S., and Cotzias, G.C. (1967). Chronic manganese poisoning. Clinical picture and manganese turnover. Neurology 17:128.

106. McFarland, R.B. and Reigel, H. (1978). Chronic mercury poisoning from a single brief exposure. J. Occupat. Med. 20:532.

107. Marinova, G., Cakarova, O., and Kaneva, Y. (1973). A study on the reproductive function in women working with mercury. Probl. Akush. Ginekol. 1:75.

108. Goncharuk, G.A. (1977). Problems relating to occupational hygiene of women in production of mercury. Gig. Truda. Prof. Zabol. 21:17.

109. Panova, Z. and Dimitrov, G. (1974). Ovarian function in women occupationally exposed to metallic mercury. Akush. Ginekol. 13:29.

110. Ogi, D. and Hamada, A. (1965). Case reports on fetal deaths and malformations of extremities probably related to insecticide poisoning. J. Jpn. Obstet. Gynecol. Soc. 17:569.

111. Lancranjan, I., Marcanescu, M., Rafaila, E., Klepsh, I., and Popescu, H.I. (1975). Gonadic function in workmen with long-term exposure to microwaves. Health Phys. 29:381.

112. Kallen, B., Malmquist, G., and Moritz, U. (1982). Delivery outcome among physiotherapists in Sweden: Is non-ionizing radiation a fetal hazard? Arch. Environ. Health 37:81.

113. Espir, M.L.E., Hall, J.W., Shirreffs, J.G., and Stevens, D.L. (1970). Impotence in farm workers using toxic chemicals. Br. Med. J. 1:423.

114. Veis, V.P. (1970). Some data on the status of the sexual sphere in women who have been in contact with organochlorine compounds. Pediatr. Akush. Ginekol. 32:48.

115. Marinova, G., Osmankova, D., Deremendzhieva, L., Khadzhikolev, I., Chakurova, O., and Kaneva, Y. (1973). Professional injuries: Pesticides and their effects on the reproductive functions of women working with pesticides. Akush. Ginekol. 12:138.

116. Nakazawa, T. (1974). Chronic organophosphorous intoxication in women. J. Jpn. Assoc. Rural Med. 22:756.

117. Makletsova, N.Y. (1979). Characteristics of the course of pregnancy, childbirth, and the period after birth in female workers in contact with the pesticide zineb. Pediatr. Akush. Ginekol. 41:45.

118. Blekherman, N.A. and Ilyina, V.I. (1973). Changes of ovary function in women in contact with organochlorine compounds. Pediatriya 52:57.

119. Ilyina, V.I. (1977). Status of the specific gynecological function of women exposed to polychlorpinene in the fields. Pediatr. Akush. Ginekol. 39:40.

120. Makletsova, N. Yu, and Lanovoi, I.D. (1981). Status of gynecological morbidity of women with occupational contact with the pesticide zineb. Pediatr. Akush. Ginekol. 43:60.

121. Roan, C.C., Matanoski, G.E., Mcilnay, C.Q., Olds, K.L., Pylant, F., Trout, J.R., and Wheeler, P. (1984). Spontaneous abortions, stillbirths, and birth defects in families of agricultural pilots. Arch. Environ. Health 39:56.

122. Aldyreva, M.V., Klimona, T.S., Izyumova, A.S., and Timofievskaya, L.A. (1975). The influence of phthalate plasticisers on the generative function. Gig. Truda. Prof. Zabol. 19:25.

123. Robertson, D.S.F. (1970). Selenium—a possible teratogen? Lancet 1:518.

124. Pokrovskii, V.A. (1967). Peculiarities of the effect produced by some organic poisons on the female organism. Gig. Truda. Prof. Zabol. 11:17.

125. Zlobina, N.S., Izyumova, A.S., and Ragule, N.Y. (1975). The effect of low styrene concentrations on the specific functions of the female organism. Gig. Truda. Prof. Zabol. 19:21.

126. Harkonen, H. and Holmberg, P.C. (1982). Obstetric histories of women occupationally exposed to styrene. Scand. J. Work Environ. Health 8:74.

127. Vurdelja, N., Farago, F., Nikolic, V., and Vuckovic, S. (1967). Clinical experience with intoxications of fuel containing lead-tetraethyl. Folia Faculatatis Medicae, Universitas Comenianae 5:133.

128. Neshkov, N.C. (1971). The influence of chronic intoxication of ethylated benzene on the spermatogenesis and sexual function of man. Gig. Truda. Prof. Zabol. 15: 45.

129. Stevens, W.J. and Barbier, F. (1976). Thalliumintoxicatie Gedurende de Zwangerschap. Acta Clinica Belgica 31:188.

130. Hamill, P.V.V., Steinberger, E., Levine, R.J., Rodriguez-Rigau, L.J., Lemeshow, S., and Avrunin, J.S. (1982). The epidemiologic assessment of male reproductive hazard from occupational exposure to TDA and DNT. J. Occup. Med. 24:985.

131. Syrovadko, O.N., Skornin, V.F., Pronkova, E.N., Sorkina, N.S., Isyumova, A.S., Gribova, I.A., and Popova, A.F. (1973). Effect of working conditions on the health

status and some specific functions of women handling white spirit. Gig. Truda. Prof. Zabol. 17:5.

132. Syrovadko, O.N. (1977). Working conditions and health status of women handling organosilicon varnishes containing toluene. Gig. Truda. Prof. Zabol. 21:15.

133. Euler, H.H. (1967). Animal experimental studies of an industrial noxa. Arch. Gynakol. 204:258.

134. Toutant, C. and Lippmann, S. (1979). Fetal solvents syndrome. Lancet 1:1356.

135. Hersh, J.H., Podruch, J.H., Rogers, G., and Weisskopf, B. (1985). Toluene embryopathy. J. Pediatr. 106:922.

136. Walker, A.E. (1975). A preliminary report of a vascular abnormality occurring in men engaged in the manufacture of vinyl chloride. Br. J. Dermatol. 93:22.

137. Infante, P.F. (1976). Oncogenic and mutagenic risks in communities with polyvinyl chloride production facilities. Ann. N.Y. Acad. Sci. 271:49.

138. Infante, P.F., McMichael, A.J., Wagoner, J.K., Waxweiler, R.J., and Falk, H. (1976). Genetic risks of vinyl chloride. Lancet 1:734.

139. Matysyak, V.G. and Yaroslavskii, V.K. (1973). Specific female organism functions in women engaged in polymer production. Gig. Truda. Prof. Zabol. 17:105.

140. Hemminki, K., Fransula, E., and Vainio, H. (1980). Spontaneous abortions among female chemical workers in Finland. Int. Arch. Occup. Environ. Health 45:123.

141. Alekperov, I.I., Sultanova, A.N., Palii, E.T., Elisuiskaya, R.V., and Lobodina, V.V. (1969). The course of pregnancy, birth and the postpartum period in women working in the chemical industry: A clinical-experimental study. Gig. Truda. Prof. Zabol. 13:52.

142. Nordstrom, S., Birke, E., and Gustavsson, L. (1983). Reproductive hazards among workers at high voltage substations. Bioelectromagnetics 4:91.

143. Czernielewska, I., Chrominska, H., and Bankowiak, D. (1976). The effect of working conditions of pregnant women on the development of fetus and the fates of newborn. Zdrow. Publiczne 87:174.

144. Hemminki, K., Mutanen, P., Luoma, K., and Saloniemi, I. (1980). Congenital malformations by the parental occupation in Finland. Int. Arch. Occup. Environ. Health 46:93.

145. Strandberg, M., Sandback, K., Axelson, O., and Sundell, L. (1978). Spontaneous abortions among women in hospital laboratory. Lancet 1:384.

146. Hansson, E., Jansa, S., Wande, H., Kallen, B., and Ostlund, E. (1980). Pregnancy outcome for women working in laboratories in some of the pharmaceutical industries in Sweden. Scand. J. Work Environ. Health 6:131.

147. Heidam, L.Z. (1984). Spontaneous abortions among laboratory workers, a follow-up study. J. Epidemiol. Comm. Health 38:36.

148. Yager, J.W. (1973). Congenital malformations and environmental influence: The occupational environment of laboratory workers. J. Occup. Med. 15:724.

149. Ericson, A., Kallen, B., Meirik, O., and Westerholm, P. (1982). Gastrointestinal atresia and maternal occupation during pregnancy.J. Occup. Med. 24:515.

150. Meirik, O., Kallen, B., Gauffin, U., and Ericson, A. (1979). Major malformations in infants born of women who worked in laboratories while pregnant. Lancet 2: 91.

151. Oleson, J. (1983). Risk of exposure to teratogens amongst laboratory staff and painters. Dan. Med. Bull. 30:24.

152. Clarke, M. and Mason, E.S. (1985). Leatherwork: A possible hazard to reproduction. Br. Med. J. 290:1235.
153. Hemminki, K., Niemi, M.-L., Koskinen, K., and Vainio, H. (1980). Spontaneous abortions among women employed in the metal industry in Finland. Int. Arch. Occup. Environ. Health 47:53.
154. Loshenfeld, R.A. and Ivakina, N.P. (1973). Nature of the menstrual cycle in workers engaged in the production of polymers. Sb. Nauch. Tr. Rostov. Gos. Med. Inst. 62:149.
155. Panova, Z., Stamova, N., and Gincheva, N. (1977). Menstrual, generative function, and gynecological morbidity in women working in the production of polyamide fibers. Khig. Zdrav. 20:523.
156. Chobot, A.M. (1979). Menstrual function in workers of the polyacrylonitrile fiber industry. Zdrav. Belor. 2:24.
157. Holmberg, P.C. (1977). Central nervous defects in two children of mothers exposed to chemicals in the reinforced plastics industry. Chance or a causal relation? Scand. J. Work Environ. Health 3:212.
158. Blomqvist, U., Ericson, A., Kallen, B., and Westerholm, P. (1981). Delivery outcome for women working in the pulp and paper industry. Scand. J. Work Environ. Health 7:114.
159. Beskrovnaya, N.I., Khrustaleva, G.F., Zhigulina, G.A., and Davydkina, T.I. (1979). Gynecological illness in rubber industry workers. Gig. Truda. Prof. Zabol. 23:36.
160. Anon. (1982) NIOSH to probe births to VDT users: Panel recommends 5-hour VDT-day. Guild Reporter 49:20.
161. Kurppa, K., Holmberg, P.C., Rantala, K., and Nurminen, T. (1984). Birth defects and video display terminals. Lancet 2:1339.
162. Morgan, R., Kheifets, L., Obrinsky, D.L., Whorton, M.D., and Foliart, D.E. (1984). Fetal loss and work in a waste water treatment plant. Am. J. Publ. Health 74:499.
163. Hemminki, K., Saloniemi, I., Luoma, K., Salonen, T., Partanen, T., Vainio, H., and Hemminki, E. (1980). Transplacental carcinogens and mutagens: Childhood cancer, malformations and abortions as risk indicators. J. Toxicol. Environ. Health 6:1115.
164. Plummer, G. (1952). Anomalies occurring in children exposed in utero to the atomic bomb in Hiroshima. Pediatrics 10:687.
165. Kitamura, S., Hirano, Y., Noguchi, Y., Kojima, T., Kakita, T., and Kuwaki, H. (1959). The epidemiological survey on Minamata disease (No. 2). J. Kumamoto Med. Soc. 33(Suppl. 3):569.
166. Wasserman, M., Wasserman, D., Cucos, S., and Miller, H.J. (1979). World PCBs map: Storage and effects in man and his biologic environment in the 1970s. Ann. N.Y. Acad. Sci. 320:69.
167. Kuratsune, M., Yoshimura, T., Matsuyaka, J., and Yamaguchi, A. (1972). Epidemiologic study on Yusho, a poisoning caused by ingestion of rice-oil contaminated with commercial brand of polychlorinated biphenyls. Environ. Health Perspect. 1:119.
168. Rogan, W.J. (1982). PCB's and cola-colored babies: Japan 1968, and Taiwan, 1979. Teratology 26:259.

169. Galston, A.W. (1970). Herbicides, no margin of safety. Science 167:237.
170. Funazaki, Z. (1971). Herbicides and deformities in Vietnam. Jpn. J. Publ. Health Nurse 27:54.
171. Laporte, J.R. (1977). Effects of dioxin exposure. Lancet 1:1049.
172. Cutting, R.T., Phuoc, T.H., Ballo, J.M., Benenson, M.W., and Evans, C.H. (1970). Congenital Malformation, Hydatiform Moles, and Stillbirths in the Republic of Vietnam 1960–1969. Washington, D.C.: GPO.
173. Stevens, K.M. (1981). Agent Orange toxicity: A quantitative perspective. Human Toxicol. 1:31.
174. Norman, C. (1983). Vietnam's herbicide legacy. Science 219:1196.
175. Donovan, J.W., MacLennan, R., and Adena, M. (1984). Vietnam service and the risk of congenital anomalies. A case-control study. Med. J. Austral. 140:394.
176. Tung, T.T., Anh, T.K., Tuyen, B.Q., Tra, D.X., and Hugen, N.X. (1971). Clinical effects of massive and continuous utilization of defoliants on civilians. Vietnamese Stud. 29:53.
177. Sare, W.M. and Forbes, P.L. (1972). Possible dysmorphogenic effects of an agricultural chemical: 2,4,5-T. NZ Med. J. 75:37.
178. Lowry, R.B. and Allen, A.B. (1977). Herbicides and spina bifida. Can. Med. Assoc. J. 117:580.
179. EPA, Epidemiology Studies Division. U.S. EPA. (1979). Six years spontaneous abortion rates in Oregon areas in relation to forest 2,4,5-T spray practices.
180. Anon. (1979). EPA halts most use of herbicide 2,4,5-T. Science 203:1090.
181. Regenstein, L. (1982). America the Poisoned. Washington, D.C.: Acropolis Books.
182. Nelson, C.J., Holson, J.F, Green, H.G., and Gaylor, D.W. (1979). Retrospective study of the relationship between agricultural use of 2,4,5-T and cleft palate occurrences in Arkansas. Teratology 19:377.
183. O'Neill, L. (1979). A letter from Alsea. EPA J. 5:4.
184. Field, B. and Kerr, C. (1979). Herbicide use and incidence of neural-tube defects. Lancet 1:1341.
185. Brogan, W.F., Brogan, C.E., and Dadd, J.T. (1980). Herbicides and cleft lip and palate. Lancet 2:597.
186. Thomas, H.F. (1980). 2,4,5-T use and congenital malformation rates in Hungary. Lancet 2:214.
187. Smith, A.H., Matheson, D.P., Fisher, D.O., and Chapman, C.J. (1981). Preliminary report of reproductive outcomes among pesticide applicators using 2,4,5-T. NZ Med. J. 93:177.
188. Hanify, J.A., Metcalf, P., Nobbs, C.L., and Worsley, K.J. (1981). Aerial spraying of 2,4,5-T and human birth malformations: An epidemiological investigation. Science 212:349.
189. Chen, E. (1979). PBB: An American Tragedy. Englewood Cliffs, NJ, Prentice-Hall.
190. Humble, C.G. and Speizer, F.E. (1984). Polybrominated biphenyls and fetal mortality in Michigan. Am. J. Public Health 74:1130.
191. Townsend, J.C., Bodner, K.M., VanPeenen, P.F.D., Olson, R.D., and Cook, R.R. (1982). Survey of reproductive events of wives of employees exposed to chlorinated dioxins. Am. J. Epidemiol. 115:695.

192. Remotti, G., De Vibianco, V., and Candiani, G.B. (1981). The morphology of early trophoblast after dioxin poisoning in the Seveso area, Italy. Placenta 2:53.

193. Reggiani, G. (1978). Medical problems raised by the TCDD contamination in Seveso, Italy. Arch. Toxicol. 40:161.

194. Commoner, B. (1977). Seveso: The tragedy lingers on. Clin. Toxicol. 11:479.

195. Hay, A. (1977). Dioxin damage. Nature 266:7.

196. Abate, L., Basso, P., Belloni, A., Bisanti, L., Borgna, C., and others (1982). Mortality and birth defects from 1976 to 1979 in the population living in the TCDD polluted area of Seveso. In: Chlorinated Dioxins and Related Compounds: Impact on the Environment. Edited by O. Hutzinger, R.W. Frei, E. Merian, and F. Pocchiari. Oxford: Pergamon Press, pp. 571–587.

197. Tarlton, F. and Cassidy, J.J. (Eds.). (1981). Love Canal: A Special Report to the Governor and Legislature. N.Y. State Dept. of Health.

198. Vianna, N.J. (1980). Adverse pregnancy outcomes-potential endpoints of human toxicity in the Love Canal. Preliminary results. In: Human Embryonic and Fetal Death. Edited by I.H. Porter and E.B. Hook. New York: Academic Press, pp. 165–168.

199. Budnick, L.D., Sokal, D.C., Falk, H., Logue, J.N., and Fox, J.M. (1984). Cancer and birth defects near the Drake Superfund Site, Pennsylvania. Arch. Environ. Health 39:409.

200. Johnson, C. (1984). Spontaneous abortions following Three-Mile Island accident. Am. J. Publ. Health 74:520.

201. Dixon, R.L. (1985). Regulatory aspects of reproductive toxicity. In: Reproductive Toxicology. Edited by R.L. Dixon. New York: Raven Press, pp. 321–328.

202. Hagen, D.R. and Dziuk, P.J. (1981). Detection of the effects of ingested caffeine on fertility of cocks by homospermic and heterospermic insemination. J. Reprod. Fertil. 63:11.

203. Collins, T.F.X. (1978). Multigeneration studies of reproduction. In: Handbook of Teratology, Vol. 4. Edited by J.G. Wilson and F.C. Fraser. New York: Plenum Press, pp. 191–214.

204. U.S. Environmental Protection Agency (1984). Series 83. Pesticide Assessment Guidelines, Subdivision F. Hazard Evaluation: Human and Domestic Animals (rev. ed.), Office of Pesticide Programs, Final Rule, Part 158.

205. U.S. Environmental Protection Agency (1985). 40 CFR, Part 798—Health Effects Testing Guidelines (TSCA). Fed. Regist. 50(188):39412–39434 and 52(97): 19056–19078.

206. Goldenthal, E.I. (1966). Guidelines for Reproduction Studies for Safety Evaluation of Drugs for Human Use, Drug Review Branch, Division of Toxicological Evaluation, Bureau of Science, FDA.

207. Guidance on Toxicology Study Data for Application of Agricultural Chemical Registration (1985). Ministry of Agriculture, Forestry and Fisheries (MAFF). 59 Nohsan No. 4200.

208. Chemicals—Ministry of International Trade and Industry (MITI). (1987). Guideline for Toxicity Testing of Chemicals.

209. OECD Guideline for Testing of Chemicals (1981, 1983). Organization for Economic Cooperation and Development, Paris, Fr.

210. Fitzhugh, O.G. (1968). Reproduction tests. In: Modern Trends in Toxicology Ed-

ited by E. Boyland & R. Goulding, New York: Appleton-Century Crofts, pp. 75–85.

211. FDA (1982). Toxicological Principles for the Safety Assessment of Direct Food Additives and Color Additives Used in Food, Bureau of Foods.

212. U.S. Environmental Protection Agency (1998). Health Effects Test Guidelines. OPPTS 870.3800 Reproduction and Fertility Effects. EPA 712-C-98-208, August.

213. Heinrichs, W.L. (1985). Current laboratory approaches for assessing female reproductive toxicity. In: Reproductive Toxicology. Edited by R.L. Dixon. New York: Raven Press, pp. 95–108.

214. Food and Drug Administration (1970). Advisory Committee on protocols for safety evaluations: Panel on reproduction. Report on reproduction studies in the safety evaluation of food additives and pesticide residues. Toxicol. Appl. Pharmacol. 16:264.

215. Marks, T.A. (1985). Animal tests employed to assess the effects of drugs and chemicals on reproduction. In: Male Fertility and Its Regulation. Edited by T.J. Lobl and E.S.E. Hafez. Boston: MTP Press, Ltd., pp. 245–267.

216. Christian, M.S. and Voytek, P.E. (1983). In: vivo reproductive and mutagenicity tests. In: A Guide to General Toxicology. Edited by F. Homburger, J.A. Hayes, and E.W. Pelikan. Basel: S. Karger, pp. 294–325.

217. Christian, M.S. and Hoberman, A.M. (1985). Current in vivo reproductive toxicity and teratology methods. In: Safety Evaluation and Regulation of Chemicals. Basel: Karger, pp. 78–88.

218. Lamb, J.C. and Chapin, R.E. (1985). Experimental models of male reproductive toxicology. In: Endocrine Toxicology. Edited by J.A. Thomas, K.S. Korach, and J.A. McLachlan. New York: Raven Press, pp. 85–116.

219. Christian, M.S. (1986). A critical review of multigeneration studies. J. Am. Coll. Toxicol. 5:161.

220. Palmer, A.K. (1981). Regulatory requirements for reproductive toxicology: Theory and practice. In: Developmental Toxicology. Edited by C.A. Kimmel and J. Buelke-Sam. New York: Raven Press, pp. 259–287.

221. Wright, P.L. (1978). Test procedures to evaluate effects of chemical exposure on fertility and reproduction. Environ. Health Perspect. 24:39.

222. Schwetz, B.A., Rao, K.S., and Park, C.N. (1980). Insensitivity of tests for reproductive problems. J. Environ. Pathol. Toxicol. 3:81.

223. Christian, M.S. (1983). Reproduction and teratology studies: Unique requirements for generation, interpretation, and reporting. Drug Inform. J. 17:163.

224. Baeder, C., Wickramaratne, G.A.S., Hummier, H., Merkle, J., Schon, H., and Tuchmann-Duplessis, H. (1985). Identification and assessment of the effects of chemicals on reproduction and development (reproductive toxicology). Food Chem. Toxicol. 23:377.

225. Palmer, A.K. (1993). Methods of testing for reproductive toxicity. In: Reproductive Toxicology, Edited by M. Richardson, New York: VCH Publishers, pp. 197–212.

226. Kimmel, G.L., Clegg, E.D., and Crisp, T.M. (1994). Reproductive toxicity testing: a risk assessment perspective. In: Reproductive Toxicology, Second Edition, Edited by R.J. Witorsh. N.Y.: Raven Press, pp. 75–98.

227. Lamb, J.C. (1989). Design and use of multigeneration breeding studies for identification of reproductive toxicants. In: Toxicology of the Male and Female Reproductive Systems. Edited by P.K. Working, N.Y.: Hemisphere Publishing, pp. 131–155.

228. Lamb, J.C., Gulati, D.K., Russell, V.S., Hommel, L., and Sabharwal, P.S. (1984). Reproductive toxicity of ethylene glycol (EG) studied by a new continuous breeding protocol. Toxicologist 4:136.

229. Reel, J.R., Lawton, A.D., Wolkowski-Tyl, R., Davis, G.W., and Lamb, J.C. (1985). Evaluation of a new reproductive toxicology protocol using diethylstilbestrol (DES) as a positive control compound. J. Am. Coll. Toxicol. 4:147.

230. Lamb, J.C. (1985). Reproductive toxicity testing: Evaluation and developing new test systems. J. Am. Coll. Toxicol. 4:163.

231. Lamb, J.C., Maronpot, R.R., Gulati, D.K., Russell, V.S., Hommel-Barnes, L., and Sabharwal, P.S. (1985). Reproductive and developmental toxicity of ethylene glycol in the mouse. Toxicol. Appl. Pharmacol. 81:100.

232. NTP (1986). Fiscal Year 1985, Annual Plan, Dept. of Health and Human Services and U.S. Public Health Service.

233. Lamb, J.C. (1985). Personal communication.

234. Bateman, A.J. (1973). The dominant lethal assay in the mouse. Agents Actions 3:73.

235. Green, S. and Springer, J.A. (1973). The dominant lethal test: Potential limitations and statistical considerations for safety evaluation. Environ. Health Perspect. 6:37.

236. Green, S., Auletta, A., Fabricant, J., Kapp, R., Manandhar, M., Sheu, C., Springer, J., and Whitefield, B. (1985). Current status of bioassays in genetic toxicology—the dominant lethal assay. Mutat. Res. 150:49.

237. Saacke, R.G., Vinson, W.E., O'Connor, M.L., Chandler, J.E., Mullins, J., Amann, R.P., Marshall, C.E., Wallace, R.A., Vincell, W.N., and Kellgren, H.C. (1980). The relationship of semen quality and fertility: A heterospermic study. Proc. 8th Tech. Conf. Artif. Insem. Reprod. Columbia, MO: Natl. Assn. Anim. Breeders, pp. 71–78.

238. Szabo, K.T., Free, S.M., Birkhead, H.A., and Gay, P.E. (1969). Predictability of pregnancy from various signs of mating in mice and rats. Lab. Anim. Care 19:822.

239. Wilson, J.R., Adler, N., and LeBoeuf, B. (1965). The effects of intromission frequency on successful pregnancy in the female rat. Proc. Nat. Acad. Sci. 53:1392.

240. Zenick, H., Blackburn, K., Hope, E., Oudiz, D., and Goeden, H. (1984). Evaluating male reproductive toxicity in rodents: A new animal model. Teratog. Carcinog. Mutag. 4:109.

241. Mercier, O., Perraud, J., Stadler, J., and Kessedjian, M.J. (1985). A standardized method to test the copulatory behavior of male rats: A basis of evaluation of drug effect. Teratology 32:28A.

242. Eliasson, R. (1978). Semen analysis. Environ. Health Perspect. 24:81.

243. Cannon, D.C. (1974). Examination of seminal fluid. In: Clinical Diagnosis 15th ed. Edited by I. Davidson and J.B. Henry. Philadelphia: W.B. Saunders, pp. 1300–1306.

244. MacLeod, J. (1965). The semen examination. Clin. Obstet. Gynecol 8:115.

245. Amann, R.P. (1970). Sperm production rates. In: The Testis, Vol. 1. Edited by A.D. Johnson, W.R. Gomes, and N.L. VanDermark. New York: Academic Press, pp. 433–482.

246. Amann, R.P. (1981). A critical review of methods for evaluation of spermatogenesis from seminal characteristics. J. Androl. 2:37.

247. Carson, W.S. and Amann, R.P. (1972). The male rabbit, VI. Effects of ejaculation and season on testicular size and function. J. Animl. Sci. 34:302.

248. Amann, R.P., Kavanaugh, J.F., Griel, L.C., and Vogimayr, J.K. (1974). Sperm production of Holstein bulls determined from testicular spermatid reserves, after cannulation of rete testis or vas deferens, and by daily ejaculation. J. Dairy Sci. 57:93.

249. Eliasson, R. (1985). Clinical effects of chemicals on male reproduction. In: Reproductive Toxicology. Edited by R.L. Dixon. New York: Raven Press, pp. 161–172.

250. Overstreet, J.W. (1984). Assessment of disorders of spermatogenesis. In: Reproduction: The New Frontier in Occupational and Environmental Health Research. Edited by J.E. Lockey, G.K. Lemasters, and W.R. Keye. New York: Alan R. Liss, Inc., pp. 275–292.

251. Overstreet, J.W. (1983). Evaluation and control of the fertilizing power of sperm. In: The Sperm Cell. Edited by J. Andre. Boston: Martinus Nijhoff Publ., p. 1.

252. MacLeod, J. and Gold, R.Z. (1951). The male factor in fertility and infertility. II. Spermatozoan counts in 1000 men of known fertility and in 1000 cases of infertile marriage. J. Urol. 66:436.

253. Barfield, A., Melo, J., Coutinho, E., Alvaez Sanchez, F., Faundes, A., Brache, V., Leon, P., Frick, J., Bartsch, G., Weisks, W.H., Brenner, P., Mishell, D., Bernstein, G., and Oritz, A. (1979). Pregnancies associated with sperm concentrations below 10 million/ml in clinical studies of a potential male contraceptive method, monthly depot medroxyprogesterone acetate and testosterone esters. Contraception 20:121.

254. Blazak, W.F., Rushbrook, C.J., Ernst, T.L., Stewart, B.E., Spak, D., DiBiasio-Erwin, D., and Black, V. (1985). Relationship between breeding performance and testicular/epididymal functioning in male Sprague-Dawley rats exposed to nitrobenzene (NB). Toxicologist 5:121.

255. Farris, E.J. (1949). The number of motile spermatozoa as an index of fertility in man: A study of 406 semen specimens. J. Urol. 61:1099.

256. Wyrobek, A.J. (1983). Methods for evaluating the effects of environmental chemicals on human sperm production. Environ. Health Perspect. 48:53.

257. Eliasson, R. (1975). Analysis of semen. In: Progress in Infertility. Edited by S.J. Behrman and R.W. Kistner. Boston: Little Brown and Co., p. 691.

258. Mitchell, J.A., Nelson, L., and Hafez, E.S.E. (1976). Motility of spermatozoa. In: Human Semen and Fertility Regulation in Men. Edited by E.S.E. Hafez. St. Louis: C.V. Mosby, pp. 89–99.

259. Blasco, L. (1984). Clinical tests of sperm fertilizing ability. Fertil. Steril. 41:177.

260. Harvey, C. (1960). The speed of human spermatozoa and the effect on it of various diluants with some preliminary observations on clinical material.J. Reprod. Fertil. 1:84.

261. Manson, J.M. and Simons, R. (1979). Influence of environmental agents on male

reproductive failure. In: Work and the Health of Women. Edited by V.R. Hunt. Cleveland: CRC Press, pp. 155–179.

262. Wyrobek, A.J. and Bruce, W.R. (1975). Chemical induction of sperm abnormalities in mice. Proc. Nat. Acad. Sci. (USA) 72:4425.

263. Wyrobek, A.J. and Bruce, W.R. (1978). The induction of sperm-shape abnormalities in mice and humans. In: Chemical Mutagens. Principles and Methods for Their Detection, Vol. 5. Edited by A. Hollaender and F.J. deSerres. New York: Plenum Press, pp. 257–281.

264. Wyrobek, J., Gordon, L.A., Burkhart, J.G., Francis, M.W.,Kapp, R.W., Letz, G., Malling, H.V., Topham, J.C., and Whorton, M.D. (1983). An evaluation of mouse sperm morphology test and other sperm tests in nonhuman mammals. Mutat. Res. 115:1.

265. Lock, L.F. and Soares, E.R., (1980). Increases in morphologically abnormal sperm in rats exposed to CO^{60} irradiation. Environ. Mutag. 2:125.

266. Byran, J.H.D. (1970). An eosin-fast green-naphthol yellow mixture for differential staining of cytologic components in mammalian spermatozoa. Stain Tech. 45:231.

267. Cassidy, S.L. (1981). Rodent testicular sperm head count—a useful method of detecting cytotoxic agents in reproductive toxicology. Teratology 24:35.

268. MacLeod, J. (1971). Human male infertility. Obstet. Gynecol. Surv. 26:335.

269. Setchell, B.P. (1978). The Mammalian Testis. Ithaca: Cornell University Press.

270. Johnson, M.H. and Everitt, B.J. (1996). Testicular function. In: Essential Reproduction, Fourth Edition. London: Blackwell Science, pp. 45–59.

271. Obasanjo, I.O. and Hughes, C.L. (1997). Biology of reproduction and methods in assessing reproductive and developmental toxicity in humans, in Handbook of Human Toxicology, Edited by E.J. Massaro, J.L. Schardein, Section Editor, Boca Raton, FL: CRC Press, pp. 929–959.

272. Foote, R.H., Berndtson, W.E., and Rounsaville, T.R. (1986). Use of quantitative testicular histology to assess the effect of dibromochloropropane (DBCP) on reproduction in rabbits. Fund. Appl. Toxicol. 6:638.

273. Potashnik, G., Yanai-Inbar, I., Sacks, M.I., and Israeli, R. (1979). Effect of dibromochloropropane on human testicular function. Isr. J. Med. Sci. 15:438.

274. Lobl, T.J., Bardin, C.W., and Change, C.C. (1980). Pharmacological agents producing infertility by direct action on the male reproductive tract. In: Research Frontiers in Fertility Regulation. Edited by G.I. Zatuchni. Hagerstown, MD: Harper and Row.

275. Chellman, G.J. and Working, P.K. (1989). Importance of assessing multiple endpoints in reproductive toxicology studies. In: Toxicology of the Male and Female Reproductive Systems, Edited by P.K. Working, New York: Hemisphere Publ., Co., pp. 257–271.

276. Hurtt, M.E. (1989). Quantitative assessment of spermatogenesis. In: Toxicology of the Male and Female Reproductive Systems, Edited by P.K. Working, New York: Hemisphere Publ., Co., pp. 187–198.

277. Blazak, W.F. (1989). Significance of cellular end points in assessment of male reproductive toxicity. In: Toxicology of the Male and Female Reproductive Systems, Edited by P.K. Working, New York: Hemisphere Publ., Co., pp. 157–172.

278. Moghissi, K.S. (1976). Postcoital test: Physiologic basis, technique and interpretation. Fertil. Steril. 27:117.

279. Ulstein, M. and Fjallbrant, B. (1976). In: vitro tests of sperm penetration in cervical mucus. In: Human Semen and Fertility Regulation in men. Edited by E.S.E. Hafez, St. Louis: C.V. Mosby, p. 383.

280. Kremer, J. (1965). A simple sperm penetration test. Int. J. Fertil. 10:209.

281. Katz, D.F., Overstreet, J.W., and Hanson, F.W. (1980). A new quantitative test for sperm penetration into cervical mucus. Fertil. Steril. 33:179.

282. Yanagimachi, R., Yanagimachi, H., and Rogers, B.J. (1976). The use of zona-free animal ova as a test-system for the assessment of the fertilizing capacity of human spermatozoa. Biol. Reprod. 15:471.

283. Rogers, B.J., VanCampen, H., Ueno, M., Lambert, H., Bronson, R., and Hale, R. (1979). Analysis of human spermatozoal fertilizing ability using zona-free ova. Fertil. Steril. 32:664.

284. Karp, L.E., Williamson, R.A., Moore, D.E., Sky, K.K., Plymate, S.R., and Smith, W.D. (1981). Sperm penetration assay: Useful test in evaluation of male fertility. Obstet. Gynecol. 57:620.

285. Prasad, M.R.N. (1984). The in vitro sperm penetration test: A review. Int. J. Androl. 7:5.

286. Pearson, P.L., Bobrow, M., and Vosa, C.G. (1970). Technique for identifying Y chromosomes in human interphase nucleus. Nature 226:78.

287. Kapp, R.W. (1979). Detection of aneuploidy in human sperm. Environ. Health Perspect. 31:27.

288. Propping, D., Tauber, P.F., and Zaneveld, L.J.D. (1978). An improved assay technique for the proteolytic activity of individual human spermatozoa. Int. J. Fertil. 23:24.

289. Ginsberg, L.C., Johnson, S.C., Salama, N., and Ficsor, G. (1981). Acrosomal proteolytic assay for detection of mutagens in mammals. Mutat. Res. 91:415.

290. Phadke, A.M., Samant, N.R., and Deval, S.D. (1973). Significance of seminal fructose studies in male infertility. Fertil. Steril. 24:894.

291. Marmar, J.L., Katz, S., Praiss, D.E., and De Benedictis, T.J. (1975). Semen zinc levels in infertile and post-vasectomy patients and patient with prostatitis. Fertil. Steril. 29:539.

292. Fair, W.R., Clark, R.B., and Wehner, N. (1972). A correlation of seminal polyamine levels and semen analysis in the human. Fertil. Steril. 23:38.

293. Crabbe, M.J.C. (1977). The development of a qualitative assay for male fertility from a study of enzymes in human semen. J. Reprod. Fertil. 51:73.

294. Beck, K.J., Schonhofer, P.S., Rodermund, O.E., Dinnendahl, V., and Peters, H.D. (1976). Lack of relationship between cyclic nucleotide levels and spermatozoal function in human sperm. Fertil. Steril. 27:403.

295. Homonnai, Z.T., Matzkin, H., Fairman, N., Paz, G., and Kracier, P.F. (1978). The cation composition of human seminal plasma and prostatic fluid and its correlation to semen quality. Fertil. Steril. 29:539.

296. Comhaire, F., Vermuelen, L., Ghedira, K., Mas, G., and Irvine, S. (1983). Adenosine triphosphate (ATP) in human semen: A marker of its potential fertilizing capacity. Am. Soc. Androl. (Abstr.).

297. Gray, L.E., Ferrell, J., Gray, K., and Ostby, J. (1986). Alterations in reproductive development in hamsters induced by methoxychlor (M). Toxicologist 6:294.
298. Chapin, R.E. and Heindel, J.J. (ed.) (1993). Methods in Toxicology, Vol. 3. Part A. Male Reproductive Toxicology, San Diego: Academic Press.
299. Christian, M.S., Diener, R.M., Hoar, R.L., and Staples, R.E. (1980). Reproduction, teratology and pediatrics. PMA Guidelines.
300. Bottomley, A.M. and Leeming, N.M. (1981). Effect of maternal bodyweight and age on outcome of mating. Teratology 24:35A.
301. Committee of Safety of Medicines (1979). Notes for Guidance on Reproduction Studies (of Applicants for Product Licenses and Clinical Trial Certificates), Medicines Act 1968, Revised 1974 and subsequently (MAL 2). Department of Health and Social Security.
302. Guidelines of Toxicity Studies (1984). Notification No. 118 of the Pharmaceutical Affairs Bureau, Ministry of Health and Welfare. Yakugyo Jiho Co., Ltd., Tokyo, Japan.
303. ICH Harmonized Tripartite Guideline. Detection of Toxicity to Reproduction for Medicinal Products. June, 1993.
304. Omenn, G.S. (1984). A framework for reproductive risk assessment and surveillance Teratog. Carcinog. Mutag. 4:1.
305. Clegg, D.J. (1979). Animal reproduction and carcinogenicity studies in relation to human safety evaluation. Dev. Toxicol. Environ. Sci. 4:45.
306. McLachlan, J.A., Newbold, R.R., Shah, H.C., Hogan, M., and Dixon, R.L. (1981). Reduced fertility in female mice exposed transplacentally to diethylstilbestrol. Fertil. Steril. 38:364.
307. McLachlan, J.A. and Dixon, R.L. (1976). Transplacental toxicity of diethylstilbestrol: A special problem in safety evaluation. In: Advances in Modern Toxicology: New Concepts in Safety Evaluation. Edited by M.A. Mehlman, R.E. Shapiro, and H. Blumenthal, Washington, D.C.: Hemisphere Publ. Co., Vol. I, Part I, pp. 423–448.
308. Gerall, A.A. and McCrady, R.E. (1970). Receptivity scores of female rats stimulated either manually or by males. J. Endocrinol. 46:55.
309. McClintock, M.K. and Adler, N.T. (1978). The role of the female during copulation in the wild and domestic Norway rat. Behavior 67:67.
310. Christian, M.S., Galbraith, W.M., Voytek, P., and Mehlman, M.A. (1983). Advances in modern environmental toxicity. In: Assessment of Reproductive and Teratogenic Hazards. Princeton, NJ, Princeton Sci. Publ., Vol. III, p. 160.
311. Tuchmann-Duplessis, H. and Mercier-Parot, L. (1961). Diminution de la fertilite du rat soumis a un traitement chronique de niamide. C. R. Acad. Sci. [D] (Paris) 253:712.
312. Greene, R. R., Burrill, M.W., and Ivy, A.C. (1939). Experimental intersexuality: The effect of antenatal androgens on sexual development of female rats. Am. J. Anat. 65:415.
313. Gray, L.E., Ferrell, J., Gray, K., and Ostby, J. (1986). Alterations in reproductive development in hamsters induced by methoxychlor (M). Toxicologist 6:294.
314. Tutak, L.S. and Arthur, A.T. (1986). Disruption of the reproductive process in female rats resulting from constant exposure to light. Toxicologist 6:99.

315. Rasmussen, E.W. and Kaada, B.R. (1965). Variation in length of heat periods in albino rats according to age.J. Reprod. Fertil. 10:9.

316. Gellert, R.J., Heinrichs, W.L., and Swerdloff, R. (1974). Effects of neonatally administered DDT homologs on reproductive function in male and female rats. Neuroendocrinology 16:84.

317. Faddy, M.J., Jones, E.C., and Edwards, R.G. (1976). An analytical model for follicular dynamics. J. Exper. Zool. 197:173.

318. Heindel, J.J. and Chapin, R.E. (ed.) (1993). Methods in Toxicology. Vol. 3B. Female Reproductive Toxicology, San Diego, CA: Academic Press.

319. Nisbet, I.C.T. and Karch, N.J. (1983). Chemical Hazards to Human Reproduction. Park Ridge, NJ: Noyes Data Corp.

320. Barlow, S.M. and Sullivan, F.M. (1982). Reproductive Hazards of Industrial Chemicals, An Evaluation of Animal and Human Data. London: Academic Press.

321. Klassen, R.W. and Persaud, T.V.N. (1978). Influence of alcohol on the reproductive system of the male rat. Int. J. Fertil. 23:176.

322. Schardein, J.L. (1993). Chemically Induced Birth Defects, Second Edition, New York: Marcel Dekker.

323. Bradley, W.R. and Frederick, W.G. (1941). The toxicity of antimony in animal studies. Indust. Med. 10. Indust. Hyg. Sec. 2:15.

324. Jackson, H., Fox, B.W., and Craig, A.W. (1959). The effect of alkylating agents on male rat fertility. Br. J. Pharmacol. 14:149.

325. Hood, R.D. and Bishop, S.L. (1972). Teratogenic effects of sodium arsenate in mice. Arch. Environ. Health 24:62.

326. Beaudoin A.R. (1974). Teratogenicity of sodium arsenate in rats. Teratology 10: 153.

327. Avilova, G.G. and Ulanova, I.P. (1975). Comparative characteristics of the effect of benzene on the reproductive function of adult and young animals. Gig. Truda. Prof. Zabol. 19:55.

328. Bouissou, H. and Castagnol. R. (1965). Action of boric acid on the testicle of the rat. Arch. Mal. Profess. Med. Travail. Secur. Soc. 26:293.

329. Weir, R.J. and Fisher, R.S. (1972). Toxicologic studies on borax and boric acid. Toxicol. Appl. Pharmacol. 23:351.

330. Barr, M. (1973). The teratogenicity of cadmium chloride in two stocks of Wistar rats. Teratology 7:237.

331. Agranovskaya, B.A. (1973). Effect of prophylactic trace element-vitamin feedings on the generative function of white rats exposed to carbon disulfide. Tr. Leningr. Sanit.-gig. Med. Inst. 103:118.

332. Tepe, S.J. and Zenick, H. (1982). Assessment of male reproductive toxicity due to carbon disulfide: Use of a new technique. Toxicologist 2:77.

333. Larson, P.S., Egle, J.L., Hennigar, G.R., Lane, R.W., and Borzelleca, J.F. (1979). Acute, subchronic, and chronic toxicity of chlordecone. Toxicol. Appl. Pharmacol. 48:29.

334. Epstein, S.S. (1978). Kepone-hazard evaluation. Sci. Tot. Environ. 9:1.

335. Hammond, B., Bahr, J., Dial, O., McConnel, J., and Metcalf, R. (1978). Reproductive toxicology of Mirex and Kepone. Fed. Proc. 37:501.

336. Huber, J.J. (1965). Some physiological effects of the insecticide Kepone in the laboratory mouse. Toxicol. Appl. Pharmacol. 7:516.

337. vonOettingen, W.F., Hueper, W.C., Deichmann-Gruebler, W., and Wiley, F.H. (1936). 2-Chloro-butadiene (chloroprene): Its toxicity and pathology and the mechanism of its action. J. Indust. Hyg. Toxicol. 18:240.

338. Salnikova, L.S. and Fomenko, V.N. (1973). Experimental investigation of the influence produced by chloroprene on the embryogenesis. Gig. Truda. Prof. Zabol. 17:23.

339. Winters, S.J., Banks, J.L., and Loriaux, D.L. (1979). Cimetidine is an antiandrogen in the rat. Gastroenterology 76:504.

340. Kabra, S.P. and Prasad, M.R. (1967). Effect of clomiphene on fertility in male rats. J. Reprod. Fertil 14:39.

341. Hart, M.M., Adamson, R.H., and Fabro, S. (1971). Prematurity and intrauterine growth retardation induced by DDT in the rabbit. Arch. Int. Pharmacodyn. Ther. 192:286.

342. Heinrichs, W.L., Gellert, R.J., Bakke, J.L., and Lawrence, N.L. (1971). DDT administered to neonatal rats induces persistent estrus syndrome. Science 173:642.

343. Coulston, F., Beyler, A., and Drobeck, H. (1960). The biologic actions of a new series of bis(dichloracetyl)-diamines. Toxicol. Appl. Pharmacol. 2:715.

344. Torkelson, T.R., Sadek, S.E., Rowe, V.K., Kodama, J.K., Anderson, H.H., Loquvam, G.S., and Hine, C.H. (1961). Toxicologic investigation of 1,2-dibromo-3-chloropropane. Toxicol. Appl Pharmacol. 3:545.

345. Rao, K.S., Murray, F.J., Crawford, A.A., John, J.A., Potts, W.J., Schwetz, B.A., Burek, J.D., and Parker, C.M. (1979). Effects of inhaled 1,2-dibromo-3-chloropropane (DBCP) on the semen of rabbits and the fertility of male and female rats. Toxicol. Appl. Pharmacol. 48:A137.

346. McLachlan, J.A., Newbold, R.R., and Bullock, B. (1975). Reproductive tract lesions in male mice exposed prenatally to diethylstilbestrol. Science 190:991.

347. Vorherr, H., Messer, R.H., Vorherr, U.F., Jordan, S.W., and Kornfeld, M. (1979). Teratogenesis and carcinogenesis in rat offspring after transplacental and transmammary exposure to diethylstilbestrol. Biochem. Pharmacol. 28:1865.

348. Wadsworth, P.F. and Heywood, R. (1978). The effect of prenatal exposure of Rhesus monkeys (Macaca mulatta) to diethylstilbestrol. Toxicol. Lett. 2:115.

349. Walker, B.E. (1980). Reproductive tract anomalies in mice after prenatal exposure to DES. Teratology 21:313.

350. Baggs, R.B. and Miller R.K. (1983). Induction of urogenital malformation by diethylstilbestrol in the ferret. Teratology 27:28A.

351. Gilloteaux, J.P., Steggles, R.J., and Alan, W. (1982). Upper genital tract abnormalities in the Syrian hamster as a result of in utero exposure to diethylstilbestrol. Virchows Arch. A: Pathol. Anat. Histopathol. 2:163.

352. Hendrickx, A.G., Benirschke, K., Thompson, R.S., Ahern, J.K., Lucas, W.E., and Oi, R.H. (1979). The effects of prenatal diethylstilbestrol (DES) exposure on the genitalia of pubertal Macaca mulatta. I. Female offspring. J. Reprod. Med. 22: 233.

353. Short, R.D., Minor, J.L., Winston, J.M., Seifter, J., and Lee, C.C. (1978). Inhalation of ethylene dibromide during gestation by rats and mice. Toxicol. Appl. Pharmacol. 46:173.

354. Chang, M.C., Gu, Z., and Saksena, S.K. (1980). Effect of gossypol on the fertility of male rats, hamsters and rabbits. Contraception 21:461.

355. Hahn, D.W., Rusticus, C., Probst, A., Homm, R., and Johnson, A.N. (1981). Anti-fertility and endocrine activities of gossypol in rodents. Contraception 24:97.

356. Shandilya, L., Clarkson, T.B., Adams, M.R., and Lewis, J.C. (1982). Effects of gossypol on reproductive and endocrine functions of male cynomolgus monkeys (Macaca fascicularis). Biol. Reprod. 27:241.

357. Ehling, U.H. (1971). Comparison of radiation—and chemically-induced dominant lethal mutations in male mice. Mutat. Res. 11:35.

358. Singhal, R.L. and Thomas, J.A. (Eds.). (1980). Lead Toxicity. Baltimore: Urban and Schwazenberg.

359. Gray, L.E. and Laskey, J.W. (1980). Multivariate analysis of the effects of manganese on the reproductive physiology and behavior of the male house mouse. J. Toxicol. Environ. Health 6:861.

360. Chandra, S.V. (1971). Cellular changes induced by manganese in the rat testis-preliminary results. Acta Pharmacologica et Toxicologica 29:75.

361. Chandra, S.V., Ara, R., Nagar, N., and Seth, P.K. (1973). Sterility in experimental manganese toxicity. Acta Biol. Med. Germanica 30:857.

362. Lee, I.P. and Dixon, R.L. (1975). Effects of mercury on spermatogenesis studies by velocity sedimentation cell separation and serial mating. J. Pharmacol. Exp. Therap. 194:171.

363. Lach, H. and Srebro, Z. (1972). The oestrous cycle of mice during lead and mercury poisoning. Acta Biologica Cracoviensia. Series Zoologica 15:121.

364. Baranski, B. and Szymczyk, I. (1973). Effects of mercury vapours upon reproductive function on white female rats. Medcyna Pracy 24:249.

365. Lamperti, A.A. and Printz, R.H. (1973). Effects of mercuric chloride on the reproductive cycle of the female hamster. Biol. Reprod. 8:378.

366. Fish, S.A. (1966). Organophosphorus cholinesterase inhibitors and fetal development. Am. J. Obstet. Gynecol. 96:1148.

367. Smith, D.J. and Joffe, J.M. (1975). Increased neonatal mortality in offspring of male rats treated with methadone or morphine before mating. Nature (London) 253:202.

368. George, R. (1971). Hypothalamus: Anterior pituitary gland. In: Narcotic Drugs: Biochemical Pharmacology. Edited by D. Clouet. New York: Plenum, pp. 283–296.

369. Davies, A.G. (1980). Effects of Hormones, Drugs and Chemicals on Testicular Function, Vol. 1. St. Albans, VT: Eden Press.

370. Orberg, J., Johansson, N., Kihlstrom, J.E., and Lundberg, C. (1972). Administration of DDT and PCB. Ambio 1:148.

371. Barsotti, D.A., Marlar, R.J., and Allen, J.R. (1976). Reproductive dysfunction in rhesus monkeys exposed to low levels of polychlorinated biphenyls (Aroclor 1248). Food Cosmet. Toxicol. 14:99.

372. Gellert, R.J. (1978). Uterotrophic activity of polychlorinated biphenyls (PCB) and induction of precocious reproductive aging in neonatally treated female rats. Environ. Res. 16:123.

373. Izyumova, A.S. (1972). The action of small concentrations of sytrol on the sexual function of albino rats. Gig. Sanit. 37:29.

374. Gibson, J.E. and Becker, B.A. (1970). Placental transfer, embryotoxicity and tera-

togenicity of thallium sulphate in normal and potassium-deficient rats. Toxicol. Appl. Pharmacol. 16:120.

375. Younoszai, M.K., Peloso, J., and Haworth, J.C. (1969). Fetal growth retardation in rats exposed to cigarette smoke during pregnancy. Am. J. Obstet. Gynecol. 104: 1207.

376. Schoeneck, F.J. (1941). Cigarette smoking in pregnancy. N.Y. State J. Med. 41: 1945.

377. Hudak, A., Rodics, K., Stuber, I., and Ungvary, G. (1977). Effects of toluene inhalation on pregnant CFY rats and their offspring. Munkavedelem 23:(1–3 Suppl.) 25.

378. John, J.A., Smith, F.A., Leong, B.K.J., and Schwetz, B.A. (1977). The effects of maternally inhaled vinyl chloride on embryonal and fetal development in mice, rats and rabbits. Toxicol. Appl. Pharmacol. 39:497.

379. Hogue, C.J.R. (1984). The effect of common exposures on reproductive outcomes. Teratog. Carcinog. Mutag. 4:45.

380. Foote, R.H., Schermerhorn, E.C., and Simkin, M.E. (1986). Measurement of semen quality, fertility, and reproductive hormones to assess dibromochlorpropane (DBCP) effects in live rabbits. Fund. Appl. Toxicol. 6:628.

381. Koeter, H.B.W.M. (1983). Relevance of parameters related to fertility and reproduction in toxicity testing. In: Reproductive Toxicity. Edited by D.R. Mattison. New York: Alan R. Liss, pp. 81–86.

382. Clegg, E.D. and Zenick, H. (1986). Issues in male reproductive risk assessment. Toxicologist 6:31.

383. Levine, R.J., Blunden, P.B., DalCorso, R.D., Starr, T.B., and Ross, C.E. (1983). Superiority of reproductive histories to sperm counts in detecting infertility at a dibromochloropropane manufacturing plant. J. Occup. Med. 25:591.

384. Omenn, G.S. (1983). Environmental risk assessment: Relation to mutagenesis, teratogenesis, and reproductive effects. J. Am. Coll. Toxicol. 2:113.

385. Varma, D. R. (1987). Epidemiological and experimental studies on the effects of methyl isocyanate on the course of pregnancy. Environ. Health Perspect. 72: 151–155.

386. Guidelines for Pesticide Toxicology Data Requirements (1981). Health Protection Branch, Health and Welfare, Canada.

11

Developmental Toxicology

Julia D. George
Research Triangle Institute, Research Triangle Park, North Carolina

I. INTRODUCTION

The field of developmental toxicology has grown out of the study of teratology, or the study of birth defects. Birth defects (terata) may be caused by prenatal exposure to pharmaceutical agents or environmental chemicals (xenobiotics), through genetic defects, or as a result of an interaction between the environment and the genetics of the individual. There are 3,000–5,000 different birth defects identified today, affecting 150,000 infants each year (1). The etiology of 60% of these birth defects is unknown. Developmental toxicology is no longer limited to the identification of morphological birth defects, as it once was in the 1970s (2,3). Although the identification of morphological defects associated with exposure to toxic agents during development is still central to the study of developmental toxicity, the field has expanded to include many areas of inquiry both in basic scientific research, to elucidate mechanisms of action, and in hazard and risk assessment. In addition, developmental toxicity can now be defined to include not only morphological alterations, but also more subtle changes in biochemical parameters and behavior. As defined by the U.S. Environmental Protection Agency (EPA), developmental toxicology is "the study of adverse effects on the developing conceptus from prior to conception through the time of sexual maturation (4)." This chapter will focus on the current approach to in vivo developmental toxicity testing (Phase II or Segment II) with regard to government requirements for pharmaceutical agents and environmental chemicals, and how these study protocols are currently acting as springboards for more in-depth studies. Additional areas such as peri- and postnatal toxicity (Phase III or Segment III), developmental neurotoxicity, male-mediated effects, toxicokinetics, molecular mechanisms, and in vitro studies will also be addressed, as will the use of developmental toxicity data in hazard and risk assessment. Finally, areas of focus for future research in developmental toxicology will be identified.

II. HISTORY

The current testing guidelines for reproductive and developmental toxicity in the United States can trace their origins to the 1960s. Prior to that time, government-regulated reproductive toxicity testing was limited to drugs specifically targeted for women of child-bearing potential, or ones that might directly alter the endocrine system. In the late 1950s and early 1960s, the use of thalidomide for the treatment of nausea during pregnancy resulted in the birth of thousands of malformed babies in more that 25 countries, and is commonly known as "the thalidomide disaster." Although thalidomide was not marketed in the United States, the reproductive toxicity test, or "litter" test, in use by the U.S. Food and Drug Administration (FDA) at the time, had in fact failed to detect the teratogenic potential of thalidomide, although it did reveal a reduction on offspring viability (5–7). The litter test, using a single species of rodent, involved continuous exposure of both male and female animals for 60 days prior to a first mating and through a second mating to scheduled necropsy. Developmental toxicity was evaluated primarily through litter size and survival. Only in retrospect would it become evident that the litter test had failed since the single species used, rats, were resistant to the teratogenic effects of thalidomide.

Subsequent to the thalidomide disaster, the FDA assumed responsibility for and expanded the testing procedures used in the U.S. to evaluate the safety of drugs used during pregnancy. The resulting testing guidelines, known as the *Guidelines for Reproductive Studies for Safety Evaluation of Drugs for Human Use*, were published in 1966 (8). These guidelines provided for the evaluation of fertility, reproductive performance, teratogenicity, and peri- and postnatal development through the use of three study designs (Figures 1, 2, and 3). The Phase I or Segment I study (Figure 1) includes chemical exposure of both the male and female animals prior to mating (premating exposure, PME) and during mating (M), and the female animals during gestation and lactation. F_1 animals are exposed indirectly through transplacental exposure and/or translactational exposure, and then directly just prior to weaning. This protocol provides information on reproductive competence: breeding, fertility, nidation, and parturition, in addition to lactation and neonatal development. The Phase II or Segment II study (Figure 2) directly addresses the effect of exposure on the morphological development and *in utero* survival and growth of the embryo and fetus, with exposure of the pregnant female during the period of major organogenesis. The third protocol (Phase III or Segment III, Figure 3) provides information on the effect of exposure on late fetal, perinatal, and postnatal development, with expo-

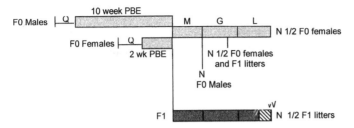

Figure 1   Segment I: Single-generation fertility study (Courtesy of Ref. 15).

sure of the pregnant females from gestational day 15 through lactation to postnatal day 21.

The reproductive and developmental toxicity testing of environmental agents in the United States by the EPA and the testing of pharmaceutical and environmental agents in other countries have followed similar protocols (9–16), yet differences in the testing requirements have existed in the past that were

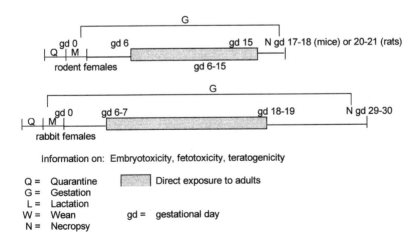

Figure 2   Segment II: Developmental toxicity study (Courtesy of Ref. 15).

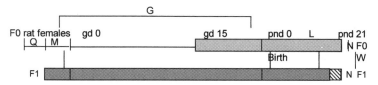

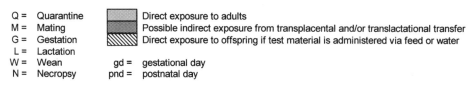

Information on: Parturition, lactation, peri- and neonatal effects

Q =   Quarantine   ▓▓▓   Direct exposure to adults
M =   Mating   ▓▓▓   Possible indirect exposure from transplacental and/or translactational transfer
G =   Gestation   ▨▨▨   Direct exposure to offspring if test material is administered via feed or water
L =   Lactation
W =   Wean   gd = gestational day
N =   Necropsy   pnd = postnatal day

Figure 3   Segment III: Perinatal and postnatal study (Courtesy of Ref. 15).

significant enough to require retesting of compounds for registration in different
countries.Of the three study protocols, it is the Segment II or "teratology" study
design that has been most closely adhered to for the testing of environmental
agents by the EPA and for testing in other countries (9–12,14–19). Testing
guidelines recently promulgated by the International Conference on Harmonization, designed to provide consistent testing protocols for the registration of pharmaceutical agents in the U.S., Japan, and Europe, include versions of the Segment I, II, and III studies which are similar to those used by the FDA, with the
Segment II study design being identical (20). In addition, the EPA requires
developmental neurotoxicity testing after exposure during gestation and early
lactation.

III. DEVELOPMENTAL TOXICITY TESTING (PHASE II OR SEGMENT II)

The primary purpose of the Segment II study, as conducted under government
regulations (21–23) is to ensure a consistent, quality-controlled approach to providing information on the effect of exposure to an exogenous agent on the in
vivo prenatal development of a mammalian embryo and fetus. The study design
assesses the effect of the treatment in the whole animal, such that the observed
toxicity (or lack thereof) represents the results of the interaction of both the
maternal and embryofetal processes that comprise development. To this end,
study design parameters have been somewhat standardized (15). These parameters include the handling of the test compound, species selected, animal husbandry and identification, route of administration and duration of exposure, and
endpoints of maternal and developmental toxicity.

A. Test Compound

The test compound should be fully characterized with respect to purity, and chemical and physical properties. Depending on the way in which the drug or chemical is used, a pure grade, technical grade, or pharmaceutical formulation may be tested. Records of these parameters, in addition to traceable records of the test chemical's origin (supplier, lot number, batch number, etc.) are part of the study records. Procedures and analysis of dosing formulations (gavage, feed, drinking water, etc.) are also part of the study records.

B. Test Species

The three most common species used for regulatory developmental toxicity testing are mice, rats, and rabbits. The FDA and EPA testing requirements for developmental toxicity (Segment II) require the use of one rodent and one nonrodent species. Thus, the rabbit satisfies the nonrodent testing requirement. The animals should be obtained from an experienced and reliable supplier. Inbred or outbred strains of animals may be chosen, depending on the desired sensitivity to general or specific chemical toxicity. Sprague-Dawley rats are most frequently used for regulatory testing, with New Zealand White rabbits the most frequent strain of choice for the nonrodent species. Mice are not routinely chosen for developmental toxicity studies since the fetuses are smaller that those of the rat and are therefore more difficult to evaluate. The CD-1 Swiss mouse is the most frequently used outbred strain, although some inbred strains are useful due to their specific sensitivity, i.e., increased tendency to exhibit a particular response in response to chemical insult or well-characterized xenobiotic metabolizing ability. In addition, in instances where other toxicity tests have been performed for a particular test chemical specific strains of animals (rats, mice, or rabbits) may be chosen to provide developmental toxicity data from animals that match those used in other tests.

C. Animal Husbandry, Identification, and Mating

All animals should be handled in accordance with the *Guide for the Care and Use of Laboratory Animals* (24). Single housing of animals during the study allows for the determination of food and water consumption. Bedding, when used, should be well characterized and from a consistent supply, with no components that may affect xenobiotic metabolism. Feed should be analyzed for contents and contaminant, and water analyzed for contaminants. Complete records of bedding, feed, water, and other aspects of animal husbandry, including light cycle, temperature and relative humidity, and ventilation should be kept in a traceable and transparent format. Animals should be uniquely identified by tail tattoo, ear tag, implanted microchip, or other methods, and these identities recorded and maintained from receipt to necropsy.

Rodents may be monogamously or polygamously mated. Vaginal lavage, performed the morning after cohabitation, provides evidence of the presence of sperm, and mating. Sperm-negative females may be cohabited with a male again until vaginal sperm are detected. Copulation plugs, observed in the vagina of mice, or a dropped plug observed after monogamous cohabitation of rats also indicates mating. Rabbits may be naturally mated or artificially inseminated. Vendor-mated rabbits are also available. The day of determination of vaginal sperm or copulation plugs (rodents) or insemination or natural mating (rabbits) is designated gestational day (gd) 0 according to the study design (Figure 2).

D. Route of Administration and Duration of Exposure

Compounds may be administered by gavage, in the diet or drinking water, by injection (intravenous, subcutaneous, intraperitoneal, or intramuscularly), by inhalation, subcutaneous implant, or dermally. The choice of the route of administration generally follows the expected route of exposure of humans to the test chemical. Any vehicles used in the dose formulation are administered to the control group of animals.

Exposure occurs during the period of major organogenesis, which corresponds to gd 6 through 15 for rodents, and gd 6 through 18 or gd 7 through 19 for rabbits if gd 0 designates the day of observation of sperm or copulation plug (rodents) or mating (rabbits). However, other periods of exposure have been specified in newer regulatory documents. In addition, the characteristics of the test compound may dictate a slightly altered period of administration.

E. Endpoints

The endpoints of maternal and developmental toxicity that are routinely collected for developmental toxicity studies are listed in Table 1 (25). The observation and documentation of maternal effects in a developmental toxicity study are critical to the interpretation of observed effects on the embryo or fetus. Much has been written regarding the relative importance of maternal toxicity in relation to developmental toxicity, and although there are some differences of opinion as to how to interpret these data, the importance of documenting maternal effects, can not be disputed (26–32). Clinical observations, timed to determine any treatment-related effects, body weight, and feed and water consumption provide information on the general health status of the maternal animal. Since exposure occurs at or around the time of implantation, fertility data provide a background against which to judge the overall reproductive performance of the mothers. Corrected maternal body weight, organ weights, and gross necropsy findings also point to the general condition of the maternal animals during the time of embryofetal development. Endpoints of developmental toxicity provide information on the result (if any) of treatment, but not on the mechanism

Table 1 Endpoints of Maternal and Developmental Toxicity

Maternal Toxicity
Fertility index (number with seminal plugs or sperm/number mated)
Gestation index (number with implants/number with seminal plugs)
Gestation length
Body weight (treatment, sacrifice)
Body weight change (gestation, treatment, posttreatment to sacrifice)
Corrected maternal body weight change (body weight change throughout gestation minus gravid uterine weight)
Organ weights (i.e., liver, kidney, organs of specific toxicity) absolute and relative to body weight
Food and water consumption
Clinical observations (during treatment and at sacrifice)
Gross necropsy
Histopathology

Developmental Toxicity
Litters with implantation sites
    Number of implantation sites per dam
    Number of corpora lutea per dam
    Percent preimplantation loss
    Number and percent live offspring per litter
    Number and percent resorptions per litter
    Number and percent litters with resorptions
    Number and percent late fetal deaths per litter
    Number and percent nonlive (late fetal deaths and resorptions) per litter
    Number and percent litters with nonlive implants
    Number and percent adversely affected (nonlive and malformed) implants per litter
    Number and percent litters with adversely affected implants
    Number and percent litters with total resorptions
    Number and percent stillbirths per litter
Litters with live offspring
    Number and percent litters with lives fetuses
    Number and percent live fetuses per litter
    Sex ratio per litter
    Mean fetal body weight per litter (male, female, sexes combined)
    Number and percent externally malformed fetuses per litter
    Number and percent viscerally malformed fetuses per litter
    Number and percent skeletally malformed fetuses per litter
    Number and percent malformed fetuses per litter
    Number and percent litters with malformed fetuses
    Number and percent malformed male fetuses per litter
    Number and percent fetuses with variations per litter
    Number and percent litters with fetuses with variations
    Incidence and description of individual malformations
    Incidence and description of individual variations
    Individual listing of fetuses and malformations (by litter within dose groups)

Source: From Ref. 25.

or possible interaction with maternal factors. Methods for the evaluation of morphological changes in external, visceral, and skeletal structures are well known (2,33–45). The favored method for thoracic and abdominal visceral examination is the fresh tissue dissection technique, which provides an excellent opportunity to view and manipulate visceral organs in situ, and allowed detailed examination of the heart and minor vessels (34). In addition, fetuses examined by this method may then be processed for skeletal evaluation. Visceral examination may also be conducted using fixed and decalcified fetuses that have been serially sectioned (2,35,36). The disadvantages of this technique for visceral examination include the inability to process the same fetus for both visceral and skeletal evaluations, the inability to observe the visceral organs their natural color and pliable state, and technical difficulties in consistent sectioning and visualizing the organs from a fixed slice. This technique, however, is still used for evaluation of the craniofacial structures (15). Skeletal examination is most effectively done after double staining with alcian blue (for cartilage) and alizarin red S (for ossified bone) (40,41), although evaluation of single-stained skeletons (alizarin red S) has been the accepted technique in the past (42,43). Double-staining of the skeleton to reveal changes in both the cartilage and ossified bone has the advantage of revealing the underlying cartilaginous structure of the skeleton to help distinguish true malformations of skeletal system from changes that may be more indicative of delayed ossification (44,45).

G. Statistics

Data from developmental toxicity studies should be analyzed using the pregnant animal as the unit of comparison, with the individual litter treated as a unit (15). Data should be analyzed to reveal trends of treatment-related effects, overall effects of treatment, and pairwise effects of treatment groups compared to the concurrent control group.

IV. PERI- AND POSTNATAL TOXICITY TESTING (PHASE III OR SEGMENT III)

The Phase III or Segment III study design (Figure 3) evaluates the effect of exposure of pregnant rats to a toxicant from the end of organogenesis (gd 15) through the end of gestation, parturition, and lactation, to weaning of the offspring (postnatal day 21). Exposure of the offspring occurs either transplacentally prior to birth, and/or via lactation. Study conditions are the same as for the Segment II studies, with a vehicle control and three treatment groups, 20 pregnant animals per group. Endpoints are listed in Table 2. Information obtained from this study design characterizes the effect of treatment on the last portion of gestation, parturition, maternal care and behavior toward the offspring, and pup growth and development to weaning.

Table 2 Endpoints of Peri- and Postnatal Toxicity

Maternal Toxicity
Body weight (gestation, lactation, sacrifice)
Body weight change (gestation, lactation)
Food and water consumption (gestation, lactation)
Clinical observations (gestation, lactation)
Reproductive and lactational indices
Gross necropsy
Organ weights (i.e., liver, kidney, organs of specific toxicity)
   absolute and relative to body weight
Histopathology

Developmental Toxicity
Live litter size
Pup body weight (pnd 0 through 21)
Developmental Landmarks (preweaning)
   surface righting reflex
   pinna detachment
   incisor eruption
   eye opening
   auditory startle
   midair righting reflex
Developmental Landmarks (postweaning)
   vaginal patency
   testis descent
   preputial separation
   motor activity
   learning and memory
Pup Gross Necropsy

Source: From Ref. 15.

V. DEVELOPMENTAL NEUROTOXICITY TESTING

The study design for the developmental neurotoxicity test is similar to that of the Segment III study (Figure 3), except dosing occurs from gestation day 6 through postnatal day 10 (46,47). Endpoints for this study design are presented in Table 3. This study design provides for the evaluation of the effect of treatment on the development of the central nervous system throughout the embryonic, fetal, and postnatal period.

A. Male Mediated Effects

The Segment II or Phase II study as described above evaluates the effect of toxicants given to the maternal animal on the development of the embryo and

Table 3   Endpoints of Developmental Neurotoxicity

Maternal Toxicity
Body weight (gestation, lactation to pnd 11, sacrifice)
Body weight change (gestation, lactation to pnd 11)
Food and water consumption (gestation, lactation to pnd 11)
Clinical observations (gestation, lactation to pnd 11)
Reproductive and lactational indices
Gross necropsy
Organ weights (i.e., liver, kidney, organs of specific toxicity)
    absolute and relative to body weight
Histopathology

Developmental Neurotoxicity
Live litter size
Pup body weight (pnd 1 through 11)
Developmental landmarks (postweaning)
    vaginal patency
    preputial separation
    motor activity
    learning and memory
Pup gross necropsy
Neuropathological assessment

Source: From Refs. 21, 22.

fetus. However, the possibility of developmental toxicity as the result of paternal exposure to a toxicant does exist, and has received increasing interest in recent years, both from epidemiologists and toxicologists (48–50). Most studies in the male have focused on adverse effects on fertility. In animals, a number of protocols address male mediated effects, although none address the effect of the toxicant on the male independent of the female (20,51).

Male mediated effects on development are generally thought of as occurring in three ways: those that occur as a result of genetic damage or toxicity to DNA of the male germ cells, those that occur through nongenetic damage to other components of the sperm (mitochondria or plasma membrane), and those nongenetic effects that occur via transfer of the toxicant in the semen (52). Endpoints of male mediated developmental toxicity include those involving the male reproductive system and germ cells, and those involving the processes of fertilization and development (53). With regard to effects on the male reproductive system, research has focused on toxicants in the semen, changes in the male reproductive tract including effects on sperm, and the hormonal control of reproduction. Methods exist to distinguish genetic from nongenetic effects, and also the contribution of the DNA in the sperm to the development of the offspring (52). Direct evidence of male-mediated developmental toxicity after a toxic exposure includes male infertility, diminished quality or quantity of the sperm, viable sperm with cytogenetic abnormalities, embryofetal chromosomal abnormalities of paternal origin, and epidemiological evidence of an association between paternal occupational exposure to toxicants and an increased risk of birth defects or childhood cancer (54,55). However, the research on male mediated effects on the male reproductive system has not yet fully investigated the interrelationship of any of these effects with changes in male reproduction. Defects in fertilization and development that are of paternal origin may result from exposure to exogenous agents that cause damage to either pre- or postfertilization processes. Agents that have been shown to cause adverse developmental effects after paternal exposure include anesthetic gases, cyclophosphamide, alcohol, smoking, lead, and ionizing radiation (50).

B. Pharmacokinetics and Pharmacodynamics

In order to understand the potential risk of a drug or environmental chemical to the developing fetus we must understand and characterize the actual exposure of the embryofetus to the toxicant. The study of pharmacokinetics gives us just this information. Several excellent references describing the current status of the use of toxicokinetics in developmental toxicology are available (56–59). Pharmacokinetics may be defined to include "(1) characterization of the pattern of metabolism and quantitation of the metabolites formed and the conditions under which they are formed, (2) identification of the chemical moieties active in the production of developmental abnormalities, (3) the pattern and amount of the active chemical appearing at the target sites in the embryo or fetus, and (4) species differences in these processes. (59)"

In the past, kinetic models have been limited with regard to the accuracy of the fit of experimental data, and thus overall predictive ability, by the fact that the mathematical models used to describe the movement and fate of the compound in the body assumed that the body was made up of so many boxes or compartments. These compartments were limited in number and were assumed to behave as discrete entities (57,59). Application of this type of model to developmental toxicology resulted in a description of the maternal–fetal unit that treated the maternal system as the central compartment, and the fetus as a peripheral compartment. The maternal body was described as several related compartments, whereas the fetal compartment may have been represented as a single compartment, or several related compartments communicating with the maternal compartment. Useful concepts that have been derived from these classical models have been summarized by O'Flaherty and Scott (59), and O'Flaherty and Clarke (57) and include the volume that the drug or chemical is distributed into in a particular compartment, total dose measured as total concentration as a function of time, the biological half-life or the time for one-half of the compound to leave the body, the volume of body fluid that is cleared of the drug or chemical in a certain period of time (clearance), the maximum concentration reached in a tissue or plasma, and the time when the maximum concentration is reached. The source of these parameters was an empirical model, designed to most closely describe the expected absorption, distribution, metabolism, and excretion of the drug or chemical in the body.

Physiologically based models redefined the compartments and the parameters to represent real tissues and groups of tissues, with characteristic blood flow rates, metabolism rates, and other physiological process and anatomical considerations. Parameters are obtained from experimental values. The application of these models to the maternal–fetal unit required further allowance for the extensive changes in absorption, perfusion, metabolism, tissue volume, and excretion of both the maternal and the fetal unit during pregnancy (56,57). As a result, for the rodent, a model can be derived that includes maternal tissues that are well- and poorly perfused tissues that increase in volume during pregnancy (uterus, mammary glands, fat, and liver), and the kidney (58). The embryo/fetus is described in terms of the circulation and tissues, with separate compartments accounting for the number of fetuses in the litter, and the type of placenta which is dominant during the period of interest (yolk sac or chorioallantoic). Physiologically based models for pregnancy have been developed for rodents (60–66). In addition, models are being prepared for humans and other primates (67,68). Although changes during pregnancy may be similar for different mammalian species, the changes may not occur at the same relative point in the development of the fetus (57). Therefore, the models must be species-specific. Using these models, kinetic models have been developed for methadone and trichloroethylene in the pregnant rat (61,64), for weak acids in rodents and monkeys (60,67), and 2-methoxyethanol in the mouse (69). These pharmacokinetic models can be used to predict the dose of chemical that the fetus is exposed to, in addition to steady-state concentrations, half-life, and other classic kinetic parameters.

Pharmacodynamics describes the relationship of the exposure of the target tissue (fetus) to the toxicant and the resulting effect, and may be defined as the "relationship between the . . . toxicant–tissue interaction and the subsequent sequence of events that manifest altered biochemical or physiological function, leading to either growth retardation, dysmorphogenesis, functional deficit, or lethality (60)." Whereas pharmacokinetics describes absorption, distribution, and elimination of the compound, pharmacodynamics characterizes the nature and extent of effect caused by exposure to a certain amount (concentration) of chemical. The development of pharmacodynamic models for pregnancy and development is just beginning (see O'Flaherty and Clarke (60) for a summary of current areas of interest). When developed, this approach will be a powerful predictive tool in the study of mechanisms of developmental toxicity.

VI. MECHANISMS OF TOXICITY

Elucidating the mechanism of teratogenesis or developmental toxicity has been of primary interest in recent years, expanding the goal of developmental toxicology from merely identifying an effect to understanding the processes that caused the effect, with the ultimate goal (still in the future) being the prediction, prevention, or reversal of a developmentally toxic event. In addition, information about normal processes of development can be obtained through the study of a disrupted process. Wilson (70) proposed 6 general categories of teratogenic mechanisms that included mitotic interference, altered membrane function/signal transduction, altered energy sources, enzyme inhibition, altered nucleic acid synthesis, and mutations. Mechanisms of developmental toxicity range from the molecular level through the cellular and tissue mechanisms, to more complex mechanisms involving the malfunctioning of whole organ or tissue systems, or purely mechanical aberrations that may interfere with the developmental process (71).

On the molecular level, the concept of a developmentally toxic event proceeding from the interaction of a drug or chemical with a cellular receptor has been investigated, and has been reviewed (72–74). Examples of this mechanism include the action of glucocorticoids on the palatal cells of fetal mice, resulting in cleft palate (74). Other examples of malformations caused by the interaction of a chemical with receptors in the sensitive tissue include opiates and central nervous system tissue in mice (74), and beta-sympathomimetic drugs and rib malformations in rats (75). Cellular mechanisms include changes in the rates of cell death or proliferation (76–78), alterations in other cellular attributes including shape, adhesion, or migration (76–80). Other theories suggest that tissues interactions may occur (81), or that merely a disruption of the tissue in a developmental field by a variety of teratogens may lead to the same malformation (82).

Other mechanistic theories are summarized by Hood (71), and include species and strain-specific, generalized, single, multiple, direct, and indirect mechanisms.

An excellent summary of documented experimental approaches to determining mechanisms of toxicity as suggested by the 6 categories of Wilson has been written by Faustman et al. (83). In this summary, the authors put forth guidelines for the assessment of mechanisms in teratogenesis. They include temporal association, relationship to dose, structure–activity relationship, strength and consistency of association of effect, and coherence (scientific basis for mechanism). In addition, they add litter responses (response of the litter within the maternal unit) to the list of levels of mechanistic investigation. By applying these guidelines to the process of investigating mechanisms of developmental toxicity, the relationship of the event (malformation) and the cause (mechanism) will be more consistently understood.

A. In Vitro Tests

The use of in vitro tests for the evaluation of developmental toxicity has been of interest to scientists for various reasons for more than 25 years. The two major thrusts of research in developmental toxicology using in vitro methods have been as screening studies to identify potential developmental toxicants, and for mechanistic studies. The use of in vitro methods for these purposes has been thoroughly reviewed elsewhere (3,84–87). Mammalian and nonmammalian methods have been developed, and can be divided into different categories. Methods include whole embryo culture, organ culture, and cell culture.

1.   Mammalian Whole Embryo Culture

Whole embryos have been proposed for use both for the screening of compounds for teratogenic potential and in mechanistic studies (88–90). In vitro systems using whole embryos can be categorized based on the developmental stage of the starting material, i.e., preimplantation, periimplantation, or postimplantation. Each of these approaches has advantages and disadvantages, and potentially answers different questions about the developmental process. Preimplantation embryos are most commonly obtained from rats, mice, rabbits, or hamsters (90,91). The method of superovulation and synchronization is used to obtain either unfertilized or fertilized (in conjunction with mating after superovulation) preimplantation embryos (92). Embryos are flushed from the oviducts, separated according to developmental stage, and cultured individually. Because of their specific stage of development, preimplantation embryos lend themselves to certain types of manipulation, and thus provide unique information about the early developmental process. Cell metabolism, uptake of macromolecules and xenobiotics, toxic effects on gametes, and cell proliferation and differentiation with respect to embryogenesis are a few of the areas well served by the use of preimplantation embryos in culture. Morphological development, and functional development assayed through biochemical methods are also accessible through the use of embryo culture. Periimplantation embryo culture can be used to provide information on the effect of the uterine environment on the process of implantation and early embryonic growth, including the effect of exogenous chemicals (93). The presence of a visceral yolk sac in the postimplantation rodent embryo makes it well suited for the study of teratogenic effects of xenobiotics during organogenesis. Although the period of useful observation is limited to prior to conversion of the embryo to the nutritional requirement for placentation, cultured postimplantation embryos are the most complex and organized in vitro systems for the study of mammalian development, and successful culture methods are well established (94–97). During the approximately 48 hours in culture (beginning on gd 8 in mice or gd 9.5 in rats), the embryo can be observed to go through stages of head fold and early somite development through closure of the neural tube and development functional cardiovascular system (95).

2. Nonmammalian Whole Embryo Culture

Methods for culturing embryos from the chick, amphibians, fish, insects, planaria, and hydra have been used for either mechanistic studies or screening studies (98–105). Advantages to the use of nonmammalian embryos include accessibility (chick), development through fetogenesis (chick, frog), and ease of manipulation (Hydra, planaria).Extrapolation to mammalian systems can be problematic, however, due to intrinsic differences in mammalian and nonmammlian systems.

3. Tissue and Organ Culture

In vitro test systems using cells, intact tissues, and functioning organs have also been used in the evaluation of developmental toxicants. The most widely used system is the cultured limb bud (106–111). Limb teratogenesis as investigated by means of the limb bud assay has focused on the differentiation of the cells that make up the limb bud, and organization of those cells. These processes involve controlled gene expression, altered cellular organization to establish morphological form, and programmed cell death. The limb bud culture has been used for the evaluation of numerous compounds (107). Studies of compounds in limb bud culture have served to provide information on the origin of toxicity, including alterations in gene expression, receptors, electrolyte balance, and mitochondral function. An overview of mechanisms that may be evaluated by means of the limb bud culture may be found in other reviews (107,108).

Because cleft palate, caused by incomplete closure of the palatal shelves, is a common malformation in both humans and experimental animals, the study of intact palatal shelves *in vitro* has been useful in understanding the etiology of these malformations. TCDD, phenytoin, retinoic acid, and glucocorticoids have been shown to interrupt palatal growth and differentiation (112–115). Culture methods have been developed and improved to the point that complex aspects of palatal shelf growth and differentiation, including fusion, elevation, cell movement, and functional interactions can be evaluated in vitro (116,117).

Other tissues and organs have been grown in culture and exposed to teratogens, including the visceral yolk sac, eye and lens, spinal cord, and lung buds (118–122).

4. Cell Culture

The study of teratogenic mechanisms has revealed that adverse effects may be the result of the sensitivity of a particular cell type to the teratogen or developmental toxin. Thus, the study of the behavior of single cell types in the presence of these toxins in vitro can be an important aid in understanding how the cells react in vivo, provided the behavior can be shown to be similar in both cases. Cranial neural crest cells, cartilage, retina, lens, midbrain, and limb bud cells have been studied this way (123–127).

The use of in vitro methods to study the mechanisms of teratogenesis and developmental toxicity provides a unique opportunity to isolate and examine the behavior of the organism at differing levels of complexity, from the single cell to a complete embryo. The use of these methods, in conjunction with *in vivo* investigations, will further the understanding of processes of both normal and abnormal development.

VII. RISK ASSESSMENT

The process of risk assessment for developmental toxicity evolved through discussions of risk assessment evaluation for reproductive toxicity and cancer in the 1980s, and is currently defined as a regulatory process by the EPA (128–130). The process may be defined to include hazard characterization and dose-response analysis, characterization of the data and quantitative risk assessment, exposure assessment, and risk characterization (129,130) and has been summarized by Kimmel and Kimmel (131,132) and Kavlock and Kimmel (133). Animal and human data are used in hazard characterization and dose-response analysis. A compound is generally considered to cause a hazard or adverse effect if it causes a dose-related change in an animal study. The relevance of this change to humans depends on many things including species differences, pharmacokinetics, etc. The data available for a compound may be characterized as sufficient or insufficient with respect to hazard assessment, and if sufficient, a developmental toxicity reference dose (RfD_{DT}) or reference concentration (RfC_{DT}, for inhalation) is derived, reflecting the dose at which critical adverse effects cannot be detected (No Observed Adverse Effect Level, or NOAEL), and various uncertainty factors to account for species differences, sensitivity, etc. Exposure assessment involves the evaluation of human exposure in different situations. For developmental toxicity, this would include parental exposure prior to conception, maternal exposure during pregnancy (duration and stage of gestation), and developmental exposure of the offspring from birth through sexual maturity. Risk characterization integrates all of this information, including strengths and weaknesses of the data, to allow for the calculation of a margin of exposure (MOE), an indicator of the level of concern for human developmental health safety in various exposure situations. This characterization is then used in conjunction with the risk characterization for other adverse effects (cancer, etc.) to determine which endpoint for which a critical adverse effect occurs at the lowest dose. This information is then used to derive the reference dose or concentration (RfD or RfC) for chronic exposure, based on the assumption that risk evaluation for chronic exposure using the most sensitive indicator (lowest NOAEL) will provide the most protection from adverse effects. Compounds for which the RfD or RfC is based on developmental effects include carbon disulfide, phenol, dinoseb, ethylbenzene, and methyl ethyl ketone. Other agencies such as the Consumer Product Safety Commission and the FDA use slightly different approaches to risk assessment for developmental toxicity (131).

The area of risk assessment for developmental toxicity, and other areas of risk assessment, like the discipline of developmental toxicology, itself, has experienced a shift in focus to more physiologically relevant quantitative approaches. Areas of inquiry include dose-response modeling, exposure–duration relationships, use of mechanistic data, and the use of human data (131). Dose-response modeling, based on statistical models and biologically-based models derived from experimental data have received much attention. Calculation of a benchmark dose (134) for developmental toxicity has the advantage of using all of the doses and data in the experimental range, and is not limited to one dose or effect. In addition to the general method for the calculation of the benchmark dose, specific models for developmental studies have also been derived (135–138). Evaluation of which developmental endpoints are the most important is also in progress (139,140). Validation of these models using experimental data indicate that the benchmark dose can be calculated using developmental toxicity data, and that incorporation of specific endpoints as variables is appropriate for enhanced fit of the model (141–144). However, the fine-tuning of this approach to risk assessment is in its beginning stages, and much more work will be required to evaluate the most appropriate modeling approach.

The development of biologically-based dose response (BBDR) models represents the other area of major focus in risk assessment for developmental toxicity. These models include extensive mechanistic and pharmacokinetic data, and may incorporate additional factors such as litter size, etc. (131–133,138). Prototype chemicals, 5-fluorouracil and dexamethasone have been used to develop models, under the sponsorship of the U.S. EPA (133,145–150). The effects of methylmercury on rat brain development has also been used to illustrate a BBDR model for developmental toxicity (151).

Additional research is being carried out in the effort to delineate the contribution of exposure duration (152) and mechanisms of toxicity (153) to developmental toxicity risk assessment. In addition to the references already cited, two excellent books, which summarize current issues in risk assessment for developmental toxicity, are available (154,155).

VIII.   FUTURE DIRECTIONS FOR DEVELOPMENTAL TOXICOLOGY

The study of developmental toxicology prompts the asking of more questions than it can currently answer, thus suggesting many areas for future investigation. A concise summary of pertinent research needs, with emphasis on how these topics may be used to further clarify risk assessment, may be found in Hood (156). Topics of importance include mechanisms of developmental toxicity, interaction of chemicals (exposure to mixtures and exposure to a single chemical in the presence of others), preimplantation effects, the relative importance of maternal and developmental toxicity, paternally mediated effects, behavioral effects, and pharmacokinetic and pharmacodynamic effects. Future research programs in these areas promise to illuminate the unresolved issues in developmental toxicology to allow the identification and control of developmental toxicants.

REFERENCES

1. March of Dimes. (1997). March of Dimes Birth Defects Foundation Home Page, Birth Defects Information, http://www.modimes.org/index.htm. Accessed on March 4, 1998.
2. Wilson, J.G. (1973). Environment and Birth Defects. New York: Academic Press.
3. Wilson, J.G. and Fraser, F.C. (Eds.). (1977). Handbook of Teratology. New York: Plenum Press.
4. U.S. Environmental Protection Agency. (1989). Proposed amendments to the guidelines for the health assessment of suspect developmental toxicants. Fed. Regist. 51:34028.
5. Palmer, A.K. (1981). Regulatory requirements for reproductive toxicology: theory and practice. In: Developmental Toxicology. Edited by C. Kimmel and J. Buelke-Sam. New York: Plenum Press, pp. 259–287.
6. Palmer, A.K. (1976). Assessment of current test procedures. Environ. Health Perspect. 18:97–104.
7. Bignami, G., Bovett-Nitti, F., and Rosnati, V. (1962). Drugs and congenital abnormalities. Lancet 2:1333.
8. Goldenthal, E.I. (1966). Guidelines for Reproduction Studies for Safety Evaluation of Drugs for Human Use. U.S. Food and Drug Administration, Washington, D.C.
9. U.S. Environmental Protection Agency. (1987). Toxic Substances Control Act (TSCA) test guidelines: final rule. Fed. Regist. 50:39412.
10. U.S. Environmental Protection Agency. (1984). Pesticide Assessment Guidelines (FIFRA), Subdivision F Hazard Evaluation: Humans and Domestic Animals (Final Rule). NTIS (PB86-108958), Springfield, VA.
11. U.S. Environmental Protection Agency. (1988). Pesticide Assessment Guidelines, Subdivision F Hazard Evaluation: Humans and Domestic Animals, Series 83-3, Rat or Rabbit Developmental Toxicity Study, June 1986 (NTIS PB86-248184), as amended in Fed. Regist. 53(86)m/sect, 158.340, May 1988.

12. Ministry of Health and Welfare. (1984). Japanese Guidelines of Toxicity Studies, Notification No. 118 of the Pharmaceutical Affairs Bureau, Ministry of Health and Welfare. 2. Studies of the Effects of Drugs on Reproduction, Yakagyo Jiho Co., Ltd. Tokyo.

13. Department of Health and Social Security. (1974). United Kingdom, Committee on Safety of Medicines: Notes for Guidance on Reproductive Studies. Department of Health and Security, Great Britain.

14. U.S. Environmental Protection Agency. (1996). OPPTS, Health Effects Test Guidelines, OPPTS 870.3700, Prenatal Developmental Toxicity Study, Public Draft, U.S. Government Printing Office, Washington, D.C., February, 1996.

15. Tyl, R.W. and Marr, M.C. (1997). Developmental Toxicity Testing. In: Handbook of Developmental Toxicology. Edited by R.D. Hood. Boca Raton, FL: CRC Press, Chapter 7.

16. Manson, J.M. (1994). Testing of Pharmaceutical Agents for Reproductive Toxicity. In: Developmental Toxicology. Edited by C.A. Kimmel and J. Buelke-Sam. New York: Raven Press, Chapter 15.

17. Canadian Ministry of Health and Welfare. (1973). Health Protection Branch. The Testing of Chemicals for Carcinogenicity, Mutagenicity, and Teratogenicity, Ministry of Ottawa.

18. Organization for Economic Cooperation and Development. (OECD). (1981). Guideline for Testing of Chemicals: Teratogenicity. Director of Information, OECD, Paris, France.

19. European Economic Community. (1983). Council recommendation of 26 October 1983 concerning tests relating to the placing on the market of proprietary medicinal products. Official Journal of the European Communities. No. L332(83/571/EEC).

20. International Conference on Harmonization (ICH). (1994). Guideline on detection of toxicity to reproduction for medicinal products. Fed. Regist. 59(183):48746–48752, September 22, 1994.

21. U.S. Food and Drug Administration. (1988). Good Laboratory Practice Regulations for Nonclinical Laboratory Studies, Code of Federal Regulations (CFR), 229, Washington, D.C., April 1, 1988.

22. U.S. Environmental Protection Agency. (1989). Federal Insecticide, Fungicide, and Rodenticide Act (FIFRA) good laboratory practice standards; final rule. Fed. Regist. 54:34051 (40-CRF-792), August 17, 1989.

23. U.S. Environmental Protection Agency. (1989). Toxic Substances Control Act (TSCA), good laboratory practice standards; final rule. Fed. Regist. 54:34033, August 17, 1989.

24. NRC. (1996). National Research Council. Guide for the Care and Use of Laboratory Animals. Washington, D.C.: National Academy Press, 125 pp.

25. U.S. Environmental Protection Agency. (1986). Guidelines for the health assessment of suspect developmental toxicants. Fed. Regist. 51:34028–34040.

26. Khera, K.S. (1984). Maternal toxicity—A possible factor in fetal malformations in mice. Teratology 29:411–416.

27. Khera, K.S. (1985). Maternal toxicity: A possible etiological factor in embryo-fetal death and fetal malformations of rodent-rabbit species. Teratology 31:129–153.

28. Khera, K.S. (1987). Maternal toxicity in humans and animals: Effects on fetal development and criteria for detection. Teratogenesis Carcinogen. Mutagen. 7: 287–295.

29. Skalko, R.G., Johnson, E.M., et al. (1987). Concensus workshop on the evaluation of maternal and developmental toxicity. Work Group I report: Endpoints of maternal and developmental toxicity. Teratogenesis Carcinogen. Mutagen. 7:307–310.

30. Palmer, A.K., Kavlock, R.J., et al. (1987). Concensus workshop on the evaluation of maternal and developmental toxicity. Work Group II report: Study design considerations. Teratogenesis Carcinogen. Mutagen. 7:311–319.

31. Schardein, J.L. (1987). Approaches to defining the relationship of maternal and developmental toxicity. Teratogenesis Carcinogen. Mutagen. 7:255–271.

32. DeSesso, J.M. (1987). Maternal factors in developmental toxicity. Teratogenesis Carcinogen. Mutagen. 7:225–240.

33. Edwards, J.A. (1968). The external development of the rabbit and rat embryo. In: Advances in Teratology. Edited by D.H.M. Woolham. New York: Academic Press, Vol. 3, p. 239.

34. Staples, R.E. (1974). Detection of visceral alterations in mammalian fetuses. Teratology 9:37.

35. Wilson, J.G. (1965). Embryological considerations in teratology. In: Teratology: Principles and Techniques. Edited by J.G. Wilson and J. Warkany. Chicago: University of Chicago Press, p. 251.

36. Wilson, J.G. and Fraser, F.C. (Eds.). (1977). Handbook of Teratology. New York: Plenum Press, Vol. 4.

37. Barrow, M.V. and Taylor, W.J. (1969). A rapid method for detecting malformations in rat fetuses. J. Morphol. 127:291.

38. Stuckhardt, J.L. and Poppe, S.M. (1984). Fresh visceral examination of rat and rabbit fetuses used in teratogenicity testing. Teratogen. Carcinogen. Mutagen. 4m: 181.

39. Van Julsingha, E.B. and Bennett, C.G. (1977). A dissecting procedure for the detection of anomalies in the rabbit foetal head. In: Methods in Prenatal Toxicology. Edited by D. Neubert, H.J. Merker, and T.E. Kwasigrouch. Littleton, MA: PSG Publishing, p. 126.

40. Inouye, M. (1976). Differential staining of cartilage and bone in fetal mouse skeleton by alcian blue and alizarin red S. Congen. Anom. 16:171.

41. Kimmel, C.A. and Trammel, C. (1981). A rapid procedure for routine double staining of cartilage and bone in fetal and adult animals. Stain Technol. 56:271.

42. Peltzer, M.A. and Schardein, J.L. (1966). A convenient method for processing fetuses for skeletal staining. Stain Technol. 41:300.

43. Crary, D.D. (1962). Modified benzyl alcohol clearing of Alizarin-stained specimens without loss of flexibility. Stain Technol. 37:124.

44. Marr, M.C., Myers, C.B., George, J.D., and Price, C.J. (1988). Comparison of single and double staining for evaluation of skeletal development: the effects of ethylene glycol (EG) in CD$^®$ rats. Teratology 37:476.

45. Marr, M.C., Price, C.J., Myers, C.J., and Morrissey, R.E. (1992). Developmental stages of the CD$^®$ (Sprague-Dawley) rat skeleton after maternal exposure to ethylene glycol. Teratology 46:169.

46. U.S. Environmental Protection Agency. (1991). Pesticide Assessment Guidelines—Subdivision F, Hazard Evaluation: Human and Domestic Animals, Addendum 10, Neurotoxicity Series 81, 82, and 83: PB 91-154617, National Technical Information Service, Springfield, VA, March 1991.

47. Bates, H.K., Cunny, H.C., and Kebede, G.A. (1997). Developmental Neurotoxicity Testing Methodology. In: Handbook of Developmental Toxicology. Edited by R.D. Hood. Boca Raton, FL: CRC Press, Chapter 9.

48. Hood, R.D. (1989). Paternally Mediated Effects. In: Developmental Toxicology. Risk Assessment and the Future. Edited by R.D. Hood. New York: Van Nostrand Reinhold, Chapter 8, p. 77.

49. Mattison, D.R. and Olshan, A.F. (Eds.). (1994). Male-Mediated Developmental Toxicity. New York: Plenum Press.

50. Friedler, G. (1993). Developmental toxicology: male-mediated effects. In: Occupational and Environmental Reproductive Hazards: A Guide for Clinicians. Mary Ingraham Bunting Inst., Radcliff Coll., Cambridge, MA, Chapter 5, p. 52.

51. NTP (1989). Reproductive toxicity testing by continuous breeding test protocol in Swiss (CD-1®) mice. National Toxicology Program Technical Document. NTIS Accession No. PB89 15425/AS.

52. Shelby, M.D., Russell, L.B., Woychik, R.P., Allen, J.W., Wiley, L.M., and Favor, J.B. (1994). Laboratory research methods in male-mediated developmental toxicity. In: Male-Mediated Developmental Toxicity. Edited by D.R. Mattison and A.F. Olshan. New York: Plenum Press, p. 379.

53. Wyrobek, A.J., Anderson, D., Lewis, S., Nagao, T., Perreault, S., Robaire, B., and Schrader, S. (1994). Biomarkers and health endpoints of developmental toxicology of paternal origin: summary of working group discussions. In: Male-Mediated Developmental Toxicity. Edited by D.R. Mattison and A.F. Olshan. New York: Plenum Press, p. 359.

54. Wyrobek, A.J. (1994). Methods and concepts in detecting abnormal reproductive outcomes of paternal origin. In: Male-Mediated Developmental Toxicity. Edited by D.R. Mattison and A.F. Olshan. New York: Plenum Press, p. 1.

55. Olshan, A.F. and Schnitzer, P.G. (1994). Paternal occupation and birth defects. In: Male-Mediated Developmental Toxicity. Edited by D.R. Mattison and A.F. Olshan. New York: Plenum Press, p. 153.

56. O'Flaherty, E.J. (1994). Physiologically based pharmacokinetic models in developmental toxicology. Risk Analysis 14:605–611.

57. O'Flaherty, E.J. and Clarke, D.O. (1994). Pharmacokinetic/Pharmacodynamic approaches for developmental toxicology. In: Developmental Toxicology, 2nd Edition. Edited by C.A. Kimmel and J. Buelke-Sam. New York: Raven Press, Chapter 8, p. 215.

58. Clarke, D.O. (1993). Technology Review: pharmacokinetic studies in developmental toxicology: practical considerations and approaches. Toxicol. Methods 3: 223–251.

59. O'Flaherty, E.J. and Scott, W. (1997). Use of toxicokinetics in developmental toxicology. In: Handbook of Developmental Toxicology. Edited by R.D. Hood. Boca Raton, FL: CRC Press, Chapter 13.

60. O'Flaherty, E.J., Scott, W., Schreiner, C., and Beliles, R.P. (1992). A physiologi-

cally based kinetic model of rat and mouse gestation: disposition of a weak acid. Toxicol. Appl. Pharmacol. 112:245–246.

61. Fisher, J.W., Whittaker, T.A., Taylor, D.H., Clewell, H.J. III, and Andersen, M.E. (1989). Physiologically based pharmacokinetic modeling of the pregnant rat: a multiroute exposure model for trichloroethylene and its metabolite, trichloroacetic acid. Toxicol. Appl. Pharmacol. 99:395–414.

62. Olanoff, L.S. and Anderson, J.M. (1980). Controlled release of tetracycline-III: a physiological pharmacokinetic model of the pregnant rat. J. Pharmacokinet. Biopharm. 8:599–620.

63. Gabrielsson, J.L., Johanson, P., Bondesson, U., and Paalzow, L.K. (1985). Analysis of methadone disposition in the pregnant rat by means of a physiological flow model. J. Pharmacokinet. Biopharm. 13:355–372.

64. Gabrielsson, J.L. and Paalzow, L.K. (1983). A physiological pharmacokinetic model for morphine disposition in the pregnant rat. J. Pharmacokinet. Biopharm. 11:147–163.

65. Gabrielsson, J.L., Paalzow, L.K., and Nordstrom, L. (1984). A physiologically based pharmacokinetic model for theophylline disposition in the pregnant and nonpregnant rat. J. Pharmacokinet. Biopharm. 12:149–165.

66. Gabrielsson, J.L. and Groth, T. (1988). An extended physiological pharmacokinetic model of methadone disposition in the rat: validation and sensitivity analysis. J. Pharmacokinet. Biopharm. 16:183–201.

67. O'Flaherty, E.J., Scott, W.J., Nau, H., and Beliles, R.P. (1992). Simulation of valproic acid kinetics in primate and rodent pregnancy by means of physiologically-based models. Teratology 43:457.

68. O'Flaherty, E.J. and Andriot, M.D. (1992). Predicting blood lead during human pregnancy. Toxicologist 12:212.

69. Clarke, D.O., Elswick, B.A., Welsch, F., and Conolly, R.B. (1993). Pharmacokinetics of 2-methoxyethanol and 2-methoxyacetic acid in the pregnant mouse: a physiologically-based mathematical model. Toxicol. Appl. Pharmacol. 121:239–252.

70. Wilson, J.G. (1977). Current status of teratology: general principles and mechanisms derived from animal studies. In: Handbook of Teratology: General Principles and Etiology. Edited by J.G. Wilson and F.C. Fraser. New York: Plenum Press, Vol. 1, p. 47.

71. Hood, R.D. (1989). Mechanisms of Developmental Toxicity. In: Developmental Toxicology: Risk Assessment and the Future. Edited by R.D. Hood. New York: Van Nostrand Reinhold, Chapter, 4, p. 51.

72. Kimmel, G.L. (1981). Developmental aspects of chemical interaction with cellular receptors. In: Developmental Toxicology. Edited by C. Kimmel and J. Buelke-Sam. New York: Plenum Press, pp. 115–130.

73. Pratt, R.M. (1985). Hormones, growth factors, and their receptors in normal and abnormal prenatal development. In: Issues and Reviews in Teratology. Edited by H. Kalter. New York: Plenum Press, Chapter 2, pp. 189–217.

74. Jurand, A. (1985). The interference of naloxone hydrochloride in the teratogenic activity of opiates. Teratology 31:235–240.

75. Stertz, H., Sponer, G., Neubert, P., and Hebold, G. (1985). A postulated mecha-

nism of beta-sympathomimetic induction of rib and limb anomalies in rat fetuses. Teratology 31:401–412.

76. Bernfeld, M. (1983). Mechanisms of congenital malformations. In: The Biological Basis of Reproductive and Developmental Medicine. Edited by J.B. Warshaw. New York: Elsevier Biomedical, pp. 143–154.

77. Scott, Jr., W.J. (1977). Cell death and reduced proliferative rate. In: Handbook of Teratology: Mechanisms and Pathogenesis. Edited by J.G. Wilson and F.C. Fraser. New York: Plenum Press, Vol. 2, pp. 81–98.

78. Wise, L.D. and Scott, Jr., W.J. (1982). Incorporation of 5-bromo-2'deoxyuridine into mesenchymal limb-bud cells destined to die: relationship to polydactyly induction in rats. J. Embryol. Exp. Morph. 72:125–141.

79. Yamada, K.M. (1977). Cell morphometric movements. In: Handbook of Teratology: Mechanism and Pathogenesis. Edited by J.G. Wilson and F.C. Fraser. New York: Plenum Press, Vol. 2, pp. 199–230.

80. Pratt, R.M., Goulding, E.H., and Abbott, B.D. (1987). Retinoic acid inhibits migration of cranial neural crest cells in the cultured mouse embryo. J. Craniofacial Genet. Devel. Biol. 7:205–217.

81. Saxon, L. (1977). Abnormal cellular and tissue interactions. In: Handbook of Teratology: Mechanisms and Pathogenesis. Edited by J.G. Wilson and F.C. Fraser. New York: Plenum Press, Vol. 2, pp. 171–197.

82. Opitz, J.M. (1979). The developmental field concept in clinical genetics. In: Developmental Aspects of Craniofacial Dysmorphology. Edited by M. Melnick and R. Jorgensen. New York: Alan R. Liss, pp. 107–112.

83. Faustman, E.M., Ponce, R.A., Seeley, M.R., and Whittaker, S.G. (1997). Experimental Approaches to Evaluate Mechanisms of Developmental Toxicity. In: Handbook of Developmental Toxicology. Edited by R.D. Hood. Boca Raton, FL: CRC Press, Chapter 2.

84. Schwetz, B.A., Morrissey, R.E., Welsch, F., and Kavlock, R.A. (1991). In vitro teratology. Environ. Health Perspect. 94:265–268.

85. Kimmel, G.L. and Kochhar, D.M. (1990). In Vitro Methods in Developmental Toxicology. Boca Raton, FL: CRC Press.

86. Welsch, F. (1992). In vitro approaches to the elucidation of mechanisms of chemical teratogenesis. Teratology 46:3.

87. Daston, G.P. and D'Amato, R.A. (1989). In vitro techniques in teratology. In: Benchmarks: Alternative Methods in Toxicology. Edited by M.A. Mehlman. Princeton, NJ: Princeton Scientific, pp. 79–109.

88. Fantel, A.G. (1982). Culture of whole rodent embryos in teratogen screening. Teratogen. Carconogen. Mutagen. 2:231.

89. Sadler, T.W., Horton, W.E., and Warner, C.W. (1982). Whole Embryo culture: a screening technique for teratogens? Teratogen. Carconogen. Mutagen. 2:243.

90. Spielman, H. and Vogel, R. (1989). Unique role of studies on preimplantation embryos to understand mechanisms of embryotoxicity in early pregnancy. Crit. Rev. Toxicol. 20:51.

91. Lawitts, J.A. and Biggers, J.D. (1993). Culture of preimplantation embryos. Methods Enzymol. 225:153.

92. Pratt, H.P.M. (1987). Isolation, culture, and manipulation of preimplantation

mouse embryos. In: Mammalian Development: A Practical Approach. Edited by
M. Monk. Washington, D.C.: IRL Press, p. 13.

93. Kimber, S.J., Waterhouse, R., and Lindenberg, S. (1993). In vitro models for
implantation of the mammalian embryo. In: Preimplantation Embryo Development. Edited by B.A. Bavister. New York: Springer-Verlag, p. 244.

94. Freeman, S.J., Coakley, M.E., and Brown, N.A. (1987). Postimplantation embryo
culture for studies of teratogenesis. In: Biochemical Toxicology: A Practical Approach. Edited by K. Snell and B. Mullock. Oxford: IRL Press, p. 4.

95. Kaufman, M.H. (1990). Morphological stages of postimplantation embryonic development. In: Postimplantation Mammalian Embryos: A Practical Approach. Edited by A.J. Copp and D.L. Cockroft. Oxford: IRL Press, pp. 4 and 81.

96. New, D.A.T. (1971). Methods for the culture of postimplantation embryos of rodents. In: Methods in Mammalian Embryology. Edited by J.C. Daniel, Jr. San
Francisco: W.H. Freeman, p. 305.

97. Cockroft, D.L. (1990). Dissection and culture of postimplantation embryos. In:
Postimplantation Mammalian Embryos: A Practical Approach. Edited by A.J.
Copp and D.L. Cockroft. Oxford: IRL Press, pp. 1 and 15.

98. Johnson, E.M. (1980). A subvertebrate system for rapid determination of potential
teratogenic hazards. J. Environ. Pathol. Toxicol. 2:153.

99. Johnson, E.M., Gorman, R.M., Gabel, B.E.G., and George, M.E. (1982). The hydra attenuata system for detection of teratogenic hazards. Teratogen. Carcinogen.
Mutagen. 2:263.

100. Dumont, J.N., Schultz, T.W., Buchanan, M., and Kao, G. (1983). Frog embryo
teratogenesis assay: Xenopus (FETAX)—a short-term assay applicable to complex environmental mixtures. In: Short-Term Bioassays in the Analysis of Complex Environmental Mixtures III. Edited by M.D. Waters, S.S. Sandu, J. Lewtas,
L. Claxton, N. Chernoff, and S. Nesnow. New York: Plenum Press, p. 393.

101. Bournias-Vardiabasis, N. and Teplitz, R.L. (1982). Use of Drosophila embryo cell
cultures as an in vitro teratogen assay. Teratogen. Carcinogen. Mutagen. 2:333.

102. Cameron, I.L., Lawrence, W.C., and Lum, J.B. (1985). Medaka eggs as a model
system for screening potential teratogens. Prog. Clin. Biol. Res. 163C:239–243.

103. Goss, L.B. and Sabourin, T.D. (1985). Utilization of alternative species for toxicity testing: an overview. J. Appl. Toxicol. 5(4):193–219.

104. Sabourin, T.D., Faulk, R.T., and Goss, L.B. (1985). The efficacy of three nonmammalian test systems in the identification of chemical teratogens. J. Appl. Toxicol. 5(4):227–233.

105. Baumann, M. and Sander, K. (1984). Bipartite axiation follow incomplete epiboly
in zebrafish embryos treated with chemical teratogens. J. Exp. Zool. 230(3):363–
376.

106. Shepard, T.H. and Pious, D. (1978). Cell, tissue and organ culture as teratologic
tools. In: Handbook of Teratology. Edited by J.G. Wilson and F.C. Fraser. New
York: Plenum Press, pp. 4 and 71.

107. Friedman, L. (1987). Teratological research using in vitro systems: II. Rodent
limb bud culture system. Environ. Health Perspect. 72:211.

108. Neubert, D. and Barrach, H.J. (1977). Techniques applicable to study morphometric differentiation of limb buds in organ culture. In: Methods in Prenatal Toxicol-

ogy. Edited by D. Neubert, H.J. Merker, and T.E. Kwasigrouch. Littleton, MA: PSG Publishing, p. 241.

109. Aydelotte, M.B. and Kochhar, D.M. (1972). Development of mouse limb buds in organ culture: chondrogenesis in the presence of a proline analog. 1-azetidine-2-carboxylic acid. Dev. Biol. 28:191.

110. Manson, J.M. and Simons, R. (1979). In vitro metabolism of cyclophosphamide in limb bud culture. Teratology 19:149–158.

111. Kochhar, D.M. and Aydelotte, M.B. (1974). Susceptible stages and abnormal morphogenesis in the developing mouse limb, analyzed in organ culture after transplacental exposure to vitamin A (retinoic acid). J. Embryol. Exp. Morphol. 31:721.

112. Pratt, R.M., Dencker, L., and Diewert, V.M. (1984). 2,3,7,8-Tetrachlorodibenzo-p dioxin-induced cleft palate in the mouse: evidence for alterations in palatal shelf fusion. Teratogen. Carcinogen. Mutagen. 4:427.

113. Pratt, R.M. (1985). Receptor-dependent mechanisms of glucocorticoid and dioxin-induced cleft palate. Environ. Health Perspect. 61:35.

114. Mino, Y., Mizusawa, H., and Shiota, K. (1994). Effects of anticonvulsant drugs on fetal mouse palates cultured in vitro. Reprod. Toxicol. 8:225.

115. Abbott, B.D., Harris, M.W., and Birnbaum, L.S. (1989). Etiology of retinoic acid-induced cleft palate varies with the embryonic stage. Teratology 40:533.

116. Abbott, B.D. and Buckalew, A.R. (1992). Embryonic palatal response to teratogens in serum-free organ culture. Teratology 45:369.

117. Shiota, K., Kosazuma, T., Klug, S., and Neubert, D. (1990). Development of the fetal mouse palate in suspension organ culture. Acta Anat. 137:59.

118. Stevenson, G.B. and Williams, K.E. (1987). Ethanol-induced inhibition of pinocytosis and proteolysis in rat yolk sac in vitro. Development 99:247.

119. Lerman, S., Koszalka, T.R., Jensen, M., Andrew, C.L., Beckman, D.A., and Brent, R.L. (1986). In vitro studies on the effect of yolk sac antisera on the functions of the visceral yolk sac. I. Pinocytosis and transport of small molecules. Teratology 34:335.

120. Armstrong, R.C. and Elias, J.J. (1968). Development of embryonic rat eyes in organ culture. II. An in vitro approach to teratogenic mechanisms. J. Embryol. Exp. Morphol. 19:407.

121. Fisher, K.R.S. and Fedoroff, S. (1978). The development of chick spinal cord in tissue culture. In Vitro, 14, 878.

122. Serra, R., Pelton, R.W., and Moses, H.L. (1994). TGFb1 inhibits branching morphogenesis and N-myc expression in lung bud organ cultures. Development 120: 2153.

123. Coon, H.G. (1966). Clonal stability and phenotypic expression of chick cartilage cells in vitro. Proc. Natl. Acad. Sci. 55:66.

124. Cahn, R.D. and Cahn, M.B. (1966). Heritability of cellular differentiation: clonal growth and expression of differentiation in retinal pigment cells in vitro. Proc. Natl. Acad. Sci. 55:106.

125. Eguchi, G. and Okada, T.S. (1973). Differentiation of lens tissue from the progeny of chick retinal pigment cells cultured in vitro: a demonstration of a switch of cell types in clonal cell culture. Proc. Natl. Acad. Sci. 70:1495.

126. Davis, W.L., Crawford, L.A., Cooper, O.J., Farmer, G.R., Thomas, D.L., and

Freeman, B.L. (1990). Ethanol induces the generation of reactive free radicals by neural crest cells in vitro. J. Craniofac. Genet. Dev. Biol. 10:277.

127. Flint, O.P. and Orton, T.C. (1984). An in vitro assay for teratogens with cultures of rat embryo midbrain and limb bud cells. Toxicol. Appl. Pharmacol. 76:383.

128. Kimmel, C.A., Kimmel, G.L., and Frankos, V. (Eds.). (1986). Interagency Regulatory Liaison Group workshop on reproductive toxicity risk assessment. Environ. Health Perspect. 66:193–211.

129. National Research Council. (1983). Risk Assessment in the Federal Government: Managing the Process. Washington, D.C.: National Academy Press.

130. U.S. Environmental Protection Agency. (1991). Guidelines for developmental toxicity risk assessment: notice. Fed. Regist. 56:63798–63826.

131. Kimmel, C.A. and Kimmel, G.L. (1994). Risk assessment for developmental toxicity. In: Developmental Toxicology. Edited by C.A. Kimmel and J. Buelke-Sam. New York: Raven Press, Chapter 17, pp. 429–453.

132. Kimmel, C.A. and Kimmel, G.L. (1997). Principles of developmental toxicity risk assessment. In: Handbook of Developmental Toxicology. Edited by R.D. Hood. CRC Press, Inc., Boca Raton, FL, Chapter 21.

133. Kavlock, R.J. and Kimmel, C.A. (1992). New approaches to developmental toxicity risk assessment at the U.S. Environmental Protection Agency. In: Risk Assessment of Prenatally-Induced Adverse Health Effects. Edited by D. Neubert, R.J. Kavlock, H.-J. Merker, and J. Klein. Berlin, Germany: Springer-Verlag, pp. 113–126.

134. Crump, K.S. (1984). A new method for determining allowable daily intakes. Fundam. Appl. Toxicol. 4:854–871.

135. Kodell, R.L., Howe, R.B., Chen, J.J., and Gaylor, D.W. (1991). Mathematical modeling of reproductive and developmental toxic effects for quantitative risk assessment. Risk Anal. 11:583–590.

136. Kupper, L.L., Portier, C., Hogan, M.D., and Yamamoto, E. (1986). The impact of litter effects on dose-response modeling in teratology. Biometrics 42:85–98.

137. Rai, K. and Van Ryzin, J. (1985). A dose response model for teratological experiments involving quantal responses. Biometrics 41:1–10.

138. Williams, P.L. and Ryan, L.M. (1997). Dose-response models for developmental toxicity. In: Handbook of Developmental Toxicology. Edited by R.D. Hood. Boca Raton, FL: CRC Press, Chapter 20.

139. Ryan, L.M., Catalano, P.J., Kimmel, C.A., and Kimmel, G.L. (1991). On the relationship between fetal weight and malformation in developmental toxicity studies. Teratology 44:215–223.

140. Catalano, P.J., Scharfstein, D.O., Ryan, L.M., Kimmel, C.A., and Kimmel, G.L. (1993). A statistical model for fetal death, fetal weight, and malformation in developmental toxicity studies. Teratology 47:281–290.

141. Faustman, E.M., Allen, B.C., Kavlock, R.J., and Kimmel, C.A. (1994). Dose-response assessment for developmental toxicity: I. Characterization of data base and determination of NOAELs. Fundam. Appl. Toxicol. 23:478–486.

142. Allen, B.C., Kavlock, R.J., Kimmel, C.A., and Faustman, E.M. (1994). Dose-response assessment for developmental toxicity: II. Comparison of generic benchmark dose estimates with NOAELs. Fundam. Appl. Toxicol. 23:487–495.

143. Allen, B.C., Kavlock, R.J., Kimmel, C.A., and Faustman, E.M. (1994). Dose-response assessment for developmental toxicity: III. Statistical models. Fundam. Appl. Toxicol. 23:497.

144. Kavlock, R.J., Allen, B.C., Kimmel, C.A., and Faustman, E.M. (1995). Dose-response assessment for developmental toxicity: IV: Benchmark doses for fetal weight changes. Fundam. Appl. Toxicol. 26:211.

145. U.S. Environmental Protection Agency. (1990). Research to improve health risk assessments (RIHRA) program. EPA Report No. EPA/600/9-90/038. Washington, D.C., Office of Research and Development.

146. Lau, C.S., Cameron, A.M., Rogers, J.M., Shuey, D.L., and Kavlock, R.J. (1992). Development of biologically-based dose-response models: correlations between developmental toxicity of 5-fluorouracil (5-FU) and its inhibition of thymidylate synthetase (TS) activity in the rat embryo. Teratology 45:457.

147. Rogers, J.M., Setzer, R.W., Shuey, D.L. et al. (1992). Development of biologically-based dose-response (BBDR) models: 5-fluorouracil (5-FU) dose response based on fetal outcome and linkage to mechanistic endpoints. Teratology 45:457.

148. Shuey, D.L., Zucker, R.M., Elstein, K.H., and Rogers, J.M. (1993). Biologically-based dose-response (BBDR) modeling in developmental toxicity: fetal anemia following exposure to 5-fluorouracil (5-FU) in utero. Toxicologist 13:255.

149. Shuey, D.L., Setzer, R.W., Lau, C., Zucker, R.M., Elstein, K.H., Narotsky, M.G., Kavlock, R.M., and Rogers, J.M. (1995). Biological modeling of 5-fluorouracil developmental toxicity. Toxicology 102:207–213.

150. LaBorde, J.B., Hansen, D.K., Young, J.F., Sheehan, D.M., and Holson, R.R. (1992). Prenatal dexamethasone exposure in rats: effects of dose, age at exposure and drug-induced hypophagia on malformations and fetal organ weights. Fundam. Appl. Toxicol. 19:545–554.

151. Lerous, B.G., Leisenring, W.M., Moolgavkar, S.H., and Faustman, E.M. (1996). A biologically-based does-response model for developmental toxicity. Risk Analysis 16:449–458.

152. Kimmel, G.L., Williams, P.L., Ryan, L.M., Kimmel, C.A., and Tudor, N. (1993). The effects of temperature and duration of exposure on in vitro development and response-surface modeling of their interaction. Teratology 47:401.

153. Kimmel, C.A., Generoso, W.M., Thomas, R.D., and Bakshi, K.S. (1993). A new frontier in understanding the mechanisms of developmental abnormalities. Toxicol. Appl. Pharmacol. 119:159–165.

154. Neubert, D., Kavlock, R.J., Merker, H.-J., and Klein, J. (Eds.). (1992). Risk Assessment of Prenatally-Induced Adverse Health Effects. Berlin, Germany: Springer-Verlag.

155. Hood, R.D. (Ed.). (1989). Developmental Toxicology. Risk Assessment and the Future. New York: Van Nostrand Reinhold.

156. Hood, R.D. (1989). Summary of Research Needs. In: Developmental Toxicology. Risk Assessment and the Future. Edited by R.D. Hood. New York: Van Nostrand Reinhold, Chapter 3, p. 11.

12

Assessment and Modeling of the Biological Hazards of Combustion Products

Shayne Cox Gad
Gad Consulting Services, Raleigh, North Carolina

John L. Orr
Purdue Pharma L.P., Ardsley, New York

Walter G. Switzer
Consultant, San Antonio, Texas

I. INTRODUCTION

Synthetic polymers, because of their chemical composition and the chemistry of additives included in them, have the potential, when burned, to release smoke and gases that are qualitatively different from those commonly produced by such natural polymers as wood, cotton, and wool (1,2). Also, the rates of thermal decomposition (and production of decomposition products) of such synthetic materials in a fire may be greater than those of natural materials.

Yet since the Second World War synthetic polymers have been used increasingly in modern society. Buildings, home furnishings, aircraft interiors, and automobiles all readily reflect this trend. All synthetic polymers may be the site of, or contribute to, a fire. Thus, evaluating the health hazards of the decomposition products formed when plastics are heated (though a relatively new field) is very important. Though early work on simple pyrolysis product toxicity is as much as 35 years old, the oldest true references to combustion toxicology go back only to the early 1950s (3). Yet today it has become a high priority area for testing within toxicology, which is itself a high priority field. It has had its own annual conferences, a multitude of study committees (both in industry and

409

government), it is the subject of various foreign, national, state, and municipal regulations, and stands on the verge of becoming the subject of federal regulation. Why?

The are currently some 5,575,000 unintentional fires annually in the U.S. alone, of which only 10% require action by fire departments. Currently, more than 4,700 people die each year in these fires and, as will be demonstrated later, there is good reason to believe that some 80% of these deaths have smoke inhalation (and not the flames themselves) as the primary cause of death (4,5). We also have a good deal of data to suggest that the proportion dying due to the product inhalation is increasing annually.

It should be remembered, however, that annual fatality rates from fires have actually been going down. In 1933 about 10,000 people lost their lives because of fires. It was observed and commented upon that many of these victims were not burned but succumbed to the effects of "smoke" and gases, but when deaths from this source were reported, it is notable that almost never was it determined if poisonous gas or gases caused the fatality (6).

Large fires with multiple toxic inhalant-caused deaths (such as the MGM Grand, White Plains Stouffers, Houston Westchase Hilton, and Sao Paulo Brazil high-rise fires) have renewed public concern, but should be recognized as not being unique since 1978. Four earlier large fires with similar patterns come to mind:

- Newport, Kentucky night club (1978)
- Maury County, Tennessee jail (1977)
- Coconut Grove night club (1942)
- Cleveland Clinic (1929)

Additionally, fire-resultant deaths have occurred in 21 postcrash commercial aircraft since 1965. Most recently, an aircraft fire with resulting smoke led to the September 1998 crash of a Swiss Air flight off Nova Scotia with the loss of all aboard.

The world has turned increasingly to synthetic polymers for use in clothes, furnishings, appliances, wall coverings, furniture, carpets, and homes. Not only are these materials less expensive, but in many cases they are more durable, lighter, and stronger than the natural products that were used in earlier days. With the addition of fire and flame retardants, their fire performance in buildings is superior. The problem is that when they burn, they can generate gas phase decomposition products that are considerably more toxic than natural products (primarily wood).

Wood generates a multitude of decomposition products when burned. When the combustion is incomplete, the major product in terms of toxicity is carbon monoxide (CO). CO acts in biological systems by competing with oxygen for binding with hemoglobin. When so bound carboxyhemoglobin (COHb) is formed. As CO has a greater affinity than oxygen for hemoglobin, it competes favorably with and is difficult for oxygen to displace.

Carbon monoxide is the most prevalent toxic component of smoke, and is responsible for the majority of deaths attributed to inhalation in fires or to asphyxia. Other highly toxic gases and aerosols are also produced, however, depending on the composition of the material and the combustion conditions.

The body depends on hemoglobin (in the form of a complex with oxygen called oxyhemoglobin) to transport oxygen to its tissues: if too much hemoglobin (50% or more) is tied up as carboxyhemoglobin then the results, in progressive order, are drowsiness, unconsciousness, and finally death.

The major concern, however, is that the synthetic polymers will either generate a greater amount of carbon monoxide (than wood) under fire conditions or that they will generate quantitatively worse toxic materials (hereafter called for the purposes of this book, toxicants) than wood. Concern initially centered largely on the generation of hydrogen cyanide or of isocyanates (7), particularly by the various nitrogen containing polymers. Cyanide is of such great concern because it causes death (by a mechanism called histotoxic hypoxia, which involves interference with the cytochrome system in the cells, therefore starving the body of oxygen on a molecular level) at very low levels (1 microgram per mL being a lethal level in the blood).

There now exists a fair body of information both on which gases people are exposed to in fires and what causes kill people in fires. The results of nine of these studies are detailed in Table 1.

The picture from all of these reports is not clear, especially when the results of experimental large scale fires conducted on purely plastic environments (such as the study of Boudene et al. (1978) on a primarily polyvinylchloride (PVC) fire) show that HCl can be a significant threat on its own. What is clear is that (1) decomposition products are a threat; (2) at this point carbon monoxide is the chief life threatening toxicant encountered in fires; and (3) the threat is not, however, limited to carbon monoxide, cyanide, and HCl.

Additionally, fires (or different stages of a fire) can produce vastly different products depending on temperature, rates of temperature change, available oxygen, and size. Table 2 presents one classification of fire types, as derived by an ISO (International Standards Organization) panel.

II. BACKGROUND

Combustion toxicology has advanced significantly in recent years. In the past, combustion focused on estimates of lethal potency of individual materials and different methodologies vied for supremacy as the method of choice for the assessment of toxic potency. Now there is a better understanding of the role of combustion toxicology in the overall process of fire hazard assessment. In general, the combustion toxicity potency of a material is seen not as a fixed intrinsic property of a material, but as a property whose manifestation is a function of several other factors. Many of these factors are parameters of combustion such

Table 1 Human Exposures and Autopsy Data from Fires

Subject Population	References	Findings
New York City Fire Fatalities	8,9	83% of all casualties resulted from toxicant inhalation. 70% of the deaths resulting from toxicant inhalation were due to carbon monoxide.
State of Maryland Fatalities	9	Of those dying within six hours, 50% died from CO inhalation; HCN and HCl did not appear to be the causes of death in a significant number of cases. In males 40 to 60 years of age, there was a high correlation between death and blood alcohol levels.
Boston City Fire Fighters	10	Analysis of multiple samples of the atmospheres firefighters were exposed to showed CO to be an acute hazard and oxygen depletion not to be significant. HCl was present in only 8 or 90 samples, while HCN (at low concentration) was present in half the samples. CO_2 and NO_2 were not present in significant amounts.
Glasgow, Scotland Fire Fatalities	11	Blood samples from fatalities identified more than 60 volatile neutral organics. Propriontrile was identified as being present in measurable quantities in many victims.
Maury County, Tennessee Jailhouse Fire	12	High levels of both NCN and CO were present in victims, but in no case was HCN present in a concentration high enough to be lethal on its own.
English Fire Fatalities (1957–1974)	13	The proportion of fire casualties due to smoke and toxic gas inhalation had tripled over this 17 year period, and now represents more than half of all fire causalities.

Table 1 Continued

Subject Population	References	Findings
Munich Fire Fatalities	14	Studied cyanide concentrations in blood of fire victims. The importance of HCN has increased over the years.
Cleveland, City Flash Fire Fatalities	15	From a small pool of flash fire victims, investigators determined that in this special case carboxyhemoglobin was not connected with the deaths.
Houston Westchase Hilton Fire Fatalities	16	Placement and autopsies on twelve fatalities from this 1982 fire indicated multiple contributing factors in deaths.

as the type of ignition, oxygen levels, adjacent materials, and time–temperature profile. Figures 1, 2, and 3 illustrate the influence of the three most common factors in a fire (carbon monoxide, temperature, and oxygen deprivation) on incapacitation and lethality in a number of test species. Note that there are not great differences between species. Other factors include the test species, and in the case of polytetrafluoroethylene (PTFE), the geometry of the combustion apparatus.

Table 2 Classification of Fires

Fire	Oxygen in Fire Plume Near Fire	CO_2/CO Ratio*	Temperature*	Irradiance onto Sample** kW/m^2
Decomposition				
Smoldering (self-sustained)	21	N/A	<100	N/A
Nonflaming (oxidative)	5–21	N/A	<500	<25
Nonflaming (pyrolytic)	<5	N/A	<1000	N/A
Developing fire (flaming)	10–15	100–200	400–600	20–40
Fully developed (flaming)				
Relatively low ventilation	1–5	<10	600–900	40–70
Relatively high ventilation	5–10	<100	600–1200	50–150

*General environmental condition (average) with compartment.
**Incident irradiance on to sample (average).
Source: ISO, 1989.

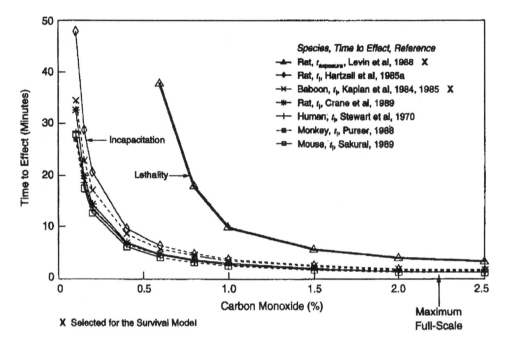

Figure 1 The influence of carbon monoxide in combustion test atmospheres on times-to-incapacitation and death in seven studies performed on five different species.

Modeling of combustion toxicity has advanced and now the concept of the fractional effective dose (FED) and multiple contributions to the toxic effect are embodied in the so-called N-gas models that endeavor to account for combustion toxicity as the sum of contributions of the major fire gases. The major fire gases are: carbon monoxide (CO), carbon dioxide (CO_2), hydrogen cyanide (HCN), lack of oxygen (O_2), and the halogen acids hydrochloric acid (HCl), hydrobromic acid (HBr), and hydrofluoric acid (HF). As in most inhalation situations, toxicity is influenced not just by what gases are present and at what concentration, but also by how long an exposure lasts. The concept of incremental dose over time, illustrated in Figure 4, is central to understanding the hazard presented by a fire situation.

In the past couple of years, there has been movement on the standards front and there are now very similar standards from the American National Standards Institute (ANSI), the International Standards Organization (ISO), and the National Fire Protection Association (NFPA).

The contemporary toxicologist working on a combustion toxicity related issue needs to understand the general role of toxicity assessment in the hazard

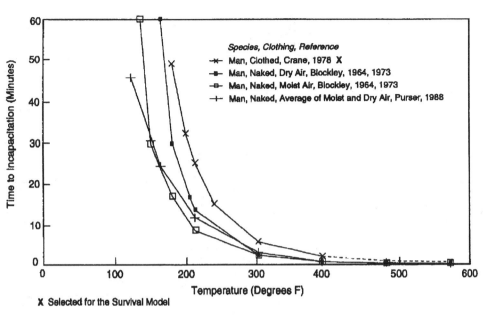

X Selected for the Survival Model

Figure 2   The influence of temperature of combustion test atmospheres on time-to-incapacitation in man under different conditions of clothing and humidity.

assessment process and practical aspects of the execution and interpretation of the tests outlined in the various standards organization documents.

A. Rules of Combustion Toxicology

The purpose of this chapter is to summarize the approaches to and uses of contemporary combustion toxicology. The following rules are generalizations based on the authors' experience and assessment of the combustion toxicology literature.

There is not a combustion toxicology issue with materials that do not pyrolyze, burn, or outgas.

Combustion toxicology is only part of the fire hazard assessment process.

There is not a single "combustion toxicity test" that is optimal for all situations.

Effective assessment is likely to involve biologists, chemists, and engineers, and, perhaps, other types of researchers as well.

All combustion research program sponsors have agendas. These agendas can include: 1) protection of existing markets, 2) penetration of new

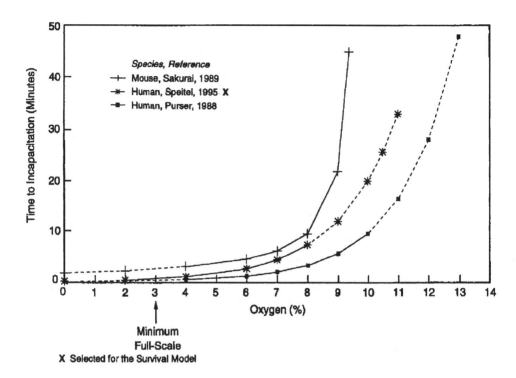

Figure 3 The influence of oxygen concentration in combustion test atmospheres on time-to-incapacitation in humans and mice.

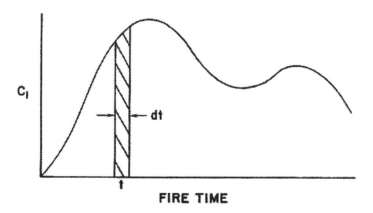

Figure 4 Concept of incremental dose ($C_i dt$).

markets, 3) protection of the potentially involuntarily exposed public, 4) litigation defense.

The scale of combustion toxicology research performed is usually related to the size of the issue under investigation. In other words, only matters that research sponsors considered to have a large potential impact, either economic or public safety, include full-scale fire testing.

There is a low but real possibility that a material may have an idiosyncratic unexpected toxicity. The only technical protection against this situation is biological testing in animal model systems. The best legal protection against legal claims following human exposure (and injury) to this combustion product is to have an extremely well-documented comprehensive assessment program, i.e., to have demonstrated "due diligence." This is particularly important in our age of legal inquiry into not only "What did you know and when did you know it?" but also, "What could you have known if you were duly diligent?"

B. Range of Toxicity Concerns

The range of concern for possible health effects of the products of thermal decomposition of plastics is very wide, almost as wide as the entire scope of toxicology. The concerns are outlined in a number of reviews (17,18), and in some cases are as broad as the incineration of plastics in dumps being a major contributor to air pollution in general (19,20).

The most significant of these concerns are those which are acute and short-term—death and incapacitation. These will be the major focus of the remainder of this book, so we will only briefly discuss them here. The two are related—indeed the real concern with whether a material generated during a fire will incapacitate someone is that an incapacitated person will not be able to escape a fire, and therefore will die in it. Death from combustion products is primarily a concern only if it occurs during the course of exposure or shortly thereafter, for a person surviving until this point (say one hour after a fire) would receive medical attention (in the form of life support, if necessary) sufficient to see him or her through a slower-developing crisis. Incapacitation can (as we will discuss later) occur in several ways. Though most of those doing research in the field are concerned with effects that cause a loss of consciousness, there are others with concerns about effects such as sensory irritation (21), which would serve to incapacitate by making a person unable to escape a fire but would not directly alter consciousness.

The second set of concerns centers on what one must consider intermediate health effects, intermediate in the sense that they are not immediately life threatening and are not apparent at the time of exposure, but rather develop or appear over a period of days or weeks. This group includes effects on the cardiovascular system (22), alterations in the activity levels of liver enzymes (23), biochemical and specific morphological changes in the lungs (24), and a condition known as polymer fume fever. All of these concerns are based on effects that have been demonstrated to occur, at least in experimental animals under laboratory conditions. Polymer fume fever, a flu-like, seemingly immuno-logic-based respiratory condition is associated at least primarily with PTFE or polyvinyl chloride (PVC) at only slightly elevated temperatures. Fume fever has been recognized for a number of years, but is believed to be a serious problem in only a few cases (25).

The third and final group of concerns center on long-term, genetically involved health effects. A number of authors have identified known mutagenic compounds present either in decomposition product streams or in the parent plastics (26,27), or upon testing decomposition products in the Ames test system have found them to be mutagenic (28,29). The concern with the presence of mutagenic components is primarily that they will be teratogenic or carcinogenic. Withey (27) has, in fact, proposed that they represent definite hazards in these two areas, while Graf has independently proposed that a carcinogenic risk is present.

Intermediate and long-term hazards are, however, continue to be a much lower priority than acute lethality or incapacitation. Because of these priorities, the main stream of research has been directed at short-term effects. To begin to understand and to evaluate these tests and the results to date, we shall first define some terms and survey the study designs which are currently being uti-lized.

As should be apparent by this point, combustion toxicology has grown to the point where it is approaching a transformation. To this point, as is the case with much of toxicology, the field has progressed in the manner of a descriptive science—data has been collected that describes what happens under a variety of situations, but does not explain why things happen. This second step (the development of models that explain why things happen and serve to predict as yet unobserved happenings) is the mechanistic phase of a science. Progress in combustion toxicology stalled on the verge of its mechanistic phase. The authors hope this volume will help in this process.

The first question that must be addressed is that of the relationship be-tween the large scale (or "real") fire and the various laboratory models currently being employed. Measurements of what goes on in the different regions of a real fire and studies of how particular materials behave in a full scale situation have been made. But only a very few attempts have been made to study the biological effects of large scale fire atmospheres, and these have not been pub-lished. Some of the laboratory-scale models attempt to address this problem indirectly by incorporating evaluations of several diverse thermolysis conditions (flaming, nonflaming, and 440°C, for example) into the evaluations. But a true validation of any of the proposed test systems will require a series of parallel experiments (large scale and laboratory scale) directly comparing results of defined loads of test materials. Only this will verify where the laboratory test results are valid predictors and where they are not. The mathematical modeling efforts for fires, which have been a primary objective of much of the large scale fire testing to day, have (unfortunately) progressed only to the stage of accounting for very simple gas mixture cases, and those not in a fire situation. These modeled situations are even less real-life than the laboratory scale tests themselves.

This brings us to the final point to be raised in considering why combustion toxicology has become such a pressing issue. This is the matter of present and (more important) future regulation of polymers based on the real or perceived hazard posed by their combustion gases. Currently, the International Organization for Standardization (ISO) (30) and the State of New York (31) regulate what may be used in buildings based on the results of combustion toxicity tests. The French regulate purely on the basis of having allowable limits on the amounts of N and Cl present in the structure of a building (believing that in so doing they are limiting the amounts of HCN and HCl that may be released in a fire). In an effort stretching over six years a committee gathered by the National Bureau of Standards (NBS) has produced a "standard" test and protocol that several agencies (FAA and CPSC, to name only two) are considering for use as the basis for Federal regulation of polymers in certain uses. New York, however, selected yet another test method.

What must be kept firmly in mind are the limits of these models and tests and their results. Although combustion product toxicity is an important consideration, it should not be the only (or even the most important) factor in regulation; and consideration of toxicity should not be limited to a simple question of acute lethality. The use of combustion toxicity data must be tempered with a knowledge of ignition temperatures and of what portions of the fuel load they would comprise in a fire. The remainder of this volume should serve to aid in these objectives.

C. Stakeholders

Many different types of organizations are involved and concerned with issues related to combustion toxicology.

1. Mass Transit (Rapid Railways, Subways, Buses)

Many factors, including their political implications, governmental or quasigovernmental involvement, and high conspicuity of catastrophes, make the combustion toxicity of materials used in mass transit systems an important issue. The combustion toxicity related issues were addressed in a report by a committee of the U.S. National Materials Advisory Board of the National Research Council (Anon), which summarized of fires per se, contemporary methods for smoke toxicity testing and some limitations, hazard assessment engineering models, and an outline for fire risk assessment.

2. Foam, Cable Coatings, and Plastics Industries

The producers of raw material (plastics) and of the products made from these materials (particularly electrical cable coatings and foam for upholstery) have economic, moral, and legal cause for understanding and minimizing the potential hazard of their products, particularly in aircraft, hotel, and mass transit uses. This is expressed through the actions of the trade associations of these industries (i.e., Society of Plastic Industries, Upholstered Foam Action Council, American Textiles Manufacturers Institute, etc.)

3. NIST

The National Institute of Standards and Technology (formerly the NBS) continues to be the lead federal agency charged with developing material standards to bring about reduced deaths and injuries due to fires.

4. Aviation Industry

In 1965, a Boeing 727 crashed at Salt Lake City but the cabin remained relatively intact. A fire from a ruptured fuel line spread into the cabin upon first impact and the contribution of the cabin materials was believed to have contributed to the heavy loss of life in the crash. This incident has been characterized as a pivotal initial event in the development of concern and discussion of such enclosures constructed of synthetic materials (32). This concern has led to a long running combustion toxicology activity at the FAA involving a combustion toxicity test systems (33), tests of cabin materials (32), exposure to pure chemical components of combustion mixtures (Crane et al. 1989), and reviews of the current status of aircraft toxicity, smoke toxicity, and survival (34).

5. Fire Risk Assessors

There are a wide range of NGOs (nongovernmental organizations) involved in the assessment and management of risks associated with fires and combustion toxicity. These range from standard setting and testing groups (such as Underwriters Laboratories) to insurance companies to organizations specifically focused on fire safety (such as NFPA, the National Fire Protection Association). These are heavily involved in acceptance and utilization of testing systems and methods. NFPA (35) has developed and published a standard test method for use in fire hazard modeling.

III. SMOKE

Though most people characterize all the products of combustion as smoke, a rigorous definition is quite different. Smokes include both solid and liquid particulates, the latter usually being the aerosols formed by condensation of supersaturated vapors. These range in size (aerodynamic diameter) from 0.01 to 1.0 micron, and for our purposes also include the materials absorbed onto the surface of these aerosols. Smoke, by this definition, is a critical (but largely ignored) part of the combustion toxicity hazard problem.

Smoke is also an important fire-response characteristic because visibility is a factor in the ability of occupants to escape from a burning structure, and in the ability of firefighters to locate and suppress a fire.

All fires produce smoke, which may be thick or thin, light or dark. Any appreciable quantity of smoke invariably is irritating and obscures light and vision. A number of methods for measuring smoke obscuration have been suggested or used during the last few years. No universal, or even general, standard exists at present, but preference has been shown in the United States for the NBS Smoke Chamber Test (36). Flame retardants increase carbon in the pyrolysis residue and decrease the yield of volatile aromatic products.

Smoke in the early stages of a fire does not contain a high enough concentration of dangerous materials to be acutely lethal. However, the initially generated smoke, by its irritant properties and obscuration of normal visibility, immobilizes the occupants within the area of the building where they are located. They are then "trapped" within the building, and unless rescued promptly, may be killed by lethal heat and gases that follow. Smoke is the primary escape problem in building fires, in spite of the fact that heat, CO, and gases are the major short term lethal components in the fire environment. Recent large-scale enclosure and occupancy tests suggest that heat, not CO or other toxicants, is the most likely second survivability criterion to be reached, usually 10 minutes after smoke bars the escape route.

Observations of the physical aspects of the smoke-forming characteristics of various polymers include the following:

> Structures containing the aliphatic carbon backbone, such as polyolefins, nylons, acetal, and PMMA, are low in smoke density. Most of these polymers melt and burn away in 1–2 minutes. PMMA is very low in smoke density, melting in about 1 minute. These resins are generally not self-extinguishing, and additives to increase the oxygen index usually increase smoke.
>
> Polymers containing aromatic rings, e.g. polystyrene, NORYL, SAN, and ABS have high smoke densities.
>
> Resins of high thermal stability, such as polysufone, polycarbonate, PPO,

PET, etc. are intermediate in smoke density, polysulfone in general having the lower values.

Alloys or blends, such as Arylon® and Kydene® (acrylic/PVC) show smoke density behavior intermediate between those of the base resins, but shifted slightly toward higher optical densities. The generation of smoke from some of the aromatic polymers is so voluminous that smaller standard samples or a larger test compartment would be preferred for accurately measuring smoke generation under laboratory conditions.

Although polyethylene (PE) is very low in smoke density, substitution of a chlorine for a hydrogen atom increases smoke density to a very high degree (compare PE with PVC).

In the case of polyolefins, as the melting point (and number of carbons) increases (from LDPE to poly-4-methylpentene), the smoke density increases. This observation may reflect the longer time in the flame for the higher melting resins before melting and dripping through the screen.

Chlorinating PE results in very high smoke densities, compared to chlorinating PVC. On the other hand, substituting a chlorine for hydrogen in polyethylene (i.e. PVC) effects a substantial increase in smoke density.

Ethylene-ethyl acrylate and ethylene vinyl acetate copolymers have low smoke densities and melt through the screen in about $1\frac{1}{2}$ min.

Smoke particles also provide a vehicle for deep lung penetration of highly reactive molecular entitites. These tend to cause damage that is not immediately lethal but nevertheless extremely serious (37). Such a mechanism may be involved in the case of those materials that are associated with seemingly unexplainable delayed deaths.

IV. HISTORY

A. Major Reviews of Combustion Toxicology

The books Combustion Toxicology Principles and Test Methods (38) and Combustion Toxicology (39) contain detailed reviews of combustion toxicity assessment methods.The NRC guidelines for evaluation of toxic hazards from fires in mass transit vehicles (Anon) include a review of approaches to lab scale combustion toxicology. The FAA hosted a meeting in 1993 that produced a full volume review of the field (40).

B. Diverse Apparatus and Approaches

1. Analytical Chemistry Approaches

There are approaches to evaluating the potential biological hazards of fire gases other than testing with laboratory animals. Most important among these are the analytical chemistry approach and the mathematical modeling approach. Both of these have been actively pursued for more than twenty years in various attempts to derive broad general answers to the problems at hand. The mathematical modeling approach depends on a number of factors or fields of research external to itself, but it is essential to have adequate analytical data to be able to construct a model and the analytical approach has turned out to be enormously complicated (41,42,43).

Chemical analyses serve a number of purposes in both large and laboratory scale combustion tests. The first and most important purpose of these measurements is to allow the determination of whether observed toxic effects are produced by carbon monoxide or by other toxic decomposition products. Because some studies have indicated a discrepancy between quantities of CO and mortality, the NMAB has recommended that CO levels be monitored in both the combustion atmosphere and in the blood of animals. Another function of these analyses is to provide an indication of the reproducibility and validity of the combustion of the material. Because of the inherent limitations of some combustion device designs, the intended combustion of a material, particularly with larger quantities, does not always occur. Measurements of CO and CO_2 generation can provide evidence of an improper combustion condition and the necessity to repeat an experiment. for example, changes in the CO to CO_2 ratio during an experiment may indicate whether or not the desired combustion mode is occurring in a satisfactory manner. Analyses are also needed to insure that excessive oxygen depletion does not occur during the exposure of animals.

Additionally, of course, accurate analytical measurements of both small and large scale fire test atmospheres are essential to allow any general case analysis of toxicity (as opposed to the special case of the material being tested under the conditions of test) or for there to be any modeling.

It has been found that simple alpha-cellulose results in approximately one hundred and seventy-five different organics under a single thermal decomposition condition (44). The decomposition products of PVC alone vary tremendously in both nature and proportions of composition with small changes in decomposition temperatures. The problem of adequately generating, sampling, and analyzing gas phase products from a fire is not an easy one (45). The common gases generated in a fire are CO, HCN, NO_2, NH_3, HC1, SO_2, other halogenated species, isocyanates, acrolein, and formaldehyde. But unless one wants to limit evaluations, as in the concept of a limiting toxicant (i.e., make a judgment purely on the basis of the most toxic gas present, as was once suggested by Petajan et al. (46,47), one has to come to the conclusion that it is not possible to make a valid assessment purely on the basis of the principal gases evolved, considered one-by-one. The contributions of heat and of O_2 deprivation, recognized for some time by a number of authors (48) and by the National Academy of Sciences Committee which studied the problem (49), are such that they must be "zeroed out" of all test systems or the studies will become enormously complex. Recently, Morihawa and Yanai (50) evaluated a limited number of materials in a series of room scale fires, looking at oxygen and heat levels and the concentrations of just eleven toxicants. Carbon monoxide alone was not found adequate to explain lethality and the study was considered a major one. When one then considers that several authors (51,52) have published studies establishing large effects on test results with changes in single variables (such as heating rate) in the combustion situation, the complexity becomes apparent.

2. Laboratory Scale Test Models

Over the years a number of test systems have been developed and utilized to evaluate the toxicity of polymer thermolysis products. Most of the data reviewed later in this chapter come from eight of these systems, which will be described and discussed in some detail. There are (or have been) a number of other systems which, due to their not having generated as large an available database, we will not consider in detail here. But it should be noted, in passing at least, that other systems (53,54,55,56) have been developed and utilized.

    a.   Potts Pot: National Bureau of Standards (NBS, now the NIST—National Institute for Standards and Technology) Method.   This test method, under development since 1976 at the U.S. National Bureau of Standards, has been described in detail in a Bureau report entitled "Further Development of a Test Method for the Assessment of the Acute Inhalation Toxicity of Combustion Products" (59). An ad hoc working committee, consisting of members from approximately 20 academic, industrial, or government organizations engaged in relevant work, was formed in 1977 for the purpose of providing a forum for exchanging technical information to assist the Bureau in the development of the test method (12). Eight labs from the ad hoc working group also participated in a "round-robin" evaluation of the test method as it evolved, with the examination of 12 materials, both natural and synthetic. The announced objectives of the intralab evaluation were to determine the operability of the procedure and to determine the reproducibility of test results from different laboratories, with many of the participants believing other test systems would also be evaluated and a "best" system selected based on the results. Currently, this test system, with variations, is the most widely used test system in the field (though the State of New York's endorsement of the University of Pittsburgh system has made that a close second).

    According to the NBS report, the test method

> . . . provides a means of assessing the acute inhalation toxicity of the combustion products of materials under specified laboratory conditions and is primarily intended for research and preliminary screening purposes. Additional factors must be considered in evaluating the potential toxic hazard

posed by a material in a given situation . . . Therefore the results of this test
method must be combined with other information when making decisions
about the suitability of materials for specified uses. (59)

The basic components of the NBS test method consist of the following:
The furnace originally employed in this system is the "Potts pot" (60), a
conductive box heater as shown in Figure 5. The sample is held in a quartz
beaker in the middle of this box heater, the temperature being controlled (in an
off/on, all-or-none manner) from the sensed temperature of the beaker. The
furnace operates in the temperature range of 300–900°C (±15°C without sample—there is a somewhat greater variation with the sample in place). The protocol employed calls for heating the furnace to the desired target temperature,
then dumping the sample into the furnace and sealing the system. As can be
seen from Figure 6, the furnace is located in the floor of the exposure chamber.
The drawbacks to this decomposition system are substantial and numerous. Control over the decomposition conditions (both in terms of temperature and oxygen
availability) is minimal. A strong case can be made that the pot can only perform destructive distillation and pyrolysis of samples and connecting the furnace
directly to the animal exposure chamber adds a heat load to the system, which
forces other design factors in compensation.

Analytical monitoring is by continuous IR spectrophotometric measurements of CO, O_2, and CO_2. The overall concentration achieved is calculated,
assuming that the entire sample is decomposed, by dividing the weight of the
fuel load by the total volume of the system. This approach to calculating concen-

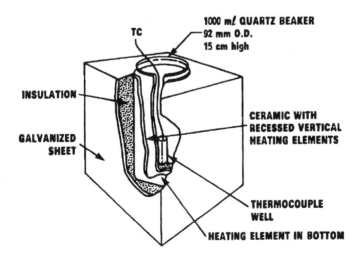

Figure 5 NBS furnace ("Pott's pot").

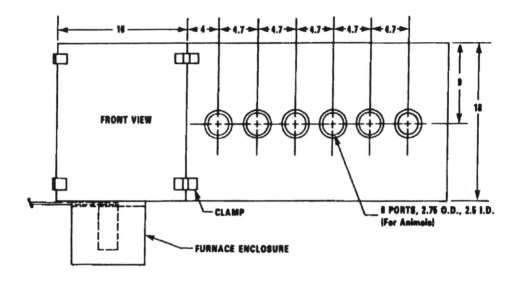

Figure 6   Schematic of NBS combustion-toxicity-testing setup.

tration tends to favor those polymers containing fillers or otherwise act to leave large residues.

The chamber, as shown in Figure 7, is a lexiglas rectangular shaped box, having a total volume of 200 l, and ports through which the head only exposure of animals can be accomplished. The shape of the chamber is such that though adequate mixing is accomplished in a short period (several minutes) for gases, a visible layering of aerosols for periods of several minutes is frequently observed.

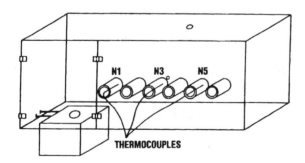

Figure 7   NBS exposure chamber.

Six male Sprague-Dawley rats are used for each 30 min of exposure, with two of these animals being terminated immediately at the end of the exposure (to obtain blood samples to determine COHb, O_2Hb, and total Hb). Incapacitation during exposure is evaluated in terms of loss of ability to keep the hind feet off a plate, the touching of which induces an electrical shock. The animals that survive exposure are observed for 14 days after exposure or until death (whichever comes first).

The protocol employing this system calls for determinations of concentration response curves (with death as the response) at each of three sample temperatures (at autoignition temperature and at 25°C above and below it).

A major disadvantage of the original NBS test method relates directly to the combustion device, a type of crucible furnace. Since heat transfer with this furnace is intended to be largely conductive, contiguous contact of a sample with the beaker surface must be maintained. Thus, the furnace is most suitable for thermoplastic materials or samples in a powder or pellet form which will melt and conform to the shape of the beaker. Considering this, it is interesting that the NBS method utilizes a block of char-forming and nonmelting material, Douglas fir, as its reference material. Use of a commercial, pelletized thermoplastic material might be more appropriate.

Problems have been encountered with low density foam samples, which filled the beaker and restricted the movement of air around the sample. Furthermore, large samples, such as are needed with low density materials, are subjected to a wide range of temperatures, since the air temperature decreases near the top of the beaker. It is not surprising, therefore, that the reproducibility of results in the case of such foams is not as good as with many other materials. The NBS combustion technique also does not satisfactorily combust, in a consistent manner, other materials such as laminates, coated specimens, carpeting/backing, one-surface fire barriers, foamed thermosets, and many other real-world materials.

One response to the limitations of the original NBS method was to utilize a radiant heat energy thermal decomposition device in place of the Pott's furnace, and to include a measure of incapacitation. In this variation, developed by S.C. Packham, the same 200-L exposure chamber and analytical devices are utilized. However, both the combustion furnace and the experimental protocol are considerably different. The combustion furnace (Figure 8) was developed by H.W. Stacy in the laboratories of the Weyerhaeuser Company. It has an elongated, trapezoidal shape with quartz windows forming the nonparallel sides. The frame is constructed of stainless steel. The radiant heat source consists of tubular quartz, tungsten-filament lamps housed in parabolic reflectors. Using lamps with a 2,000-Watt power rating, heat fluxes up to 5 W/cm^2 can be obtained. A sample holding tray is suspended from a load cell into the combustion zone of the furnace. The furnace configuration allows testing based on exposed

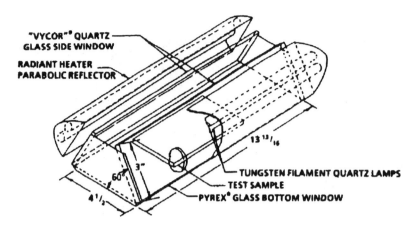

Figure 8   Quartz-windowed radiant heat furnace.

surface area for many materials such as composites, laminates, tiles, fabrics and coatings. Procedural dosages are expressed in terms of specimen surface area exposed to a designated heat flux. Incapacitation is monitored using the leg-flexion shock avoidance method.

Materials are evaluated for both acute toxic potency and general toxic potency on the following bases: acute toxic potency is based on average times to incapacitation (T_is) determined from tests on sample specimens having a surface area of 100 cm^2; general toxic potency reports are based on 14-day lethality and gross lung and respiratory tract pathology determined from tests on sample specimens having a surface are of 20 cm^2. This test method employs radiant heat for combustion of a material, a process occurring in most fires and fire test procedures. Thus, selection of parameters can be made in order to be of use in fire scenario modeling, e.g., ramped heat flux, fixed heat flux, flaming, nonflaming, etc. One advantage of the test method is that it permits the evaluation of many end-use materials (e.g., composites, laminates, coatings, films, etc.) that cannot be appropriately accommodated in most of the other test methods. Also, the surfaces of materials are exposed to heat, which is the way materials are likely to be exposed in certain stages of a real fire. The method expresses toxic potency on the basis of surface area (LA_{50}) rather than weight. Another advantage is that the method provides a measurement of time-to-incapacitation.

A disadvantage of this method is that different samples may have variable absorptivities to radiant heat due to surface color, char formation, or other characteristics. This may result in different surface temperatures among materials, when the same heat flux is applied. Also, smoke buildup in the combustion chamber may reduce the heat flux at the surface of the sample during the course of the test. Radiant heating may cause a greater temperature buildup in the animal exposure chamber than that produced by other combustion devices. Finally, the selection of a 10-min incapacitation time as the criterion to differentiate between two different types of test reports is arbitrary and needs further evaluation when sufficient data from the test method becomes available.

   b.   DIN Method.   This test method was developed in the Federal Republic of Germany and has been used by a number of German investigators, including G. Kimmerle, H.T. Hoffman, H. Oettel, J.J. Klimisch, H. Hollander and others (61,62,63,64,65). The method was developed in response to the German Commission of Standards desire for a standardized test method for generating combustion products in toxicity studies of smoke produced by materials. The standardized method has been designated DIN 53 436.

   The basic components of test protocols used in conjunction with the DIN method consist of the following (61). The system is illustrated in Figure 9.

   1.   Combustion Apparatus.   The combustion apparatus and procedure are used for generation of thermal decomposition products. The apparatus consists of a 1300-mm long quartz combustion tube with an outside diameter of 39 mm and a moveable, circular electric oven which tightly encloses a section of the tube. The procedure permits variable thermal exposure of the test material in a controlled air stream. Air enters the tube at a rate of approximately 100 l per hour in the direction opposite to the movement of the oven. The test specimens, cut so as to have an equal volume or weight per unit length, are heated in the quartz tube at different constant furnace temperatures between 200°C and 600°C. The mixture of air and combustion products from the tube is cooled and

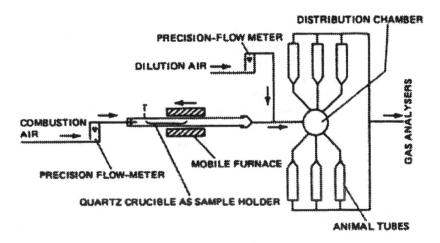

Figure 9   DIN 53436 apparatus. (Courtesy of Refs. 64, 65.)

further diluted by a secondary stream of air, controlled by a flowmeter, prior to passage into and through an animal exposure chamber.

2. Exposure Chamber. The animal chamber is operated in the dynamic mode for exposure of rats to the diluted combustion mixture. A variety of animal exposure chambers of different sizes and configurations have been used with the DIN apparatus to provide both head-only and whole-body exposures of animals, but usually the latter. At least 5, but usually 20, animals are used in each test. In most tests, the duration of exposure is 30 min.

3. Biological End Points. Toxicological measurements consist of mortality as the primary end point, exposure and postexposure observations of toxic signs, animal body weight determinations, and gross pathological examinations.

4. Atmosphere Analysis. Chemical analyses, consisting of continuous monitoring of CO, CO_2, and O_2, periodic measurements of HCN or other selected gases, and measurements of blood COHb in animals at the termination of exposure are performed.

The DIN method may be used to assess the relative toxicities of combustion products of a material under different temperatures or to compare the relative toxicities of combustion atmospheres produced by different materials. Toxicity may be expressed in terms of mortality as the ratio of the number of dead animals to the number of animals exposed. Mortality values may also be related to the total air flow and to either the volume of the specimen heated during the 30-min period or to the mass or mass loss of the specimen. A dose–response relationship and LC_{50} may also be determined for each material by varying the volume of diluting air in order to vary to concentration of the combustion mixture to which the animals are exposed.

A defined critical temperature (T_C) has been used in a number of studies with the DIN method to assess the relative toxicity of the pyrolysis products of plastics. In addition to the critical temperature, Kimmerle and Prager (1980) have used a number of other parameters to compare relative toxicities.

One of the advantages of the DIN method is the reported excellent reproducibility of the method, when used by different laboratories to generate combustion atmospheres for acute toxicity studies. This reproducibility was evaluated in recent studies by Klimisch and coworkers (62,64,65). Three laboratories participated in the evaluation which consisted of 1) measurements of toxicity in animals exposed to thermal decomposition products 2) measurements of carbon monoxide and carbon dioxide in inhalation chambers; and 3) measurements of total volatile organic substances in inhalation chambers. The results for each of the three parameters by the three laboratories demonstrated clearly that reproducible results may be obtained in different laboratories using the DIN method. Another advantage of this method is its versatility in allowing both whole-body and head-only exposures of test animals.

There are two features of the DIN combustion device and technique which are unique. One is that the tube furnace moves along the test material at a fixed rate, thermally decomposing a constant quantity of material per unit time. This enables the generation of a defined concentration of thermal products that can be kept steady during the whole period of exposure. The second is that concentrations of combustion products can be obtained for determining dose–response relationships by diluting the combustion mixture while maintaining the same proportion of individual components.

One limitation of the DIN method is that furnace temperatures are limited to 600°C, although temperatures in real fires can exceed this temperature. Additionally, time-to-incapacitation is not measured.

C. Rotorod Boxes.

1. Carnegie Mellon Institute of Research System.   This system was developed over the period 1977 to 1979 by J.B. Reid, T.F. Brecht, and S.C. Gad with funding from Union Carbide Corporation. It has been described by Gad and Smith (51).

The furnace utilized is shown in Figure 10. A focused infrared heater serves to heat a sample on a quartz plate on a thermogravimetric analysis (TGA) device. A thermocouple directly in the sample serves to monitor sample temperature and can control this for a range from 150°C to 1500°C (±5°C). Alternatively, the system can control the heat flux from the IR heater. As shown in Figure 11, the furnace is not directly in the animal exposure chamber. Rather, it is connected by a series of glass tubes that serve to close the entire system. A sealed fan acts to circulate and mix the chamber contents and the changer contents. Warming tapes about the glass tubing prevent condensation and collection of aerosols. A Data Trak 5600 microprocessor controls the entire system, allowing complete and precise reproducibility and ability to alter sample temperature in any desired manner (5°C/min, 10°/min, etc.). The furnace is also configured to allow complete control over the initial atmosphere of the furnace (by adding O_2, N_2, or CO_2), and a propane torch acts as an ignition source when necessary. Concentrations are calculated based on the weight of sample volatized.

Analytical monitoring in this system is based primarily on continuous measurement (and recording) of O_2, CO, CO_2, NO/NO_X (all by IR spectrophotometry), total hydrocarbons (by flame protometry), and HCN (by a specific electrode). Periodic measurements of other, special interest gases can be made by draw tubes.

The animal exposure system is a glass cylinder with stainless steel ends, having a motor driven activity wheel suspended on a stainless steel shaft through the chamber. The volume of the complete system is 55 l.

Six male Sprague Dawley rats are utilized for each 30 min exposure. Incapacitation is evaluated as occurring once an animal is incapable of walking on the wheel, but rather tumbles. A high intensity lamp placed behind the chamber provides the ability to observe animals when even a heavy smoke is gener-

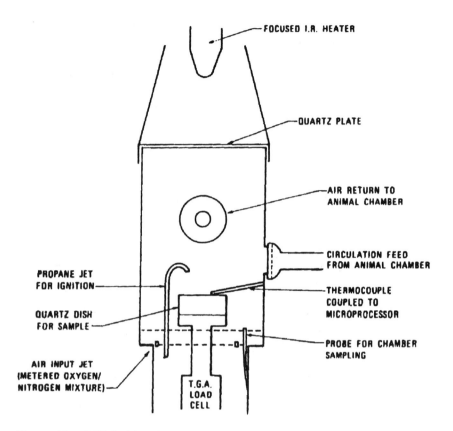

Figure 10   CMIR ignition-chamber system.

ated. A disadvantage is that this incapacitation model can be called a subjective one, and indeed it requires some degree of observer training. One approach to adding an objective measure to the system is to monitor the torque or drag on the turning wheel, but this effort has not been pursued to completion. End points are time to incapacitation, lethality, and (with blood taken from one animal, by heart puncture after the exposure) COHb, O_2Hb, and total Hb.

The protocol employed calls for determining concentration response curves for both death and incapacitation at each of three temperatures (these temperatures normally being achieved by raising the sample temperature at the rate of 40°C per minute). The three temperatures are 10°C below the AIR, 10°C above the AIT, and 440°C.

The major drawback to this system is the capital equipment cost. It is, however, probably the most versatile and reproducible of the existent systems.

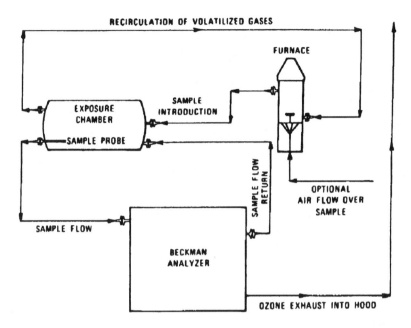

Figure 11   CMIR combustion-toxicity-testing system.

2.   United States Testing System.   This U.S. Testing System was developed by Eugene Rider at U.S. Testing during 1976. It utilized as a furnace a conductive heated tube furnace with an on/off controller, controlled from a thermocouple contained in the wall of the quartz furnace tube. The furnace has the capability of heating a sample within the range 200°C to 800°C (±25°C). Analytical monitoring is by continuous IR monitoring for O_2, CO, CO_2 and NO/NO_X.

The animal chamber is a 52 l glass cylinder with a motor driven activity wheel in it. The system is sealed (and therefore technically "static"), with a fan serving to circulate the atmospheric contents. No provision is made to avoid condensation or collection of volatiles for aerosols at bends and "cold spots" in the system. 6 male Sprague-Dawley rats are exposed for 30 min (then held for 14 days postexposure) at levels sufficient to establish concentration lethality curves under each of two sets of decomposition conditions (25°C above and below the AIT). Incapacitation is evaluated in terms of the inability to continue walking on the motor driven wheel.

3.   University of Pittsburgh System (UPITT).   Originally developed by Y. Alarie and C.S. Barrow (66) from 1973 to 1976 (under a contract from the National Bureau of Standards), then later modified to its present design (67,68),

this method is based on a method for studying the sensory irritation response of rodents (69).

The decomposition source is a conductively heated vertical tube furnace controlled by a linear programmer to increase temperature at 20°C per minute. The sample is held in a crucible in the furnace, with the crucible being on a Stanton Redcraft recording thermobalance. The furnace is connected to the exposure chamber by tubing which is cooled to reduce heat stress in the animals.

The 2.3 l glass chamber, shown in Figure 12, is a glass cylinder with parts fitted for the dose-only exposure of 4 mice at a time. The system is an open or dynamic one. Air flows in a single pass through the furnace and chamber and out of the system at 20 l/minute. 4 male Swiss Webster mice are exposed for 30 min in this system. During exposure, everything but their noses is mounted in a plethysmograph—sensitive device designed to monitor respiration by measuring changes in air pressure. In this system, changes in respiration rates and volumes are utilized to determine if sensory or pulmonary irritation (which are, in this usage, held to be equivalent to incapacitation) are induced. Animals are not held for observation after exposure.

Analytical support consists of GC monitoring for O_2, CO, and CO_2.

The protocol used here is based on the premise that a sample will, under these conditions, pass through each of the possible decomposition temperatures. Times to incapacitation and a concentration-lethality curve are determined.

Each material is evaluated for the toxic effects of its combustion products by the use of 5 toxicity indices or end points. Sensory irritation is evaluated in the same manner as in the previous method. A concentration-response relation-

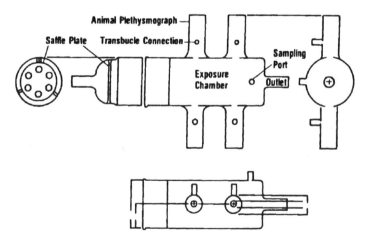

Figure 12 Pittsburgh mouse exposure chamber.

ship for sensory irritation and an RD_{50} value are obtained by measuring the average maximal decrease in respiratory rate within 10 min of the initiation of exposure to the smoke produced by a series of increasing sample weights. According to Alarie and his coworkers, the RD_{50} concentration in mice is equivalent to an intolerable level of sensory irritation in humans and is predicted to be incapacitating within 3–5 min (70,71,72).

A secondary toxicity end point used in this test method is the stress index (SI), also referred to as the sensory irritation stress index (SISI). According to Alarie and his coworkers, sensory irritants evoke a series of reflex responses, apart from the decrease in respiratory rate, to compensate for the reduced breathing and apneic periods. The adjustments, which include changes in heart rate, blood pressure and blood vessel size, are representative of the total stress on the animal. The intensity of this stress is proportional to the decrease in respiratory rate, but the exact relationship has not been defined (73). A mathematical approximation of this relationship was proposed by the investigators for calculation of a stress index for the decomposition products of materials (74). This index takes into consideration the rate of onset and recovery for the respiratory effect as well as the degree of depression of the respiratory rate.

Concentration–response relationships may be obtained by graphing SI values as a function of sample size. From these relationships, the sample size of a material associated with an SI value of 10 is selected for comparison of potency among materials and is termed the SI100 value.

For screening purposes, investigators desire a simple test to reveal materials having unusually high toxicity. For this test, they propose the use of only the lethality end point of their complete protocol. The LC_{50}, designed by them as the sample weight that causes death of half of the exposed animals within a fixed time, is selected as the lethality end point. Exposure of the four mice in plethysmographs, with heads extended into the chamber, begins with decomposition of the sample, as evidenced by weight loss, and continues for either 10 or 30 min. A 5-min recovery period follows 10-min exposures and a 10-min recovery period follows 30-min exposures. Lethality is determined by recordings of respiration and is defined as apnea (absence of breathing) persisting for 17 sec. Any animal that dies during the exposure or the recovery period is counted in the LC_{50} calculation. Dose–response lethality curves of materials are prepared by graphing percent mortality as a function of the logarithm of sample weight and a classification system to rate the acute lethal potential of each material on the basis of its LC_{50} value is proposed. It is arrived at by placing the LC_{50} value of Douglas fir (taken as the reference material) at the middle of an order of magnitude on a logarithmic scale. Materials with LC_{50} values within this order of magnitude are classified "as toxic as wood." Those materials with LC_{50} values within one order of magnitude lower than this are classified "more toxic than wood"; similarly, materials with LC_{50} values within one order of magnitude higher than this are designated "less toxic than wood." The LC_{50} values determined by this test method were incorporated into a formula developed by Alarie and his coworkers for comparing the toxicological hazard of materials (75).

Other variables used to calculate an acute lethal hazard (ALH) of a material are the temperature at 1% weight loss and the density of the material. The initial decomposition temperature was predicted to have an inverse relationship and the material density a direct relationship with the acute lethal hazard. Thus, a material requiring a high temperature for decomposition would tend to have a lower ALH value. Also, if the density of this material were low, these investigators made the assumption that less weight of material would be used and the hazard (ALH) would be less. Additionally, when comparing materials intended for the same structural function, other variables to define the amount of material used are incorporated into the formula. For example, for materials intended for insulation, the thermal conductivity (K) was used in addition to the density because both parameters define the total amount of material used for a particular insulating function. The thermal conductivity was predicted to have a direct relationship with the ALH. Under this assumption, a material with high thermal conductivity would be a poor insulator and require greater quantities, thereby resulting in a larger ALH value. Thus, the ALH for comparing the acute toxicological hazard of insulating materials was expressed as:

$$\text{ALH} = \frac{K \cdot D}{T \cdot LC_{50}}$$

where K is the thermal conductivity, D is the density, T is the temperature at which the material begins to decompose and LC_{50} is the sample weight lethal to half of the animals.

There are a number of strong objections to this system. The single pass nature of exposure permits the animals to conceivably avoid exposure to some extremely irritating decomposition stream components by holding their breath. No provision is made to avoid volatiles or particulates being condensed out prior to reaching the animals; and the assumption that the respiratory irritation model is in all cases equivalent to incapacitation models is not accepted by everyone. Additionally, materials with the same intended use, but with different thermal stabilities, are not evaluated under the same temperature conditions. There is also some question regarding the use of the RD_{50} value as an indicator of the incapacitating concentration of sensory irritants in man. The results of a study by Potts and Lederer (1978) do not support the predictions of Alarie and his coworkers that the RD_{50} concentration of thermal decomposition products of a material would be rapidly incapacitating to man. In this study, mice and human volunteers were simultaneously exposed in a room to the decomposition products of a quantity of red oak calculated to produce an RD_{50} sensory irritation level for mice. Although the mice exhibited a greater than 50% decrease in respiratory rate, the human subjects complained of no ill effects, did not exhibit a greater than 50% decrease in respiratory rate, and were definitely not incapacitated. However, strain differences in sensory irritation response by mice do exist and Potts and Lederer did not use the same strain of mouse as Alarie.

Advantages of the Pittsburgh method are that it provides the following: 1) an in-depth evaluation of toxic effects of the thermal decomposition products of a material by the use of 5 distinct end points; 2) determination of an LT_{50} value; 3) quantification of sensory irritation by determination of dose–response relationships and RD_{50} values; 4) determination of the asphyxiant range; and 5) detailed information relevant to the rates of thermal decomposition of a material and its release of toxicants. The method is also unique in its standard usage of ramped heating of the tube furnace (although this heating mode is an alternative procedure in the USF and improved FSS methods), and in the quantification of stress and the histopathological examination of exposed animals.

4. Federal Aviation Agency System. This test system was developed from 1974 on by a group led by C.R. Crane (33) at the FAA facility in Oklahoma City. The decomposition device utilized is a Lindberg conductive tube furnace, preheated to 600°C (±1°C) before the sample (in a quartz tube) is placed in the furnace and the system is sealed. The system as diagrammed in Figures 13 and 14, is a closed loop "static" system.

Analytical monitoring consists of periodic determinations of HCN, CO, O_2, and CO_2 by 2 gas chromatographs.

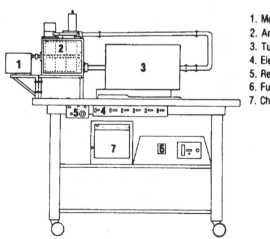

1. Motor to drive activity wheel
2. Animal exposure chamber
3. Tube Furnace
4. Electrical outlet strip
5. Recirculating fan controller
6. Furnace temperature controller
7. Chamber temperature recorder

Figure 13 FAA exposure system.

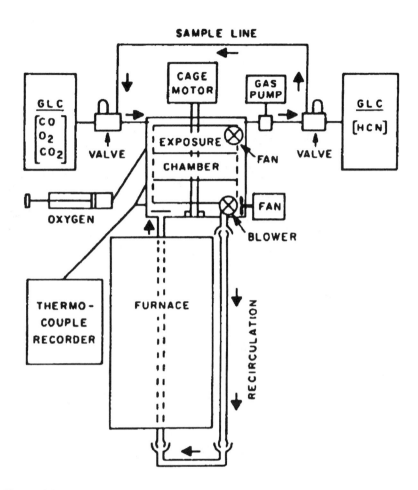

Figure 14 FAA exposure system.

For each trail, 3 male Sprague-Dawley rats are placed in a motor drive activity wheel, the wheel being in a plexiglass box with a volume of 12.6 l. Exposure is for 30 min, but the furnace is connected for only 10 min of this period. Both time-to-death and time-to-incapacitation are determined by observation. Surviving animals are watched for 14 days postexposure.

Samples consisting of a low density material are cut into 1 cm cubes before being placed in a furnace. The protocol calls for determination only at different concentrations (the concentrations being determined by calculating a nominal concentration based on the weight of sample volatized) achieved by heating the sample to 600°C. This is adequate for most materials but: (1) there are some which only decompose at higher temperatures and (2) higher temperatures are achieved in a real fire. And decomposition, in many materials, progresses over a period exceeding 10 min. The relatively small number of animals utilized per trial also serves to reduce somewhat the sensitivity of the system.

There were several marked limitations to the use of the first FAA test system for the evaluation of materials. The 10-min decomposition time at 600°C might not produce complete decomposition of some materials. Recirculation of the thermal decomposition products between the furnace and chamber could possibly cause further degradation of these produces and/or loss of products by reaction or absorption. The test method did not quantify toxic potency by determination of dose–response relationships and LC_{50} values. Finally, determination of time-to-incapacitation and time-to-death by observation might be obscured in dense smoke-containing atmospheres. This latter possibility was eliminated by modification of the rotating wheel to enable electronic monitoring of animal responses. However, it was reported that rotation of the wheel cannot be stopped until the last animal is incapacitated and, consequently, $T_d s$ occurring prior to the final T_i cannot be recorded (78).

Most of these limitation have been circumvented by modifications to the system, which now allows fixed or ramped heating to 800°C and variation of sample size to quantify toxic potency. However, the improved test system also is a recirculating system, with the inherent potential limitations described. Advantages of the improved system are 1) its versatility in providing fixed or ramped heating and nonflaming or flaming combustion, and 2) its provision of time-to-incapacitation and time-to-death data in addition to the quantification of toxic potency.

d. NASA/USF. C.J. Hilado developed this system under contract for NASA. It has been extensively described in the literature (79,80).

Decomposition is achieved by a conductively heated tube furnace attached by a noninsulated tube to a polymethylmethacrylate exposure chamber which is 4.2 l in volume and hemispherical in shape (see Figure 15). Analytical support consists of continuous oxygen and temperature monitoring (but without continuous recording). 4 male Swiss albino rats are free to move about the exposure chamber during the course of the 30 min test. An observer judges both incapacitation and death of animals, recording a time to each of these end points. The system is a dynamic, open one; decomposition products make a single passage through the chamber and out of the system.

There are a number of serious problems with this system. The control over decomposition conditions is extremely limited. Animals have ample opportunity to avoid breathing toxic chemical species that are present for only short periods. Finally, the analytical measurements in this system are just too minimal

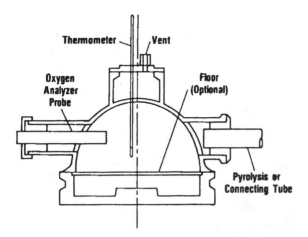

Figure 15   USF/NASA exposure chamber.

to allow any real evaluation of relationships to toxicant concentration to be made.

The USF test method has been recommended by Hilado as a simple, economical and rapid screening test. However, the method provides only limited toxicological and analytical data. It is unique in its flexibility to operate the tube furnace under either fixed or ramped temperature conditions and in either a static or dynamic flow mode.

One of the limitations of the USF test protocol is that it does not quantify toxic potency of the decomposition products of a material. As a consequence, the USF method is the only system which did not identify PTFE as producing highly toxic smoke.

The extreme toxicity of the decomposition products of this material has been demonstrated by several other test methods. The modified protocol, the Dome Chamber Toxicity Test method, does provide for determination of dose-response lethality relationships and LC_{50} and LT_{50} values.

The USF method evaluates incapacitation and death by visual, and therefore subjective, measurements. Although these seem to be reproducible and require no animal training, more objective end points would be preferable. The use of three end points (staggering, convulsions, and collapse) by Hilado to provide insight into the nature of the toxic species is also subjective, is not supported by any explanation of mechanisms of action, and has not been confirmed by any other researchers. The fact that the animals are allowed to run free is an advantage in setup costs and maintenance but may be a disadvantage because the rodents can huddle together and "protect" one another from irritant gases.

Identification of the cause of incapacitation or death is an important aspect of combustion toxicology that has been emphasized in studies by numerous authors. This capability is limited in the USF methodology, primarily because of the small sample size and small chamber volume (which preclude extracting many samples for analysis). In his more recent studies, however, Hilado made measurements of carbon monoxide in an effort to relate the cause of death to CO concentration–time (C · t) relationships. Although these data appear to be reasonable, conclusions based on a single point measurement and an assumption of the pattern of CO evolution with time could easily be in error by 50 percent or more in the C · t product. More extensive studies of CO evolution from various materials should be conducted to verify the conclusions reached. Another unknown factor in the USF methods that influences the combustion atmosphere is the length of travel of products down the combustion tube without the aid of air flow. It would seem that some of the combustion products could remain in the tube long after they were released.

e. SwRI Primate. Research studies were being conducted by the Department of Fire Technology of the Southwest Research Institute to assess the potential of irritant combustion gases to impair escape from postcrash aircraft fires. These studies are being sponsored by the Federal Aviation Administration (FAA) of the Department of Transportation (DOT).

The objectives of this program are to: (1) determine the potential of representative combustion atmosphere irritant gases to impair human escape from a fire environment, and (2) evaluate the validity and relevance of behavioral tasks that are presently used for material evaluation in laboratory smoke toxicity tests with rodents. A nonhuman primate model (the juvenile baboon) and operant behavioral methodology are used in these studies. The protocol is designed to determine the threshold concentration for escape impairment when these animals are exposed to irritant gases for the short periods of time relevant to escape from postcrash fire scenarios. A behavioral escape task of equivalent complexity will be used with rodents under similar exposure conditions in order to compare the sensitivity and response of the two species of animals and evaluate current methodology used for measurement of escape impairment or incapacitation in laboratory smoke toxicity tests.

A Beckman diesel analyzer serves to continuously measure and record levels of CO, CO_2, O_2, NO/NO_X, and hydrocarbons, while a gas chromatograph/ mass spectrophotometer arrangement is available for specialty gases. The system is otherwise just like the NBS system and the protocol utilized is the same. SwRI also performed large scale testing using a facility illustrated in Figure 16. This facility produced an understanding of the complexity of combination toxicity events, as illustrated in Figure 17.

f. University of Michigan System. Developed by a group led by Boetner and Hartung under a Society of Plastics Industry contract from 1975 to

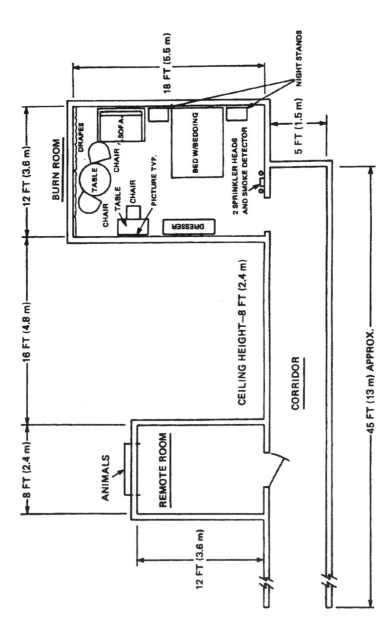

Figure 16 A diagram of the layout of the SWRI large scale fire-testing facility.

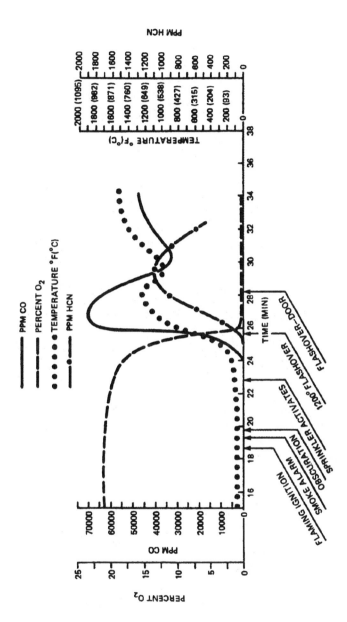

Figure 17 The relationships between various events occurring during a large scale fire test (at SWRI) and changes in CO, O₂, and HCN concentrations and room temperatures.

1978, several configurations of systems were evaluated by this group, but the one finally adapted is described in Hartung et al. (81). A radiant panel heater is used to decompose samples in this closed system.

Analytical support consists of infrared measurement of carbon monoxide and, when needed, calorimetric or gas chromatographic analysis of special interest gases.

The exposure system is a 370 l plexiglass cube with a rotarod mounted in it. The entire system is static with recirculation within the chamber.

Each trial consists of a 30 min exposure of 4 male Sprague-Dawley rats, with inability to stay on the rotarod being evaluated as incapacitation. Concentration lethality and time to incapacitation curves are determined at 10°C below and above the auto ignition temperature.

g. Utah Flammability Research Center System. Developed under contract to the NBS, this system (82) is the product of a team at the FRC in Salt Lake City. It uses the Pott's pot as a decomposition device, with the furnace having its open upper face flush with the bottom of a 64 l, octagonal polymethylmethacrylate exposure chamber. The system is a closed, "static" system, with a flexible bag attached to allow for expansion of total gas volume.

4 male Long Evans rats receive 30 min, head only exposure to concentrations (calculated based on weight volatized) of test materials, with 14 days of postexposure observation for survivors. The leg flexion model is utilized here to evaluate incapacitation. An extensive analytical support package based on a GC mass spectrophotometric system is included and a wide range of blood parameters (total hemoglobin, COHb, O_2Hb, and blood gases) is determined. The protocol utilized requires concentration response curves for each of two sample decomposition modes (just below auto ignition and just above auto ignition). The small number of animals utilized does serve to reduce sensitivity to some degree.

C. Summary

These systems still need critical evaluation in terms of being (as discussed earlier) a primary (pass/fail), secondary (ranking), or tertiary (total evaluation) level system. Most, if not all, of these systems can operate as primary level systems—they will identify those materials that have a high probability of generating extremely toxic degradation materials. Several of the systems (with some weaknesses) can act as secondary level evaluations, while the NBS, CMIR, SWIR, FAA, and University of Michigan systems can be utilized to generate comparative hazard data. What is needed for a tertiary level system will be discussed later. One universal weakness in all existing systems is that they do not quantitate and evaluate smokes and other aerosols. And they all allow at least some possibility that the hazards associated with aerosols will not be adequately evaluated.

D. Increase in On-line Analysis

Across the board there has been an almost complete shift of the analytical aspects of combustion toxicity testing. Prompted by the belief that the probability of exotic "supertoxicants" being other than rare events is low, virtually all analysis of combustion atmospheres has gone to continuous on-line monitoring of a range of "standard" gases "O_2, CO_2, CO, NO_x and CN).

This shift is a reflection of the belief that the combustion toxicity issue has been "solved."

E. Decline in Activity in the 90s

The belief that the questions around combustion toxicity have been solved is reflected in an almost complete cessation of research and testing activity in the field. Only one contract testing firm remains in the business of testing, and the UPITT testing system has largely become the standard (despite its known limitations) largely by default. Likewise, such research that continues is in the nonexperimental realm of modeling.

V. MATHEMATICAL MODELS

Recent years have witnessed the return of some individuals to supporting mathematical models as an effective way to deal with combustion toxicity here and now. Before looking at these recent efforts and models, however, at least two aspects of the underpinnings of such models should be reviewed.

Mathematical models in combustion toxicology are a special case of structure activity relationship (SAR) models. Combustion toxicology itself is a special case of the problem of evaluating the toxicity of mixtures. The problems and principles involved with these two general cases (SAR models and mixtures toxicology) apply equally well to this special case.

Structure activity relationship (SAR) methods have become a legitimate and useful part of toxicology over the last fifteen years or so. These methods are composed of various forms of mathematical or statistical models that seek to predict the adverse biological effects of chemicals based on their structure. The prediction may be of either a qualitative (irritant/nonirritant) or quantitative (LD_{50}) nature, with the second group usually being denoted as QSAR (quantitative structure activity relationship) models. It should be obvious at the outset that the basic techniques utilized to construct such models are mathematical modeling and reduction of dimensionality methods, as discussed in Gad (83).

Starting with the initial assumption that there is a relationship between

Table 3 Combustion Products, Sources, and Biological Effects

Toxicant	Combustion sources	Primary toxicologic effect	Estimate of short-term (10-Min) lethal concentration (PPM)
Hydrogen cyanide (HCN)	Wool, silk, polyacrylonitrile, nylon, polyurethane, and paper	Cellular level asphyxiant	350
Nitrogen dioxide (NO_2) and other oxides of nitrogen	Fabrics and in larger quantities from cellulose nitrate and celluloid	Respiratory irritant	>200
Ammonia (NH_3)	Wood, silk, nylon, and melamine; concentrations generally low in ordinary building fires	Sensory irritant	>1000
Hydrogen chloride (HCl)	PVC (polyvinylchloride) and some fire-retardant treated materials	Respiratory irritant toxicity potential of HCl and other halogen acid gases may be significantly greater when they are coated on particulates achieving deep long penetration	>500, if particulate is absent
Carbon monoxide (CO)	Carbon-containing materials. CO_2/CO ratio dependent on oxygen supply	Hypoxia	NA—very time and concentration dependent
Other halogen acid gases (HF and HBr)	Fluorinated resins or films and some fire-retardant materials containing bromine	Respiratory irritants	HF = 400 HBR > 500
Neurotoxic phosphorous compounds (apparently rare)	Materials containing phosphorous. Hydraulic fluids and some fire-retardant treated materials	Neurotoxicity	
Sulfur dioxide (SO_2)	Materials containing sulfur	Irritant	>500
Isocyanates	Urethane polymers	Respiratory irritants	100 (TDI)
Acrolein	Pyrolysis of polyolefins and cellulose containing material	Respiratory irritant	30–100
Other organic compounds (small quantities)	Many	Potentially genotoxic, and/or carcinogenic	

Source: Ref. 9.

structure and biological activity, we can proceed to more readily testable assumptions.

First, the dose of a chemical species is subject to a number of modifying factors (such as membrane selectivity and selective metabolic action) that are each related in some manner to chemical structure. Indeed, absorption, metabolism, pharmacologic activity, and excretion are each subject not just to structurally determined actions, but also to (in many cases) stereospecific differential handlings.

Given these assumptions, actual elucidation of SARs requires the following:

1. Knowledge of the biological activities of existing structures.
2. Knowledge of structural features that serve to predict activity (also called molecular parameters of interest).
3. One or more models that relate 2 to 1 with some degree of reliability.

There are a number of approaches to using structural and substructural data and correlating these to biological activity. Such approaches are generally classified as regression analysis methods, pattern recognition methods, and miscellaneous other (such as factor analysis, principal components, and probabilistic analysis).

The regression analysis methods that use structural data have been, as we will see when we survey the state of the art in toxicology, the most productive and useful. "Keys" or fragments of structure are assigned weights as predictors of an activity, usually in some form of the Free–Wilson model developed at virtually the same time as the generally better known Hansch. According to this method, the molecules of a chemical series are structurally decomposed into a common moiety (or core) that may be substituted in multiple positions. A series of linear equations are constructed.

The favorable aspects of Free–Wilson type models are:

1. Any set of quantitative biological data may be employed as the dependent variable.
2. No independently determined substituent constants are required.
3. The molecules comprising a sample of interest may be structurally dismembered in any desired or convenient manner.
4. Multiple sites of variable substitution are readily handled by the model.

There are also several limitations: a substantial number of compounds with varying substituent combinations is required for a meaningful analysis; the derived substituent contributions are given no reasonable basis for extrapolating predictions from the substituent matrix analyzed; and the model will break down if nonlinear dependence on substituent properties is important or if there are interactions between the substituents.

Pattern recognition methods comprise yet another approach to examining structural features and/or chemical properties for underlying patterns that are associated with differing biological effects. Accurate classification of untested molecules is again the primary goal. This is carried out in two stages. First, a set of compounds, designated the training set, is chosen for which the correct classification is known. A set of molecular or property description features is generated for each compound. A suitable classification algorithm is then applied to find some combination and weight of the descriptors that allows perfect classification. Many different statistical and geometric techniques for this purpose have been presented elsewhere (83). The derived classification function is then applied in the second step to compounds not included in the training set to evaluate test performance in terms of accuracy of prediction. In published work these have generally been other compounds of known classification also. Performance is judged by the percentage of correct predictions. Stability of the classification function is usually tested by repeating the procedure several times with slightly altered, but randomly varied, sets or samples.

The main difficulty with these methods is in "decoding" the QSAR in order to identify particular structural fragments responsible for the expression of a particular activity; and even if identified as "responsible" for activity, far harder questions for the model to answer are whether the structural fragment so identified is "sufficient" for activity, whether it is always "necessary" for activity, and to what extent its expression is modified by its molecular environment. Most pattern recognition methods use as weighting factors either the presence or absence of a particular fragment or feature (coded 1 or 0), or the frequency of occurrence of a feature. They may be made more sophisticated by coding the spatial relationship between features.

None of our past or current test systems in toxicology work well for predicting effects in the case of mixtures (84). We have data on either pure materials or fairly simple mixtures with a fixed ratio of components. While predicting over a limited range for single structures based on current data can generally be performed with reasonable comfort, the interactions between mixture components as both total amounts and relative proportions vary is beyond our current understanding, especially since many commercially or environmentally encountered mixtures are very complex, containing in some cases hundreds of components. And, frequently, we are faced with a desire to explore mixtures with a range of amounts of the same components, or with alterations (substitutions) in components.

There can be four general categories of interactions between components—additivity (effect A + effect $B = A + B$), antagonism (effect A and effect $B = A - B$, synergism (effect A and effect $B = AB$) or a combined effect which is qualitatively very different from that of the individual components. Such interactions may also be very time dependent.

Our current understanding of human health and the real world effect of toxicants is a reflection of what is called the multiple causation theory of disease. This holds that each input into the status of an individual's physiological and psychological condition (whether that input is a xenobiotic chemical or a "susceptibility factor"), is a component cause of that status.

Pozzani et al. (85) published data on the toxicity of 36 simple (2 component or "binary") mixtures of vapors to rats, and found that in only two of the cases did the results differ by more than 1.96 standard errors of the estimate from the predictions of Finney's model for additive/joint action. This model calculates the harmonic mean of the LD_{50} of mixture components as:

$$1/\text{predicted } LD_{50} - P_A/LD_{50} \text{ of component A} + P_B/LD_{50} \text{ of component } B$$

Where P_A and P_B are the proportions of components A and B in the mixture. Smyth et al. (86) later found much the same result for the oral LD_{50}s of 27 pairs of chemical in rats, and, indeed, for many binary (two component) mixtures the system works well (and is not limited to LD_{50}s). But most mixtures of concern are multicomponent. It has been proposed that some form of multiple logistic regress model be used for such extrapolations. All of this requires knowledge of the components of the toxicant mixture—in our current case, the combustion atmosphere.

A. Concept of Exposure Dose

In a static system where the volume is constant, the nominal concentration of the material in the "smoke" consumed is the mass consumed and the volume of exposure.

$$C_{FL} = \frac{m_0}{V} \tag{1}$$

For a static exposure system where the volume is constant this corresponds to:

$$C_{WL} = \frac{m_0 - m_T}{V} \tag{2}$$

In a dynamic or flow-through system, the volume is not fixed and is expressed as a rate:

$$C_{FL} = \frac{m_0}{q_v \cdot t} \tag{3}$$

For a dynamic or flow-through system, the numerator is unchanged, but the denominator must now reflect the flow

$$C_{WL} = \frac{m_0 - m_T}{q_v \cdot t} \tag{4}$$

In "mass-lost" models, there is an experimental linkage between the amount of material consumed and an LC_{50} for a given time period. If the rate of mass loss changes during the test scenario, the mass lost can be summed up for different parts of the exposure period. For example, for a static exposure volume:

$$\text{exposure dose} = \sum_{i=1}^{n} \frac{(\Delta m)_i \cdot (\Delta t)_i}{V} \tag{5}$$

And, assuming a constant flow rate, for a dynamic system:

$$\text{exposure dose } eq \sum_{i=1}^{n} \frac{(\Delta m)_i}{q_v} \tag{6}$$

1. Concept of LC_{50}

The LC_{50} is the concentration that produces lethality in half of the exposed animals after a given period of exposure, often 30 min.

2. Haber's Rule

Haber's Rule holds if the effect produced is proportional to the total dose, not the dose rate or peak dose. If Haber's Rule holds and the LC_{50} for 30 min is 1000 ppm (30,000 ppm*min), then the LC_{50} for 10 min will be 3,000 ppm which is also 30,000 ppm*minutes. Haber's Rule is often an appropriate description of empirical data obtained under specified conditions. Table 4 presents a study

Table 4 Distribution of Fire Victims According to Blood CO Saturation Levels

COHb (%)	Number of Victims	Percent
0–9	48	9
10–19	42	8
20–29	37	7
30–39	38	7
40–49	43	8
50–59	58	11
60–69	79	15
70–79	111	21
880	74	14
Total	530	100

Source: (89).

of the distribution of fire deaths in relation to their levels of carboxyhemoglobin, an example of how the concept does not precisely work.

3. Concept of Fractional Exposure Dose

The concept of fractional exposure dose is important because it is a key element of most of the contemporary models. It has also been incorporated into the NFPA (National Fire Protection Association) and ISO standards (35,87) and is illustrated in Figure 18.

The FED is the fraction of an LC_{50} determined at a particular time period.

$$FED = \frac{\text{exposure dose*exposure duration}}{LC_{50}\text{*exposure duration}_{LC_{50}}} = \frac{500 \text{ ppm*30 min}}{1000 \text{ ppm*30 min}} = 0.5 \quad (7)$$

If the LC_{50} and the test exposure are the same duration, 30 min in the example above, the times in the numerator and denominator cancel and the FED is the ratio of the exposure dose to the LC_{50}.

The fundamental model for the effects of exposure to multiple materials is to sum the FED for each component to obtain an overall FED for n materials:

$$FED = \sum_{i}^{n} FED_i \quad (8)$$

When there is LC_{50} as a function of exposure time available, the concept of FED can be generalized by integrating over time.

$$FED_i = \int_{t(bi)}^{t} \frac{C_i \, ms \, b_i}{K_i} dt \quad (9)$$

The combination of these two equations gives the Hartzell-Emmons (94) model:

$$FED = \sum_{i=1}^{n} \int_{t(b_i)}^{t} \frac{C_i - b_i}{K_i} dt \quad (10)$$

4. N-Gas Model

Babrauskas et al. (98) have proposed what they call the N-gas model. This model assumes the following: that toxicity of fire smoke is determined mainly by a small number of gases and that these may act additively, synergistically, or antagonistically.

Deviations from this postulate will occur infrequently and can be detected using a limited number of animal tests.

The steps in implementing and using this approach are then proposed to be:

Identifying the initial set of gases to be considered.
Determining the toxicity of these gases, individually and in combination.
Combusting samples of test materials under conditions appropriate to the

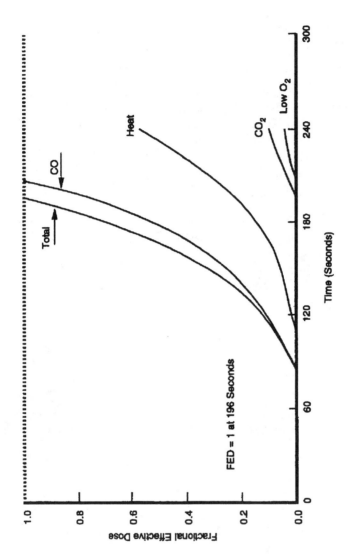

Figure 18 The relationship between the fractional effective dose (the FED, as incorporated into NFPA and ISO standards) and its constituent components (CO, CO_2, low O_2, and heat) over the period of the first 240 seconds of a fire.

fire scenarios of concern, and measuring the concentrations of the N evolved gases, either continuously or as batch samples.

Computing the toxicity, usually taken as the LC_{50}, the concentration of combustion products needed to cause 50 percent of the test animals to die after a specified exposure time.

Running one or two animal tests at that smoke concentration, minus a confidence interval, to ascertain whether an additional, important toxicant is contributing.

Adding a limited number of new gases as they are shown to have relevance to commercial products.

Creating and maintaining a publicly available database of mixed gas toxicities.

The interaction assumption is that of linear additivity, i.e. that the effective concentration to reach some endpoint, which may be the LC_{50} or some other measure, should be evaluated as:

$$= \frac{1}{C_{eff}} - \sum_i \frac{1}{C_i}$$

where C_i is the LC_{50} or other toxic level value for the individual component i. This simple method does not account for any nonlinearities, such as synergisms or antagonisms. In practice, a more general formulation is used, which has been termed the fractional summation approach, but still has the same limitations.

Tsuchiza and Nakaya (90) have proposed a version of this linear multiple gas interaction model, and have presented some experimental data supporting its validity in the case of mixtures containing up to 3 component gases. Tsuchiza (90) has also published an analysis of various sets of data on carbon monoxide–hydrogen cyanide mixtures showing the effects to be linearly additive. He has proposed that, based on this data, the case of synergistic interactions can be disregarded.

The group of researchers at Southwest Research Institute have published a series of five articles (91–96) on modeling the toxicity of fire gases. Based on sets of data on two component gas mixtures, they have proposed what they call the fractional effective dose (FED) model. It starts with the assumption that time-to-effect/concentration experimental data for a toxicant can be plotted as concentration vs. the reciprocal of time ($1/t$). A linear plot is obtained, from which the slope (K) and intercept (b) can be used to calculate EC_{50} or LC_{50} values for any exposure time from the equation

$$C - K \frac{1}{t} b$$

Components can then be simply summed as to exposure time/concentration product, and a result in effect predicted based on the totals resulting from such a near-linear combination. Again, only two component models of simple gases (CO, HNC, and HCI) have been evaluated under nonfire situations. Current N-gas models differ from the mass–loss models in the calculation of the FED. In the N-gas models, the FED is based on the concentration of component gases and the LC_{50} for the component gases.

For example, assuming the same exposure duration for the test and the LC_{50} determination so time cancels from the equation:

$$FED_i = \frac{component\ gas_i}{LC_{50}\ component\ gas_i} \tag{11}$$

Because CO is not well approximated by Haber's Rule, in part because increased CO_2 increases respiratory rate and thus CO uptake, the FED is obtained by using a piecewise approximation from a fitted function where different constants are used if the concentration of CO_2 is >5%:

$$\frac{m[CO]}{[CO_2] - b} \tag{12}$$

The basic N-gas equation includes the concentrations of gases that are related to oxygen uptake, the asphyxiant gases: CO, CO_2, HCN, and O_2:

$$N - gas\ value = \frac{m[CO]}{[CO_2] - b} + \frac{[HCN]}{LC_{50}HCN} + \frac{21 - [O_2]}{21 - LC_{50}O_2} \tag{13}$$

$$N - gas\ value = \frac{m[CO]}{[CO_2] - b}$$
$$+ \frac{[HCN]}{LC_{50}HCN}$$
$$+ \frac{21 - [O_2]}{21 - LC_{50}O_2} + \frac{[HCl]}{LC_{50}HCl} + \frac{[HBr]}{LC_{50}HBr} \tag{14}$$

And in its most developed form:

$$N - gas\ value = \frac{m[CO]}{[CO_2] - b}$$
$$+ \left(\frac{[HCN]}{LC_{50}HCN} \times \frac{0.4[NO_2]}{LC_{50}NO_2} \right) + 0.4 \left(\frac{[NO_2]}{LC_{50}NO_2} \right) + \frac{[HCN]}{LC_{50}HCN} \tag{15}$$

$$+ \frac{2 - [O_2]}{21 \text{ ms } LC_{50}O_2} + \frac{[HCl]}{LC_{50}HCl} + \frac{[HBr]}{LC_{50}HBr}$$

VI.   EGREGIOUS FAILURES TO PREDICT

The dependence on the functional dose leads to some occasional catastrophic failures to predict hazard. Two well known examples of this—of the occurrence of extremely toxic combustion products—occur with PTFE (Teflon™) under certain conditions and of the "bird cage" cyclic phosphate neurotoxicants.

VII.   THE DILEMMA OF LABORATORY SCALE TESTS

In 1980, Punderson (97) identified what he characterized as "a fundamental dilemma" which is that " . . . from extensive studies using animal exposure tests is the fact that toxicity test rankings vary widely depending on both test procedures and test conditions." More recently, in 1996, Purser commented in a panel discussion (Toxicology p. 216) that, "I think we all agree that one should never use a toxicity test as a reason for selecting or deselecting a material. We have to be very careful in addressing kinds of fire conditions and in defining material responses. . . . We should never use data in isolation and say, 'Oh! This is a great material and this is a bad one,' just on the basis of toxicity tests."

The difference between the two statements above reflects the progress that has been made in combustion toxicology over the time period. Instead of the earlier quest for a clearly superior laboratory scale test that could supplant all others, the present and future utility of combustion toxicology is to become more and more integrated into the overall process of hazard assessment.

The various FED models are a step in this direction of integration with hazard assessment. The FED models use analytic concentration measurements to predict the level of biological hazards. The ANSI/ISO guideline uses an animal test to assess the reasonableness of the model and to serve as a backstop to prevent missing unexpected toxicity and is literally "more than the sum of the parts (FEDs)."

VIII.   STAGED APPROACH TO COMBUSTION TOXICITY
HAZARD ASSESSMENT

The question of whether or not to use a particular polymer material in an application really is a fairly complex one, even when only issues related to potential fire hazards are of concern. Ultimately the central question comes down to is there an unacceptable incremental increase in risk associated with such a use. A series of questions must be considered in making such a decision, including:

- Is the plastic a replacement for a noncombustible?
- Does the plastic contain only H, C, and/or O?
- What is the similarity to current material?
- Does the plastic add N, F, Cl, Br, I, P, or S to the construction?
- Is the material a modification to add fire retardant properties?
- What is the potential for involuntary exposure in case of a fire?
- What is the number of people potentially exposed in a fire?
- What is your risk aversion level?
- Is the use in a regulated transportation or construction industry?

If the answer to these questions is such that use of the material is still being considered, then a stepwise approach should be taken to assessing the combustion toxicity associated risks. The steps involved include:

1. Assessing the chemical properties of the polymer
2. Performing a bench scale test, such as the UPITT
3. Analyzing the combustion products generated in bench scale testing
4. Assessing the results of the above in the context of an approach such as that of ASTM
5. If necessary, performing special studies

IX. CONCLUSION

Comprehensive assessment of the combustion toxicity of a material, a component, or an entire system requires the contributions from multiple technical fields, biology, chemistry, and engineering. The scale of the assessment should match the scale of the driving factor, whether the driver is, for example, the number of people potentially exposed or the degree of public concern. Single simple tests provide only a small amount of information about a large set of potential combustion scenarios and should be used as a component in the assessment, not as the only element of assessment. Animal tests are required to verify that the model is adequate and correctly applied. Skipping the animal test process leaves one vulnerable to the possibility that a relatively more toxic unanticipated combustion product renders all the modeling effort invalid.

ACKNOWLEDGMENTS

The authors gratefully acknowledge the assistance of Diane Erwin, Norma Cantu, and Robert Garay of Southwest Research Institute, the staff of Rogers Word Service (Raleigh, NC), and Dr. Gordon Hartzell in the preparation of this manuscript.

REFERENCES

1. Cullis, C.F. and Hirschler, M.M. (1981). The Combustion of Organic Polymers. Oxford: Clarendon, p. 420.
2. Landrock, A.H. (1983). Handbook of Plastics Flamability And Combustion Toxicology. Principles, Materials, Test, Safety and Smoke Inhalation Effects. Park Ridge, NJ: Noyes, p. 308.
3. Zapp, J.A. (1951). The Toxicity of Fire. Chemical Corps., Army Chemical Center, Maryland. Medical Division Sp.
4. Alexeeff, G. and Packham, S.C. (1984). Evaluation of Smoke Toxicity using Concentration-Time Products. J. Fire Sci. 2:3 62.
5. Alarie, Y. (1985). The Toxicity of Smoke from Polymeric Materials During Thermal Decomposition. Ann. Rev. Pharmacol. Toxicol. 25:35.
6. Ferguson, G.E. (1933). Fire Gases. Quarterly of the National Fire Protection Association 27:110.
7. Napier, D.H. and Wong, T.W. (1972). Toxic Products from the Combustion and Pyrolysis of Polyurethane Foams. Br. Polym. J. 4:45–52.
8. Zikria, B.A., Ferrer, J.M., and Floch, H.F. (1972). The Chemical Factors Contributing to Pulmonary Damage in 'Smoke Poisoning,' Surgery 71:704–709.
9. Terrill, J.B., Montgomery, R.R., and Reinhardt, C.F. (1978). Toxic Gases from Fires. Science 200:1343–1347.
10. Gold, A., Burgess, W.A., and Clougherty, E.V. (1978). Exposure of Firefighters to Toxic Air Contaminants. Am. Ind. H. Assoc. J. 39:534–539.
11. Harland, W.A. and Woolley, W.D. (1979). Fire Fatality Study-University of Glasgow, Information Paper IP 18/79, Glasgow, Scotland: Building Research Establishment.
12. Birky, M.M., Paabo, M., and Brown, J.E. (1980). Correlation of Autopsy Data and Materials Involved in the Tennessee Jail Fire. J. Fire Saf. 2:17–22.
13. Bowes, P.C. (1974). Smoke and Toxicity Hazards of Plastics in Fire. Ann. Occup. Hyg. 17:143–157.
14. Von Meyer, L., Drasch, G., and Kauert, G. (1979). Significance of Hydrocyanic Acid Formation During Fires. Z. Rechtsmed. 84:69–73.
15. Hirsch, C.S., Bost, R.O., Gerber, S.R., Cowan, M.E., Adelson, L., and Sunshine, I. (1977). Carboxyhemoglobin Concentrations in Flash Fire Victims Without Elevated Carboxyhemoglobin. Amer. J. Clin. Path. 68:317–320.
16. NFPA. (1983). Twelve Die in Fire at Westchase Hilton Hotel, Houston, Texas. Fire Journal January, 1983, 10–56.
17. Echardt, R.E. and Hindin, R. (1973). The Health Hazards of Plastics. J. Occup. Med. 15:808–819.
18. Barry, T.J. and Newman, B. (1976). Some Problems of Synthetic Polymers at Elevated Temperatures. Fire Technol. 12:186–192.
19. Van Grimbergen, M., Reybrouck, G., and van de Voorde, H. (1971). Development of Impurities in the Air by Burning Thermoplastics, Zentralbl. Bakteriol. Parasitenk Infektionskr. Hyg. 155:123–130.
20. Boettner, E.A. and Hartung, R. (1978). The Analysis and Toxicity of the Combus-

tion Products of Natural and Synthetic Materials. Final Report to the Society of the Plastics Industry, Inc. and the Manufacturing Chemists Association.

21. Barrow, C.S., Alaire, Y., and Stock, M.F. (1978). Sensory Irritation and Incapacitation Evoked by Thermal Decomposition Products of Polymers and Comparisons with Known Sensory Irritants. Arch. Environ. Health 33:79.

22. Thomas, W.C. and O'Flaherty, E.J. (1982). The Cardiotoxicity of Carbon Monoxide as a Component of Polymer Pyrolysis Smokes. Tox. Appl. Pharmacol. 63:363–372.

23. Thomas, W.C., O'Flaherty, E.J., Bell, R.H., and Stemmer, K.L. (1978). The Effect of Polymer Pyrolysis Fumes on the Activity of Rat Hepatic Cytochrome C Oxidase. Toxicol. Appl. Pharmacol. 45:98.

24. Heimann, R., Skornik, W., and Jaeger, R. J. (1979). Biochemical Changes in Guinea Pig Lungs Following Exposure to Plastic Combustion Products, Paraqual, or ANTU. Toxicol. Appl. Pharmacol. 48:A58.

25. Williams, N., Atkinson, G.W., and Patchesky, A.S. (1974). Polymer Fume Fever; Not So Benign. J. Occup. Med. 16:519–526.

26. Critterdan, B.D. and Long R. (1976). The mechanisms of Formation of Polynuclear Aromatic Compounds in Combustion Systems. In: Polynuclear Aromatic Hydrocarbons; Chemistry, Metabolism and Carcinogenesis. A Comprehensive Survey. (R. Frendenthal and P. W. Jones, eds.), pp. 209–223.

27. Withey, J.R. (1977). Mutagenic, Carcinogenic, and Teratogenic Hazards Arising from Human Exposure to Plastics Additives. In: Origins of Human Cancer Vol. 4 (H.H. Hiatt, J.D. Watson and J.A. Winsten, eds.), 219–241.

28. Zitting, A., Pfaffli, P., and Vainio, H. (1978). Effects of Thermal Decomposition Products of Polystyrene on microsomal Enzymes and Glutathione Levels in Mouse Liver. In: Proceedings of the International Symposium on Styrene: Occupational and Toxicological Aspects, pp. 16–17.

29. Parent, R.A., Dilley, J.V., and Simmon, V.F. (1979). Mutagenic Activity of Smoke Condensates from the Non-Flaming Combustion of Ten Flexible Polyurethane Foams Using the Salmonella/Microsome Assay. J. Combus. Toxicol. 6:256–264.

30. ISO. (1995). ISO 13344: Determination of the Lethal Toxic Potency of Fire Effluents, International Standards Organization, Geneva, Switzerland.

31. New York State. (1986). New York State Uniform Fire Prevention and Building Code, Article 15, Part 1120, Combustion Toxicity Testing, Office of Fire Prevention and Control, Department of State, New York State, Albany, NY.

32. Sarkos, C.P., Spurgeon, J.C., and Nicholas, E.B. Laboratory fire testing of cabin materials used in commercial aircraft. J. Aircraft. 1979 Feb; 16(2):78–89.

33. Crane, C.R., Sanders, D.C., Endecott, B.R., Abbott, J.K., and Smith, P.W. (1977). Inhalation Toxicology: I. Design of a Small-Animal Test System. II. Determination of the Relative Toxic Hazards of 75 Aircraft Cabin Materials. Report No. FAA-AM-77-9, Department of Transportation, Federal Aviation Administration. Washington, DC: Office of Aviation Medicine.

34. Chaturvedi, A.K. and Sanders, D.C. (1996). Aircraft fires, smoke toxicity, and survival. Aviat. Space Environ. Med. 67:275–278.

35. NFPA. (1996). NFPA 269: Standard Test Method for Developing Toxic Potency Data for Use in Fire Hazard Modeling. Quincy, MA: NFPA.

36. ASTM. (1995). ASTM E1678: Standard Test Method for Measuring Smoke Toxicity for use in Fire Hazard Analyses. Philadelphia, PA: American Society for Testing and Materials.
37. Alexeeff, G.V., Lee, Y.C., Thorning, D., Howard, M.L., and Hudson, L.D. (1986). Pulmonary Tissue Reactions in Response to Smoke Injury. J. Fire Sci. 4:427–442.
38. Kaplan, H.L., Grand, A.F., and Hartzell, G.E. (1983). Combustion Toxicology: Principles and Test Methods. Lancaster, PA, Technomic Publishing Company, Inc., pp. 1–174.
39. Gad, S.C. and Anderson, R.C. (1990). Combustion Toxicology, Boca Raton, FL: CRC Press.
40. Gad, S.C., Hartzell, G.E., Pursur, D.A., Roux, H.J., and Sarkos, C.P. (1996). Smoke toxicity standard test method for materials. Toxicology 115:201–222.
41. Rasbash, D.J. (1967). Smoke and Toxic Products Produced at Fires. Plast. Inst. Trans. J. 2:55–60.
42. Taylor, W. and Scott, C.A.C. (1979). Toxic Gases in Plastics Fires. Plast. Rubber. Inst. 95:259–266.
43. Bott, B., Firth, J.G., Jones, T.A. (1969). Evolution of Toxic Gases from Heated Plastics. Brit. Polym. J. 1:203–4.
44. Sumi, K. and Tsuchiya, Y. (1975). Toxicity of Decomposition Products. JFFIComb. Tox. 2:213.
45. Boettner, E.A. and Ball, G.L. (1973). Combustion Products from the Incineration of Plastics. Springfield, VA: NTIS.
46. Petajan, J.H., Baldwin, R.C., Rose, R.F., Jeppsen, R.B. (1976). Assessment of the Relative Toxicity of Materials; Concept of a Limiting Toxicant. ASTM Spec. Tech. Publ. STD 614:285–99.
47. Petajan, J.H., Voorhees, K.J., Packham, S.C., Baldwin, R.C., Einhorn, L.N., Grunnet, M.L., Dinger, B.G., and Birky, M.M. (1975). Extreme Toxicity from Combustion Products of a Fire-Retarded Polyurethane Foam. Science 187:742–7.
48. Chisnall, B. (1978). Toxic Gases in Fires. Fire Prev. Sci. Sc. Tech. 19:16–19.
49. National Materials Advisory Board. (1978). Smoke and Toxicity (Combustion Toxicology of Polymers). Vol. 3. Publication No. NMAB 318-3, Washington, DC: National Academy of Sciences, pp. 1–55.
50. Morikawa, T. and Yanai, E. (1986). Toxic Gases Evolution from Air-Controlled Fires in a Semi-Full Scale Room. J. Fire Science 4:299–314.
51. Gad, S.C. and Smith, A.C. (1983). Influence of Heating Rates on the Toxicity of Evolved Combustion Products: Results and a System for Research. J. Fire Science 1:465–479.
52. Grand, A.F. (1985). Effect of Experimental Conditions on the Evolution of Combustion Products using a modified University of Pittsburgh Toxicity Test Apparatus. J. Fire Science 3:280–304.
53. Hoffmann, H. Jr. and Oettel, H. (1969). Relative Toxicity of Plastics Combustion Products, Particularly Rigid Polystyrene Foam. KunststRundsch 15:261–8.
54. Kishitani, K. and Nakamura, K. (1974). Toxicities of Combustion Products. J. Fire Flam. Combust. Toxicol. Suppl. 1:104–123.
55. Wright, P.L. and Adams, C.H. (1977). Toxicity of Combustion Products from

Burning Polymers: Development and Evaluation of Methods. Environ. Health Perspect. 17:75–83.

56. Rodkey, F.L. and Jenkins, L.J. (1979). Toxicity of Shipboard Fire Combustion Products. Toxicol. Res. Proj. Direct. 4.

59. National Bureau of Standards. (1982). Further Development of a Test Method for the Assessment of the Acute Inhalation Toxicity of Combustion Products. NBSIR 82-2532 (June 1982).

60. Potts, W.J. and Lederer, T.S. (1977). A Method for Comparative Testing of Smoke Toxicity. J. Comb. Toxicol. 4:114–162.

61. Kimmerle, G. and Prager, F.C. (1980). The Relative Toxicity of Pyrolysis Products. Part II. Polyisocyanate Based Foam Materials. Journal of Combustion Toxicology 7:54.

62. Klimisch, H. (1980). Generation of Constant Concentrations of Thermal Decomposition Products in Inhalation Chambers. A Comparative Study with a Method According to DIN 53 436. 11. Measurement of Concentrations of Total Volatile Organic Substances in Inhalation Chambers. Journal of Combustion Toxicology 7: 257.

63. Hoffmann, H. and Sand, H.E. (1976). Evaluation of the Acute Toxicity Hazard of Combustion Products Given Off by Organic materials. In: Proceedings: International Symposium on Toxicity and Physiology of Combustion Products. National Academy of Sciences Committee on Fire Research, National Research Council, Salt Lake City, Utah (March 22–26, 1976).

64. Klimisch, H., Hollander, H.W.M., and Thyssen, J. (1980). Generation of Constant Concentrations of Thermal Decomposition Products in Inhalation Chambers. A Comparative Study with a Method According to DIN 53 436. I. Measurement of Carbon Monoxide and Carbon Dioxide in Inhalation Chambers. Journal of Combustion Toxicology 7:243.

65. Klimisch, H., Hollander, H.W.M., and Thyssen, J. (1980). Comparative Measurements of the Toxicity of Laboratory Animals of Products of Thermal Decomposition Generated by the Method of DIN 53 436. Journal of Combustion Toxicology 7:209.

66. Alarie, Y. and Barrow, C.S. (1977). Toxicity of Plastic Combustion Products. Toxicologic to Assess the Relative Hazards of Thermal Decomposition Products from Polymeric Materials. National Technical Information Service Publication PB267 23; 286 pp.

67. Anderson, R.C., Dierdorf, J., Stock, M.F., Matijak, M., Sawin, R., and Alaire, Y. (1978). Use of Experimental Materials to Assess Toxicological Tests for Rating Polymeric Materials Under Thermal Stress. Fire Mater. 2:136–140.

68. Anderson, R.C. and Alarie, Y.C. (1978). Screening Procedure to Recognize "Supertoxic" Decomposition Products From Polymeric Materials Under Thermal Stress. Journal of Combustion Toxicology 5:54–63.

69. Alarie, Y., Lin, C.K., and Geary, D.L. Sensory Irritation Evoked by Plastic Decomposition Products. Presented at the American Industrial Hygiene Conference Miami, Florida (May 15, 1974).

70. Alarie, Y. (1973). Sensory Irritation by Airborne Chemicals. CRC Crit. Rev. Toxicol. 2:299.

71. Barrow, C.S., Alarie, Y., and Stock, M.F. (1978). Sensory Irritation and Incapacitation Evoked by Thermal Decomposition Products of Polymers and Comparisons with Known Sensory Irritants. Arch. Environ. Health 33:79.

72. Kane, L.E., Barrow, C.S., and Alarie, Y. (1979). A Short-Term Test to Predict Acceptable Levels of Exposure to Airborne Sensory Irritants. Amer. Ind. Hyg. Assoc. J. 40:207–229.

73. Barrow, C.S., Lucia, H., and Alarie, Y.C. (1979). A Comparison of the Acute Inhalation Toxicity of Hydrogen Chloride Versus the Thermal Decomposition Products of Polyvinylchloride. Journal of Combustion Toxicology 6:3–12.

74. Barrow, C.S., Lucia, H., Stock, M.F., and Alarie, Y. (1979). Development of Methodologies to Assess the Relative Hazards from Thermal Decomposition Products of Polymeric Materials. J. Amer. Ind. Hyg. Assoc. 40:408–423.

75. Anderson, R.C. and Alarie, Y.C. (1978). An Attempt to Translate Toxicity of Polymer Thermal Decomposition Products Into a Toxicological Hazard index and Discussion on the Approaches Selected. Journal of Combustion Toxicology 5:476.

78. Spurgeon, J.C., Filipczak, R.A., Feher, R.E., and Sternik, S.J. (1979). A Procedure of Electronically Monitoring Animal Response Parameters Using the Rotating Wheel. Journal of Combustion Toxicology 6:198.

79. Hilado, C.J., Saxton, G.L., Kourtides, D.A., Parker, J.A., and Gilwee, W.J. (1976). Relative Toxicity of Pyrolysis Products of Some Cellular Polymers. J. Comb. Tax. 3:259.

80. Hilado, C.J. and Crane, C.R. (1977). Comparison of Results with the USF/NASA and FAA/CAMI Toxicity Screening Test Methods. J. Combust. Toxicol. 4:56–60.

81. Hartung, R., Ball, G.L., Boettner, E.A., Rosenbaum, R., and Hollingsworth, Z.R. (1977). The Performance of Rats on a Rotarod During Exposure to Combustion Products of Rigid Polyurethane Foams and wood. J. Combust. Toxicol. 4:506–522.

82. Petajan, J.H. (1977). An Approach to the Toxicology of Combustion Products of Materials. Environ. Health Perspect. 17:65–73.

83. Gad, S.C. (1998). Statistics and Experimental Design for Toxicologists. Third Edition. CRC Press, Boca Raton, FL.

84. Gad, S.C. and Chengelis, C.P. (1997). Acute Toxicology: Principles and Methods, Second Ed. San Diego, CA: Academic Press.

85. Pozzani, U.C., Weil, C.S., and Carpenter, C.P. (1959). The Toxicological Basis of Threshold Basis of Threshold Limit Values. 5. The Experimental Inhalation of Vapor Mixtures by Rats, with Notes Upon the Relationship Between Single Dose Inhalation and Single Dose Oral Data. Am. Ind. Hygiene Assoc. J. 20:364–369.

86. Smyth, H.F., Weil, C.S., West, J.F., and Carpenter, C.P. (1969). An Explanation of Joint Toxic Action: Twenty-Seven Industrial Chemicals Intubated in Rats in All Possible Pairs. Tox. Appl. Pharmacol. 14:340–347.

87. ISO. (1993). Toxicity of Fire Effluents. ISO/TR 9122 (Parts 1–5), American National Standards Institute: New York.

89. Birky, M.M., Halpin, B.M., Caplan, Y.H., Fisher, R.S., McAllister, J.M., and Dixon, A.M. (1979). Fire fatality study. Fire Materials 3:211.

90. Tsuchiya, Y. (1981). Dynamic Toxicity Factor-Evaluating Fire Gas Toxicity. J. Comb. Tax. 8:187. Waritz, R.S. (1975). Industrial Approach to Evaluation of Pyrolysis and Combustion Hazards. Environ. Health Perspect. 11:197–202.

91. Kaplan, H.L. and Hartzell, G.E. (1984). Modeling of Toxicological Effects of Fire Gases: I. Incapacitating Effects of Narcotic Fire Gases. J. Fire Science 2:286–305.
92. Hartzell, G.E., Packham, S.C., Grand, A.F., and Switzer, W.G. (1985). Modeling of Toxicological Effects of Fire Gases: III. Quantification of Post-Exposure Lethality of Rats from Exposure to HCl Atmospheres. J. Fire Science 3:195–206.
93. Hartzell, G.E., Priest, D.N., and Switzer, W.G. (1985). Modeling of Toxicological Effects of Fire Gases: II. Mathematical Modeling of Intoxication of Rats by Carbon Monoxide and Hydrogen Cyanide. J. Fire Science 3:115–128.
94. Hartzell, G.E. and Emmons, H.W. (1988). The Fractional Effective Dose Model for Assessment of Hazards Due to Smoke from Materials. J. Fire Sciences 6(5): 356–362.
95. Hartzell, G.E., Stacy, H.W., Switzer, W.G., Priest, D.N., and Packham, S.C. (1985). Modeling of Toxicological Effects of Fire Gases: IV. Intoxication of Rats by Carbon Monoxide in the Presence of an Irritant. J. Fire Science 3:263–279.
96. Hartzell, G.E., Switzer, W.G., and Priest, D.N. (1985). Modeling of Toxicologic Effects of Fire Gases: V. Mathematical Modeling of Intoxication of Rats by Combined Carbon Monoxide and Hydrogen Cyanide Atmospheres. J. Fire Science 3: 330–342.
97. Punderson, J.O. (1980). A Closer Look at Cause and Effect in Fire Fatalities—The Role of Toxic Fumes, Fire and Materials 5:41.
98. Babrauskas, V., Levin, B.C., and Gann R.G. (1986). A New Approach to Fire Toxicity Data for Hazard Evaluation. ASTM Stand. News 14:28–33.

13
Practical Statistical Analysis

Shayne Cox Gad
Gad Consulting Services, Raleigh, North Carolina

I. INTRODUCTION

This chapter is for both the practicing toxicologist and product safety individual as a practical guide to the common statistical problems encountered in toxicology and the methodologies that are available to solve them. It has been enriched by the inclusion of discussions of why a particular procedure or interpretation is suggested, and of examples of problems and pitfalls encountered in the day-to-day conduct and interpretation of studies. This chapter focuses on approaches, decisions, and issues, as opposed to techniques. Readers are directed to *Statistics and Experimental Design for Toxicologists* (1) if they wish to pursue details of actual statistical techniques.

Because of societal and regulatory requirements, studies are being designed and executed to generate increased amounts of data, which are then utilized to address various areas of concern. As the resulting problems of data analysis have become more complex due to the nature of the field, toxicology and safety evaluation have come to draw more deeply from the well of available statistical techniques. In fact, however, the field of statistics has also been very active and growing during the last 35 years; to some extent, at least, because of the very growth of toxicology. These simultaneous changes have led to an increasing complexity of data and, unfortunately, to the introduction of numerous confounding factors that severely limit the utility of the resulting data in all too many cases.

One (and perhaps the major) difficulty is that there is a very real need to understand the biological realities and implications of a problem, and to know the peculiarities of toxicological data before procedures are selected and employed for analysis. Some of these characteristics include the following.

1. The need to work with a relatively small sample set of data collected from the members of a population (laboratory animals, cultured cells, and bacterial cultures) that is not actually our population of interest (that is, people or a wildlife population).

2. Dealing frequently with data resulting from a sample that was censored on a basis other than investigator design. By censoring, of course, we mean that not all data points were collected as might be desired. This censoring could be the result of either a biological factor (the test animal being dead or too debilitated to manipulate) or a logistic factor (equipment being inoperative or a tissue being missed in necropsy).

3. The conditions for which our experiments are supposed to predict outcome are very open-ended. In pharmacology (the closest cousin to at least classical toxicology), the possible conditions of interaction of a chemical or physical agent with a person are limited to a small range of doses via a single route over a short course of treatment to a defined patient population. In toxicology however, all these things (a dose, route, time span, and subject population) are virtually wide open.

4. The time frames available to solve our problems are limited by practical and economic factors. This frequently means that there is not time to repeat a critical study if the first attempt fails. So a true iterative approach is not possible.

Unfortunately, there are very few toxicologists or product safety professionals who are also statisticians, or vice versa. In fact, the training of most toxicologists in statistics has been limited to a single introductory course concentrating on some theoretical basics. As a result, the armamentarium of statistical techniques of most toxicologists are limited and the tools that are usually present (t-tests, chi-square, analysis of variance, and linear regression) are neither fully developed nor well understood. This chapter will increase your understanding of statistical analysis.

As a point of departure toward this objective, it is essential that any data and analysis be interpreted by a professional who firmly understands three concepts: the difference between biological significance and statistical significance, the nature and value of different types of data, and causality.

For the first concept, we should consider the four possible combinations of these two different types of significance, for which we find the relationship shown below

		Statistical Significance	
		No	Yes
Biological	No	Case I	Case II
Significance	Yes	Case III	Case IV

Cases I and IV give us no problems, for the answers are the same statistically and biologically. But cases II and III present problems. In Case II (the "false positive"), we have a circumstance where there is a statistical significance in the measured difference between treated and control groups, but there is no true biological significance to the finding. This is not an uncommon happening, for example, in the case of clinical chemistry parameters. This is called type I error by statisticians, and the probability of this happening is called α (alpha) level. In case III (the "false negative"), we have no statistical significance, but the differences between groups are biologically/toxicologically significant. This is called type II error by statisticians, and the probability of such an error happening by random chance is called the β (beta) level. An example of this second situation is when we see a few of a very rare tumor type in treated animals. In both of these latter cases, numerical analysis, no matter how well done, is no substitute for professional judgment. Along with this, however, must come a feeling for the different types of data and for the value of each.

We will explore more fully the types of data (the second major concept) and their value (and the implications of value of data to such things as animal usage) in the next section.

There are many reasons why biological and statistical significance are not identical, but a central reason is certainly causality. Through our consideration of statistics, we should keep in mind that just because a treatment and a change in an observed organism are seemingly or actually associated with each other does not "prove" that the former caused the latter. Though this fact is now widely appreciated for correlation (for example, the fact that the number of storks' nests found each year in England is correlated with the number of human births that year does not mean that storks bring babies), it is just as true in the general case for significance. Timely establishment and proof that treatment causes an effect requires an understanding of the underlying mechanism and proof of its validity. At the same time, it is important that we realize that not finding a good correlation or suitable significance associated with a treatment and an effect likewise does not prove that the two are not associated—that a treatment does not cause an effect. At best, it gives us a certain level of confidence that under the conditions of the current test, these items are not associated.

II. Basic Principles

Let us first introduce (or review) a few simple terms and concepts which are fundamental to an understanding of statistics.

Each measurement we make, that is, each individual piece of experimental information we gather, is called a datum. It is extremely unusual, however, to either obtain or attempt to analyze a datum. Rather, we gather and analyze multiple pieces at one time, the resulting collection being called data.

Data are collected on the basis of their association with a treatment (intended or otherwise) as an effect (a property) that is measured in the experimental subjects of a study, such as body weights. These identifiers (that is, treatment and effect) are termed variables. Our treatment variables (those that are the researcher or nature control, and which can be directly controlled) are termed independent, while our effect variables (such as weight, life span, and number of neoplasms) are termed dependent variables because their outcome is believed to depend on the "treatment" being studied.

All the possible measures of a given set of variables in all the possible subjects that exist is termed the population for those variables. Such a population of variables cannot be truly measured. For example, one would have to obtain, treat, and measure the weights of all the Fischer-344 rats that were, are, or ever will be. Instead, we settle for dealing with a representative group or sample. If our sample of data is appropriately collected and of sufficient size, it serves to provide good estimates of the characteristics of the parent population from which it was drawn.

Two terms refer to the quality and reproducibility of our measurements of variables. The first, accuracy, is an expression of the closeness of a measured or computed value to its actual or "true" value in nature. The second, precision, reflects the closeness or reproducibility of a series of repeated measurements of the same quantity.

If we arrange all of our measurements of a particular variable in order as a point on an axis marked as to the values of that variable, and if our sample were large enough, the pattern of distribution of the data in the sample would begin to become apparent. This pattern is a representation of the frequency distribution of a given population of data, that is, of the incidence of different measurements, their central tendency, and dispersion.

The most common frequency distribution and one we will talk about throughout this chapter, is the normal (or Gaussian) distribution. This distribution is so common in nature that two-thirds of all values are within one standard deviation (defined below) of the mean (or average value for the entire population) and 95% are within 1.96 standard deviations of the mean. There are other frequency distributions such as the binomial, Poisson, and chi square, which are encountered from time to time, but none of these are as pervasive as the normal distribution.

In all areas of biological research, optimal design and appropriate interpretation of experiments require that the researcher understand both the biological and technological underpinnings of the system being studied and of the data being generated. From the point of view of the statistician, it is vitally important that the experimenter both know and be able to communicate the nature of the data, and understand its limitations. One classification of data types is presented in Table 1.

Table 1 Types of Variables (Data) and Examples of Each Type

Classified by	Type	Example[a]
Scale		
Continuous	Scalar	Body weight
	Ranked	Severity of a lesion
Discontinuous	Scalar	Weeks until the first observation of a tumor in a carcinogenicity study
	Ranked	Clinical observations in animals
	Attribute	Eye colors in fruit flies
	Quantal	Dead/alive or present/absent
Frequency distribution	Normal	Body weights
	Bimodal	Some clinical chemistry parameters
	Others	Measures of time-to-incapacitation

[a]It should be kept in mind that though these examples are most commonly of the data types assigned above, it is not always the case.

The nature of the data collected is determined by three considerations. These are the biological source of the data (the system being studied), the instrumentation and techniques used to make measurements, and the design of the experiment. The researcher has some degree of control over each of these: the least over the biological system (he/she normally has a choice of one of several models to study) and the most over the design of the experiment or study. Such choices, in fact, dictate the type of data generated by a study.

Statistical methods are each based on specific assumptions. Parametric statistics, those that are most familiar to the majority of scientists, have more stringent sets of underlying assumptions than nonparametric statistics. Among these underlying assumptions (for many parametric statistical methods, such as analysis of variance) is that the data are continuous. The nature of the data associated with a variable (as described above) imparts a "value" to that data, the value being the power of the statistical tests which can be employed.

Continuous variables are those which can at least theoretically assume any of an infinite number of values between any two fixed points (such as measurements of body weight between 2.0 and 3.0 kg). Discontinuous variables, meanwhile, are those which can have only certain fixed values, with no possible intermediate values (such as counts of 5 or 6 dead animals, respectively).

Limitations on our ability to measure constrain the extent to which the real-world situation approaches the theoretical here, but many of the variable studied in toxicology are in fact continuous. Examples of these are lengths, weights, concentrations, temperatures, periods of time, and percentages. For these continuous variables, we may describe the character of a sample with measures of central tendency and dispersion that we are most familiar with: the mean, denoted by the symbol $\overline{X}$ and also called the arithmetic average, and the standard deviation (SD, which is denoted by the symbol σ and is calculated as being equal to

$$\sqrt{\frac{\Sigma X^2 - \frac{(\Sigma X)^2}{N}}{N-1}}$$

where X is the individual datum and N is the total number of data in the group.

Contrasted with these continuous data, however, we have discontinuous (or discrete) data, which can only assume certain fixed numerical values. In these cases our selection of types of statistical tools or tests is more limited. A lot of data in toxicology fits into this category.

A. Probability

Probability is simply the likelihood that in a sufficiently large sample a particular event would occur or a particular value be found. Hypothesis testing, for example, is generally structured so that the likelihood of a treatment group being the same as a control group (the so called "null hypothesis") can be assessed as being less than a selected low level. Very frequently this is 5% (or $p \leq 0.05$), which implies that we are 95% (that is, 1.0–0.05) sure that the groups are *not* equivalent.

B. Functions of Statistics

Statistical methods may serve to do any combination of three possible tasks. The one we are most familiar with is hypothesis testing, that is, determining if two (or more) groups of data differ from each other at a predetermined level of confidence. A second function is the construction and use of models that may be used to predict future outcomes of chemical–biological interactions. This is most commonly seen as linear regression or as the derivation of some form of correlation coefficient. Model fitting allows us to relate one variable (typically a treatment or "independent" variables) to another. The third function, reduction of dimensionality, continues to be less commonly utilized than the first two. In this final category are the methods for reducing the number of variables in a system while only minimally reducing the amount of information, therefore making a problem easier to visualize and to understand. Examples of such techniques are factor analysis and cluster analysis. A subset of this last function, discussed later under descriptive statistics, is the reduction of raw data to single expressions of central tendency and variability (such as the mean and standard deviation).

There is also a special subset that is part of both the second and third functions of statistics. This is data transformation, which includes such things as the conversion of numbers to log or probit values.

C. Descriptive Statistics

Descriptive statistics are used to convey, in a summarized manner, the general nature of the data. As such, the parameters describing any single group of data have two components. One of these describes the location of the data, while the other gives a measure of the dispersion of the data in and about this location. Often overlooked is that the choice of what parameters are used to give these pieces of information implies a particular nature of distribution for the data.

Most commonly, location is described by giving the (arithmetic) mean and the dispersion by giving the standard deviation (SD) or the standard error of the mean (SEM). The calculation of the first two of these has already been described. If we again denote the total number of data in a group as N, then the SEM would be calculated as

$$\text{SEM} = \frac{\text{SD}}{\sqrt{N}}$$

1. Comparison of SD and SEM

The standard deviation and the standard error of the mean are related to each other but yet are quite different. To compare these two, let us first demonstrate their calculation from the same set of 15 observations.

	Sum (Σ)
Date Points (X_i): 1, 2, 3, 4, 4, 5, 5, 5, 6, 6, 6, 7, 7, 8, 9	78
Squares (X_i^2): 1, 4, 9, 16, 16, 25, 25, 25, 36, 36, 36, 49, 49, 49, 64, 81	472

The standard deviation can then be calculated as:

$$\text{SD} = \sqrt{\frac{472 - \dfrac{(78)^2}{15}}{15 - 1}} = \sqrt{\frac{472 - \dfrac{(6084)}{15}}{14}}$$

$$= \frac{472 - 405.6}{14} = 4.742851 = 2.1778$$

with a mean of ($\overline{X}$) of $78/15 = 5.2$ for the data group. The SEM for the same set of data, however, is

$$\text{SEM} = \frac{2.1778}{\sqrt{15}} = \frac{2.1778}{3.8730} = 0.562301$$

The SEM is quite a bit smaller than the SD, making it very attractive to use in reporting data. This relative size is due to the SEM actually being an estimate of the error (or variability) involved in measuring the data from which means are calculated. This is implied by the central limit theorem, which has three main points associated with it.

> The distribution of sample means will be approximately normal regardless of the distribution of values in the original population from which the samples were drawn.
> The mean value of the collection of all possible sample means will equal the mean of the original population.
> The standard deviation of the collection of all possible means of samples of a given size, called the standard error of the mean, depends on both the standard deviation of the original population and the size of the sample.

The SEM should be used only when the uncertainty of the estimate of the mean is of concern, which is almost never the case in toxicology. Rather, we are concerned with an estimate of the variability of the population, for which the standard deviation is appropriate.

The use of the mean with either the SD or SEM implies, however, that we have reason to believe that the data being summarized are from a population which is at least approximately normally distributed. If this is not the case, then we should rather use a set of terms that do not have such a rigid underpinning. These are the median, for location, and the semiquartile distance, for a measure of dispersion. These somewhat less commonly familiar parameters are characterized as follows.

2. Median

When all the numbers in a group are arranged in a ranked order (that is, from smallest to largest), the median is the middle value. If there is an odd number of values in a group then the middle value is obvious (in the case of 13 values, for example, the seventh largest is the median). When the number of values in the sample is even, the median is calculated as the midpoint between the $[N/2]$th and the $([N/2] + 1)$th number. For example, in the series of numbers 7, 12, 13, 19, the median value would be the midpoint between 12 and 13, which is 12.5.

3. Semiquartile Distance

When all the data in a group are ranked, a quartile of the data contains one ordered quarter of the values. Typically, we are most interested in the borders of the middle two quartiles. Q_1 and Q_2, which together represent the semiquartile distance and which contain the median as their center. Given that there are N values in an ordered group of data, the upper limit of the jth quartile (Q_j) may be computed as being equal to the $[j(N+1)/4\text{th}]$ value. Once we have used this formula to calculate the upper limits of Q_1 and Q_3, we can then compute the semiquartile distance (which is also called the quartile deviation, and as such is abbreviated as the QD) with the formula $QD = (Q_3 - Q_1)/2$.

For example, for the 15 member data set 1, 2, 3, 4, 4, 5, 5, 5, 6, 6, 6, 7, 7, 8, 9, we can calculate the upper limits of Q_1 and Q_3 as

$$Q_1 = \frac{1(15+1)}{4} = \frac{16}{4} = 4$$

$$Q_3 = \frac{3(15+1)}{4} = \frac{48}{4} = 12$$

The 4th and 12th values in this data set are 4 and 7, respectively. The semiquartile distance can then be calculated as

$$QD = \frac{12-4}{2} = 4$$

There are times when it is desired to describe the relative variability of one or more sets of data. The most common way of doing this is to compute the coefficient of variation (CV), which is calculated simply as the ratio of the standard deviation to the mean, or

$$CV = \frac{SD}{\overline{X}}$$

A CV of 0.2 or 20% thus means that the standard deviation is 20% of the mean. In toxicology, the CV is frequently between 20 and 50% and may at times exceed 100%.

D. Outliers

Outliers are extreme (high or low) values which are widely divergent from the main body of a group of data and from what is our common experience. They may arise from an instrument (such as a balance) being faulty, the seeming natural urge of some animals to frustrate research, or they may be indicative of a "real" value. Outlying values can be detected by visual inspection of the data, use of a scattergram (as will be discussed later), or (if the data set is small enough, which is usually the case in toxicology) by a large increase in the parameter estimating the dispersion of data, such as the standard deviation.

When we can solidly tie one of the above error-producing processes (such as a balance for being faulty) to an outlier, we can safely delete it from consideration. But if we cannot solidly tie such a cause to an outlier (even if we have strong suspicions), we have a much more complicated problem, for then such a value may be one of several other things. It could be a result of a particular cause that is the grounds for the entire study: that is, the very "effect" that we are looking for, or it could be because of the collection of legitimate effects which constitute sample error. As will be discussed later under exploratory data analysis, and as is now becoming more widely appreciated, in animal studies outliers can be an indication of a biologically significant effect which is not yet statistically significant. Variance inflation can be the result of such outliers, and can be used to detect them. Outliers, in fact, by increasing the variability within a sample, decrease the sensitivity of our statistical tests and actually preclude our having a statistically significant result (103).

Alternatively, the outlier may be the result of an unobserved technician error, for example, and may be such as to change the decisions that would result from a set of data.

In this last case we want to reject the data point, to exclude it from consideration with the rest of the data. But how can one identify these legitimate statistical rejection cases?

There are a wide variety of techniques for data rejection. Their proper use depends on one's understanding of the nature of the distribution of the data. For normally distributed data with a single extreme value, a simple method such as Chauvenet's criterion (2) may legitimately be employed. This states that if the probability of a value deviating from the mean is greater than $1/2N$, one should consider that there are adequate grounds for its rejection.

A second relatively straightforward approach, for when the data are normally distributed but contain several extreme values, is to "winsorize" the data. Though there are a number of variations on this approach, the simplest (called the G-1 method) calls for replacing the highest and lowest values in a set of data. In a group of data consisting of the values 54, 22, 18, 15, 14, 13, 11, and 4, we would replace 54 with a second 22 and 4 with a replicate 11. This would give us a group consisting of 22, 22, 18, 15, 14, 14, 13, 11, and 11, which we would then treat as our original data. Winsorizing should not be performed, however, if the extreme values constitute more than a small minority of the entire data set.

Yet another approach is to use Dixon's test (3) to determine if extreme values should be rejected. In Dixon's test, the set of observations is first ordered according to magnitude (as we did earlier for the data set used to demonstrate quartile deviations, though there this step was simply to make the case clearer). The ratio of the difference of an extreme value from one of its nearest neighbor values to the range of values in the sample is then calculated, using a formula that varies with sample size. This ratio is then compared to a table value, and if found to be equal or greater, is considered to be an outlier at the $p \leq 0.05$ level.

The formula for the ratio varies with sample size and according to whether it is the smallest or largest value that is suspect. If we have more information as to the nature of the data or the type of analysis to be performed, there are yet better ways to handle outliers.

E. Sampling

Sampling (the selection of which individual data points will be collected), whether in the form of selecting certain animals to collect blood from or removing a portion of a diet mix to analyze, is an essential step upon which all other efforts toward a good experiment or study are based.

There are three assumptions about sampling that are common to most of the statistical analysis techniques that are used in toxicology: 1) sample is collected without bias; 2) each member of a sample is collected independently of the others; 3) members of a sample are collected with replacements. Precluding bias, both intentional and unintentional, means that at the time of selection of a sample to measure, each portion of the population from which that selection is to be made has an equal chance of being selected. Ways of precluding bias are discussed in detail in the section on experimental design.

Independence means that the selection of any portion of the sample is not affected by and does not affect the selection or measurement of any other portion.

Finally, the assumption of sampling with replacement means that in theory, after each portion is selected and measured, it is returned to the total sample pool and thus has the opportunity to be selected again. This is a corollary of the assumption of independence. Violation of this assumption (which is almost always the case in toxicology and all the life sciences) does not have serious consequences as long as the total pool from which samples are being drawn is large enough (say 20 or greater) that the chance of reselecting that portion is small anyway.

There are four major types of sampling methods: random, stratified, systematic, and cluster. Random is by far the most commonly employed method in toxicology. It stresses the fulfillment of the assumption of avoiding bias. When the entire pool of possibilities is mixed or randomized (procedures for randomization are presented in a later section), then the preselected members of the pool are selected as they appear.

Stratified sampling is performed by first dividing the entire pool into subsets or strata, then doing randomized sampling from each strata. This method is employed when the total pool contains subsets that are distinctly different but in which each subset contains similar members. An example is a large batch of a powdered pesticide in which it is desired to determine the nature of the particle size distribution. Larger pieces or particles are on the top while progressively smaller particles have settled lower in the container. At the very bottom the material has been packed and compressed into aggregates. To determine a timely representative answer, proportionately sized subsets from each layer or strata should be selected, mixed, and randomly sampled. This method is used most commonly in diet studies.

In systematic sampling, a sample is taken at set intervals (such as every fifth container of reagent or taking a sample of water from a fixed sample point in a flowing stream every hour). This is most commonly employed in quality assurance or (in the clinical chemistry lab) in quality control.

To perform cluster sampling, the pool is already divided into numerous separate groups (such as bottles of tablets), and we select small sets of groups (such as several bottles of tablets), then select a few members from each small set. What one gets then is a cluster of measures. Again, this is a method most commonly used in quality control or in environmental studies when the effort and expense of physically collecting a small group of units is significant.

In classical toxicology studies, sampling arises in a practical sense in a limited number of situations. The most common of these are:

1. Selecting a subset of animals or test systems from a study to make some measurement (which is either destructive or stressing of the measured system or is expensive) at an interval during a study. This may include doing interim necropsies in a chronic study or collecting and analyzing blood samples from some animals during a subchronic study.
2. Analyzing inhalation chamber atmospheres to characterize aerosol distributions with a new generation system.
3. Analyzing diet in which test material has been incorporated.
4. Performing quality control on an analytical chemistry operation by having duplicate analyses performed on some materials.
5. Selecting data to audit for quality assurance purposes.

F. Generalized Methodology Selection

One approach for the selection of appropriate techniques to employ in a particular situation is to use a decision-tree method. Figure 1 is a decision tree that leads to the choice of one of three other trees to assist in technique selection, with each of the subsequent trees addressing one of the three functions of statistics that was defined earlier in this chapter. Figure 2 is for the selection of hypothesis-testing procedures, Figure 3 for modeling procedures, and Figure 4 for reduction of dimensionality procedures. For the vast majority of situations, these trees will guide the user into the choice of the proper technique. The specifics of the tests in these trees are beyond the scope of this chapter and should be pursued elsewhere (1).

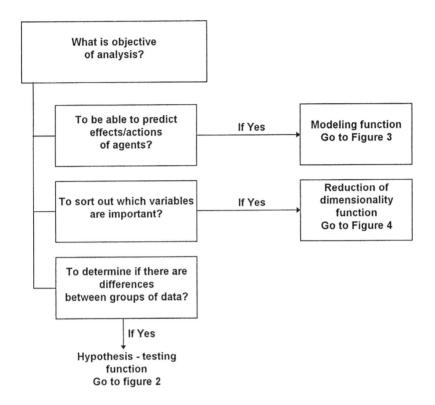

Figure 1 Overall decision tree for selecting statistical procedures.

III. EXPERIMENTAL DESIGN

In toxicology, we generally carry out experiments for a twofold purpose. The first question we ask is whether or not an agent results in an effect on a biological system. Our second question, which is never far behind, is how much of an effect is present. Both the cost to perform research to answer such questions and the value that society places upon the results of such efforts have continued to increase rapidly. Additionally, it has become increasingly desirable that the results of studies aimed at assessing the effects of environmental agents allow conclusions as straightforward as possible. As these trends seem to have little likelihood of changing in the foreseeable future, it is essential that every experiment and study yield as much information as possible, and that (more specifically) the results of each study provide possible answers to the questions it was conducted to address. The statistical aspects of such efforts, as they are aimed at structuring experiments in design to maximize the possibilities of success, are called experimental design.

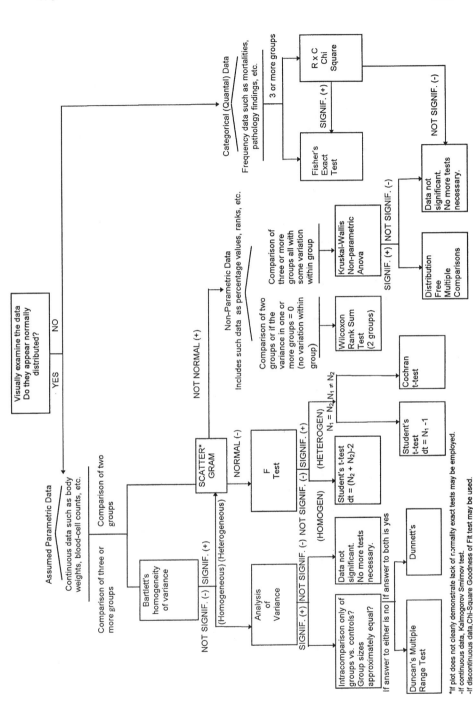

Figure 2 Decision tree for selecting hypothesis-testing procedures.

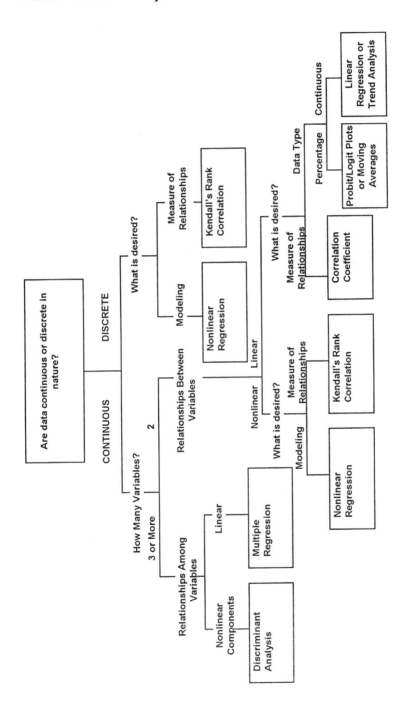

Figure 3 Decision tree for selecting modeling procedures.

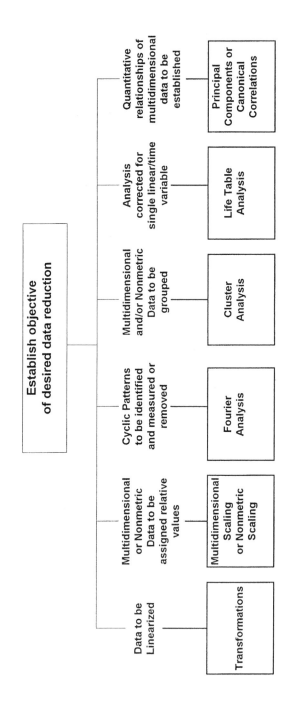

Figure 4 Decision tree for selection of reduction of dimensionality procedures.

We have now become accustomed to developing exhaustively detailed protocols for an experiment or study prior to its conduct. But, typically, such protocols do not include or reflect a detailed plan for the statistical analysis of the data generated by the study and certainly even less frequently, reflect such consideration in their design. A priori selection of statistical methodology (as opposed to the post hoc approach) is as significant a portion of the process of protocol development and experimental design as any other and can measurably enhance the value of the experiment or study. Such prior selection of statistical methodologies is essential for effective detailing of such other portions of a protocol as the number of animals per group and the sampling intervals for body weight. Implied in such a selection is that the toxicologist has both an in-depth knowledge of the area of investigation and an understanding of the general principles of experimental design, for the analysis of any set of data is dictated to a large extent by the manner in which the data are obtained.

The four basic statistical principles of experimental design are replication, randomization, concurrent ("local") control, and balance. In abbreviated form, these may be summarized as follows.

A. Replication

Any treatment must be applied to more than one experimental unit (animal, plate of cells, litter of offspring, etc.). This provides more accuracy in the measurement of a response than can be obtained from a single observation, since underlying experimental errors tend to cancel each other out. It also supplies an estimate of the experimental error derived from the variability among each of the measurements taken (or "replicates"). In practice, this means that an experiment should have enough experimental units in each treatment group (that is, a large enough "N") so that reasonably sensitive statistical analysis of data can be performed. The estimation of what is a large enough sample size is addressed in detail later in this chapter.

B. Randomization

This practice ensures that every treatment shall have its fair share of extreme high and extreme low values or of hyper- and hyporesponding individuals. It also serves to allow the toxicologist to proceed as if the assumption of "independence" is valid. That is, there is no avoidable (known) systematic basis in how one obtains data.

C. Concurrent Control

Comparisons between treatments should be made to the maximum extent possible between experimental units from the same closely defined population.

Therefore, animals used as a "control" group should come from the same source, lot, age, etc. as test group animals. Except for the treatment being evaluated, test and control animals should be maintained and handled in exactly the same manner.

D. Balance

If the effect of several different factors is being evaluated simultaneously, the experiment should be laid out in such a way that the contributions of the different factors can be separately distinguished and estimated. There are several ways of accomplishing this end by using one of several different forms of design, as will be discussed below.

There are four basic types of experimental designs that are utilized in toxicology. These are the randomized block, latin square, factorial design, and nested design. Other designs that are used are really combinations of these basic designs, and furthermore are very rarely employed in toxicology. Before examining these four basic types, however, we must first examine the basic concept of blocking.

Blocking is, simply put, the arrangement or sorting of the members of a population (such as all of an available group of test animals) into groups based on certain characteristics that may (but are not sure to) alter an experimental outcome. Such factors that may cause a treatment to give a differential effect are genetic background, age, sex, overall activity levels, and so on. The process of blocking then acts (or attempts to act), so that each experimental group (or block) is assigned its fair share of the members of each of these subgroups.

We should now recall that randomization is aimed at spreading out the effects of undetectable or unsuspected characteristics in a population of animals or some portion of this population. The merging of the two concepts of randomization and blocking leads to the most basic experimental design, the randomized block. This type of design requires that each treatment group have at least one member of each recognized characteristic group (such as age), the exact members of each block being assigned in an unbiased (or random) fashion.

A second concept and its understanding are essential to the design of experiments in toxicology, that of censoring. Censoring is the exclusion of measurements of certain experimental units, or indeed of the experimental units themselves, from consideration in data analysis or inclusion in the experiment at all, respectively. Censoring may occur either prior to initiation of an experiment (where, in modern toxicology, this is almost always a planned procedure), during the course of an experiment (when they are almost universally unplanned, resulting from, for example, the death of animals on test), or after the conclusion of an experiment (when, usually, data are excluded because of being identified as some form of outlier).

In practice, a priori censoring in toxicology studies occurs in the assignment of experimental units to test groups. The most familiar example is in the common practice of assignment of test animals to acute, subacute, subchronic, and chronic studies, where the results of otherwise random assignments are evaluated for body weights of the assigned members. If the mean weights are found not to be comparable by some pre-established criterion (such as a 90% probability of difference by analysis of variance) then members are reassigned (censored) to achieve comparability in terms of starting body weights. Such a procedure of animal assignment to groups is a censored randomization.

The first precise or calculable aspect of experimental design to be considered is determining what are sufficient test and control group sizes to allow one to have an adequate level of confidence in the results of a study. This number (N) can be calculated by using the formula

$$N = \frac{(t_1 + t_2)^2 s^2}{d^2}$$

where t_1 is the one-tailed value with N-1 degrees of freedom corresponding to the desired level of confidence, t_2 is the one-tailed t value with N-1 degrees of freedom corresponding to the probability that the sample size will be adequate to achieve the desired precision, and S is the sample standard deviation, derived typically from historical data and calculated as (with V being the variable of interest)

$$S = \sqrt{\frac{1}{N-1} \Sigma(V_1 - V_2)^2}$$

d is the acceptable range of variation in the variable of interest.

A good approximation can be generated by substituting the t values (from a table of t values) for an infinite number of degrees of freedom. This entire process is demonstrated in the following example.

Example. In a subchronic dermal study in rabbits, the principal point of concern is the extent to which the compound causes oxidative damage to the erythrocytes. To quantitate this, the laboratory will be measuring the numbers of reticulocytes in the blood. What then would be an adequate sample size to allow the question at hand to be addressed with reasonable certitude of an answer?

To do this, we use the one-tailed t value for an infinite number of degrees of freedom at 95% confidence level (that is, $p \leq 0.05$). Going to a set of t tables, we find this number to be 1.645. From prior experience, we know that the usual values for reticulocytes in rabbit blood are from 0.5 to 1.9. The acceptable range of variation, 0, is therefore equal to the span of this range, or 1.4. Likewise, examining the control data from previous rabbit studies, we find our sample standard deviation to be 0.825. When we insert all of these numbers into the equation (presented above) for sample size, we can calculate the required sample size (N) to be equal to

$$\frac{(1.645 + 1.645)^2}{(1.4)^2} \, 0.825 = \frac{10.824}{1.96} \, (0.825) = 4.556$$

In other words, in this case where there is little natural variability, measuring the reticulocyte counts of groups of only five animals each should be sufficient to answer the question.

There are a number of aspects of experimental design that are specific to the actual practice to toxicology. Before we look at a suggestion for step-by-step development of experimental designs, these aspects should first be considered.

1. Frequently, the data gathered from specific measurements of animal characteristics are such that there is wide variability in the data. Often, such wide variability is not present in a control or low dose group, but in an intermediate dosage group variance inflation may occur. That is, there may be a large standard deviation associated with the measurements from this intermediate group. In the face of such a data set, the conclusion that there is no biological effect based on a finding of no statistically significant effect might well be erroneous.

2. In designing experiments, a toxicologist should keep in mind the potential effect of involuntary censoring on sample size. In other words, though the study described in the example might start with five dogs per group, this provides no margin should any die before the study is ended and blood samples are collected and analyzed. Just enough experimental units per group frequently leaves too few at the end to allow meaningful statistical analysis, and allowances should be made accordingly in establishing group sizes.

3. It is certainly possible to pool the data from several identical toxicological studies. For example, after first having performed an acute inhalation study where only three treatment group animals survived to the point at which a critical measure (such an analysis of blood samples) was performed, we would not have enough data to perform a meaningful statistical analysis. We could then repeat the protocol with new control and treatment group animals from the same source. At the end, after assuring ourselves that the two sets of data are comparable, we would combine (or pool) the data from survivors of the second study with those from the first. The costs of this approach, however, would then be both a greater degree of effort expended (than if we had performed a single study with larger groups) and increased variability in the pooled samples (decreasing the power of our statistics).

4. Another frequently overlooked design option in toxicology is the use of an unbalanced design, that is, of different group sizes for different levels of treatment.

There is no requirement that each group in a study (control, low dose, intermediate dose, and high dose) have an equal number of experimental units assigned to it. Indeed, there are frequently good reasons in toxicology to assign more experimental units to one group than to the others, and, as we shall see later, all the major statistical methodologies have provisions to adjust for such inequalities, within certain limits. The two most common uses of the unbalanced design have larger groups assigned to either the highest dose to compensate for losses due to possible deaths during the study or to the lowest dose to give more sensitivity in detecting effects at levels close to a threshold of effect, or more confidence that there is not an effect.

5. Frequently, we are confronted in toxicology with the situation that an undesired variable is influencing our experimental results in a nonrandom fashion. Such a variable is called a confounding variable and its presence, as discussed earlier, makes clear attribution and analysis of effects at best difficult, and at worst impossible. Sometimes such confounding variables are the result of conscious design or management decisions, such as the use of different instruments, personnel, facilities, or procedures for different test groups within the same study. Occasionally, however, such confounding variables are the result of unintentional factors or actions, in which case it is called a lurking variable. Examples of such variables are almost always the result of standard operating procedures being violated: water not being connected to a rack of animals over a weekend, a set of racks not being cleaned as frequently as others, or a contaminated batch of feed or vehicle being used.

6. Finally, some thought must be given to the clear definition of what is meant by experimental unit and concurrent control.

The experimental unit in toxicology encompasses a wide variety of possibilities. It may be cells, plates of microorganisms, individual animals, litters of animals, and so forth. The importance of clearly defining the experimental unit is that the number of such units per group is the "N" used in statistical calculations or analysis resulting from studies, and there, critically affects the power of such calculations.

The experimental unit is the unit that receives treatments and yields a response which is measured and becomes a datum. What this means in practice is that, for example, in reproduction or teratology studies where we treat the parental–generation females and then determine results by counting or evaluating offspring, the experimental unit is still the parent. Therefore, the number of litters, not the number of offspring, is the N (4).

A true concurrent control is one that is identical in every manner with the treatment groups except for the treatment being evaluated. This means that all manipulations, including gavaging with equivalent volumes of vehicle or exposing to equivalent rates of air exchanges in an inhalation chamber, should be duplicated in the control groups just as they occur in the treatment.

The goal of the four principles of experimental design is good statistical efficiency and economy of resources. An alternative way of looking at this in a stepwise logical manner is to do a logic flow analysis of the problem. Such an undertaking is conducted in three steps, and should be performed every time any major study or project is initiated or indeed, at regular periods during the course of conduct of a series of "standard" smaller studies. These steps are detailed below.

1. Define the objective of the study: get a clear statement of what questions are being asked.
   A. Can the question, in fact, be broken down into a set of subquestions?
   B. Are we asking one or more of these questions repeatedly? For example, does "X" develop at 30, 60, 90+ days and/or does it progress/regress or recover?
   C. What is our model to be in answering this/these questions? Is it appropriate and acceptably sensitive?
2. For each subquestion (i.e., separate major variable to be studied):
   A. How is the variable of interest to be measured?
   B. What is the nature of the data generated by the measure? Are we getting an efficient set of data? Or are we buying too little information, and would another technique improve the quality of the information generated to the point that it becomes a higher "class" of data? Or too much information (i.e., does some underlying aspect of the measure limit the class of data obtainable within the bounds of feasibility of effort)?
   C. Are there possible interactions between measurements? Can they be separated/identified?
   D. Is our N (sample size) both sufficient and efficient?
   E. What is the control (formal or informal)? Is it appropriate?
   F. Are we needlessly adding confounding variables (asking inadvertent or unwanted questions)?
   G. Are there "lurking variables" present? These are undesired and not readily recognized differences that can affect results, such as different technicians observing different groups of animals.
   H. How large an effect will be considered biologically significant? This is a question that can only be resolved by reference to experience or historical control data.
3. What are the possible outcomes of the study, that is, what answers are possible to both our subquestions and to our major question?
   A. How do we use these answers?
   B. Do the possible answers offer a reasonable expectation of achieving the objectives that caused us to initiate the study?

C. What new questions may these answers cause us to ask? Can the study be redesigned, before it is actually started, so that these "revealed" questions may be answered in the original study?

A practical example of the application of this approach can be demonstrated in the process of designing a chronic inhalation study. Although in such a situation the primary question being asked is usually "does the chemical result in cancer by this route?," even at the beginning there are a number of other questions that it is expected that the study will answer. Two of these questions are 1) If cancer is caused, what is the relative risk associated with it? and 2) Are there other expressions of toxicity associated with chronic exposure? Several, if not all, of the above questions are actually to be asked repeatedly during the course of the study. Before the study starts, a plan and arrangement must be formed and criteria established against which to measure the answers to these questions.

The last phase of our logical analysis must start by considering each of the things which may go wrong during the study. These include the occurrence of an infectious disease (Do we continue or stop exposures? How will we now separate what portions of observed effects are due to the chemical under study and what is due to the disease process?), finding that extreme nasal and respiratory irritation was occurring in test animals, or revealing the existence of some hidden variable. Can we preclude (or minimize) the possibility of a disease outbreak by doing a more extensive health surveillance and quarantine on our test animals prior to the start of the study? Could we select a better test model, that is, one that is not as sensitive to upper respiratory or nasal irritation?

If the reader has a greater degree of interest in experimental design, there are many tests available that provide detailed guidance on the statistical aspects of experimental design. Among those that are recommended are Cochran and Cox (99); Diamond (100); Federer (101); Hicks (102); and Myers (2).

IV. DATA ANALYSIS APPLICATIONS IN TOXICOLOGY

Having reviewed the necessary basic principles and provided a set of methods for statistical handling of data, the remainder of this book will address the practical aspects and difficulties encountered in day-to-day toxicology.

As a starting point, we present an overview of data types actually encountered in toxicology (Table 2) classified by type (as presented at the beginning of this book). It should be stressed, however, that this classification is of the most frequent nature of each sort of observation (such as body weight) and will not be universally true.

There are now common practices in the analysis of toxicology data, though they are not necessarily the best. These are discussed in the remainder

Table 2 Classification of Data Commonly Encountered in Toxicology by Type

Continuous normal	Body weights
	Food consumption
	Organ weights: absolute and relative
	Mouse ear swelling test (MEST) measurements
	Pregnancy rates
	Survival rates
	Crown-rump lengths
	Hematology (some)
	Clinical chemistry (some)
Continuous but not normal	Hematology (some-WBC)
	Clinical chemistry (some)
	Urinalysis
Scalar data	Neurobehavioral signs (some)
	Primary dermal and ocular irritation scores
	Histopathology (some)
Count data	Resorption sites
	Implantation sites
	Stillborns
	Hematology (some reticulocyte counts/Howel-Jolly/ WBC differentials)
Categorical data	Clinical signs
	Neurobehavioral signs (some)
	GP sensitization scores
	Mouse ear swelling tests (MEST) sensitization counts
	Fetal abnormalities
	Dose/mortality data
	Sex ratios
	Histopathology data (most)

of this chapter, which seeks to review statistical methods on a use-by-use basis and to provide a foundation for selection of alternatives in specific situations.

A. Median Lethal and Effective Doses

For many years, the starting point for evaluating the toxicity of an agent was to determine its LD_{50} or LC_{50}, which are the dose or concentration of a material at which half of a specified dosed or exposed population of animals would be expected to die. These figures are analogous to the ED_{50} (effective dose for half a population) used in pharmacologic activities, and are derived by the same means.

To calculate either of these figures the data we have before us are, at each of several dosage (or exposure) levels, the number of animals dosed and the number that died. If we are seeking only to establish the median effective dose in a range-finding test, then 4 or 5 animals per dose level using the Thompson and Weil (5) method of moving averages is the most efficient and will give a sufficiently accurate solution. With two dose levels, if the ratio between the high and low dose is two or less, even total or no mortality at these two dose levels will yield an acceptably accurate medial lethal dose, although a partial mortality is desirable. If, however, we wish to estimate a number of toxicity levels (LD_{10}, LD_{90}) and are interested in more precisely the slope of the dose/lethality curve, the use of at least 10 animals per dosage level with the log/probit regression technique is most commonly used.

Note that in the equation $Y_i = a + bx_i$, b is the slope of the regression line, and that our method already allows us to calculate 95% confidence intervals about any point on this line. Note that the confidence interval at any one point will be different from the interval at other points, and must be calculated separately Additionally, the nature of the probit transform is such that toward the extremes (LD_{10} and LD_{90}) the confidence intervals will "balloon." That is, they become very wide. Since the slope of the fitted line in these assays has a very large uncertainty, in relation to the uncertainty of the LD_{50} itself (the midpoint of the distribution), caution must be used with calculated LD_xs other than LD_{50}s. The imprecision of the LD_{35}, a value close to the LD_{50}, is discussed by Weil (6), as is that of the slope of the log dose–probit line (7). Debanne and Haller recently reviewed the statistical aspects of different methodologies for estimating a median effective dose.

There have been questions for years as to the value of LD_{50} and the efficiency of the current study design (which uses large numbers of animals) for determining it. As long ago as 1953, Weil et al. (8) presented forceful arguments that an estimate having only minimally reduced precision could be made using significantly fewer animals. More recently, the last few years have brought forth an increased level of concern over the numbers and manners of use of animals in research and testing, and have produced additional strong arguments against the existing methodologies for determining the LD_{50}, or even the need to produce this estimate of lethality at all (9). In response a number of suggestions for alternative methodologies have been advanced (10–12).

These methods center around one of two techniques. The first of these (as Gad et al. (11) propose) use an approach with probes and a staggered dosing procedure. Prior to the start of an acute study comprising sufficient numbers of animals to permit conclusions to be drawn, single animals are treated on successive days at a series of dose levels. The first level probed is either the maximum level required to be tested (based on regulatory criteria, e.g., 2 g/kg in a dermal study) or at a lower level if a material is judged to have a greater potential for lethality. One or two days later, based on the observed results in the single probe animal, an additional animal is dosed. If death or severe signs of toxicity occur in the initial animal, the second animal is given a lower dose, for example, at one-third or one-tenth of the initial dose level depending on the speed of observed response. If no severe signs of toxicity are observed, the probe dose is the maximum required to be tested, and the initial dose is followed for a week postdosing. If it survives, the main study is initiated with the high dose group receiving the same dose level as the probe. If no severe toxicity is observed and the level tested was one based on judgment (i.e., not the maximum required), an additional animal is dosed at a level two or three times the initial test level. This process, a variation on the up-and-down methodology, commonly results in allowing us to state that "the LD_{50} is greater than" the highest test level we actually evaluate in the main study.

Where the lethality results are of concern for regulatory purposes (such as finding that an oral probe animal dies at 50 mg/kg, raising the possibility that the material needs to be labeled as a poison), a full group of animals is dosed at the decision-point level. Otherwise, the highest dose level tested is just below what is expected to be a 100% lethal level, as testing a full group at a higher level would only serve to confirm lethality at that level while precluding the investigation of mechanisms or other expressions of toxicity.

The actual study is performed in a staggered startup manner. That is, the high dose and vehicle control groups are dosed on one day. After two days of measurements and observations, one or two additional groups are dosed at levels based on the observed results from the high dose group. If the response in the high dose group has been minimal or unremarkable, only one additional group is dosed at a lower level such as one-half to one-third of the high dose level. If signs of toxicity were more marked, two groups are dosed at levels ranging from one-third to one-tenth of the high dose. The nature of effects observed for is modified in response to the results seen in the high dose. If the second set of groups shows signs of toxicity within two days, an additional group of animals is dosed at a yet lower level. Those animals brought in for a study but not utilized because additional dose levels are not needed provide probe animals for subsequent studies.

The second approach, the up-and-down methods, were proposed by Bruce (12). This is an adaptive procedure for conducting dose–response experiments having a yes–no endpoint. Using this strategy for acute toxicity testing, animals are dosed one at a time, starting the first animal at the toxicologist's best estimate of the LD_{50}. If this animal survives, then the next animal receives a higher dose, while if the first animal dies, the next animal receives a lower dose. Doses are usually adjusted by a constant multiplicative factor, such as 1.3 or 2. The dose for each successive animal is adjusted up or down depending upon the outcome for the previous animal. It can be seen that this method of experimentation causes the doses to be rapidly adjusted toward the LD_{50} and then to be maintained in the region of the LD_{50}. The procedure concentrates experimental effort on the region of the interest and, as a result, uses animals in a very efficient manner.

B. Body and Organ Weights

Among the sets of data commonly collected in studies where animals are dosed with (or exposed to) a chemical are body weight and the weights of selected organs. In fact, gain in body weight (also called "growth") is frequently the most sensitive parameter to indicate an adverse effect. How to best analyze this and in what form to analyze the organ weight data (as absolute weights, weight changes, or percentages of body weight) have been the subject of a number of articles in the past (4, 13–15).

Both absolute body weights and rates of body weight change (calculated as changes from a baseline measurement value which is traditionally the animal's weight immediately prior to the first dosing with or exposure to test material) are almost universally best analyzed by analysis of variance (ANOVA) followed, if called for, by a post hoc test. Even if the groups were randomized properly at the beginning of a study (no group being significantly different in mean body weight from any other group, and all animals in all groups within two standard deviations of the overall mean body weight), there is an advantage to performing the computationally slightly more cumbersome (compared to absolute body weights) changes in body weight analysis.

This advantage is an increase in sensitivity due to the adjustment of starting points (the setting of initial weights as a "zero" value) acting to reduce the amount of initial variability. In this case, Bartlett's test is first performed in ensure homogeneity of variance and the appropriate sequence of analysis is followed.

With smaller sample sizes, the normality of the data becomes increasingly uncertain and nonparametric methods such as Kruskal-Wallis may be more appropriate (16).

Analysis of relative (to body weight) organ weights is a valuable tool for identifying possible target organs (11). How to perform this analysis is still a matter of some disagreement, however.

Weil (14) presented evidence that organ weight data expressed as percentages of body weight should be analyzed separately for each sex. Furthermore, as the conclusions from organ weight data of the males differed so often from those of females, data from animals of each sex should be used in this measurement. Also, Weil (4,17), Boyd (18), and Boyd and Knight (19), have discussed in detail other factors that influence organ weights and must be taken into account.

The two competing approaches to analyzing relative organ weights call for either: 1) calculating organ weights as percentages of total body weights (at the time of necropsy) and analyzing the results by analysis of variance (ANOVA), or 2) analyzing results by analysis of covariance (ANCOVA) with body weights as the covariates as previously discussed by the author (15).

A number of considerations should be kept in mind when these questions are addressed. First, one must keep a firm grasp on the concept of biological significance as opposed to statistical significance. In the case of these particular considerations, we are particularly concerned with examining organ weights when an organ weight changes out of proportion to changes in whole body weight. Second, we are now being required to detect smaller and smaller changes while still retaining a similar sensitivity (i.e., the $p < 0.05$ level).

There are several devices to attain the desired increase in power. One is to use larger and larger sample sizes (number of animals) and the other is to utilize the most powerful test we can. The use of even currently employed numbers of animals is being vigorously questioned. The power of statistical tests must, therefore, now assume increased importance in our considerations.

The biological rationale behind analyzing both absolute body weight and the organ weight to body weight ratio (this latter as opposed to a covariance analysis of organ weights) is that in the majority of cases, except for the brain, the organs of interest in the body change weight (except in extreme cases of obesity or starvation) in a parallel manner with the body overall. And it is the cases where this is not so that we are particularly interested in detecting. Analysis of actual data from several hundred studies (published data) has shown no significant difference in rates of weight change of target organs (other than the brain) compared to those of the body itself for healthy animals in those species commonly used for repeated dose studies (rats, mice, rabbits, and dogs). Furthermore, it should be noted that analysis of covariance is of questionable validity in analyzing body weights and related organ weight changes, as it has as a primary assumption the fact that it is independent of treatment, that is, that the relationship of the two variables is the same for all treatments (20). Pointedly, in toxicology this is not true.

In cases where the differences between the error mean squares are much greater, the ratio of F ratios will diverge in precision from the result of the efficiency of covariance adjustment. These cases occur either when sample sizes are much larger or where the differences between means themselves are much larger. This latter case is one that does not occur in the designs under discussion in any manner that would leave analysis of covariance as a valid approach, because group means start out being very similar and cannot diverge markedly unless there is a treatment effect. As we have discussed earlier, a treatment effect invalidates a prime underpinning assumption of analysis of covariance (ANCOVA).

Finally, in cases where ANCOVA does reveal a difference between groups, one is somewhat hampered in determining where the difference lies if the adjustment was critical to the sensitivity of the analysis.

C. Clinical Chemistry

A number of clinical chemistry parameters are commonly determined on the blood and urine collected from the animals in chronic and subchronic (and occasionally acute) toxicity studies. In the past (and still, in some places), the accepted practice has been to evaluate these data using univariate parametric methods (primarily t tests and/or ANOVA). However, this can be shown to be not the best approach on a number of grounds.

First, such biochemical parameters are rarely independent of each other. Neither is our interest often focused on just one of the parameters. Rather, there are batteries of parameters associated with toxic actions at particular target organs. For example, increases in creatinine phosphokinase (CPK), hydroxybutyrate dehydrogenase (HBDH), and lactate dehydrogenase (LDH) occurring together are strongly indicative of myocardial damage. In such cases, we are not just interested in a significant increase in one of these, but in all three. Table 3 gives a brief overview of the association of various parameters with actions at particular target organs. More detailed coverage of the interpretation of such clinical laboratory tests can be found in Wallach (21).

Similarly, changes in serum electrolytes (sodium, potassium, and calcium) interact with each other; a decrease in one is frequently tied to an increase in one of the others. Furthermore, the nature of the data (in the case of some parameters), because of either the biological background of the parameter or the way in which it is measured, frequently is either not normally distributed (particularly because of being markedly skewed) or not continuous in nature. This can be seen in some of the reference data for experimental animals in Mitruka and Rawnsley (23) or Weil (24) in, for example, the cases of creatinine, sodium, potassium, chloride, calcium, and blood urea nitrogen. It should be remembered that both normal distribution and continuous data are underlying assumptions in the parametric statistical techniques described in this chapter. Such data has also been as termed being from "contaminated" normal distributions.

D. Hematology

Much of what we said about clinical chemistry parameters is also true for the hematologic measurements made in toxicology studies. The pragmatic approach of evaluating which test to perform by use of a decision tree should be taken until one becomes confident as to which are the most appropriate methods. Keeping in mind that both sets of values and (in some cases) population distribution vary not only between species, but also between the commonly used

Table 3 Association of Changes in Biochemical Parameters with Actions at Particular Target Organs

Parameter	ORGAN SYSTEM								Notes
	Blood	Heart	Lung	Kidney	Liver	Bone	Intestine	Pancreas	
Albumin				↓	↓				Produced by the liver. Very significant reductions indicate extensive liver damage.
ALP (Alkaline phosphatase)					↑	↑	↑		Elevations usually associated with cholestasis. Bone alkaline phosphatase tends to be higher in young animals.
Bilirubin (Total)	↑				↑				Usually elevated due to cholestasis— either due to obstruction or hepatopathy.
BUN (Blood urea nitrogen)				↑	↓				Estimates blood filtering capacity of the kidneys. Doesn't become significantly elevated until kidney function is reduced 60–75%
Calcium				↑					Can be life threatening and result in acute death.
Cholinesterase				↑	↓				Found in plasma, brain, and RBC.
CPK (Creatinine phosphokinase)		↑							Most often elevated due to skeletal muscle damage but can also be produced by cardiac muscle damage. Can be more sensitive than histopathology.
Creatinine				↑					Also estimates blood filtering capacity of kidney as BUN does. More specific than BUN.

		Comments
Glucose	↑	Alterations other than those associated with stress are uncommon and reflect an effect on the pancreatic islets or anorexia.
GGT (Gamma glutamyl transferase)	↑	Elevated in cholestasis. This is a microsomal enzyme and levels often increase in response to microsomal enzyme induction.
HBDH (Hydroxybutyric dehydrogenase)	↑	
LDH (Lactic dehydrogenase)	↑	Increase usually due to skeletal muscle, cardiac muscle, and liver damage. Not very specific.
Protein (Total)	↓	Absolute alterations are usually associated with decreased production (liver) or increased loss (kidney). Can see increase in case of muscle "wasting" (catabolism).
SGOT (Serum glutamic-oxaloacetic transaminase); also called AST (Aspartate amino transferase)	↑	Present in skeletal muscle and heart and most commonly associated with damage to these.
SGPT (Serum glutamic-pyruvic transaminase); also called ALT (alanide amino transferase)	↑	Elevations usually associated with hepatic damage or disease.
SDH (Sorbitol dehydrogenase)	↑OR →	Liver enzyme which can be quite sensitive but is fairly unstable. Samples should be processed as soon as possible.

Arrow indicates increase (↑) or decrease (↑)

strains of species (and that the "control" or "standard" values will "drift" over the course of only a few years), familiarity should not be taken for granted.

The majority of these parameters are, again, interrelated and highly dependent on the method used to determine them. Red blood cell count (RBC), platelet counts, and mean corpuscular volume (MCV) may be determined by a device such as a Coulter counter taking direct measurements, and the resulting data are usually suitable for parametric methods. The hematocrit, however, may actually be a value calculated from the RBC and MCV values and, if so, is dependent on them. If the hematocrit is measured directly, instead of being calculated from the RBC and MCV, it may be compared by parametric methods.

Hemoglobin is directly measured and is an independent and continuous variable. However, probably because at any one time a number of forms and conformations (oxyhemoglobin, deoxyhemoglobin, methemoglobin, etc.) of hemoglobin are actually present, the distribution seen is not typically a normal one, but rather may be a multimodal one. Here a nonparametric technique such as the Wilcoxon or multiple rank-sum test is called for.

Consideration of the white blood cell (WBC) and a differential count leads to another problem. The total WBC is, typically, a normal population amenable to parametric analysis, but differential counts are normally determined by counting, manually, one or more sets of 100 cells each. The resulting relative percentages of neutrophils are then reported as either percentages or are multiplied by the total WBC count with the resulting "count" being reported as the "absolute" differential WBC. It is widely believed that "relative" (%) differential data, particularly in the case of eosinophils where the distribution do not approach normality and should usually be analyzed by nonparametric methods, should not be reported because they are likely to be misleading.

Lastly, it should always be kept in mind that it is rare for a change in any single hematologic parameter to be meaningful. Rather, because these parameters are so interrelated, patterns of changes in parameters should be expected if a real effect is present, and analysis and interpretation of results should focus on such patterns of changes. Classification analysis techniques often provide the basis for a useful approach to such problems.

E. Histopathologic Lesion Incidence

In the last 20 years, there has been an increasing emphasis on histopathological examination of many tissues collected from animals in subchronic and chronic toxicity studies. While it is not true that only those lesions that occur at a statistically significantly increased rate in treated/exposed animals are of concern (for there are the cases where a lesion may be of such a rare type that the occurrence of only one or few such in treated animals "raises a flag"), it is true that, in most cases, a statistical evaluation is the only way to determine if what we are seeing in treated animals is significantly worse than what has been seen in control animals. And although cancer is not our only concern, it is the category of lesions that is of the greatest interest.

Typically, comparison of incidences of any one type of lesion between controls and treated animals are made using multiple 2×2 chi square or Fischer's exact test with a modification of the numbers as the denominators. Too often, experimenters exclude from consideration all those animals (in both groups) that died prior to the first animals being found with a lesion at that site. The special case of carcinogenicity bioassays will be discussed in detail in a later section and the last chapter.

An option which should be kept in mind is that frequently a pathologist can and will not just identify a lesion as present, but also grade those that are present as to severity. This represents a significant increase in the information content of the data, which should not be given up by performing an analysis based only on the perceived quantal nature (present/absent) of the data. Quantal data, analyzed by chi-square or Fisher's exact tests, are a subset (the 2×2 case) of categorical or contingency table data. On the case under discussion it also becomes ranked (or "ordinal") data, in other words, the categories are naturally ordered (for example, no effect > mild lesion > moderate lesion > severe lesion). This gives a $2 \times R$ table if only one treatment and one control group are involved, or an $N \times R$ ("multiway") table if there are three or more groups of animals.

The traditional method of analyzing multiple cross-classified data has been to collapse the $N \times R$ contingency table over all but two of the variables, and to follow this with the computation of some measure of association between these variables. For an N-dimensional table this results in $N(N - 1)/2$ separate analyses. The result is very crude, "giving away" information and even (by inappropriately pooling data) yielding a faulty understanding of the meaning of data. Though computationally more laborious, a multiway ($N \times R$ table) analysis should be utilized.

F. Reproduction

Reproductive implications of the toxic effects of chemicals are becoming increasingly important. Because of this, reproduction studies, along with other closely related types of studies (such as teratogenesis, dominant lethal, and mutagenesis studies, which are discussed later in this chapter), are now common companions to chronic toxicity studies.

One point that must be kept in mind with all the reproduction-related studies is the nature of the appropriate sampling unit. Put another way: What is the appropriate N in such a study—the number of individual pups or the number of litters (or pregnant females)? Fortunately, it is now fairly well accepted that the first case (using the number of offspring as the N) is inappropriate (4). The real effects in such studies are actually occurring in the female that receives the dosage or exposure to the chemical, or that is mated to a male that received a dosage or exposure. What happens to her and to the development of the litter she is carrying is biologically independent of what happens to every other female/litter in the study. This cannot be said for each offspring in each litter; the death of, or other change in, one member of a litter can and will be related to what happens to every other member in numerous ways. Or the effect on all of the offspring might be similar for all of those from one female and different or lacking in another.

As defined by Oser and Oser (22), there are four primary variables of interest in a reproduction study. First, there is the fertility index (FI) defined as the percentage of attempted matings (i.e., each female housed with a male) resulting in pregnancy, with pregnancy being determined by a method such as the presence of implantation sites in the female. Second, there is the gestation index (GI), defined as the percentage of mated females, as evidenced by a vaginal plug being dropped or a positive vaginal smear, delivering variable litters (i.e., litters with at least one live pup). Two related variables that may also be studied are the mean number of pups born per litter and the percentage of total pups per litter that are stillborn. Third, there is the viability index (VI), defined as the percentage of offspring born that survive at least 4 days after birth. Finally (in this four-variable system) there is the lactation index (LI), the percentage of those animals per litter alive at 4 days that survive to weaning. In rats and mice, this is classically taken to be until 21 days after birth. An additional variable that may reasonably be included in such a study is the mean weight gain per pup per litter.

Given that our N is at least 10 (we will further explore proper sample size under the topic of teratology), we may test each of these variables for significance using a method such as the Wilcoxon-Mann-Whitney U test, or the Kruskal-Wallis nonparametric ANOVA. If N is less than 10, then we cannot expect the central limit theorem to be operative and should use the Wilcoxon sum of ranks (for two groups) or the Kruskal-Wallis nonparametric ANOVA (for three or more groups) to compare groups.

G. Teratology

When the primary concern of a reproductive/developmental study is the occurrence of birth defects or deformations (terata, either structural or functional) in the offspring of exposed animals, the study is one of teratology. In the analysis of the data from such a study, we must consider several points.

First is sample size. Earlier in this book we reviewed the general concerns with this topic, and presented a method to estimate what a sufficient sample size would be. The difficulties with applying these methods here revolve around two points: 1) selecting a sufficient level of sensitivity for detecting an effect and 2) factoring in how many animals will be removed from study (without contributing a datum) by either not becoming pregnant or not surviving to a sufficiently late stage of pregnancy. Experience generally dictates that one should attempt to have 20 pregnant animals per study group if a pilot study has provided some confidence that the pregnant test animals will survive the dose levels selected. Again, it is essential to recognize that the litter, not the fetus, is the basic independent unit for each variable.

A more fundamental consideration, as we alluded to in the section on reproduction, is that as we use more animals, the mean of means (each variable will be such in a mathematical sense) will approach normality in its distribution. This is one of the implications of the central limit theorem; even when the individual data are not normally distributed, their means will approach normality in their distribution. At a sample size of ten or greater, the approximation of normality is such that we may use a parametric test (such as a t test or ANOVA) to evaluate results. At sample sizes less than ten, a nonparametric test (Wilcoxon rank-sum or Kruskal-Wallis nonparametric ANOVA) is more appropriate. Other methodologies have been suggested (25,26) but do not offer any widespread acceptance of usage. One nonparametric method that is widely used in the Mann-Whitney U test, which was described earlier. Williams and Buschbom (27) further discuss some of the available statistical options and their consequences, and Rai and Van Ryzin (28) have recommended a dose-responsive model.

H. Dominant Lethal Assay

The dominant lethal study is essentially a reproduction study, which seeks to study the end point of lethality to the fetuses after implantation and before delivery. The proper identification of the sampling unit (the pregnant female) and the design of an experiment so that a sufficiently large sample is available for analysis are the prime statistical considerations of concern. The question of sampling unit has been adequately addressed in earlier sections. Sample size is of concern here because the hypothesis-testing techniques that are inappropriate with small samples are of relatively low power, as the variability about the mean in such cases is relatively large. With sufficient sample size (e.g., from 30 to 50 pregnant females per dose level per week (29)), variability about the mean and the nature of the distribution allow sensitive statistical techniques to be employed.

The variables of concern that are typically recorded and included in analysis are (for each level/week): (a) the number of pregnant females, (b) live fetuses/pregnancy, (c) total implants/pregnancy, (d) early fetal deaths (early resorptions)/pregnancy, and (e) late fetal deaths/pregnancy.

A wide variety of techniques for analysis of these data have been (and are) used. Most common is the use of ANOVA after the data have been transformed by the arc sine transform (30).

Beta binomial (31,32) and Poisson distributions (33) have also been attributed to these data, and transforms and appropriate tests have been proposed for use in each of these cases (in each case with the note that the transforms serve to "stabilize the variance" of the data). With sufficient sample size, as defined earlier in this section, the Mann-Whitney U test is to be recommended for use here. Smaller sample sizes should necessitate the use of the Wilcoxon rank-sum test.

I. Diet and Chamber Analysis

Earlier we presented the basic principles and methods for sampling. Sampling is important for many aspects of toxicology, and here we address its application in diet preparation and the analysis of atmospheres from inhalation chambers.

In feeding studies, we seek to deliver desired doses of a material to animals by mixing the material with their diet. Similarly, in an inhalation study we mix a material with the air the test animals breathe.

In both cases, we must then sample the medium (food or atmosphere) and analyze these samples to determine what levels or concentrations of material were actually present and to assure ourselves that the test material is homogeneously distributed. Having an accurate picture of these delivered concentrations, and how they varied over the course of time, is essential on a number of grounds:

1.   The regulatory agencies and sound scientific practice require that analyzed diet and mean daily inhalation atmosphere levels be ±10% of the target level.

2.   Marked peak concentrations, because of the overloading of metabolic and repair systems, could result in extreme acute effects that would lead to apparent results in a chronic study that are not truly indicative of the chronic low level effects of the compound, but rather of periods of metabolic and physiologic overload. Such results could be misinterpreted if the true exposure or diet levels were not maintained at a relatively constant level.

Sampling strategies are not just a matter of numbers (for the statistical aspects), but of geometry, so that the contents of a container or the entire atmosphere in a chamber is truly sampled; and of time, in accordance with the stability of the test compound. The samples must be both randomly collected and "representative" of the entire mass of what one is trying to characterize. In the special case of sampling and characterizing the physical properties of aerosols in an inhalation study, some special considerations and terminology apply. Because of the physiologic characteristics of the respiration of humans and of test animals, our concern is very largely limited to those particles or droplets which are of respirable size. Unfortunately, "respirable size" is a somewhat complexly defined characteristic based on aerodynamic diameter, density, and physiological characteristics. A second misfortune is that while those particles with an aerodynamic diameter of less than 10 µm are generally agreed to be respirable in humans (that is, they can be drawn down to the deep portions of the lungs). In the rat this characteristic is more realistically limited to those particles below 3 µm in aerodynamic diameter. The one favorable factor is that there are now available a section of instruments that accurately (and relatively easily) collect and measure aerodynamically sized particles or droplets. These measurements result in concentrations in a defined volume of gas, and can be expressed as either a number concentration or a mass concentration (the latter being more common). Such measurements generate categorical data or concentrations measured in each of a series of aerodynamic size groups (such as >100 µm, 100–25 µm, 25–10 µm, 10–3 µm, etc.). The appropriate descriptive statistics for this class of data are the geometric mean and its standard deviation. These aspects and the statistical interpretation of the data that are finally collected should be considered after sufficient interaction with the appropriate professionals. Typically, it then becomes a matter of the calculation of measures of central tendency and dispersion statistics, with the identification of those values that are beyond acceptable limits (34).

J. Mutagenesis

Since the late 1960s a wide variety of tests (see Kilbey et al. (35) for an overview of available tests) for mutagenicity have been developed and brought into use. These tests give us a quicker and cheaper (though not as conclusive) way of predicting whether a material of interest is a mutagen, and possibly a carcinogen, than do longer term whole-animal studies.

How to analyze the results of this multitude of tests (Ames, chromosome aberations, micronucleus, mouse lymphoma, host-mediated, cell transformation, sister chromatid exchange, and so on, just to name a few) is a new and extremely important question. Some workers in the field hold that it is not possible (or necessary) to perform statistical analysis, that the tests can simply be judged to be positive or not positive on the basis of whether or not they achieve a particular degree of increase in the incidence of mutations in the test organism. This is plainly not an acceptable response, when societal needs are not limited to yes/no answers but rather include at least relative quantitation of potencies (particularly in mutagenesis, where we have come to recognize the existence of a nonzero background level of activity from naturally occurring factors and agents). Such quantitations of potency are complicated by the fact that we are dealing with a nonlinear phenomenon. For though low doses of most mutagens produce a linear response curve, with increasing doses the curve will flatten out (and even turn into a declining curve) as higher doses take the target systems into levels of acute toxicity to the test system.

Several concepts, different from those we have discussed previously need to be examined, for our concern has now shifted from how a multicellular organism acts in response to one of a number of complex actions to how a mutational event is expressed, most frequently by a single cell. Given that we can handle a much larger number of experimental units in these systems that use smaller test organisms, we can seek to detect both weak and strong mutagens.

Conducting the appropriate statistical analysis and utilizing the results of such an analysis properly, must start with understanding biological system involved and, from this understanding developing the correct model and hypothesis. We start such a process by considering each of five interacting factors (36,37):

1. α, which is the probability of our committing a type I error (saying an agent is mutagenic when it is not, equivalent to our p in such earlier considered designs as the Fisher's exact text); false positive
2. β, which is the probability of our committing a type II error (saying an agent is not mutagenic when it is); false negative
3. Δ, our desired sensitivity in an assay system (such as being able to detect an increase of 10% in mutations in a population)
4. σ, the variability of the biological system and the effects of chance errors
5. n, the necessary sample size to achieve each of these (we can only, by our actions, change this one portion of the equation) as n is proportional to:

$$\frac{\sigma}{\alpha, \beta, \text{ and } \Delta}$$

The implications of this are, therefore, that (a) the greater σ is, the larger n must be to achieve the desired levels of α, β, and Δ, (b) the smaller the desired levels of α, β, and/or Δ, if n is constant, the larger our σ is.

What is the background mutation level and the variability in our technique? As any good genetic or general toxicologist will acknowledge, matched concurrent control groups are essential. Fortunately, with these test systems large n's are readily attainable, although there are other complications to this problem we will consider later. An example of the confusion that would otherwise result is illustrated in the intralaboratory comparisons of some of these methods done to date, such as that reviewed by Weil (40).

New statistical tests based on these assumptions and upon the underlying population distributions have been proposed, along with the necessary computational background to allow one to alter one of the input variables (α, β, or Δ).

A set that shows particular promise is that proposed by Katz (38,39) in his two articles. He described two separate test statistics: ϕ for when we can accurately estimate the number of individuals in both the experimental and control groups, and θ, for when we do not actually estimate the number of surviving individuals in each group, and we can assume that the test material is only mildly toxic in terms of killing the test organisms. Each of these two test statistics is also formulated on the basis of only a single exposure of the organisms to the test chemicals. Given this, then we may compute

$$\phi = \frac{\alpha(M_E - 0.5) - K_b(M_C + 0.5)}{\sqrt{K_{ab}(M_E + M_C)}}$$

where a and b are the number of groups of control (C) and experimental (E) organisms, respectively.

N_C and N_E are the number of surviving microorganisms.

$K = N_E/N_C$

M_E and M_C are the numbers of mutations in experimental and control groups.

μ_E and μ_C are the true (but unknown) mutation rates (as μ_C gets smaller, Ns must increase).

We may compute the second case as

$$\theta = \frac{\sigma(M_E - 0.5) + (M_C + 0.5)}{ab(M_E + M_C)}$$

with the same constituents.

In both cases, at a confidence level for α of 0.05, we accept that $\mu_C = \mu_E$ if the test statistic (either ϕ or θ) is less than 1.64. If it is equal to or greater than 1.64, we may conclude that we have a mutagenic effect (at $\alpha = 0.05$).

In the second case (θ, where we do not have separate estimates of population sizes for the control and experimental groups) if K deviates widely from 1.0 (if the material is markedly toxic), we should use more containers of control organisms (tables for the proportions of each to use given different survival frequencies may be found in Katz (39)). If different levels are desired, tables for θ and ϕ may be found in Kastenbaum and Bowman (41).

An outgrowth of this is that the mutation rate per surviving cells (μ_C and μ_E) can be determined. It must be remembered that if the control mutation rate is high enough that a reduction in mutation rates can be achieved by the test compound, these test statistics must be adjusted to allow for a two-sided hypothesis (42). The levels may likewise be adjusted in each case, or tested for, if what we want to do is assure ourselves that we do have a mutagenic effect at a certain level of confidence (note that this is different from disproving the null hypothesis).

It should be noted that there are numerous specific recommendations for statistical methods designed for individual mutagenicity techniques, such as that of Berstein et al. (43) for the Ames test. Exploring each of them is beyond the scope of this chapter, however.

K. Behavioral Toxicology

A brief review of the types of studies/experiments conducted in the area of behavioral toxicology, and a classification of these into groups is in order. Although there are a small number of studies that do not fit into the following classification, the great majority may be fitted into one of the following four groups. Many of these points were first covered by one of the authors in an earlier article (44).

Observational score-type studies are based on observing and grading the response of an animal to its normal environment or to a stimulus which is imprecisely controlled. This type of result is generated by one of two major sorts of studies. Open-field studies involve placing an animal in the center of a flat, open area and counting each occurrence of several types of activities (e.g., grooming, moving outside a designated central area, rearing) or timing until the first occurrence of each type of activity. The data generated are sclera of either a continuous or discontinuous nature, but frequently are not of a normal distribution (see Tilson et al. (45) for examples). Observational screen studies involve a combination of observing behavior or evoking a response to a simple stimulus, the resulting observation being graded as normal or as deviating from normal on a graded scale. Most of the data so generated are of a rank nature, with some portions being quantal or interval in nature. Irwin (46) and Gad (47) have presented schemes for the conduct of such studies.

The second type of study is one that generates rates of response as data. The studies are based on the number of responses to a discrete controlled stimulus or are free of direct connection to a stimulus. The three most frequently measured parameters are licking of a liquid (milk, sugar water, ethanol, or a psychoactive agent in water), gross locomotor activity (measured by a photocell or electromagnetic device), or lever pulling. Work presenting examples of such studies has been published by Annau (48) and Norton (49). The data generated are most often of a discontinuous or continuous scalar nature, and are often complicated by underlying patterns of biological rhythm (to be discussed more fully later).

The third type of study generates a variety of data classified as error rates. These are studies based on animals learning a response to a stimulus or memorizing a simple task (such as running a maze or a Skinner box-type shock avoidance system). These tests or trials are structured so that animals can pass or fail on each of a number of successive trials. The resulting data are quantal, though frequently expressed as a percentage.

The final major type of study results in data that are measures of the time to an endpoint. They are based on animals being exposed to or dosed with a toxicant; then the time until an effect is observed is measured. Usually the endpoint is failure to continue to be able to perform a task. The endpoints can, therefore, be death, incapacitation, or the learning of a response to a discrete stimulus. Burt (50) and Johnson et al. (51) present data of this form. The data are always of a censored nature, that is, the period of observation is always artificially limited on one end, such as in measuring time to incapacitation in combustion toxicology data, where animals are exposed to the thermal decomposition gases of test materials for a period of 30 min. If incapacitation is not observed during these 30 min, it is judged not to have occurred. The data generated by these studies are continuous, discontinuous, or rank in nature. They are discontinuous because the researcher may check, or may be restricted to checking for the occurrence of the endpoint only at certain discrete points in time. On the other hand, they are rank if the periods to check for occurrence of the endpoint are far enough apart, in which case one may actually only know that the endpoint occurred during a broad period of time, but not where in that period.

There is a special class of test to also consider at this point: the behavioral teratology or reproduction study. These studies are based on dosing or exposing either parental animals during selected periods in the mating and gestation process or pregnant females at selected periods during gestation. The resulting offspring are then tested for developmental defects of a neurological and behavioral nature. Analysis is complicated by a number of facts: 1) the parental animals are the actual targets for toxic effects, but observations are made on offspring; 2) the toxic effects in the parental generation may alter the performance of the mother in rearing its offspring, which in turn can lead to confusion of behaviors developed at different times (which will be discussed further below).

A researcher can, by varying the selection of the animal model (species, strain, sex), modify the nature of the data generated and the degree of dispersion of these data. Particularly in behavioral studies, limiting the within-group variability of data is a significant problem and generally should be a highly desirable goal.

Most, if not all, behavioral toxicology studies depend on at least some instrumentation. Very frequently overlooked here (and, indeed, in most research) is that instrumentation, by its operating characteristics and limitations, goes a long way toward determining the nature of the data generated by it. An activity monitor measures motor activity in discrete segments. If it is a "jiggle cage" type monitor these segments are restricted so that only a distinctly limited number of counts can be achieved in a given period of time and then only if they are of the appropriate magnitude. Likewise, technique can also readily determine the nature of data. In measuring response to pain, for example, one could record it as a quantal measure (present or absent), a rank score (on a scale of 1–5 for from decreased to increased responsiveness, with 3 being "normal"), or as scalar data (by using an analgesia meter which determines either how much pressure or heat is required to evoke a response).

Study design factors are probably the most widely recognized of the factors that influence the type of data resulting from a study. Number of animals used, frequency of measures, and length of period of observation are three obvious design factors that are readily under the control of the researchers and directly help to determine the nature of the data.

Finally it is appropriate to review each of the types of studies presently seen in behavioral toxicology, according to the classification presented at the beginning of this section, in terms of which statistical methods are used now and what procedures should be recommended for use. The recommendations, of course, should be viewed critically. They are intended with current experimental design and technique in mind and can only claim to be the best when one is limited to addressing the most common problems from a "library" of readily and commonly available and understood tests.

Table 4 summarizes this review and recommendation process in a straightforward form.

Table 4 Overview of Statistical Testing for Behavioral Toxicology: Tests Commonly Used[a] as Opposed to Those Most Frequently Appropriate

Type of observation	Most commonly used procedures[a]	Suggested procedures
Observational scores	Either Student's t-test or one-way ANOVA	Kruskal-Wallis nonparametric ANOVA or Wilcoxon Rank sum
Response rates	Either Student's t-test or one-way	Kruskal-Wallis ANOVA or one-way ANOVA
Error rates	ANOVA followed by a posthoc test	Fisher's exact, or RXC Chi square, or Mann-Whitney U-test
Times to	Either Student's t-test or one-way ANOVA	ANOVA then a posthoc test or Kruskal-Wallis ANOVA
Teratology and reproduction	ANOVA followed by a posthoc test	Fisher's exact test, Kruskal-Wallis ANOVA, or Mann-Whitney U-test

[a]That these are the most commonly used procedures was established by an extensive literature review which is beyond the scope of this book. The reader need only, however, look at the example articles cited in the text of Gad and Weil (1) to verify this fact.

V. CARCINOGENESIS AND RISK ASSESSMENT

Both carcinogenesis and the broader realm of risk assessment (as it applies to toxicology) have in common that, based on experimental results in a nonhuman species at some relatively high dose or exposure level, an attempt is made to predict a result of extreme impact in humans at much lower levels. In this section we will examine the assumptions involved in these undertakings, review the aspects of design and interpretation of animal carcinogenicity studies, and present the framework on which risk assessment is based.

The reader should first understand that, contrary to popular belief, risk assessment in toxicology is not limited to carcinogenesis. Rather, it may be applied to all the possible deferred toxicologic consequences of exposure to chemicals or agents of a truly severe nature—that is, those things (such as carcinogenesis, teratogenesis, or reproductive impairment) that threaten life (either existing or prospective) at a time distant to the actual exposure to the chemical or agent. Because the consequences of these toxic events are so extreme yet are detached from the actual cause by time (unlike when a person dies from overexposure to an acutely lethal agent, such as carbon monoxide), society is willing to accept only a low level of risk while maintaining the benefits of use of the agent. Though the most familiar (and, to date, best developed) case is that of carcinogenesis, much of what is presented for risk assessment may also be applied to the other endpoints of concern.

A. Carcinogenicity Bioassays

At least in a general way, we now understand what appear to be most of the mechanisms underlying chemical- and radiation-induced carcinogenesis. A review of these mechanisms is not germane to this chapter [readers wishing a good short review are advised to read Miller and Miller (52)], but it is now clear that cancer as seen in humans is the result of a multifocal set of causes. The single most important statistical consideration in the design of bioassays in the past was based on the point of view that what was being observed and evaluated was a simple quantal response (cancer occurred or it did not), and that a sufficient number of animals needed to be used to have reasonable expectations of detecting such an effect. Though the single fact of whether or not the simple incidence of neoplastic tumors is increased due to an agent of concern is of interest, a much more complex model must now be considered. The time-to-tumor, patterns of tumor incidence, effects on survival rate, and age at first tumor all must now be included in a model.

1. Bioassay Design

As presented earlier in the section on experimental design, the first step which must be taken is to clearly state the objective of the study to be undertaken.

Carcinogenicity bioassays have two possible objectives, though (as we shall see) the second is now more important and (as our understanding of carcinogenesis has grown) increasingly crowding out the first.

The first objective is to detect possible carcinogens. Compounds are evaluated to determine if they can or cannot induce a statistically detectable increase of tumor rates over the background levels, and only happenstance is information generated which is useful in risk assessment. Most older studies have such detection as their objective. Current thought is that at least two species must be used in detection to be adequately sensitive.

The second objective for a bioassay is to provide a range of use response information (with tumor incidence being the response) that a risk assessment may be performed. Unlike detection, which requires only one treatment group with adequate survival times (to how expression of the endpoint of interest as tumors), dose response requires at least three treatment groups with adequate survival. We will shortly look at the selection of dose levels for this one. However, given that the species is known to be responsive, only one species of animals need be used for this objective.

To address either or both of these objectives, three major types of study designs have evolved. First is the classical skin painting study, usually performed in mice. A single easily detected end point (the formation of skin tumors) is evaluated in such a study (dose usually being varied by using different concentrations of test material in volatile solvent). Most often detection is the objective of such a study. Though others have used different frequencies of application of test material to vary dose, there are data to suggest that this only serves to introduce an additional variable (53). Traditionally, both test and control groups in such a study consist of 50 or 100 mice of one sex (males being preferred because of their very low spontaneous tumor rate). This design is also used in tumor initiation/promotion studies.

The second common type of design is the original National Cancer Institute (NCI) bioassay. The announced objective of these studies is detection of moderate to strong carcinogens, though the results have also been used in attempts at risk assessment. Both mice and rats were used in parallel studies. Each study used 50 males and 50 females at each of two dose levels (high and low) plus an equal sized control group. The National Toxicology Program (NTP) has currently moved away from this design because of a recognition of its inherent limitations.

Finally, there is the standard industrial toxicology design, which uses at least two species (usually rats and mice) in groups of no fewer than 100 males and females each. Each study has three dose groups and at least one control. Frequently additional numbers of animals are included to allow for interim terminations and histopathological evaluations. In both this and the NCI design, a long list of organs and tissues are collected, processed, and examined microscopically. This design seeks to address both the detection and dose-response objectives with a moderate degree of success.

Selecting the number of animals to use for dose groups in a study requires consideration of both biological (expected survival rates, background tumor rates, etc.) and statistical factors. The prime statistical consideration is reflected in Table 5, where it can be seen that if, for example, we were studying a compound which caused liver tumors, and were using mice (with a background or control incidence of 30%), we would have to use 389 animals per sex per group to be able to demonstrate that an incidence rate of 40% in treatment animals was significant compared to the controls at the $p \leq 0.05$ level.

Perhaps the most difficult aspect of designing a good carcinogenicity study is the selection of the dose levels to be used. At the start, it is necessary to consider the first underlying assumption in the design and use of animal cancer bioassays, the need to test at the highest possible dose for the longest practical period.

The rationale behind this assumption is that although humans may be exposed at very low levels, statistically detecting the resulting small increase (over background) in incidence of tumors would require the use of an impractically large number of test animals per group. This point is illustrated by Table 6 where only 46 animals (per group) are needed to show a 10% increase over a zero background (that is, a rarely occurring tumor type), 770,000 animals (per group) would be needed to detect a tenth of a percent increase above a 5% background. As we increase dose, however, the incidence of tumors (the re-

Table 5 Sample Size Required to Obtain a Specified Sensitivity at p < 0.05

Back-ground tumor incidence	p^a	Treatment Group Incidence									
		0.95	0.90	0.80	0.70	0.60	0.50	0.40	0.30	0.20	0.10
0.30	0.90	10	12	18	31	46	102	389			
	0.50	6	6	9	12	22	32	123			
0.20	0.90	8	10	12	18	30	42	88	320		
	0.50	5	5	6	9	12	19	28	101		
0.10	0.90	6	8	10	12	17	25	33	65	214	
	0.50	3	3	5	6	9	11	17	31	68	
0.05	0.90	5	6	8	10	13	18	25	35	76	464
	0.50	3	3	5	6	7	9	12	19	24	147
0.01	0.90	5	5	7	8	10	13	19	27	46	114
	0.50	3	3	5	5	6	8	10	13	25	56

[a]p = Power for each comparison of treatment group with background tumor incidence.

Table 6 Average Number of Animals Needed to Detect a Significant Increase in the Incidence of an Event (Tumors, Anomalies, etc.) Over the Background Incidence (Control) at Several Expected Incidence Levels Using the Fisher Exact Probability Test ($p \leq 0.05$)

Background incidence (%)	Expected Increase in Incidence (%)					
	0.01	0.1	1	3	5	10
0	46,000,000[a]	460,000	4,600	511	164	46
0.01	46,000,000	460,000	4,600	511	164	46
0.1	47,000,000	470,000	4,700	520	168	47
1	51,000,000	510,000	5,100	570	204	51
5	77,000,000	770,000	7,700	856	304	77
10	100,000,000	1,000,000	10,000	1,100	400	100
20	148,000,000	1,480,000	14,800	1,644	592	148
25	160,000,000	1,600,000	16,000	1,840	664	166

[a]Number of animals needed in each group, controls as well as treated.

sponse) will also increase until it reaches the point where a modest increase (say 10%) over a reasonably small background level (say 1%) could be detected using an acceptably small sized group of test animals (in Table 5 we see that 51 animals would be needed for this example case). There are, however, at least two real limitations on how high the highest dose may be. First is that the test rodent population must have a sufficient survival rate after receiving a lifetime (or two years) of regular doses to allow for meaningful statistical analysis. The second is that we really want the metabolism and mechanism of action of the chemical at the highest level tested to be the same as those at the low levels where human exposure would occur. Unfortunately, we usually must select the high dose level based only on the information provided by a subchronic or range-finding study. Selection of too low a dose will make the study invalid for detection of carcinogenicity, and may seriously impair the use of the results for risk assessment.

There are several approaches to this problem. One has been the rather simplistic approach of the NTP Bioassay Program, which is to conduct a 3-month range-finding study with sufficient dose levels to establish a level which significantly (10%) decreases the rate of body weight gain. This dose is defined as the maximum tolerated dose (MTD) and is selected as the highest dose. Two other levels, generally one half MTD and one quarter MTD, are selected for testing as the intermediate and low dose levels. In many earlier NCI studies, only one other level was used.

The dose range-finding study is a must in most cases, but the suppression of body weight gain is a scientifically questionable benchmark when dealing with establishment of safety factors. Physiologic, pharmacologic, or metabolic markers generally serve as better indicators of the systemic response than body weight. A series of well-defined acute and subchronic studies designed to determine the "chronicity factor" and to study onset of pathology can be more predictive for dose setting than body weight suppression.

Also, the NTPs MTD may well be at a level that the metabolic mechanisms for handling a compound at real-life exposure levels have been saturated or overwhelmed, bringing into play entirely artifactual metabolic and physiologic mechanisms (54). The regulatory response to the questioning of the appropriateness of the MTD as a high dose level [exemplified by Haseman (55)] has been to acknowledge that occasionally an excessively high dose is selected, but to counter that using lower doses would seriously decrease the sensitivity of the detection function.

Selection of levels for the intermediate and lower doses for a study is easy only in comparison to the selection of the high dose. If an objective of the study is to generate dose-response data, then the optimal placement of the doses below the high is such that they cover as much of the range of a response curve as possible and yet still have the lowest dose at a high enough level that one can detect and quantify a response. If the objective is detection, then having too great a distance between the highest and next highest dose creates a risk to the validity of the study. If survival in the high dose is too low, yet the next highest dose does not show none-neoplastic results (that is, cause other than neoplastic adverse biological effects) so as to support it being a high enough dose to have detected a strong or moderate carcinogen, the entire study may have to be rejected as inadequate to address its objective. Portier and Hoel (56) have proposed statistical guidelines (for setting dose levels below the high) based on response surfaces. In so doing they suggest that the lowest dose be no less than 10% of the highest.

While it is universally agreed that the appropriate animal model for testing a chemical for carcinogenicity would be one whose metabolism, pharmacokinetics, and biological responses were most similar to humans, economic considerations have largely constrained the actual choices to rats and mice. The use of both sexes of both species is preferred on the grounds that it provides for (in the face of a lack of understanding of which species would actually be most like humans for a particular agent) a greater likelihood of utilizing the more sensitive species. Use of the mouse is both advocated and defended on these grounds and because of the economic advantages and the species' historical utilization (57). There are those who believe that the use of the mouse is redundant and represents a diversion of resources while yielding little additional information (58) citing a "unique contribution" for mouse data in 273 bioassays of only 13.6% of the cases (that is, 37 cases). Others question the use of the mouse based on the belief that it gives artifactual liver carcinogenesis results. One suggestion for the interpretation of mouse bioassays is, that in those cases where there is only an increase in liver tumors in mice (or lung tumors in strain A mice) and no supporting mutagenicity findings (a situation characteristic of some classes of chemicals), the test compound should not be considered an overt carcinogen (59). This last question, however, is even more strongly focused on the strain of mouse that is used than on the use of the species itself.

The NCI/NTP (National Toxicology Program) currently recommends an F1 hybrid cross between two inbred strains, the C57Bl/6 female and the C3H male, the results being commonly designated as the B6C3F1. This mouse was found to be very successful in a large-scale pesticide testing program in the mid-1960s. It is a hardy animal with good survival, easy to breed, disease resistant, and was reported to have a relatively low spontaneous tumor incidence. Usually, up 20 24 months termination, at least 80% of the control mice are still alive.

The problem is that, contrary to what was originally believed (60), the spontaneous liver tumor incidence in male B6C3F1 mice is not 15.7%, but more like 32.1% (61). The issue of spontaneous tumor rates and their impact on the design and interpretation of studies will be discussed more fully later. Thus, use of a cross of two inbred mouse strains is also a point of controversy. Haseman and Hoel (52) have presented data to support the idea that inbred strains have lower degrees of variability of biological functions and tumor rates, making them more sensitive detectors and quantitators. These authors also suggest that the use of a cross from two such inbred strains allows one to more readily detect tumor incidence increases. On the other hand, it is argued that such genetically homogeneous strains do not properly reflect the diversity of metabolic functions (particularly ones which would serve to detoxify or act as defense mechanisms) present in the human population.

Study length and frequency of treatment are design aspects that must also be considered. These are aspects where the objectives of detection and dose-response definition conflict.

For the greatest confidence in a "negative" detection result, an agent should be administered continuously for the majority of an animal's lifespan. The NTP considers that 2 years is a practical treatment period in rats and mice, although the animals currently used in such studies may survive an additional 6–12 months. Study lengths of 15–18 months are considered adequate for shorter-lived species such as hamsters. An acceptable exposure/observation period for dogs in considered to be 7–10 years, an age equivalent to about 45–60 years in humans. For dietary treatments, continuous exposure is considered desirable and practical. With other routes, practical considerations may dictate interrupted treatments. For example, inhalation treatment for 6–8 hr/day on a 5 day/week schedule is the usual practice. Regimens requiring special handling of animals, such as parenteral injections, are usually on a 5 day/week basis. With some compounds intermittent exposures may be required because of toxicity. Various types of recovery can occur during exposure-free periods, which may either enhance or decrease chances of carcinogenicity. In view of the objective of assessing the carcinogenicity as the initial step, intermittent exposures on a 3–5 day/week basis is considered both practical and desirable for most compounds.

Following cessation of dosing or exposure, continued observation during a nontreatment period may be required before termination of the experiment. Such a period is considered desirable because 1) induced lesions may progress to more readily observable lesions, and 2) morphologically similar but noncarcinogenic proliferative lesions that are stress related may regress. Neoplastic or "neoplastic-like" lesions that persist long after removal of the stimulus are considered of serious consequence, from the hazard viewpoint. Many expert anatomical pathologists, however, feel able to diagnose and determine the biological nature of tumorous lesions existing at the time of treatment without the added benefit of a treatment-free period.

In determining the length of an observation period, several factors must be considered: period of exposure, survival pattern of both treated and control animals, nature of lesions found in animals that have already died, tissue storage and retention of the chemical, and results of other studies that would suggest induction of late-occurring tumors. The usual length of a treatment-free observation period is 3 months in mice and hamsters and 6 months in rats. An alternative would be to terminate the experiment or an individual treatment group on the basis of survival (say at the point at which 50% of the group with the lowest survival has died).

The arguments against such prolonged treatment and maintenance on study revolve around the relationship between age and tumor incidence. As test animals (or humans) become older, the background ("naturally occurring") incidence of tumors increases (63) and it becomes increasingly more difficult to identify a treatment effect apart from the background effect. Salsburg (64) has published an analysis of patterns of senile lesions in mice and rats, citing what he calls the principle of biological confounding. "If a particular lesion (e.g., pituitary tumor) is part of a larger syndrome induced by the treatment, it is impossible to determine whether the treatment has 'caused' that lesion."

This could lead to a situation where any real carcinogen would be non-identifiable. If the usual pattern of old-age lesions for a given species or strain of animals includes tumors, then almost every biologically active treatment can be expected to influence the incidence of tumors in some cluster of lesions at a sufficiently high dose.

Reconsidering our basic principles of experimental design, it is clear that we should try to design bioassays so that any carcinogenesis is a clear-cut single event, unconfounded by the occurrence of significant numbers of lesions due to other causes (such as age). One answer to this problem is the use of interim termination groups. When an evaluation of tumor incidences in an interim sacrifice (sample) of animals indicates that background incidences are becoming a souce of confounding data, termination plans for the study can be altered to minimize the loss of power. Several authors (65) have presented such adaptive sacrifice plans.

A number of other possible confounding factors can enter into a bioassay unless design precludes them. These include (a) cage and litter effects (which can be avoided by proper prestudy randomization of animals and rotation of cage locations), (b) vehicle (corn oil, for example, has been found to be a promoter for liver carcinogens), and (c) the use of the potential hazard route for humans, for example, dietary inclusion instead of gastric intubation. Other general aspects of the design of carcinogenicity bioassay may be found in Robens et al. (66).

2. Bioassay Interpretation

The interpretation of the results of even the best designed carcinogenesis bioassay is a complex statistical and biological problem. In addressing the statistical aspects, we shall have to overview some biological points (which have statistical implications) along the way.

First, all such bioassays are evaluated by comparison of the observed results in treatment groups with those in one or more control groups. These control groups include at least one group that is concurrent, but because of concern about the variability in background tumor rates, a historical control group is also considered in at least some manner.

The underlying problem in the use of concurrent controls alone is the belief that the selected populations of animals are subject both to an inordinate degree of variability in their spontaneous tumor incidence rates and that the strains maintained at separate breeding facilities are each subject to a slow but significant degree of genetic drift. The first case raises concern that, by chance, the animals selected to be controls for any particular study will be either "too high" or "too low" in their tumor incidences, leading to either a false positive or false negative statistical test result when test animals are compared to these controls. The second problem leads to the concern that over the years, different laboratories will be using different standards (control groups) against which to compare the outcome of their tests, making any kind of relative comparison between either compounds or laboratories impossible.

The last 10 years have seen at least 8 separate publications reporting on 5 sets of background tumor incidences in test animals. These 8 publications are summarized and compared in Tables 7 and 8 for B6C3F1 mice and Fischer 344 rats, respectively.

It should be kept in mind in considering these separate columns of num-

Table 7 Reported Background Tumor Incidences in B6C3F1 Mice

Organ/Tissue	(68) M	(68) F	(60, 70, 71, 72) M	(60, 70, 71, 72) F	(68) M	(68) F	(73) M (Ranges)	(73) F
Brain	.1	.1	<	0	<.1	.1		
Skin/subcutaneous	1.9	1.6	1	<1.0	<.1	.1		
Mammary gland	—	.8	—	<1.0	—	1.3		
Circulatory system	2.4	1.7	<1.0	<1.0	2.9	2.4		
Lung/trachea	11.7	4.4	9.2	3.5	13.7	5.2	10.6–21.9	3.6–7.1
Heart	.1	.1	<1.0	0				
Liver	21.9	4.0	15.6	2.5	24.6	4.7	25.0–40.1	4.6–9.7
Pancreas	.1	.1	<1.0	<1.0	2.1	<.1		
Stomach	.3	.3	1.1	<1.0	.4	.4		
Intestines	.4	.4	<1.0	<1.0	.5	.2		
Kidney	.2	.1	<1.0	<1.0	.3	<.1		
Urinary/bladder	.1	.1	0	1.0	<.1	<.1		
Preputial gland	—	—	—	—	—	—		
Testis	.5	NA	<1.0	NA	.4	NA		
Ovary	NA	.7	NA	<1.0	NA	.9		
Uterus	N	1.2	NA	1.9	NA	1.6		
Pituitary	.2	3.2	<1.0	3.5	.3	3.6		
Adrenal	.9	.7	<1.0	<1.0	1.4	.6		
Thyroid	1.0	1.3	1.1	<1.0	1.0	1.7		
Pancreatic islets	.3	.1	<1.0	<1.0	.4	.2		
Body cavities	.1	.3	<1.0	<1.0	.4	.3		
Leukemia/lymphoma	5.6	12.7	1.6	6.8	10.3	20.6	7.2–12.2	1.7–30.4
N	2355	2365	1132	1176	3543	3617	?	?

bers that there are some overlaps in the populations being reported. For example, it is almost certain that some NCI/NTP study control groups were incorporated in several separate publications. At the same time, the related survival and growth data on control animals (broken out by type of treatment and vehicle) has also been published (67), allowing for some assessment of comparability of control animal populations based on grounds other than just tumor incidences. It is interesting that in these NCI/NTP bioassay program control populations, mean survival of B6C3F1 mice was greater than that of F344 rats.

Generally, historical control group data are used primarily as a check to

Table 8 Reported Background Tumor Incidences in Fischer 344 Rats

Organ/Tissue	(68) M	(68) F	(60, 70, 72) M	(60, 70, 72) F	(74) M	(74) F	(68) M	(68) F	(73) M	(73) F
Brain	.9	.6	1.3	<0	8.1	.55	.8	.6		
Skin/subcutaneous	6.6	3.2	5.7	2.5	6.4	3.0	7.8	3.2		
Mammary gland	1.4	17.9	0	18.8	1.54	8.5	1.5	20.9		
Circulatory system	.4	.5	<1.0	<1.0	3.8	.27	.7.4			
Lung/trachea	3.1	1.8	2.4	<1.0	2.9	2.0	3.0	1.9		
Heart	.3	.1	<1.0	<1.0	.2	.2	.05			
Liver	1.8	3.1	1.2	1.3	1.74	3.9	2.2	1.9	0.7 3.4	.5 2.9
Pancreas	.2	—	<1.0	<0.16	0.2					
Stomach	.3	.2	<1.0	<1.0	.32	.2	.3	.2		
Intestines	.3	.5	<1.0	<1.0	.31	.36	.6	.3		
Kidney	.4	.2	<1.0<	1.0	.38	.16	.5	.2		
Urinary/bladder	.1.2	<1.0	<1.0	.1	.22	.1	.3			
Preputial gland	1.4	1.2	—	—	1.4	1.2	2.4	1.8		
Testis	80.6	NA	76.2	NA	80.1	NA	2.3	NA		
Ovary	NA	.3	NA	<1.0	NA	.33	NA	.4		
Uterus	NA	15.6	NA	16.8	NA	5.55	NA	17		
Pituitary	11.5	30.5	10.2	29.5	11.4	0.3	4.7	34.9	7.5– 31.2	31.0– 58.6
Adrenal	10.0	4.6	8.7	4.0	9.95	4.58	2.4	5.2		
Thyroid	7.1	6.5	5.1	5.6	7.16	6.65	8.2	6.8	3.6–	4.7–
Pancreatic islets	.8	1.0	3.2	1.3	3.89	1.05	3.9	.8		
Body cavities	1.1	.3	<1.0	<1.0	2.51	.38	2.6	.4	2.8– 9.0	1.0– 1.9
Leukemia/ lymphoma	11.7	9.1	6.5	5.4	12.3	9.9	9.9	13.4	9.1– 23.6	7.5– 15.4
N	1806	1765	846	840	1794	1754	**	**		

ensure that the statistical evaluations used in comparing treatment groups to concurrent controls have a sound starting point (68).

Dempster et al. (69) have, however, proposed a method for incorporating historical control data in the actual process of statistical analysis. A variable degree of pooling (combining) of historical with concurrent controls is performed based on the extent to which the historical data fit an assumed normal logistic (log transform) model.

Age (either animals or humans) is clearly related to both "background" cancer incidence and chemically induced carcinogenesis. Indeed, one view of chemically induced carcinogenesis is that it serves in many, if not all, cases to accelerate the rate at which developing deficiencies in the body's defense system allow cancers to be expressed. As either a carcinogen becomes more potent or a larger dose is used, neoplasms successfully overcome or evade defense mechanisms and are expressed as tumors. In some cases, clearly the effect of a test chemical has been to result in the earlier appearance of tumors in a test animal population than in nontreated members of the same population. Unless a study is designed and conducted so that a reasonably accurate measurement of time-to-tumor can be made, one is left with only the incidence of tumors found at the end of the study and the variable incidence in animals that die on study, and cannot rule out that though the terminal incidences were comparable, the test chemical resulted in an earlier development or expression of these same tumors. This is one of the strengths of the traditional skin painting studies, which allow easy detection of skin tumors as soon as they appear and tracking of their progress.

If the target organ is not the skin, the only reasonably sensitive manner of evaluating time-to-tumor (unless the tumors are rapidly life threatening and there is an accordingly high early mortality rate leading to necropsy of spontane-ous deaths in test animals) is to periodically, during the study, terminate, nec-ropsy, and histopathologically evaluate random samples of test and control ani-mals. The traditional NCI bioassay had no such interim or serial sacrifices (73) and therefore could not address such issues.

Such serial sacrifices are usually conducted on at least 20 animals per sex per group starting at one year into the study. Several statistical methods other then life table procedures are available for analysis of such data (75,76).

A related issue is the age at which to terminate the animals. We have already presented the point that as a study progresses, the rise in the background level of tumors makes it more and more difficult to clearly partition out treat-ment-effect tumors from age-effect tumors. Swenberg (77) and Solleveld et al. (78) have made the point that the incidence of many tumor types has increased from 100 to 500% when control rat results from two-year studies (rats 100–116 weeks of age) were compared to those from lifespan studies (140–146 weeks of age). If such an increase in age (25%) can result in such extreme increases in spontaneous tumors, what is the effect on interpretation of incidence rates seen in concurrent treatment groups? This is especially the case if, as Salsburg (64) has suggested, any biologically active treatment will result in a shift in the patterns of neoplastic lesions occurring in aging animals. The current practice is to interpret tumor incidence on an independent site-by-site basis (on the as-sumption that what happens at each tissue site is independent of what happens elsewhere), and no allowance or factoring is made for the fact that what may be occurring in animals over a lifespan (as expressed by tumor incidence levels at an advanced age) is merely a shifting of patterns from one tumor site to another. In other words, commonly the "significantly" increased incidence of liver tumors is focused on, while the just as statistically significant decrease in kidney tumors compared to controls is ignored. Clearly, we should not try to analyze data from animals that are advancing into senescence in the same manner that we do the data from those which lack these onfounding factors Where should a cutoff point be? This is a problem requiring some work, but clearly the data of Cameron et al. (67) suggest that the growth curves of 9,385 B6C3F1 mice and 10,023 F344 rats from control groups in NCI/NTP studies show consistent patterns of decline in body weights from these animals starting at the following ages (in weeks).

	Males	Females
B6C3F1 mice	96	101
Fischer 344 rats	91	106

A consideration of similar data on tumor incidences (unfortunately not available from NCI/NTP studies) would certainly improve confidence in selecting cutoff points for age, but the above ages merit consideration as termination points.

Having reviewed the preceding biological factors, we may now begin to directly address the statistical interpretation of carcinogenesis bioassays. Such interpretation, once believed to be a simple problem of calculating the statistical significance of increases of tumor incidences in treatment groups at each of a number of tissue sites, is now clearly of itself a more complex task. Assuming dose level and route were appropriate, at least four separate questions must still be addressed in such an interpretation of incidence.

1.   Are the data resulting from the bioassay sufficient to warrant analysis and interpretation? Factors that may invalidate a bioassay include inadequate survival in test or control groups, extreme (high or low) control group tumor incidence levels, excessive loss of tissues from autolysis, infection during the study, and the use of contaminated diet or water.

2.   Are there increases in tumor incidences in test groups compared to those in control groups? If so, then we must proceed to do an incidence comparison on some form of contingency table arrangement of the data. Such comparisons are traditionally performed using a series of Fisher's exact tests.

3.   If there is a significant increase in tumor incidence, is there a trend (dose response) in the data for these sites that concurs with what we know about biological responses to toxicants? That is, as dose increases, response should increase. A significant increase occurring only in a low dose group (with the incidence levels in the higher dose groups being comparable to controls), would be of very questionable biological significance.

4.   If significant incidence and trend are present, is there supporting evi-

dence of the material being a carcinogen? An example of this was cited earlier in the case of mouse liver tumors where the presence of positive mutagenicity findings would support a belief of biological significance and concern about real-life exposure of humans.

Two major controversial questions are involved in such comparisons: (a) Should they be based on one-tailed or two-tailed distribution? and (b) What are the effects and implications of multiple comparisons? The one- or two-tailed controversy revolves around the question of which hypothesis we are properly testing in a study such as a chronic carcinogenicity study. Is the tumor incidence different between the control and treated groups? In such cases, it is a bidirectional hypothesis and, therefore, a two-tailed distribution we are testing against. Or are we asking is the tumor incidence greater in the treated group than in the control group? In the latter case, it is a unidirectional hypothesis and we are contemplating only the right-hand tail of the distribution. The implications of the answer to this question are more than theoretical; significance is much greater (exactly double, in fact, for Fisher's exact test) in the one-tailed case than in the two-tailed. For example, a set of data analyzed by Fisher's exact test which would have a two-tailed p level of 0.098 and one-tailed level of 0.049 would be flagged, therefore, as significantly different if the one-tailed test were employed. Feinstein (79) provides excellent discussion of the background in a nonmathematical way. Determination of the correct approach must rest on a clear definition by the researcher, beforehand, of the objective of his study and of the possible outcomes (if a bidirectional outcome is possible, are we justified in using a one-tailed test statistic?).

The multiple comparisons problem is a much more lively one. In chronic studies, we test lesion/tumor incidence on each of a number of tissues, for each sex and species, with each result being flagged if it exceeds the fiducial limit of $p \leq 0.05$.

The point we must ponder here is the meaning of "$p \leq 0.05$." This is the level of the probability of our making a type I error (incorrectly concluding we have an effect when, in fact, we do not). So we have accepted the fact that there is a 5% chance of our producing a false positive from this study. Our trade-off is a much lower chance (typically 1%) of a type II error, that is, of our passing as safe a compound which is not safe. These two error levels are connected; to achieve a lower type II level inflates our type I level. The problem in this case is that when we make a large number of such comparisons, we are repeatedly taking the chance that we will "find" a false positive result. The set of lesions and/or tumor comparisons described above may number more than 70 tests for significance in a single study, which will result in a large inflation of our false positive level. The extent of this inflated false positive rate (and how to reduce its effects) has been discussed and estimated with a great degree of variability. Salsburg (80) has estimated that the typical original National Cancer Institute

(NCI) type cancer bioassay has a probability of type I error ranging between 20 and 50%. Fears and colleagues (70,71), however, have estimated it as being between 6 and 24%. Haseman and Hoel (55) have also reviewed some of Salsburg's calculations and stated that correcting for multiple counting of individual animals and adjusting for survival differences markedly reduced the false positive rate. Without some form of correction factor, the "false positive" rate of a series of multiple tests can be calculated as being equal to $1 - 0.05^N$ where N is the number of tests and the selected alpha level is 0.05. Salsburg (80) expressed the concern that such an exaggerated false positive result may cause a good compound to be banned. Though Haseman (81) challenged this on the point that a much more mature decision process than this is used by the regulatory agencies. Salsburg has pointed out at least two cases, however, where the decision to ban was based purely on such a single statistical significance. What, then, is a proper use of such results? Or, conversely, how can we control for such an inflated error rate?

There are statistical methods available for dealing with this multiple comparisons problem. One such is the use of Bonferroni inequalities to correct for successive multiple comparisons (82). This method has the drawback that there is some accompanying loss of power expressed as an inability to identify true positives properly. A method proposed by McKnight and Crowley (83), if information from frequent interim terminations is present, provides a reasonably sensitive yet unbiased means of evaluating such data. Similarly, Meng and Dempster (84) have proposed a Bayesian approach to such analysis to solve the multiple comparisons problem. In this, a logistically distributed (or log-transformed) model, which accommodates the incidences of all tumor types or sites observed in the current experiment simultaneously as well as their historical control incidences, is developed. Exchangeable normal expected values are assumed for certain linear terms in the model. Posterior means, standard deviaton, and Bayesian p values are computed for an overall treatment effect as well as for the effects on individual tumor types or tissue sites. Model assumptions are then evaluated using probability plots and the sensitivity of the parameter estimates to alternative expected values is analyzed.

The third and fourth questions presented earlier are parts of what is evolving as a second set of approaches to the interpretation of bioassay results.

These new second approaches use the information in a more mature decision making process. First, the historical control incidence rates such as given for the B6C3F1 mouse and the Fischer-344 rats in Tables 7 and 8 should be considered; as we have seen, some background incidences are so high that these tissues are "null and void" for making decisions. Second, we should look not just for a single significant incidence in a tissue, but rather for a trend. For example, we might have the following percentages of a liver tumor incidence in the female rats of a study: (a) control = 3%, (b) 10 mg/kg = 6%, (c) 50 mg/

kg = 17%, and (d) 250 mg/kg = 54%. In this study only the incidence at the 250 mg/kg level might be statistically significant. However, the trend through each of the levels is suggestive of a dose-response. Looking for such a trend is an essential step in a scientific assessment of the results, and one of the available trend analysis techniques, such as presented in Gad and Weil (1), should be utilized. Another method for determining whether statistically significant incidences are merely random occurrences is to compare the results of the quantitative variables to two or more concurrently run control groups. Often the mean of one variable will differ from only one of these controls and be numerically within the range of this same variable of the two control means. If so, the statistical significance compared to the one control must be seriously questioned as to its being associated with a biological significance. Three different such stepwise interpretative procedures are common. These are the NCI method, the weight-of-evidence method, and the Peto method. The NCI approach is somewhat complex, involving each of the four steps outlined earlier in a process overviewed by Tarone et al. (73). The statistical aspects of this are outlined below.

B. NCI Bioassay Method

1. Survival Analysis. By sex, species, and organ, exclude all animals dying prior to first incidence of tumor at that site. Do a life table analysis for survival at the same time.
2. Use Fisher exact test to obtain one-tailed p at each site using the survival adjusted ratios obtained in 1 above.
3. Utilize the Bonferroni correction using r (where r = the number of dose levels; not k = the number of total comparisons); multiply the computed p by r to maintain overall error rate. Significance is claimed only if p is less than α/r.
4. Perform tests for linear trend using Cochran-Armitage test (dose response curve must be significantly different from zero, and positive).

Notes. In 100 animal bioassays, you need 5 or more animals to have tumors achieve a one-tailed $p \geq 0.05$. With Bonferroni correction, 7 or more are needed. NCI believes and practices the rare tumor incidence flag mechanism. (See Refs. 96–98.)

The 9 possible interpretations of an analysis of tumor incidence and survival analysis are summarized in Table 9.

The weight of evidence approach consists primarily of the four steps of interpretation presented earlier, with emphasis on the last step (integration of related and supporting information into the evaluation process) as opposed to the NCI approach (which places emphasis on the two "statistical" steps). The weight of evidence approach poses difficulty in the regulatory and legal fields

Table 9 Interpretation of the Analysis of Tumor Incidence and Survival Analysis (Life Table)

Outcome Type	Tumor Association with Treatment[a]	Mortality Association with Treatment	Interpretation[b]
A	+	+	Unadjusted test may underestimate tumorigenicity of treatment.
B	+	+	Unadjusted test gives valid picture of tumorigenicity of treatment.
C	+	−	Tumors found in treated groups may reflect longer survival of treated groups. Time adjusted analysis is indicated.
D	−	+	Apparent negative findings in tumors may be due to the shorter survival in treated groups. Time-adjusted analysis and/or a retest at lower doses is indicated.
E	−	0	Unadjusted test gives a valid picture of the possible tumor-preventive capacity of the treatment.
F	−	−	Unadjusted test may underestimate the possible tumor-preventive capacity of the treatment.
G	0	+	High mortality in treated groups may lead to unadjusted test missing a possible tumorigen. Adjusted analysis and/or retest at lower doses in indicated.
H	0	0	Unadjusted test gives valid picture of lack of association with treatment.
I	0	−	Longer survival in treated groups may mask tumor-preventive capacity of treatment.

[a] + = yes, − = no and 0 = no bearing on discussion.
[b] The unadjusted test referred to here is a contingency table type of analysis of incidence, such as a Fisher's Exact test.

because it requires judgment and is not overtly quantitative. However, it does represent a scientifically valid approach for distinguishing important differences in the potential of chemicals to induce cancer. The greatest weight of evidence should be given to chemicals that induce dose-related increases in malignant tumors at multiple sites, in both sexes and in multiple species using appropriate routes of administration. At the other end of the spectrum, much less weight should be given to chemicals that induce only an increased incidence of a benign neoplasm, whose incidence is normally quite variable, and is found only in the high dose group of one sex of a single species. One must also integrate a significant amount of additional information.

For example, the shape and extent of the dose–response curve should be known in relation to factors such as the chemical's pharmacokinetics, its overwhelming of host defenses, or saturation of metabolic systems. Is the chemical genotoxic? How do the site and dose response for toxicity compare with those for carcinogenicity? This knowledge is highly relevant when attempting to understand the mechanism involved in carcinogenesis for each specific chemical, and can and should be incorporated into both hazard identification and risk assessment to improve their accuracy. It is widely believed to be appropriate to test a chemical at the MTD in order to gain assurance that it has been adequately tested. However, if a chemical is not genotoxic, but induces frank cytotoxicity in the liver only at doses at which it also induces liver tumors, it should be considered differently than a chemical that is genotoxic and induces liver tumors over a large dose range including noncytotoxic doses.

The Peto procedure (85) is actually a collection of approaches arising from the central belief that it is possible to generate an additional vital set of data from a well run bioassay, and that we should utilize these same pieces of data in interpreting results.

The data in question constitute an evaluation of the likelihood that each individual tumor would (or would not) be life threatening. The approach calls for the pathologist on a study to not only identify a mass or tumor as neoplastic or not, but also to categorize each neoplasm in one of several possible classes as to the risk it presents to the survival of the host organism. Such classification is generally in one of at least five different categories:

1. Tumor did or would definitely cause death of animal.
2. Tumor probably die or could cause death of animal.
3. Cannot be determined.
4. Tumor probably didn't or wouldn't cause death of animal.
5. Tumor didn't or wouldn't cause death of animal.

Such data can then be employed in a more precise interpretation of the meaning of the bioassay. An entire separate, sensitive set of significance tests based on such data have been proposed by Peto et al. (85).

The last point to be addressed under the topic of carcinogenicity bioassay is the use of the resulting data for the conduct of carcinogenic potency comparisons. Such a potency comparison would both be valuable in a scientific sense and provide a basis for prioritization of regulatory actions.

Potency and dose response of carcinogens for any single species of animals may be expressed in one of two manners, either as the incidence rate of tumors at the end of a set period of time or as the time lag from treatment to a specified incidence rate of tumors. This second way has also been extended to determining time to death as a result of tumors produced by a carcinogen (86).

Squire (87) has proposed a ranking system for animal carcinogens based on data from NTP bioassays (that is, in the absence of time-to-tumor information). The major considerations are:

1. Number of species affected
2. Number of different types of neoplasms induced in one or more species
3. A negative correction for the spontaneous incidence in control groups of induced neoplasms
4. Cumulative dose or exposure per kilogram body weight in affected groups
5. The proportion of induced neoplasms which were malignant
6. The degree of supporting genotoxicity (mutagenicity) data

Of course, our real interest in the potency of carcinogens is in humans, which means an interspecies comparison. Crouch and Wilson (1979), using the results of some 70 NCI/NTP bioassays where carcinogenicity was established in both rats and mice, reported that a comparison demonstrated empirically that good correlations exist between these two species for suitably defined carcinogenic potencies for various chemicals. Such a correlation would allow sufficient accuracy in extrapolating from animal data to human risk to support a logical scheme for the evaluation of such risks. More recently, however, Bernstein et al. (88) examined a larger NCI/NTP Bioassay Program data base. They observed that there is a very high correlation of the maximum doses tested (max-d) for rats and mice on a milligram per kilogram body weight per day basis. Calculating the carcinogenic potency (b-defined in their paper), they found it to be restricted to an approximately 30-fold range surrounding $\log(2)$/max-d, which has a biological as well as a statistical basis. Since the max-ds for the set of NCI/NTP test chemicals varied over many orders of magnitude, it necessarily follows statistically that the carcinogenic potencies will be highly correlated. This "artifact" of potency estimation does not imply that there is no basis for extrapolating animals results to humans. They concluded that "it does suggest, however, that the interpretation of correlation studies of carcinogenic potency needs much further thought."

On an intermediate level, others have suggested a class of Bayesian statistical methods for the combining of data from different substances and species of animals, using the results as one constructs the model to estimate interexperimental error between the different sources of data being combined.

C. Areas of Controversy in Statistics as Used for Toxicology

It should now be clear to the reader that the use of statistics in toxicology is not a cut and dried matter. There are a number of areas which are (and have been) the subject of honest controversy, and it should be expected that others will arise as the two fields advance.

There remain three areas to be addressed that are somewhat peculiar to toxicology. These are the effects of censoring on data, the direction of hypothesis testing, and the use of unbalanced designs.

1. Censoring

Censoring is practiced when not all the possible data arising from an experiment are available for or used in analysis. Though some would make the distinction that censored data are different from missing data in that the values for the former can be accurately estimated and those for missing data cannot, here the term is used to mean all data not included in analysis for whatever reasons. There are four major reasons for data being censored in toxicology studies. The degree of accuracy for which the value of such censored values can be estimated varies, depending on the reason for censoring.

1.   The most common reason for censoring in toxicology is because of death; not all the animals that start a study end it. In these cases we have no basis to accurately estimate the observations that would have been made had the animal (or animals) lived. Censoring by death is an example of "left censoring;" unplanned without recourse and generally during a period when the information lost would be of interest. Right censoring, on the other hand, generally is planned; there is recourse to get the information if needed and the information potentially lost is of minimal if any interest.

2.   Data may be censored by having samples lost to measurement at intermittent periods. Such losses are the result of occurrences such as clotting of blood samples prior to analysis, loss of tissues during necropsy, and breakdown of instruments at critical times. Usually the values of the last observations can be estimated with some accuracy. And most such cases can be remedied by resampling (collecting more blood, for example).

3.   When we judge an extreme value to be an outlier and reject it, we are censoring it. If the value is cleanly discarded, we are de facto saying we cannot accurately estimate its value. If, however, we use a procedure such as winsorizing and replace it with a less extreme value, we are in fact estimating the most probable true value of the observations.

4.   Finally, some observations may be censored because their values are beyond the range at which the instruments were used can accurately measure.

An example is in measuring rabbit methemoglobin with an instrument designed for humans. Extreme low values are not measured accurately, and are reported as negative percentage values. In this case, we can accurately estimate a censored value as being "less than" or "greater than" a known value.

What are the consequences of censoring? The answer depends on the nature and extent of the censoring process. If only a few of a large number of values are lost and the pattern of loss is randomly distributed among all groups on study, little if any harm is done. If the extent of data loss is too severe, for example, because the majority of the animals in a group die, the entire experiment may have to be discarded. An intermediate case is when the extent of censoring is low but the censoring is not random. This is not uncommon in toxicology, where censoring because of death tends to be concentrated in the high dose groups. In these cases, the experiment is not lost but rather truncated; that is, some effects cannot be addressed with reference to the treatment used in highly censored groups. And, as we will discuss a little later, it may imbalance a design.

An additional common effect of censoring that should be kept in mind is on the normality of the sample. If all values above a certain level (say of serum electrolytes) are censored because animals having such values die before the measurements are made, we are left with a truncated normal distribution. A special case of this was discussed by Gad and Smith (89) in that the time-to-incapacitation values in combustion toxicology are censored because they are only measured to 30 min, and not beyond. Such truncated populations cannot be treated as normal for purposes of statistical analysis.

Additionally, entire family of methods have been developed to address censored data sets. Bishop et al. (90) present an excellent overview of some of these.

2.   Direction of Hypothesis Testing

Which direction (or directions) we are testing a hypothesis in can be restated as asking whether we are to use a one-tailed or a two-tailed test. This is of consequence because one-tailed tests are always more sensitive (more likely to find an effect) than are two-tailed tests.

Generally, such a selection must be made prior to the start of an experiment, based on a clear statement of the question being asked (that is, the objective of the study). If we are asking if a chemical increases the incidence of cancer, then our question is one-tailed—we are not interested in the detection of any significant decrease in the incidence of cancer. Most toxicology studies, however, are of a "shotgun" nature. They are designed to detect and identify any and all effects. This is a two-tailed question: can a chemical either increase or decrease the incidence of cancer?

Feinstein (79) provides a clear discussion of questions of direction of effect as they relate to biostatistics.

3. Unbalanced Designs

One of the principles of experimental design presented earlier was that of balance. This held that group sizes should be at least approximately equal. As we have reviewed the different methods presented in this book, we have noted that a number of them have impaired performance if the sizes of the groups are not equivalent.

Yet, it is not uncommon to lose data because of censoring in toxicology studies, and if such censoring is related to a compound or treatment effect, it is very likely that the most affected groups will not be equivalent in size to our control group at the end of an experiment.

At the same time, it should be clear that it is easier to statistically detect large effects than small effects. In the vast majority of cases, larger effects occur in high dose groups (not infrequently to the extent that no statistical analysis is necessary), while it is in the lower dose groups that the guidance provided by statistical analysis is most needed.

These reasons argue for the use of unbalanced designs in toxicology. In other words, those treatments where it is expected that more statistical power will be needed or which are expected to suffer from an increased level of censoring due to death (where death itself is not the variable of interest) should be administered to larger test groups. Farmer et al. (91) have reviewed a number of options for deciding on the degree of imbalance with which to start a study.

4. Use of Computerized Statistical Packages

Finally, we must recognize that for many toxicology laboratories and researchers, the approach to statistical analysis of data is to use one of the computer-based analysis packages that automatically selects and utilizes statistical tests. It is critically important in these cases to understand the limitations and proper uses of statistical tests that are automatically employed.

5. Screens

One major set of activities in toxicology (and also in pharmacology, for that matter) is screening for the presence or absence of an effect. Such screens are almost always focused on detecting a single endpoint of effect (such as mutagenicity, lethality, neuro or developmental toxicity, etc.) and have a particular set of operating characteristics in common.

1. A large number of compounds are to be evaluated, so that ease of performance (which can also be considered efficiency) is a major desirable characteristic.

2. The screen must be very sensitive in its detection of potential effective agents. An absolute minimum of effective agents should escape detection, that is, there should be very few false negatives (in other words, the type II error rate or β should be low.)

3. It is desirable that the number of false positives be small (that is, that there be a low type I error rate or an α level).

4. Items 1–3 are all to some degree contradictory, requiring the involved researchers to agree on a set of compromises. The typically start with acceptance of a relatively high α level (0.10 or more).

5. In an effort to better serve item 1, such screens are frequently performed in batteries so that multiple endpoints are measured in the same mode. Additionally, such measurements may be repeated over a period of time in each model.

In an early screen, a relatively large number of compounds will be tested. It is unlikely that one will stand out so much as to be statistically significantly more important than all the other compounds. A more or less continuous range of activities will be found. Compounds showing the highest activity will proceed to the next assay in the series, and may be used as lead compounds in a new cycle of testing and evaluation.

Each assay can have an associated activity criterion. If the result for a particular test compound meets this criterion, the compound may pass to the next stage. This criterion could be based on statistical significance (i.e., all compounds with observed activities significantly greater than the control at the 5% level could be tagged). However, for early screens such criterion may be too strict and few compounds may go through to further testing.

A useful indicator of the efficiency of an assay series is the frequency of discovery of truly active compounds. This is related to the probability of discovery and to the degree of risk associated with a compound. These two factors in turn depend on the distribution of activities in the test series and the changes at each stage of rejecting and accepting compounds with given activities.

Statistical modeling of the assay system may lead to the improvement of the design of the system to reduce the interval between discoveries. Preliminary results suggest that in the early screens it may be beneficial to increase the number of compounds tested, decrease the numbers of animals per group, and increase the range and number of doses. The result will be less information on more structures, but an overall increase in the frequency of discovery (assuming that truly active compounds are entering the system at a steady rate).

The design of each assay and the choice of the activity criterion should therefore be adjusted bearing in mind the relative costs of retaining false positives and rejecting false negatives. Decreasing the group sizes in the early assays reduces the chance of obtaining significance at any particular level (such as 5%) so that the activity criterion must be relaxed, in a statistical sense, to allow more compounds through. At some stage, however, it becomes too expensive to continue screening many false positives and the criteria must be tightened up accordingly.

An excellent introduction to this subject is Redman's (92) interesting approach, which identifies four characteristics of an assay. It is assumed that a compound is either active or inactive, and that the proportion of actives can be estimated from past experience. After testing, a compound will be classified as positive or negative. It is then possible to design the assay to optimize the following characteristics:

Sensitivity	The ratio of true positives to total actives
Specificity	The ratio of true negatives to total inactives
Positive accuracy	The ratio of true to observed positives
Negative accuracy	The ratio of true to observed negatives

An advantage of testing more compounds is that it gives the opportunity to average activity evidence over structural classes, or study quantitative structure–activity relationships (QSARs). QSARs can be used to predict the activity of new compounds and thus reduce the chance of in vivo testing on negative compounds. It can increase the proportion of truly active compounds passing through the system.

In conclusion, it may be said that maximization of the performance of a series of screening assays requires close collaboration between the biologist, chemist, and statistician. It should be noted, however, that screening forms only part of a much larger research and development context.

Screens may thus truly be considered the biological equivalent of exploratory data analysis (EDA). EDA methods, in fact, provide a number of useful possibilities for less rigid and yet quite utilitarian approaches to the statistical analysis of the data from screens. A brief presentation of such methods comprises the final section of this chapter.

As an example of such an approach, a set of devices called quality control charts may be advantageously constructed and used during assay development and in routine screening procedures. During the development of assay methodology, for example, by keeping records of assay results, an initial estimate of the assay standard deviation is available when full-scale use starts. The initial estimate can then be revised as more data is generated.

The following example shows the usefulness of control charts for control measurements in a screening procedure. Our example test for screening potential immune suppressive agents measures reduction of edema (mouse ear volume) by test compounds compared to a control treatment. A control chart was established to monitor the performance of the control agent (a) to establish the mean and variability of the control, (b) to ensure that the results of the control for a given experiment are within reasonable limits (a validation of the assay procedure). The average ear volume difference (ear volume before treatment – ear volume after treatment) and the average range for a series of experiments are shown in Table 10.

As in quality control charts, the mean and average range of the assay were determined from previous experiments. In this example, the screen had been run 20 times previous to the data of Table 10. These initial data showed a mean ear volume difference of 40 and a mean range ($\overline{R}$) of 9. These values were used for the control charts shown in Figure 5. The subgroups are of size 4. Using the values provided in Table 11, the action limits for the $\overline{X}$ and range charts were calculated as follows:

$$\overline{X} \pm 0.73\overline{R} = 40 \pm 0.73(9) = 33.4 \text{ to } 46.6 \qquad (\overline{X} \text{ chart})$$

$$\overline{R}(2.28) = 9(2.28) = 20.5 \qquad \text{the upper limit for the range}$$

Note that the lower limit for the range of subgroups consisting of four units is zero. Six of the 20 means are out of limits. Efforts to find a cause for the large interest variation failed. The procedures were standardized and followed carefully, and the animals appeared to be homogeneous. Because different shipments of animals were needed to proceed with these tests over time, the investigators felt that there was no way to reduce the variability of the procedure. Therefore, a new control chart was prepared based on the variability between test means. A moving average was recommended using five successive averages.

Table 10 Average Paw Volume Difference and Range for Screening Procedure

Test number	Mean	Range	Test number	Mean	Range
1	38	4	11	28	12
2	43	3	12	41	10
3	34	3	13	40	22
4	48	6	14	34	5
5	38	24	15	37	4
6	45	4	16	43	14
7	49	5	17	37	6
8	32	9	18	45	8
9	48	5	19	32	7
10	34	8	20	42	13

Four guinea pigs per test group.

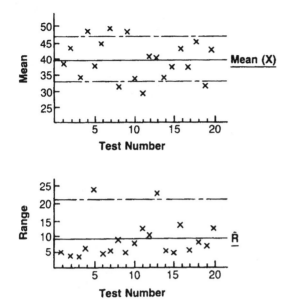

Figure 5 Quality control chart for means and range for control group in screening procedure for mouse ear swelling agents.

Table 11 Values for Determining Upper and Lower Limits for Mean $(\overline{X})$ and Range Charts

Sample size of subgroup (N)	A: Factor for $\overline{X}$ chart	Range chart factors	
		Lower limit (D_L)	Upper limit (D_U)
2	1.88	0	3.27
3	1.02	0	2.57
4	0.73	0	2.28
5	0.58	0	2.11
6	0.48	0	2.00
7	0.42	0.08	1.92
8	0.37	0.14	1.86
9	0.34	0.18	1.82
10	0.31	0.22	1.78
20	0.18	0.41	1.59

Based on historical data, $\overline{X}$ was calculated as 39.7 with an average moving range of 12.5. The limits for the moving average graph are

$$39.7 \pm 0.73(12.5) - 30.6 \text{ to } 48.8$$

The factor 0.73 is obtained from Table 2 for subgroup samples of size 4.

Such charts may also be constructed and used for proportion or count type data. By constructing such charts for the range of control data, we may then use them as a rapid and efficient tool for detecting effects in groups being assessed for that same screen endpoint.

6. Exploratory Data Analysis

Over the past 20 years, an entirely new approach has been developed to get the most information out of the increasingly larger and more complex data sets facing scientific researchers. This approach involves the use of a very diverse set of fairly simple techniques that comprise exploratory data analysis (EDA). As expounded by Tukey (93), there are four major ingredients to EDA:

Displays.   These visually reveal the behavior of the data and suggest a framework for analysis. The scatterplot (presented earlier) is an example of this approach.

Residuals.   These are what remain of a set of data after a fitted model (such as linear regression) or some similar level of analysis has been subtracted out.

Re-expressions.   These involve the questions of what scale would serve to best simplify and improve the analysis of the data. Simple transformations, such as presented earlier in this chapter, are used to simplify data behavior (such as linearizing or normalizing it) and clarify analysis.

Resistance.   This is a matter of decreasing the sensitivity of analysis and summary of data to misbehavior. This means that the occurrence of a few outliers will not invalidate or make too difficult the methods used to analyze the data. For example, in summarizing the location of a set of data, the median (but not the arithmetic mean) is highly resistant.

These four ingredients are utilized in a process falling into two broad phases: an exploratory phase and a confirmatory phase. The exploratory phase isolates patterns and features of the data and reveals them, allowing for inspection of the data before there is any firm choice of actual hypothesis testing or modeling methods.

Confirmatory analysis allows evaluation of the reproducibility of the observed patterns or effects. Its role is close to that of classical hypothesis testing, but also often includes steps such as (a) incorporating information from an analysis of another, closely related set of data and (b) validating a result by assembling and analyzing additional data (Figure 6 shows an example of this approach).

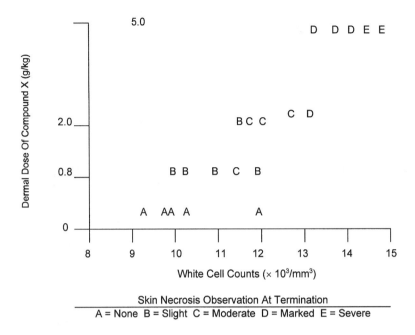

Figure 6 Explory data analysis correlative plots.

These techniques are in general beyond the scope of this text. Velleman and Hoaglin (94) and Hoaglin et al. (95) present a clear overview of the more important methods, along with the codes for their performance on the microcomputer (they have also now been incorporated into Minitab). A short examination of a single case of the use of these methods, however, is in order.

Toxicology has long recognized that no population, animal or human, is completely uniform in its response to any particular toxicant. Rather, a population is composed of a (presumably normal) distribution of individuals; some resistant to intoxication (hyporesponders), the bulk that respond close to a central value (such as an LD_{50}), and some that are very sensitive to intoxication (hyperresponders). This distribution of population can, in fact, result in additional statistical techniques. The sensitivity of techniques such as ANOVA is reduced markedly by the occurrence of outliers (extreme high or low values including hyper- and hyporesponders) which, in fact, serve to markedly inflate the variance (standard deviation) associated with a sample. Such a variance inflation effect is particularly common in small groups that are exposed or dosed at just over or under a threshold level, causing a small number of individuals in the sample (who are more sensitive than the other members) to respond mark-

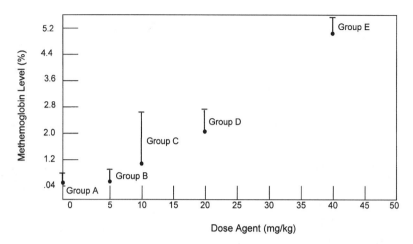

(Points Are Means - Error Bars Are + One Standard Deviation)

Figure 7   Variance inflation.

edly. Such a situation is displayed in Figure 7, which plots the mean and standard deviations of methemoglobin levels in a series of groups of animals exposed to successively higher levels of a hemolytic agent.

Though the mean level of methemoglobin in group C is more than double that of control group A, no hypothesis test will show this difference to be significant because of the large standard deviation associated with it. Yet this "inflated" variance exists because a single individual has such a marked response. Such inflation certainly indicates that the data need to be examined closely. Indeed, all tabular data in toxicology should be visually inspected for both trend and variance inflation.

A concept related (but not identical) to resistance and exploratory data analysis is that of robustness. Robustness generally implies insensitivity to departures from assumptions surrounding an underlying model such as normality.

In summarizing the location of data the median, though highly resistant, is not extremely robust. But the mean is both badly nonresistant and badly nonrobust.

REFERENCES

1. Gad, S.C. (1998). Statistical and Experimental Design for Toxicologists, 3rd Ed. CRC Press: Boca Raton, FL.
2. Myers, J.L. (1972). Fundamentals of Experimental Design. Boston: Allyn and Bacon.

3. Dixon, W.J. and Massey, F.J., Jr. (1969). Introduction to Statistical Analysis, 3rd ed. New York: McGraw-Hill.

4. Weil, C.S. (1970). Selection of the valid number of sampling units and a consideration of their combination in toxicological studies involving reproduction, teratogenesis or carcinogenesis. Food Cosmet. Toxicol. 8:177–182.

5. Thompson, W.R. and Weil, C.S. (1952). On the construction of tables for moving average interpolation. Biometrics 8:51–54.

6. Weil, C.S. (1972). Statistics vs. safety factors and scientific judgment in the evaluation of safety for man. Toxicol. Appl. Pharmacol. 21:459.

7. Weil, C.S. (1975). Toxicology experimental design and conduct as measuredby interlaboratory collaboration studies. J. Assoc. Off. Anal. Chem. 58:687–688.

8. Weil, C.S., Carpenter, C.P., and Smith, H.I. (1953). Specifications for calculating the median effective dose. Am. Indust. Hyg. Assoc. Quart. 14:200–206.

9. Zbiden, G. and Flury-Roversi, M. (1981). Significant of the LD_{50} test for the toxicological evaluation of chemical substances. Arch. Toxicol. 47:77–99.

10. DePass, L.R., Myers, R.C., Weaver, E.V., and Weil, C.S. (1984). An assessment of the importance of number of dosage levels, number of animals per dosage level, sex and method of LD_{50} and slope calculations in acute toxicity studies. In: Alternative Methods in Toxicology, Vol. 2: Acute Toxicity Testing: Alternate Approaches. Edited by A.M. Goldberg. New York: Mary Ann Liebert, Inc.

11. Gad, S.C., Smith, A.C., Cramp, A.L., Gavigan, F.A., and Derelanko, M.J. (1984). Innovative designs and practices for acute systemic toxicity studies. Drug Chem. Toxicol. 7:423–434.

12. Bruce, R.D. (1985). An up-and-down procedure for acute toxicity testing. Fund. App. Toxicol. 5:151–157.

13. Jackson, B. (1962). Statistical analysis of body weight data. Toxicol. Appl. Pharmacol. 4:432–443.

14. Weil, C.S. (1962). Applications of methods of statistical analysis to efficient repeated-dose toxicological tests. I. General considerations and problems involved. Sex differences in rat liver and kidney weights. Toxicol. Appl. Pharmacol. 4: 561–571.

15. Weil, C.S. and Gad, S.C. (1980). Applications of methods of statistical analysis to efficient repeated-dose toxicologic tests. 2. Methods for analysis of body, liver and kidney weight data. Toxicol. Appl. Pharmacol. 52:214–226.

16. Zar, J.H. (1974). Biostatistical Analysis. Englewood Cliffs, NJ: Prentice-Hall, p. 50.

17. Weil, C.S. (1973). Experimental design and interpretation of data from prolonged toxicity studies. In: Proc. 5th Int. Congr. Pharmacol. San Francisco, Vol. 2, pp. 4–12.

18. Boyd, E.M. (1972). Predictive Toxicometrics. Baltimore: Williams & Wilkins.

19. Boyd, E.M. and Knight, L.M. (1963). Postmortem shifts in the weight and water levels of body organs. Tox. Appl. Pharm. 5:119–128.

20. Ridgemen, W.J. (1975). Experimentation in Biology. New York, pp. 214–215.

21. Wallach, J. (1978). Interpretation of Diagnostic Tests. Boston: Little, Brown and Company.

22. Oser, B.L. and Oser, M. (1956). Nutritional studies in rats on diets containing

high levels of partial ester emulsifiers. II. Reproduction and lactation. J. Nutr. 60:
    429.

23. Mitruka, B.M. and Rawnsley, H.M. (1977). Clinical Biochemical and Hematologi-
    cal Reference Values in Normal Experimental Animals. New York: Masson.

24. Weil, C.S. (1982). Statistical analysis and normality of selected hematologic and
    clinical chemistry measurements used in toxicologic studies. Arch. Toxicol.
    (Suppl.)5:237–253.

25. Kupper, L.L. and Haseman, J.K. (1978). The use of a correlated binomial model
    for the analysis of certain toxicological experiments. Biometrics 34:69–76.

26. Nelson, C.J. and Holson, J.F. (1978). Statistical analysis of teratologic data: Prob-
    lems and advancements. J. Environ. Pathol. Toxicol. 2:187–199.

27. Williams, R. and Buschbom, R.L. (1982). Statistical analysis of litter experiments
    in teratology. Battelle PNL-4425. 15 pp.

28. Rai, K. and Van Ryzin, J. (1985). A dose-response model for teratological experi-
    ments involving quantal responses. Biometrics 41:1–9.

29. Bateman, A.T. (1977). The dominant lethal assay in the male mouse. In: Hand-
    book of Mutagenicity Test Procedures. Edited by B.J. Kilbey, M. Legator, W.
    Nichols, and C. Ramel. New York: Elsevier, pp. 325–334.

30. Mosteller, F. and Youtz, C. (1961). Tables of the Freeman-Tukey transformations
    for the binomial and Poisson distributions. Biometrika 48:433–440.

31. Aeschbacher, H.U., Vautaz, L., Sotek, J., and Stalder, R. (1977). Use of the beta
    binomial distribution in dominant-lethal testing for "weak mutagenic activity,"
    Part I. Mutat. Res. 44:369–390.

32. Vuataz, L. and Sotek, J. (1978). Use of the beta-binomial distribution in dominant-
    lethal testing for "weak mutagenic activity," Part 2. Mutat. Res. 52:211–230.

33. Dean, B.J. and Johnston, A. (1977). Dominant lethal assays in the male mice:
    evaluation of experimental design, statistical methods and the sensitivity of
    Charles River (CD1) mice. Mutat. Res. 42:269–278.

34. Bliss, C.I. (1965). Statistical relations in fertilizer inspection. Connecticut Agricul-
    tural Experiment Station, New Haven, CT. Bulletin, p. 674.

35. Kilbey, B.J., Legator, M., Nicholas, W., and Ramel, C. (1977). Handbook of Mu-
    tagenicity Test Procedures. New York: Elsevier, pp. 425–433.

36. Grafe, A. and Vollmar, J. (1977). Small numbers in mutagenicity tests. Arch.
    Toxicol. 38:27–34.

37. Vollmar, J. (1977). Statistical problems in mutagenicity tests. Arch. Toxicol. 38:
    13–25.

38. Katz, A.J. (1978). Design and analysis of experiments on mutagenicity. I. Minimal
    sample sizes. Mutat. Res. 50:301–30.

39. Katz, A.J. (1979). Design and analysis of experiments on mutagenicity. II. Assays
    involving micro-organisms. Mutat. Res. 64:61–77.

40. Weil, C.S. (1978). A critique of the collaborative cytogenetics study to measure
    and minimize interlaboratory variation. Mutat. Res. 50:285–291.

41. Kastenbaum, M.A. and Bowman, K.O. (1970). Tables for determining the statisti-
    cal significance of mutation frequencies. Mutat. Res. 5:61–77.

42. Ehrenberg, L. (1977). Aspects of statistical inference in testing genetic toxicity.

In: Handbook of Mutagenicity Test Procedures. Edited by B.J. Kilbey, M. Legator, W. Nichols, and C. Ramel. New York: Elsevier, pp. 419–459.

43. Bernstein, L., Kaldor, J, McCann, J., and Pike, M.C. (1982). An empirical approach to the statistical analysis of mutagenesis data from the Salmonella test. Mutat. Res. 97:267–281.

44. Gad, S.C. (1982). Statistical analysis of behavioral toxicology data and studies. Arch. Toxicol. (Suppl.) 5:256–266.

45. Tilson, H.A., Cabe, P.A., and Burne, T.A. (1980). Behavioral procedures for the assessment of neurotoxicity. In: Experimental and Clinical Neurotoxicology. Edited by P.S. Spencer and N.H. Schaumburg. Baltimore, Williams & Wilkins, pp. 758–766.

46. Irwin, S. (1968). Comprehensive observational assessment. In: Systematic, quantitative procedure for assessing the behavioral and physiologic state of the mouse. Psychopharmacologia 13:222–257.

47. Gad, S.C. (1982). A neuromuscular screen for use in industrial toxicology. J. Toxicol. Env. Health 9:691–704.

48. Annua, Z. (1972). The comparative effects of hypoxia and carbon monoxide hypoxia on behavior. In: Behavioral Toxicology. Edited by B. Weiss and V.G. Laties. New York: Plenum Press, pp. 105–127.

49. Norton, S. (1973). Amphetamine as a model for hyperactivity in the rat. Physiol. Behav. 11:181–186.

50. Burt, G.S. (1972). Use of behavioral techniques in the assessment of environmental contaminants. In: Behavioral Toxicology. Edited by B. Weiss and V.G. Laties. New York: Plenum Press, pp. 241–263.

51. Johnson, B.L., Anger, W.K., Setzer, J.V., and Xinytaras, C. (1972). The application of a computer controlled time discrimination performance to problems. In: Behavioral Toxicology. Edited by B. Weiss and V.G. Laties. New York: Plenum Press, pp. 129–53.

52. Miller, E.C. and Miller, J.A. (1981). Mechanisms of chemical carcinogenesis. Cancer 47:1055–1064.

53. Wilson, J.S. and Holland, L.M. (1982). The effect of application frequency on epidermal carcinogenesis assays. Toxicology 24:45–53.

54. Gehring, P.J. and Blau, G.E. (1977). Mechanisms of carcinogenicity: Dose response. J. Environ. Pathol. Toxicol. 1:163–179.

55. Haseman, J.K. and Hoel, D.G. (1979). Statistical design of toxicity assays: Role of genetic structure of test animal population. J. Toxicol. Environ. Health 5:89–101.

56. Portier, C.J. and Hoel, D.H. (1984). Design of animal carcinogenicity studies for goodness-of-fit of multistage models. Fund. Appl. Toxicol. 4:949–959.

57. Grasso, P. and Crampton, R.F. (1972). The value of the mouse in carcinogenicity testing. Fund. Cosmet. Toxicol. 10:418–426.

58. Wittenau, M.S. and Estes, P. (1983). The redundancy of mouse carcinogenicity bioassays. Fund. Appl. Toxicol. 3:631–639.

59. Ward, J.M., Griesemer, R.A., and Weisburger, E.K. (1979). The mouse liver tumor as an endpoint in carcinogenesis tests. Toxicol. Appl. Pharmacol. 51:389–397.

60. Page, N.P. (1977). Concepts of a bioassay program in environmental carcinogenesis. In: Environmental Cancer. Edited by H.F. Kraybill and M.A. Mehlman. New York: Hemisphere Publishing, pp. 87–171.

61. Nutrition Foundation. (1983). The Relevance of Mouse Liver Hepatoma to Human Carcinogenic Risk. Washington, DC: Nutrition Foundation.

62. Haseman, J.K. (1985). Issues in carcinogenicity testing: Dose selection. Fund. Appl. Toxicol. 5:66–78.

63. Dix, D. and Cohen, P. (1980). On the role of aging in cancer incidence. J. Theor. Biol. 83:163–173.

64. Salsburg, D. (1980). The effects of lifetime feeding studies on patterns of senile lesions in mice and rats. Drug. Chem. Tox. 3:1–33.

65. Ciminera, J.L. (1985). Some issues in the design, evaluation and interpretation of tumorigenicity studies in animals. Presented at the Symposium on Long-term Animal Carcinogenicity Studies: A Statistical Perspective, March 4–6, 1985, Bethesda, MD.

66. Robens, J.F., Joiner, J.J., and Schueler, R.L. (1982). Methods in testing for carcinogenesis. In: Principles and Methods of Toxicology. Edited by A.W. Hayes. New York: Raven Press, pp. 79–105.

67. Cameron, T.P., Hickman, R.L., Korneich, M.R., and Tarone, R.E. (1985). History, survival and growth patterns of B6C3F1 mice and F344 rats in the National Cancer Institute carcinogenesis testing program. Fund. Appl. Toxicol. 5:526–538.

68. Chu, K. (1977). Percent Spontaneous Primary Tumors in Untreated Species Used at NCI for Carcinogen Bioassays. NCI Clearing House.

69. Dempster, A.P., Selwyn, M.R., and Weeks, B.J. (1983). Combining historical and randomized controls for assessing trends in proportions. J. Am. Stat. Assoc. 78: 221–227.

70. Fears, T.R., Tarone, R.E., and Chu, K.C. (1977). False-positive and false-negative rates for carcinogenicity screens. Cancer Res. 27:1941–1945.

71. Fears, T.R. and Tarone, R.E. (1977). Response to "Use of Statistics When Examining Life Time Studies in Rodents to Detect Carcinogenicity," J. Tox. Environ. Health 3:629–632.

72. Gart, J.J., Chu, K.C., and Tarone, R.E. (1979). Statistical issues in interpretation of chronic bioassay tests for carcinogenicity, J. Natl. Cancer Inst. 62:957–974.

73. Tarone, R.E., Chu, K.C., and Ward, J.M. (1981). Variability in the rates of some common naturally occurring tumors in Fischer 344 rats and (C57BL/6NXC3H/ HEN)F[1] (B6C3F1) mice. J. Natl. Cancer Inst. 66:1175–1181.

74. Goodman, D.G., Ward, J.M., Squire, R.A., Chu, K.C., and Linhart, M.S. (1979). Neoplastic and nonneoplastic lesions in aging F344 rats. Toxicol. Appl. Pharmacol. 48:237–248.

75. Bratcher, T.L. (1977). Bayesian analysis of a dose-response experiment with serial sacrifices. J. Environ. Pathol. Toxicol. 1:287–292.

76. Dinse, G.E. (1985). Estimating tumor prevalence, lethality, and mortality. Presented at the Symposium on Long-term Animal Carcinogenicity Studies: A Statistical Perspective, March 4–6, 1985. Bethesda, MD.

77. Swenberg, J.A. (1985). The interpretation and use of data from long-term carcinogenesis studies in animals. CIIT Activities 5(6):1–6.

78. Solleveld, H.A., Haseman, J.K., and McConnel, E.E. (1984). Natural history of body weight gain, survival, and neoplasia in the F344 rat. J. Natl. Cancer Inst. 72: 929–940.

79. Feinstein, A.R. (1975). Clinical biostatistics XXII: Biologic dependency, hypothesis testing, unilateral probabilities, and other issues in scientific direction vs. Statistical duplexity. Clin. Pharmacol. Ther. 17:499–513.

80. Salsburg, D.S. (1977). Use of statistics when examining life time studies in rodents to detect carcinogenicity. J. Toxicol. Environ. Health 3:611–628.

81. Haseman, J.K. (1977). Response to use of statistics when examining life time studies in rodents to detect carcinogenicity. J. Toxicol. Environ. Health 3:633–636.

82. Wilks, S.S. (1962). Mathematical Statistics. New York: John Wiley, pp. 290–291.

83. McKnight, B. and Crowley, J. (1984). Tests for differences in tumor incidence based on animal carcinogenesis experiments. J. Am. Stat. Assoc. 79:639–648.

84. Meng, C. and Dempster, A.P. (1985). A Bayesian approach to the multiplicity problem for significance testing with binomial data. Presented at the Symposium on Long-term Animal Carcinogenicity Studies: A Statistical Perspective, March 4–6, 1985, Bethesda, MD.

85. Peto, R., Pike, M., Day, N., Gray, R., Lee, P., Parish, S., Peto, J., Richards, S., and Wahrendorf, J. (1980). Guidelines for Simple, Sensitive Significance Tests for Carcinogenic Effects in Long-Term Animal Experiments. In: IARC Monographs on the Evaluation of the Carcinogenic Risk of Chemicals to Humans, Supplement 2, Long-Term and Short-Term Screening Assays for Carcinogens: A Critical Appraisal. Lyon, International Agency for Research in Cancer, pp. 311–346.

86. Lijinsky, W., Reuber, M.D., and Riggs, C.W. (1981). Dose response studies of carcinogenesis in rats by nitrosodiethylamine. Cancer Res. 41:4997–5003.

87. Squire, R.A. (1981). Ranking animal carcinogens: A proposed regulatory approach. Science 214:877–880.

88. Bernstein, L., Gold, L.S., Ames, B.N., Pike, M.C., and Hoel, D.G. (1985). Some tautologous aspects of the comparison of carcinogenic potency in rats and mice. Fund. Appl. Toxicol. 5:79–86.

89. Gad, S.C. and Smith, A.C. (1984). Influence of heating rates on the toxicity of evolved combustion products: Results and a System for Research. J. Fire Sci. 1(6):465–479.

90. Bishop, Y., Fujii, K., Arnold, E., and Epstein, S.S. (1971). Censored distribution techniques in analysis of toxicological data. Experientia 27:1056–1059.

91. Farmer, J.H., Uhler, R.J., and Haley, T.J. (1977). An unbalanced experimental design for dose response studies. J. Environ. Pathol. Toxicol. 1:293–299.

92. Redman, C.E. (1981). Screening compounds for clinically active drugs. In: Statistics in the Pharmaceutical Industry. Edited by C.R. Buncher and J. Tsay. New York: Marcel Dekker, pp. 19–42.

93. Tukey, J.W. (1977). Exploratory Data Analysis. Reading, MA: Addison-Wesley Publishing Co.

94. Velleman, P.F. and Hoaglin, D.C. (1981). Applications, Basics and Computing of Exploratory Data Analysis. Boston, MA: Duxbury Press.

95. Hoaglin, D.C., Mosteller, F., and Tukey, J.W. (1983). Understanding Robust and Explanatory Data Analysis. New York: John Wiley.

96. Miller, R.G. (1966). Simultaneous Statistical Inference. New York: McGraw-Hill, pp. 6–10.
97. Tarone, R.E. (1975). Tests for trend in life tables analysis. Biometrika 62:679–682.
98. Armitage, P. (1955). Tests for linear trends in proportions and frequencies. Biomet. II:375–386.
99. Cochran, W.G. and Cox, G. M. (1975). Experimental Designs. New York: John Wiley.
100. Diamond, W.J. (1981). Practical Experimental Designs. Belmont, CA: Lifetime Learning Publications.
101. Federer, W.T. (1955). Experimental Design. New York: Macmillan.
102. Hicks, C.R. (1982). Fundamental Concepts in the Design of Experiments. New York: Holt, Rinehart and Winston.
103. Beckman, R.J. and Cook, R.D. (1983). Outliers, Technometrics 25:119–163.

14

Placing and Monitoring Testing at External Facilities

Shayne Cox Gad
Gad Consulting Services, Raleigh, North Carolina

I. INTRODUCTION

Companies needing to evaluate the toxicity of their materials (products, raw materials, intermediates, etc.) may not have the capability to perform the required testing. Alternatively, although the capability may exist, the company's laboratory schedule may not be able to accommodate a rush study. At some time, for various reasons, industry will need to contract studies to external facilities, whether they are commercial contract laboratories, university laboratories, or even a member company's laboratory as in the case of a consortium study. As with all contractual arrangements, thorough preparation is required in order to obtain the desired product or service, to avoid confusion and misunderstanding, and to produce a timely result. This chapter is a practical guide for sponsors who need to place their studies at external laboratories. The information provided is drawn from a number of readily available sources as well as from the author's experience gained from visiting numerous laboratories in this country and abroad.

II. DEFINING THE STUDY

A. Development of the Study Record

The objective of a study or any research is to evaluate theories and produce results. The written record of this work is called the study record and includes all records, documentation, and results of the research. Let us now consider the logical progression of research activities and the development of the study record.

B. Research Plan

The research project begins with developing the research plan, or simply thinking through what will be done. Whether the worker is performing independent research, grant work, or research in support of regulatory requirements, this plan should be written down. When written, the research plan becomes the protocol for the project and includes the hypothesis, the proposed methods, observations to be made, and the expected results. Researchers should pay special attention to the level of detail in this plan. For example, in certain research environments there are requirements for inclusion of particular details in the protocol and a specified format. Optional experimental methods may be included in the protocol or amended into it as needed, but (again) must be recorded. Even if a written protocol is not specifically required for your research project, it is useful to develop the habit of producing a protocol because it requires you and your colleagues to think clearly through the experimental design. It also provides guidance for the actual conduct of the work and promotes consistency in performance (Figure 1).

C. Standard Operating Procedures

Some of the procedures performed during the study are routine for the laboratory. Formalize the documentation of these routine procedures into written standard operating procedures (SOPs). SOPs are detailed descriptions of such things as equipment operation, methods for taking and recording data, and procedures for reagent receipt, storage, and preparation—the types of procedures that are common to all laboratory operations. Write SOPs in sufficient detail to promote consistency in performing the procedures. Having SOPs and insisting that they are followed provides the researcher with a measure of control over potential variables in the experiment.

D. Data Recording

The experiment begins. You perform a procedure, write down what you did, and record the observed results. The level of detail of this written record should

| Research Plan or Protocol |
| Standard Operation Procedures (SOPs) |
| Recording Observations -- Data Generation |
| Evaluation of Data |
| Report of Data, Results and Conclusion |

Figure 1   Progression of a research project.

enable someone else with equivalent technical training to perform your experiment exactly as you did. Why? *Reproducibility*. That experimental results must be reproducible is a basic rule of science. It is the process through which scientific conclusions and discoveries are confirmed. Reproducibility is promoted by the specific data-recording requirements for data that are submitted to FDA, EPA, and other government agencies. Reproducibility is required in research performed to support a patent request.

For now, I wish to introduce you to the concept of "if you didn't write it down you didn't do it." You, the researcher, have the burden of proof in regulated research, in protection of patent rights, and in defense of your work in professional circles. The issue is *completeness* of your records. The study record must be a complete record of all data and procedures performed. If you didn't write it down, you didn't do it. In the experimental record, there are some accepted shortcuts. Here some of the hard preparatory work pays off. In your written record, you may include references to previously described methods and SOPs, state that they were followed exactly, or describe deviations from them. And efficient ways of collecting data may be developed to encourage the complete recording of all required data. Later in this chapter, methods for recording procedures and observations will be discussed in detail.

The accuracy of recorded data is another important consideration because any observed result, if not recorded immediately, may not be recorded accurately. Don't lose data because of some rationalization about time, money, or your ability to remember what happened. All data should be recorded directly into a notebook or onto a worksheet at the time of the observation. Also, transcribed data— data copied by hand or entered by a person into a computer—often is subject to errors. If data are copied to a table or a spreadsheet, the entered data should be checked against the original data to ensure accuracy.

E. Analysis of the Data

When the laboratory work is done, the researcher's analysis of the data begins. Observed data are entered into formulas, calculations are made, and statistical analysis is performed. All these manipulations must be carefully recorded, for from these data the conclusions will be drawn. The manipulations of the data are the link between the original observation and the conclusions. Consistency between the data and the result is controlled by monitoring all transcription, manipulation, and correlations of the data in generation of the final manuscript.

F. Reporting of Results and Conclusions

Finally, the manuscript or draft final report is submitted for peer review, to the publisher, or to the client. It will receive critical review before publication. The final version will then be published and again will receive critical review by your peers or some skeptical governmental or public audience. In all cases, it will be essential to be able to justify the data. The methods, initial data, the calculations and statistical analysis, and the conclusions must be defensible, meaning complete, accurate, internally consistent, and repeatable to withstand scientific criticism.

G. Types of Data

Earlier, I mentioned different elements of the study record: research plan or protocol, observations, calculations and statistical output, and conclusions. For ease of explanation, the terminology from the EPA's Good Laboratory Practice (GLP) regulations—protocol, raw data, statistical analysis, and final report—will be used to describe the components of the study record.

From the GLPs, the protocol is a written document that is approved by the study director (person responsible for the technical conduct of the study) and sponsoring organization. The protocol is the research plan, the approved grant proposal, the project plan in a management sense. It clearly indicates the objectives of the research project and describes all methods for the conduct of the work. It includes a complete description of the test system, the text article, the experimental design, the data to be collected, the type and frequency of tests, and planned statistical analysis.

The protocol will be strictly followed during research. "What," you say, "no experimental license, no free expression of scientific inquiry?" Of course there is, as long as the changes in procedures or methods are documented. If the work you are doing is governed by strict contractual or regulatory guidelines, you may not be able to express much creativity, but remember, the objective, in this case, is to provide consistent reliable comparisons for regulatory purposes. Even the GLPs make provisions to amend the protocol and document deviations from it. During all research, except perhaps during the most routine analysis, there may be changes in experimental methods and procedures, rethinking of design, decisions to analyze data in new or different ways, or unexpected occurrences that cause mistakes to be made. An important concept to apply here is that these variances from the plan must be documented.

1. Raw Data

"Raw data" is the term used to describe the most basic element of experimental observations. It is important to understand fully the concept of raw data. There are unique standards for recording raw data that do not apply to other types of data. These will be discussed later in the chapter. For now, let us look at what constitutes raw data. In the FDA and EPA GLPs,

> ... raw data means any laboratory worksheets, records, memoranda, notes or exact copies thereof that are the result of original observation and activi-

ties of the study and are necessary for the reconstruction and evaluation of the report of that study.

All terms must be taken in the most literal sense and must be interpreted collectively to apply this definition to the data generated during an experiment. There are two key phrases: "are the result of original observations and activities of the study," and "are necessary for the reconstruction and evaluation of the report of that study." Raw data include visual observations, measurements, output of instrumental measurements, and any activity that describes or has an impact on the observations. Anything that is produced or observed during the study that is necessary to reconstruct (know what happened) and evaluate (analyze or, for regulatory purposes, assess the quality of) the reported results and conclusions is raw data. This definition of raw data has been carefully designed to encourage the development of data that are defensible.

Included in the scope of raw data may be data that result from calculations that allow the data to be analyzed, for example, the results of gas chromatography where the raw data are defined as the curve that was fitted by the instrument software from individual points. The individual points on the curve are essentially meaningless by themselves, but the curve provides the needed basic information. The area under the curve, which is used to calculate the concentration, is an interpretation of the curve based on decisions made about the position of the baseline and the height of the peak. This is not "raw data" since it is not the original observation and may be calculated later and, practically, may be recalculated. For the researcher to completely understand the results, the curve with the baseline, the area under the curve, and the calculations are required and recorded, but only the curve itself is "raw data." The distinction is that the curve is the original observation and must be recorded promptly.

2. Other Types of Data

Other types of data that are not thought of as raw data may be included here. For example, correspondence, memoranda, and notes that may include information that is necessary to reconstruct and evaluate the reported results and conclusions. While these are not records of original experimental observations, they do represent documentation of the activities of the study. They often contain approvals for method changes by study management or sponsoring organizations, instructions to laboratory staff for performing procedures, or ideas recorded during the work. Here are some examples of raw data that are generated during a toxicology study:

Test article receipt documents	Equipment use and calibration
Animal receipt documents	Equipment maintenance
Records of quarantine	Transfer of sample custody
Dose formulation records	Sample randomization

Sample collection records   Animal or sample identification
Dosing records   Assignment to study
Animal observations   Necropsy records
Blood collections and analysis   Analytical results
Euthanasia records   Histology records
Pathologist's findings

For government-regulated research, all records that are documentation of the study conduct are treated as raw data. From the perspective of the scientific historian, the original notes, correspondence, and observations tell the story of the life and thought processes of the scientist being studied. From the mundane to the extreme, these records are important.

3. Computerized Data Collection

Special attention must be dedicated to computer-generated raw data. Automated laboratory instrumentation has come into widespread use. In hand-recorded data, the record of the original observation is raw data. But what is considered raw data in computerized systems? In this case, raw data are the first recorded occurrence of the original observation that is human readable. This definition treats computer-generated data as hand-recorded data. It documents the "original observations and activities of the study and is necessary for reconstruction and evaluation of the report of that study" (FDA, 1987; EPA, 1989). However, we must pay special attention to this type of data. The validity of hand-recorded data is based on the reliability of the observer and on well-developed and validated standards of measurement. For computer-generated data, the observer is a computerized data collection system, and the measurements are controlled by a computer program. These are complex systems that may constrain complex flaws. Just as the principles behind measurements with a standard thermometer were validated centuries ago and are verified with each thermometer produced today, so must modern computerized instrumentation be validated and its operation verified. This causes a real dilemma for many scientists who are proficient in biomedical research but not in computer science. Because of the size and scope of this issue, I can only call your attention to the problem and refer you to the literature for additional guidance. I will discuss special issues in recording raw data, including computer-generated raw data, later in this chapter.

4. Statistical Data

Statistical data result from descriptive processes, summarization of raw data, and statistical analysis. Simply put, these data are not raw data but represent manipulation of the data. However, during this analysis process, a number of situations may affect the raw data and the final conclusions. For example, certain data may be rejected because they are shown to be experimentally flawed, an outlier believed to have resulted from an error, or not plausible. I will leave it to other texts to discuss the criteria by which decisions like these are made. Here, I will say only that any manipulating of raw data is itself raw data. For example, a series of organ weights is analyzed. One of the weights is clearly out of the usual range for the species, and no necropsy observations indicated the organ was of unusual size. The preserved tissues are checked, and the organ appears to be the same size as others in the group. The statistician then may decide to remove that organ weight from the set of weights. This record of this action is raw data. The analysis is not, because it can be replicated. It is a fine distinction that matters only in the context of recording requirements for raw data since both the analyses and record of the data change are required to reconstruct the report.

Statistical analysis is part of the study record. Documentation of the methods of statistical analysis, statistical parameters, and calculations is important. Critical evaluation of conclusions often involves discussion of the statistical methods employed. Complete documentation and reporting of these methods, calculations, and results allows for constructive, useful critical review.

5. Results and Conclusions

The study record includes the results and conclusions made from review of the data produced during the scientific investigation. The data are summarized in abstracts, presented at meetings, published in journals, and, with all previously discussed types of data, are reported to government agencies. However, it is the scientist's interpretation of the data that communicates the significance of the experimentation. In all scientific forums, scientists present their interpretation of the data as results and conclusions. Results and conclusions are separate concepts. This is an important distinction not only because it is the required format for journal articles and reports, but because it is important to separate them in one's understanding. Results are a literal, objective description of the observations made during the study, a statement of the facts. Conclusions, on the other hand, represent the analysis of the significance of these observations. They state the researcher's interpretation of the results. If results are presented clearly and objectively, they can be analyzed by any knowledgeable scientist, thereby testing the conclusions drawn. This is the process by which the body of scientific knowledge is refined and perfected.

For regulatory purposes, the results presented to the regulatory agencies (FDA or EPA) must be complete. Included in the reports submitted are tables of raw data, all factors that affect the data, and summaries of the data. In journals, the results section usually is a discussion with tabular or graphical presentations of what the researcher considers relevant data to support the conclusions. Conclusions presented in either case interpret the data, discuss the significance of the data, and describe the rationale for reaching the stated conclusions. In both cases, the results are reviewed and the conclusions analyzed by scientific peers. The function of the peer review process is to question and dispute or confirm the information gained from the experiment. Objective reporting of results and clear discussion of conclusions are required to successfully communicate the scientist's perspective to the scientific community.

H. Development of Study Data

Above we have discussed the types of data that make up the study record. The following discussion addresses: quality characteristics for the study record, requirements for recording raw data, and methods for fulfilling the quality characteristics and raw data requirements by using various record keeping formats.

1. Quality Characteristics

There are four characteristics the study record must have: completeness, consistency, accuracy, and reconstructability. Completeness means the information is totally there, self-explanatory, and whole. Consistency in the study record means that there is "reasonable agreement between different records containing the same information (DeWoskin, 1995)." *Accuracy* is agreement between what is observed and what is recorded. The final characteristic is *reconstructability*. Can the data record guide the researcher or someone else through the events of the study? These characteristics are goals to meet in developing the study record and will be used in Chapter 4 to evaluate the quality of these records. They must be built into the study from the beginning. Considerable attention to these goals will be required as the study progresses to produce a complete, consistent, accurate, and reconstructable study record.

2. Recording Raw Data

Raw data may be recorded by hand in laboratory notebooks and worksheets or entered into a computerized data management system. Today, more and more data are computer generated and recorded as paper outputs or are electronically written to magnetic media, microfiche, or other storage media. This section will discuss how raw data in both forms are recorded.

a. General Requirements for Raw Data Recording. Raw data must be recorded properly to preserve and protect them. The following is excerpted from the FDA GLPs:

> All data generated during the conduct of a study, except those that are generated by automated data collection systems, shall be recorded directly, promptly, and legibly in ink. All data entries shall be dated on the date of entry and signed or initialed by the person entering the data. [Emphasis added.]

All introductory laboratory courses teach these basic techniques for recording raw data. Even though these standards are published as regulations for only certain types of research, I believe that there is never an instance when these minimum standards do not apply. There may be researchers who "get by" writing in pencil or scribbling data on paper towels, but they often suffer the consequences of their carelessness when data are lost or their records are unintelligible. Too, if these same researchers attempt to patent a product or method, or to submit their data to regulatory agencies, their data are not acceptable. In fact, if the regulatory data are incomplete or obscured in some way, the scientist involved may be subject to civil or criminal penalties. Chapter 1 discusses many related instances. It is always best to establish good habits early, especially for scientific record keeping.

For hand-recorded data, "directly, promptly, and legibly in ink" means to write it down in the notebook or on the worksheet as soon as you see it, so it is readable and in ink. The purpose is to preserve accurately the observation. Notes on paper towels or scratch paper may be lost. Prompt recording promotes accuracy. Legibility assures that later you will understand what is written. This does not necessarily mean neat. If you are recording directly and promptly, neatness may have to be forgone. It does, however, mean readable and understandable.

The use of ink preserves the record from being erased or smeared. It is commonly understood that the ink should be indelible, meaning it cannot be erased and can withstand water or solvent spills. Some organizations may require a specific color of ink to be used, usually black or dark blue. This requirement originated because black ink was the most permanent and could be photocopied. Without such requirements, the ink used in the lab should be tested to see how it withstands common spills and to see if it copies on the standard photocopier. Some colors of ink (such as blue) and some thin line pens may not copy completely. There are a number of reasons why data may need to be copied, and that they are copied exactly becomes a very practical issue. Inks should not fade with time. Some analytical instruments produce printed data on heat sensitive paper. To preserve these data, laboratories will make photocopies. See Chapter 3 for a more detailed discussion.

The requirements to sign and date the data record flow from practical and legal considerations; it is often useful to know who made and recorded the observation. In many research labs, graduate assistants or research technicians are responsible for recording the raw data. If questions arise later, the individual responsible may be sought out and asked to clarify an entry. For GLP studies, the signature represents a legal declaration meaning the data recorded here are correct and complete. The data must be dated at the time of entry. This attests to the date of the recording of the observation and the progression in time of the study conduct. Some lab work is time dependent and in this case the time and date must be recorded. There is no instance when data or signatures may be backdated or dated in advance.

Signatures and dates are crucial when documenting discovery and in supporting a patent claim. For studies conducted under the GLPs, the signature and date are legal requirements for the reconstruction of the study conduct. Falsely reported data may then result in civil or criminal penalties to the person recording the data and his/her management for making false and misleading statements.

In some types of research, additional signatures and dates may be required. Data used to support a patent and data generated during the manufacture of drugs or medical devices must be signed and dated by an additional person—a witness or reviewer thus corroborating the stated information.

b. Error Correction in Data Recording.   What happens when there is a mistake in recording data or an addition that must be made to the data at a later time? The FDA and EPA GLPs address this.

> Any changes to entries shall be made so as not to obscure the original entry,
> shall indicate the reason for such change, and shall be dated and signed at
> the time of the change.

All changes to the written record of data must be explained and signed and dated. Doing so provides justification for the correction and again provides testimony as to who made the change and when it was done. To make corrections to the data, the original entry is not obscured. A single line is drawn through the entry. Then, the reason for the change is recorded with the date the change is made and the initials of the person making the change. A code may be established and documented to explain common reasons for making corrections to data. A simple example may be a circled letter designation like:

S = sentence error
E = entry error
X = calculation error

This is easy to remember and use. Any other types of errors or corrections must be described in sufficient detail to justify the change.

Raw data may be generated by computer programs and stored on paper or magnetic media. Most laboratories approach this kind of data as they would hand-generated data. The GLPs state:

> In automated data collection systems, the individual responsible for direct
> data input shall be identified at the time of the data input. Any changes to
> automated data entries shall be made so as not to obscure the original entry,
> shall indicate the reason for the change, shall be dated and the responsible
> individual shall be identified.

For automated data collection systems, there are standards similar to hand-recorded data (FDA, 1987; EPA, 1989). All raw data should be recorded promptly and directly. Whereas the requirement for hand-collected data is that records be written legibly and in ink, permanence and security of computer-collected data is the requirement. However, there may be special considerations for how signatures and dates are recorded. Physical signature of data may not be possible when using electronic storage media. Electronic signature or the recording of the operator's name and the date are often a function provided in the software and are recorded with the data. When the data are printed in a paper copy, this information should be included. Some labs have adopted a policy requiring that the paper printout must be signed and dated by the operator. Some instruments produce a continuous printout or strip chart. In this case, the chart should be signed by the operator and dated on the date the data are retrieved. If the data are maintained on electronic media, the operator's name and date must be recorded on that medium.

Because computer security and risk of corruption or destruction of computer-stored data are a major concern, many laboratories maintain computer-generated data in paper printouts because the means for maintaining the data are traditional and easy to implement. As long as the printout represents a verified exact copy of the original raw data, it is acceptable and often even preferable to designate the printout as the raw data.

When changes to the electronically stored raw data are made, the original observation must be maintained. This is accomplished in several ways. Newer software packages allow these changes to be made and properly documented. To do this, the original entry is not erased, and there is a way of recording the reason for the change along with the electronic signature of the person authorized to make the change and the date of the change. However, some data collection systems still do not have this capability. If this is the case, the original printout may be retained with the new printout that contains the change, the reason for the change, the signature of the person authorized to make the change, and the date of the change. Some computer programs allow for footnotes and addenda to be added to the record. These additions to the record, if made later, should also include a handwritten or computer-recorded signature and date.

I. Formats for Recording Data

We will now begin to construct the study record. The format for the study record may be determined by the preferences of the researcher. Some researchers prefer to maintain all study records in laboratory notebooks. In private industry, research and development labs may be required to use lab notebooks because of potential patent documentation requirements. Many chemists have become accustomed to the use of lab notebooks. However, handwritten data may be maintained in laboratory notebooks, on worksheets and forms, or one may use computer-generated printouts and electronic storage media. The remainder of this section discusses guidelines for recording data using all formats.

A. Laboratory Notebooks

Laboratory notebooks are usually bound books with ruled or gridded pages that are used to record the events of an experiment. Organizations may order specially prepared notebooks that are uniquely numbered on the cover and spine. They have consecutively numbered pages, and some come with additional carbonless pages to make exact copies of the entries. Organizations may have procedures in place for issuing notebooks to individuals for use on specific research projects. After the glassware is cleaned, all that remains of a study is the notebook; its value is the cost of repeating all the work. Therefore, SOPs should be written to control the assignment, use, and location of these records.

The pages may be designed to contain formats for recording information. In the header, there may be space for the title and date. In the footer, space may be allocated for signature and date of the recorder, and signature and date of a reviewer or witness. When beginning to use a laboratory notebook, set aside the first few pages for the table of contents. Then a few pages may be held in reserve for notes, explanations, and definitions that are generally applicable to the contents.

The remainder of this section discusses the rules for recording data in the notebook. First, each page should contain a descriptive title of the experiment that includes the study designation and the experimental procedure to be performed. The date the procedure was performed is also recorded. Often a complete description of the experiment will require several pages. After the first page, subsequent pages should indicate, at least, an abbreviated title and cross reference to the page from which it was continued.

The body of the experimental record should include the following sections:

- Purpose of the experiment
- Materials needed, including instruments, equipment and reagents
- Reagent and sample preparation
- Methods and procedures
- Results

The *purpose* may be recorded in a few sentences. The *materials section* is a list of all the things you need for the experiment—the instruments to be used, the equipment, and chemicals. When recording the analytical instruments, include the make, model number, and serial number; the location of the instrument; and all settings and conditions for the use of the instrument. The description of the chemical used should include a complete description including name, manufacturer, lot or serial number, and concentration. *Reagent and solution* preparation must be described in detail with a record of all weights and measurements. It is extremely important that sample identification and sample preparation be com-

pletely documented. The *methods and procedures* section is a step-by-step description of the conduct of the experiment.

If SOPs are in place that describe any of the above information in sufficient detail, they may be referenced. Then information recorded in the notebook
is all weights and measurements and any information that is unique to this
experiment or not specifically discussed in the SOP. SOPs often are written for
more general applications. An SOP may state that the pH will be adjusted using
a buffer or acid as required. The notebook should indicate what was used to
adjust the pH and how much was used. An SOP may describe the formulation
of a compound in a certain amount when the experiment requires a different
amount. The mixing procedures may be cross-referenced, but it will be necessary to describe in detail the conversion of the SOP quantities and any changes
in procedure resulting from the change in quantity.

The *experimental results* section must contain all observations and any
information relating to those results. It should include any deviation from established methods, from SOPs, and from the protocol. Failed experiments must be
reported even though the procedure was successfully repeated. Justification for
repeating the procedure and a description of what may have gone wrong is
recorded. All calculations should include a description of the formula used.

Remember, all entries are recorded directly and promptly into the notebook at the time of the experiment and are recorded legibly in ink. Some information may be entered at the beginning of the day, some entered at the end of
the day, but all weights, measurements, and recorded observations must be entered into the notebook directly and promptly.

For a complete record, it is often necessary to insert such information as
shipping receipts, photographs, and printouts into the lab notebook. In doing so,
do not obscure any writing on the page. The following are tips for inserting
information into the notebook.

> Glue the loose paper in place. (I do not recommend using tape because
> tape over time loses its holding power.)
>
> Inserts may be signed, dated, and cross-referenced to the notebook and
> page so that they can be replaced if they become loose.
>
> Make verified copies of data that are too large for the page, shrinking it
> to fit the notebook page.
>
> If by some chance data are accidentally recorded on a paper towel or other
> handy scrap of paper, these should be signed, dated, and glued into the
> notebook. It is not wise to transcribe data, introducing the possibility of
> error and the distasteful possibility of data tampering.

The bottom of each page must be signed by the person entering the data
and dated at the time of entry. The date at the top of the page—the date of the
activity—in most cases will be the same as the date at the bottom of the page.

A few exceptions are appropriate. The most legitimate exception to this rule occurs when a page is reserved for the results printout. The printout may not be available to insert until the following day. The printout should indicate the date when the data were first recorded, which should in turn match the top date. The date at the bottom of the page indicates when it was glued into the notebook.

Occasionally, a scientist will forget to sign and date the page. When this happens, there is no quick fix. The only remedy is to add a notation: "This page was not signed and dated on _____, the time of entry," Then, sign and date this statement.

This discussion has been detailed because the signature and dates on the pages are very important. They are legally required for regulatory purposes. Data used to support patents and some data produced under the FDA current Good Manufacturing Practices (cGMPs) require the signature and date of a witness or reviewer. For example, the cGMPs require that all materials weighed or measured in the preparation of the drug be witnessed, signed, and dated. Patent applications are supported by witnessed experimental records. Some institutions may require supervisory review of notebook entries with accompanying signature and date. This is to say that you should be aware of the uses your data and any requirements for this additional signature.

An important concept to remember is that bound, consecutively page-numbered notebooks are used to demonstrate the progression of the research and to document the dates of data entry and when the work was performed. To prevent the corruption of this record, unused and partially used pages may be marked out so no additions may be made. A suggested method is to draw a "Z" through the page or portion of the page not used. At the end of the project, there may be used notebook pages. These may be "Z'd," or the last page may indicate that this is the end of the experimental record and no additional pages will be used.

B. Forms and Worksheets

While many analytical laboratories continue to use lab notebooks, other labs may use forms and worksheets to record their data. The purpose is to provide an efficient format for recording data that are routine in nature. Gad and Taulbee (1996) contains guidelines for the preparation of forms. The basic concept is that forms and worksheets should be designed to be easy to use and to provide a complete record of all relevant data. They may be used in combination with lab notebooks as described above or kept in files or loose-leaf binders. Explanatory footnotes may be preprinted or added to explain abbreviations and/or the meaning of symbols. Additional space for comments and notes should be incorporated into the format.

Computer spreadsheets and word processing make forms and worksheets easy to design and produce.

The advantages of using forms and worksheets include the following:

They may be formatted to prompt for all necessary information.
They are easy to follow and complete.
Header information, title, study designation, sample numbers, etc. may be filled out in advance, thus saving time.
Cross-references to applicable SOPs may be included on the worksheet.
They help to standardize data collection.

Disadvantages of using forms and worksheets include the following:

They must be carefully designed and should be pretested for completeness and ease of use.
They may encourage a tendency not to write more information than is specifically requested. Space should be allotted for notes and comments.
Forms and worksheets that are designed for general use may contain blanks that are not necessary for the current study. Yet all blanks must be completed. If not needed, "n/a" (not applicable) should be written in the blank or a dash put in the space.
Forms and worksheets create a routine that can become mindless; take care to properly complete the form.
Example 1: Necropsy forms often contain a complete list of tissues to be checked by the technician. When only some tissues are inspected or retrieved, it may be too easy to check inappropriate boxes.
Example 2: Animal behavioral observation forms contain blanks to record all observations. The observer must record something in the blank space. A check or "OK" may be used for normal behavior if defined on the form or in an SOP. A problem occurs when these designations are used automatically without proper attention to observing and recording the behavior of each animal, particularly when most animals are behaving normally.

In discussing the above disadvantages, I'm not trying to discourage the use of worksheets. However, institute procedures and practices assure that forms and worksheets are properly used.

As in any data record, the signature and the date of entry are recorded at the time of the entry and represent and attest to the accuracy of the information. Any changes to the data or additional notes made after completion of the form or worksheet are made as previously described. Any unused lines on the form or worksheet should be crossed or "Z'd" out. If the signature of a witness or reviewer is required, there should be a line allocated for this purpose.

Forms and worksheets can be a useful and practical way to record and preserve raw data—if you pay attention to the rules of data recording.

1. Automated Data Collection Systems

This is the hottest and most difficult topic of this book. Application of data collection rules to computer systems has been the topic of seminars, books, journal articles, government policy committees, and regulatory interpretation. As an example of the policy difficulties, the FDA has spent the last several years trying to reach consensus on a policy for electronic signatures. This policy may be published in the Federal Register by the time this book is published.

Two major issues surround automated data collection systems: validation of the system and verification of the system's proper operation.

Validation asks whether the system is properly designed and tested so that it performs as it should to measure and record data accurately, completely, and consistently. In other words, are all the bugs worked out so that the system does not lose, change, or misrepresent the data you wish to obtain? I recall, from many years ago, a software program for recording animal weights. If a particular animal had died on study and was not weighed at a weigh session, a "0" was entered for the weight. It was discovered that the software would automatically reject the 0 and record in its place the next animal's weight. This was totally unacceptable. The system was inadequately designed to properly handle commonly occurring data collection exceptions.

The second issue is the verification of the system's operation. Have you tested and proven that the data produced and recorded by the system are accurate, complete, and consistent, meeting all the date quality standards discussed under handwritten data?

Validation and verification are processes that involve hardware and software development, and acceptance testing, laboratory installation procedures and testing, computer security, and special record keeping procedures, to name a few. There are numerous publications on this topic. If you are working in a research area subject to FDA or EPA, I suggest starting with the following: the FDA Computerized Data Systems for Nonclinical Safety Assessment—Current Concepts and Quality Assurance, known as the Red Apple Book; the FDA Technical Reference on Software Development Activities; and the EPA's Good Automated Laboratory Practices (GALPs).

The following sections will discuss the defining of raw data for automated data collection systems, what should be recorded in the raw data, electronic signatures, and report formats and spreadsheets.

2. Computer-Generated Raw Data

It was my privilege to work with the author of the EPA's GALPs and a team of experts during the later stages of finalization of the GALPs. One of the most difficult tasks was deciding how to define raw data for laboratory information management systems (LIMS). Hours and days were spent on this issue alone. Here is the definition that was ultimately used:

LIMS Raw Data are original observations recorded by the LIMS that are needed to verify, calculate, or derive data that are or may be reported. LIMS raw data storage media are the media to which LIMS Raw Data are first recorded.

From these discussions, I have developed a broader-based alternative definition of computer-generated raw data. For automated data collection systems, "raw data" mean the first record on the system of original observations that are human readable and that are needed to verify, calculate, or derive data that are or may be reported. The GALP definition was designed to fit the scope of the GALPs and applicability to EPA's LIMS.

The real issue is how to apply the definition. Hand-recorded raw data are easy to define. What you see is what you write. Automated systems are much more complex. Analytical instruments may perform several functions—a transmitted light beam is measured, is converted into an electronic signal, this signal is transmitted to a computer, the software on the computer converts the signal to a machine-readable representation, this representation is translated into a value, this value is recorded into a report format that performs calculations and a summary of the input data, and the report is sent to an electronic file or to a printer.

The question is when do we have raw data? It is when an understandable value is first recorded. If the human-readable value is saved to a file prior to formatting, this is raw data. If the first recording of the data is in the report format, this is raw data. Some labs have declared the signal from the instrument to the computer to be raw data, but it is then very difficult to use the signal as a means for verification of the report of the data. This example represents only one situation of the possible variations in instrumentation. Each automated data collection system must be assessed to determine when the output is "raw data."

Why is the definition of raw data for computer applications so important? One obvious reason is to meet regulatory requirements. Behind these requirements are the same data quality characteristics that apply to hand-recorded data: accuracy, completeness, consistency, and reconstructability; as mentioned earlier, transcription of data can cause errors. Each time data are translated or reformatted by a software application, there is a potential for the data to be corrupted or lost. When the data are recorded and human readable before these operations, these "raw data" can then be used to verify any subsequent iterations.

Here is the type of information that should be included in the automated raw data record:

- The instrument used to collect the data
- The person operating the instrument
- The date (and time) of the operation

- All conditions or settings for the instrument
- The person entering the data (if different from the operator)
- The date and time entered or reported
- The study title or code
- Cross-reference to a notebook or worksheet
- The measurements with associated sample identification
- All system-calculated results

If the system does not allow the input of any of the above information, it may be recorded by hand on the printout or on cross-referenced notebook pages or worksheets.

Automated raw data may be scored in soft copy (e.g., magnetic media) or in hard copy (e.g., paper printout, microfiche, microfilm). However soft copy storage of raw data presents a unique set of problems that are often avoided by printing it in hard copy. Many labs choose to print out raw data, because it assures the data are available and unchanged.

Many software applications for instruments record the data in a worksheet format. The same rules as those for hand-generated worksheets should apply for automated formats. However, some raw data may not yet be formatted when they are first recorded. In this case, a key to format of the raw data must accompany the data.

Why do we not designate the final formatted report as raw data in all cases? Remember, in the definition of raw data, the phrase, "first recorded occurrence of the original observation." This is important because the data should have undergone as little manipulation and transfer as possible over different software applications. This prevents corruption and loss and allows the raw data to be used to verify additional operations performed on it. Also, why not designate the signal read by the instrument or transmitted by the instrument as the raw data? Simply because it cannot be understood by humans and therefore is not useful to verify the results and conclusions. Testing should be performed on this signal, however, to validate the operation of the instrument and its communication functions.

3. Electronic Signatures

Electronic signatures are the recorded identity of the individual entering data and are input through on-log procedures—presumed to be secure. One of the issues regarding electronic signatures is the validity of a computer-entered signature because it is not traceable by handwriting analysis to the signer, and presumably anyone could type in a name. One of the charges against Craven Labs was that the lab changed the clock on the computer to make it appear that samples were analyzed on an earlier date. Currently the FDA is accepting electronically recorded names or initials as signatures although the policy has not been made official at this writing.

Until a policy statement is made, two criteria may be used to justify the use of electronic signatures. All individuals who operate the instruments or associated software must be aware of the meaning and importance of the entry of their name (or unique personal code) and the computerized date stamp. That is what constitutes a legal signature. Second, the electronic signature is best justified when access to the system is strictly controlled. Controlled access usually involves some sort of password or user identification system that must be activated before an authorized person may perform an operation. Some automated systems have levels of access that may control different operations by allowing only certain individuals to perform certain tasks. Access levels may include read only, data entry, data change authorization, and system level entry or change. When these controls are in place, the system may automatically record the persons name into the file based on the password entered. Some systems use voice recognition or fingerprint recognition. This discussion only begins to touch on the complexities of issues related to computer security.

4. Spreadsheets

Spreadsheet use to the modern lab is what the invention of the printing press was to publication. Although spreadsheets make recording, processing, and reporting data easy and quick, some special considerations are important to the use of these powerful programs. Whether data are keyed into spreadsheets or electronically transferred to them from existing data files, the entry of the data must be checked to assure the data record is complete and correct. Commonly, mistakes occur in calculations and formulas, in designating data fields, and in performing inappropriate operations on the data. Because of the versatility of spreadsheets, take special care in validating the spreadsheet. When you perform calculations, check the spreadsheet formulas and be sure that the arithmetic formula is defined on the spreadsheet. The way the program rounds numbers and reports significant digits is important to the calculation of results and the reporting of the data. When you try to recalculate or evaluate the processes performed by the spreadsheet program, be sure to define all functions.

J. Reporting the Data

This final section suggests ways to generate data tables and figures for the final report or manuscript. Here are some guidelines:

- The title of the table or figure should be descriptive of the data.
- Column and row headings should be understandable, avoiding undefined abbreviations.

- Units of measure should be included in the column headings or axes of charts.
- For individual data, all missing values must be footnoted and explained.
- All calculations used to derive the data should be defined and, when the calculation is complex or nonstandard, given in a footnote.
- Statistical summaries or analyses should be clearly defined including the type of process performed. Statistically significant values may be identified with a unique symbol that is footnoted.
- All but the most common abbreviations should be defined.
- Continuing pages should contain at least a descriptive portion of the title and indicate "continued."
- The data should be easy to read and be uncluttered.
- Charts should contain a legend of any symbols or colors used, and the labels of the axes should be descriptive and easily understood.
- The text of the report should include references to the tables or figures when the data is presented.
- The text of the report should exactly match the data in the tables or figures. Any generalization, summarization, or significant rounding should be designated as such in the text.

1. Distinguishing Essential from Negotiable Study Elements

An important step is to determine which parts of the study must be included. It is desirable to maximize the amount of information to be obtained, while also considering time, number of animals, and use of other resources. It may not be realistic to try to accomplish all the objectives that can be stated during the early stages of study design. This distinction of essential and negotiable study elements is a critical step that will enable the study sponsor to select a suitable laboratory as well as to negotiate the specific components of the study.

2. Designating the Study Monitor

Another early aspect to consider in external placement concerns personnel, specifically, the study's director. It is not uncommon that the employee who functions as a study monitor on behalf of the sponsor is called the "study director." This is a difficult concept to grasp, since the responsibilities of the study director imply being intimately involved with and overseeing the day-to-day activities of the study and can therefore be discharged only by an employee of the laboratory contracted to perform the study. Regardless of what the on-site study director is called, the sponsor needs to provide sufficient authority to allow important decisions to be made without prolonged discussions on the telephone, or worse yet, emergency site visits by the sponsor.

For complex or long-term studies, the laboratory should provide an alternate study director to ensure both continuing internal oversight as well as a contact for the sponsor if the primary study director is unavailable.

Having defined the work to be done, ranked the elements of the study as essential or negotiable, and selected a study monitor from within the sponsor's organization, a laboratory must be found that can do the necessary work.

III. IDENTIFYING COMPETENT LABORATORIES

The first step is to obtain a list of laboratories engaged in contract toxicological testing. Although other opportunities exist, for example, university laboratories, laboratories of a consortium member's company, and, in some cases, government laboratories, the vast majority of externally placed studies involve the contracting party (the "sponsor") placing a study in a "contract laboratory." Therefore, this situation will be used as the model for the rest of this chapter. The CRO (contract research organization) industry has become truly international. Laboratories can be selected based on a range of factors, as we shall see.

A. Published Lists

Several lists of contract laboratories exist (1,2) but the most current available should be utilized. These lists are updated from time to time, since the contract laboratory industry is dynamic and the capabilities of an individual laboratory change over time. Also, it must be recognized that the contract research industry has become an international one.

These compendia serve as a basic information for finding laboratories capable of performing a specific study. More detailed information can be obtained by writing to the individual laboratories.

B. Information Available at Meetings

A great deal of information about contract laboratories can be obtained at scientific and industry meetings. Brochures explaining the types of study the laboratory is capable of conducting, and descriptions of facilities, staff, and price ranges for standard studies are displayed at such meetings by many contract laboratories. Laboratory sales representatives attend these meetings frequently to discuss specific study needs with prospective sponsors.

A second source of information available at meetings is the experience of professional colleagues, who may be able to provide advice on where to have certain kinds of studies conducted, having had similar work done previously. Of particular importance is information about where their work was done, its perceived quality, and how to avoid mistakes or misunderstandings in dealing with a particular contract laboratory.

This latter source of information needs to be taken with the proverbial "grain of salt." Almost anyone who has contracted studies has had some problems; those who have contracted many studies have had at least one study with a major problem; and probably every good contract laboratory has been inappropriately criticized for poor work at least once. A distorted evaluation is altogether possible if, for example, uncontrollable events (power shutdowns, shipping strikes, etc.) might have affected study results and the sponsor's overall impression of the laboratory.

For highly specialized studies, choices in laboratories may be very limited. Phytotoxicity testing, for example, is still a relative rarity. Reproductive and developmental toxicity evaluations, although offered by many laboratories, are tricky, demanding and performed well by only a few. Genetic toxicity testing is in similar circumstances. An even more complex situation involves tests requiring several kinds of relatively unusual expertise or equipment. A developmental toxicity study requiring inhalation exposure, for example, may limit laboratory selection to only a few facilities. Contract laboratories will usually provide information on the availability of services in specialized areas, if they are unable to provide such testing themselves.

C. "Freedom of Information" Requests

Copies of reports of laboratory inspections conducted by federal agencies are available under the Freedom of Information (FOI) Act. These reports generally follow the format of the laboratory inspection guidance given to Food and Drug Administration (FDA) or Environmental Protection Agency (EPA) investigators, and provide a great deal of information of varying utility. Since they are purged of references to proprietary activities, trademarks, specific sponsorship of studies, and much other information, it is sometimes difficult to understand the intent of the report. In addition, they present the opinions of individual investigators concerning isolated activities and events and therefore may not be truly representative of a laboratory's usual practices.

On the other hand, since the laboratory inspection procedures used by a particular agency are consistent, the FOI reports permit some comparison among laboratories. This information, coupled with other inputs, is therefore valuable and should not be ignored.

FOI requests should be made to the specific agency that conducted the inspection. Since FDA's inspection program has been in existence for some time, they are the logical first agency to call in seeking inspection reports on particular laboratories.

Having developed a list of laboratories able to do the study in question, the most critical part of getting a good job done is in selecting the laboratory at which to place the study. The rest of this chapter will be spent reviewing selection criteria in detail.

IV. LABORATORY SELECTION CRITERIA

A number of criteria serve as guides in selecting a laboratory. Particular studies might require additional selection criteria. What follows is a minimal list of aspects of the laboratory that will have to be evaluated. Presumably there exists in the sponsor's company a standard against which all individual laboratories will be evaluated. Certain aspects may be more important that others, but all laboratories will have to meet this minimum standard.

A. Physical Resources

An essential element in producing a good product is the availability of sufficient physical resources at a contract laboratory to ensure the uninterrupted progress of the study from beginning to end. The complex array of personnel, materials, and financial resources for successful progression of the study begins with consideration of the physical resources of the laboratory. Elements to consider include: space, fuel and water supply, power (with backup), heating, ventilation and air conditioning, equipment needed to run the study, etc. Financial resources should be sufficient to run the study from the creation of the draft protocol to the production of the final report and beyond, if revisions are needed. Laboratory failures do occur so the prudent study sponsor must select carefully. One of the aims is to obtain a stable laboratory that will still be in business beyond study termination.

Laboratory animal care facilities may be accredited by the American Association for Accreditation of Laboratory Animal Care (AAALAC). This is a voluntary body that accredits laboratories based on its own standards as supplemented and reinforced by those of other organization. Accreditation is based on elements of several major activities, programs or capabilities of the individual laboratory, such as veterinary resources, physical resources, administrative matters and the presence and activity of an animal care and use (animal welfare) committee. AAALAC accreditation is frequently the only objective symbol of the general compliance of the laboratory with standards of good practice in animal use and care, veterinary, physical plant, and administrative areas. Although no guarantee that the laboratory does good testing, AAALAC accreditation represents a worthwhile first step toward excellence.

B. Personnel and Technical Expertise

Does the laboratory employ personnel trained in the needed specialty? What about ancillary expertise (pathology, statistics)? If not directly employed by the laboratory, are trained specialists available on a consulting basis? For example, if the major emphasis of a study is the determination of the inhalation toxicity of a test agent, but a minor component concerns teratogenic effects, the selected laboratory will require skilled, experienced inhalation toxicologists on staff. The laboratory does not necessarily have to employ its own teratologists, however, since coverage of these evaluations may reasonably be done by consultants in this specialty.

A skilled, competent staff will be necessary to the conduct of the work. Prospective laboratories' personnel environments should be scrutinized for signs of frequent or rapid staff turnover, difficulties in recruiting and retaining new staff and lack of career pathways for staff currently employed.

Many laboratories rely on independent organization certification to demonstrate a standard of achievement and competence on the part of their technical and scientific staff. For example, both the American Board of Toxicology and the American College of Toxicology have certification programs for toxicologists. Likewise, the American Association of Laboratory Animal Sciences (AALAS) has three stages for certification of laboratory animal technical staff. Other specialties have similar certification programs based on some combination of experience and achievement demonstrated by written and practical testing.

Hand in hand with personnel availability is the selection criterion of technical expertise. Many different specialties are brought to bear on a particular study. The more complex the study, the greater the difficulty in finding a contract laboratory with all the necessary expertise.

In attempting to evaluate the qualifications of contract laboratory staff, organizational charts and curricula vitae should be obtained. These documents are standard tools that are used by contract laboratories as marketing aids. Both FDA's and EPA's GLP regulations (5–8) require laboratories to maintain documentation of the training, experience and job descriptions of personnel. This is usually done by means of compilations of curricula vitae.

Another important point in evaluating staff capabilities is the number of people employed by the laboratory. The proposed study staff should be sufficient to perform all the work required. Attention should be directed to the laboratory's overall workload relative to available staff.

C. Standard Operating Procedures

A large portion of the initial visit to prospective contract laboratories can usefully be spent in reviewing standard operating procedures (SOPs). These should be written for all routinely performed activities.

GLPs require that SOPs be established in the following general areas: animal room preparation, animal care, test and control substance management, test system (animal) observations, laboratory tests, management of on-study dead or moribund animals, necropsy, specimen collection and identification, histopathology, data management, equipment maintenance and calibration, identification of animals, and quality assurance. Although not specifically required by GLP regulations, the laboratory should also have SOPs for archiving activities. In each of these areas, numerous individual SOPs should be in place. For example, in the area of histopathology, SOPs should be available to describe tissue selection, preparation, processing, staining, and coverslipping; slide labeling and packaging; and storage and retention of wet tissues, blocks, and slides. Similarly, SOPs should be available for maintenance and calibration of all equipment and instrumentation requiring these activities.

The laboratory's SOPs should be clear, understandable, and sufficiently detailed to permit a technically experienced person to perform them. They should be up to date, and the method for keeping them current should be described. They should have the sanction of facility management, usually provided by the signature of the person responsible for the pertinent laboratory activity.

To be effective, SOPs should be available to those who need them. For example, animal care SOPs should be available to vivarium workers, as analytical and clinical chemistry SOPs should be available in these laboratories. Compendia of SOPs, which sit pristinely on shelves in offices, may not reflect what is actually occurring in the laboratories and animal quarters. Likewise, SOPs that have not been reviewed or revised in several years should be viewed with suspicion. Improvement in actual methods occur frequently, and should be reflected in the written procedures.

If the laboratory has contracts with other laboratories, SOPs should be available for the secondary laboratories as well. Both the SOPs and these contracts should be reviewed in the same way.

D. Cost

A key factor in laboratory selection for most sponsors is the cost of the study. This single element can largely affect the quality of a study. "Caveat emptor" applies equally to the toxicologist as to the home consumer. Many of the negotiable elements of a carefully defined study will not be performed in a similarly titled study at a different laboratory for a lower cost. Conversely, some of the extras offered for a higher priced study should not be included for extra cost if they are neither necessary nor desirable. The objective in considering the cost of a study is to select the laboratory that offers all the essential study elements at the lowest cost consistent with good quality. Good quality in turn relies on the other criteria previously discussed. When a laboratory is found that can perform all desired elements of the study, does high quality work, and offers a low price for the study than its competitors, this is probably the laboratory to choose to perform the study.

In discussing costs, the sponsor should attempt to determine whether the laboratory will be able to add elements to the study if this appears desirable as the study progresses. The laboratory should have the capability to expand the original study design. Sponsor and laboratory should attempt to foresee how the cost of such additions would be determined.

E. Ease of Monitoring

A consideration in selection of contract laboratories is the sponsor's ease of monitoring the study, which is largely a function of distance between the sponsor and the laboratory. In some studies, this may be a major consideration; in others, not worthy of mention. If the study is complex and requires frequent oversight, a trade-off may need to be made between the best laboratory relative to the previously mentioned selection criteria and monitoring ease.

On the other hand, sponsors do not plan complex studies unless they anticipate substantial product safety evaluation concerns, and therefore, considerable potential profit. If this is the case, the relatively small additional sum spent in the increased cost of frequent or distant monitoring may be minuscule in the eyes of those selecting the laboratory.

F. Reputation

The reputation held by particular contract laboratories is clearly a guide in laboratory selection. Although not an absolutely reliable indicator of the worth of a contract laboratory's efforts, by and large laboratories earn their reputations over time. Beware of laboratories that submit low bids for studies and either cut corners to stay within their quoted cost or include add-ons at the sponsor's expense through the course of the study. Study additions can significantly increase the actual cost if the contract requires the sponsor to pay for them.

Other laboratories try to foresee likely additional aspects of the study, which may increase the quoted cost but yield a much better product. Producing the study at the price quoted is only one part of a contract laboratory's reputation. Quality, professional qualifications of staff, activity in scientific professional societies, accreditation, regulatory interface, and many other issues are important as well.

G. Protection of Client Confidentiality

Most contract laboratories expend considerable effort in trying to maintain confidentiality on behalf of their clients. In walking through a laboratory, clients should not be able to see proprietary labels on test material containers, or cage labels that state company names. A contract laboratory concerned about client confidentiality will be careful not to allow visible evidence to be seen by other potential clients. Confidentiality is usually of significant concern and should be discussed with laboratory management. The laboratory's master schedule should maintain client confidentiality as well.

H. Prior Experience

Prior experience with specific contract laboratories simplifies the task of selecting a laboratory. Establishing a continuing relationship with one or several laboratories in the case of routine testing provides an opportunity to fine tune study protocols. This will be discussed in greater detail in Section X below.

I. Scheduling

Undoubtedly, starting the study as soon as possible is important. The ability of the laboratory to begin the study soon may well determine where the study is performed. Most of the larger contract houses can start all but very large studies within 4–6 weeks. Some studies may be able to be initiated on even shorter notice. Certainly for shorter studies, less complicated protocols are needed and generally less lead time is required to begin the study. The converse is equally true, so if the study is large, long-term, or complicated, a fairly long time before study initiation will be needed to get the details of the study worked out with the laboratory. As a result, a laboratory that is willing to start a lengthy or complex study before the details have been settled should generally be avoided.

J. Special Capabilities

As the science of toxicology and the questions society, regulatory agencies, and companies seek to answer become more complex, hard-to-find technical skills and equipment become more in demand. Such special capabilities are frequently found in smaller or university laboratories where procedures, documentation, and adherence to regulatory standards may not be as rigorous as either one's own corporation or larger contract laboratories. One may even have to help investigators develop protocols, standard operating procedures, and record keeping systems.

   Evaluating technical competency for specialized procedures is obviously difficult, as one is usually dependent on others to initially identify such specialists and they may have to also get outside help to evaluate the appropriateness and quality of the results. A not uncommon case of special capabilities is when human testing (such as repeat insult patch testing (RIOT) must be performed). Here one must understand the special regulatory, legal, and ethical strictures on work with human subjects, and generally deal with an ORB (institutional review board) which must review, approve, and oversee any such human studies from the perspective of subject protection and ethics.

K. Reliability

When considering contract laboratories for selection, reliability is hard to objectively evaluate in advance and very frequently underrated in importance. In this author's opinion, being able to depend on a laboratory to precisely execute protocols, meet agreed upon deadlines, and inform the study monitor of any study-related issues or problems in a timely manner is as important as any other aspect of a contract laboratory.

V. SITE VISITS OF PROSPECTIVE CONTRACT LABORATORIES

In scheduling site visits with contract laboratories, the objectives should be clearly defined. Meeting those people who will be directing and contributing importantly to the study provides an opportunity to evaluate their understanding of the nature of the potential questions or problems. Ancillary contributors (pathologists, statisticians) should be interviewed carefully as well, since their contributions can be fundamentally significant to the quality and outcome of the study.

The facilities should be inspected for appropriate size, construction, spacing and design. GLP regulations as promulgated under the Food, Drug, and Cosmetic Act, the Toxic Substances Control Act, or the Federal Insecticide, Fungicide, and Rodenticide Act provide guidance as to the general facility, equipment and operational requirements of laboratories.

Storage areas for extra racks and cages, feed and bedding, and so forth are frequently inadequate in laboratories, and these facilities should be inspected and evaluated.

Both EPA and FDA provide their field investigators who conduct laboratory inspections for compliance with GLPs with "Compliance Guidance Manuals" (9,10). These are comprehensive documents using a checklist approach to inspect a laboratory for adherence to all the elements of GLP regulations. They can be obtained from the agencies, and can be used as guidance for study sponsors in evaluating prospective laboratories. An advantage of using this approach is that the sponsor will not omit an important element in inspecting a prospective laboratory. However, the sponsor should not get so bogged down in reviewing checklist items that actual observation of the laboratory is abbreviated.

VI. THE CONTRACT

A sound contract is an important element in placing a study at an external laboratory. If negotiated carefully, it will pay off in improved communication at all stages of the study and should reduce the possibility of misunderstanding.

A. General Terms

General terms of the contract should address such aspects as timeliness, proprietary rights, confidentiality, adherence to regulatory requirements (in the research effort and in the laboratory's practices in waste disposal, workers' protection, and safety, etc.), type and frequency of reports, communications between parties, conditions under which the study may be aborted and restarted, timing and method of payment, and the like. Such a contract " . . . should be negotiated by a team of lawyers and scientists who have a thorough understanding of the problems to be investigated, including both the scientific issues and the potential business implications . . . Armed with this . . . understanding, the lawyers can then proceed to develop a contract that is appropriate to the situation. . . . Much of the language will be routine or "boiler plate," the type commonly found in agreements of various kinds (11)."

The contract should specify who does what in the furtherance of the study. For example, if analysis is necessary, the sponsor may wish to retain the responsibility to analyze the test material as a means of keeping its identify confidential. The derivative concern about documentation of the analysis is presumably also retained by the sponsor, but the contract should be clear on the responsibilities of both parties.

When discussing study personnel, various degrees of authority are vested in contract laboratory study staff by the sponsor. The study contract should define as clearly as possible the degree of authority vested in the contract laboratory staff and at what point the sponsor would be consulted for a decision when unforeseen situations arise. In general terms, then, the contract should define the rights and responsibilities of both parties.

The contract should also address financial matters, such as the cost of the study and the method and timing of payment. Certain unanticipated activities not directly related to the study may increase the cost to the laboratory; the contract should attempt to anticipate these events and establish reasonable incremental costs to the sponsor to deal with them. For example, study-specific inspections by agencies authorized to review a study (FDA or EPA) may add to the cost to the laboratory for additional staff time to accompany inspectors, copy documents, and otherwise field the inspections. If the sponsor wishes to be present at such inspections, additional direct costs will be incurred. Although many readers would view this simply as part of the laboratory's cost of doing business, the contract should anticipate how each party is expected to respond financially if the inspection becomes very time consuming or onerous.

Likewise, poststudy activities and responsibilities should be defined in the contract. Who will archive tissue and other samples and specimens? For how long? If statistical analysis is to be performed, of what does it consist? Who decides? If further analysis appears desirable after evaluation of the data, will the sponsor incur extra costs?

B. The Study Protocol

The most important part of site visits to laboratories will be the discussion of the study and establishment of the protocol. Extensive prior experience of the sponsor in conducting the contemplated study is helpful although many elements may still have to be negotiated. If the sponsor has limited experience, the importance of the protocol increases, since it contains the specific language of the contract, which governs the conduct of the study, between sponsor and laboratory.

To write a protocol with little flexibility may preclude the study director's judgment and may actually compromise the quality of the study. Each party must feel comfortable that the study protocol provides sufficient detail to specify what is to be done, when, and under what conditions. However, the protocol must not be so rigid that the study director is hampered in responding to changing conditions and events as they occur. Since unanticipated events almost always occur, the objective is to provide a protocol that permits the study to be conducted as closely as possible to the original study plan and to answer all the important study questions.

C. Other Terms

1. Authorship

The question of authorship of publications resulting from the proposed study should be covered in the contract. Not all work is worthy of publication nor do contract laboratory staff often get an opportunity to author papers. But if the laboratory has contributed significantly to the work, and a publication is contemplated, help in writing portions of the manuscript should be solicited from members of the study staff, for which coauthorship is a deserved award.

2. Reports

The contract should specify the nature and frequency of reports that the laboratory will make to the sponsor. For example, a short-term study (two weeks or less) may require only telephone confirmation of study start, status of the animals at the halfway point, confirmation of termination, and the usual draft and final report (see Section VIII below).

For a longer study, the sponsor may request written status reports at regular intervals. In the case of chronic studies the sponsor may wish to have formal interim reports prepared by the laboratory. The contract should clearly specify the expectations of both parties concerning reports.

3. Inspections by the Sponsor

Most contract laboratories do not like the thought of unscheduled site visits by study sponsors, for understandable reasons. Under ordinary circumstances, a large amount of staff time is spent escorting visitors through the laboratory. Unscheduled visitors therefore place an additional burden on already stretched resources.

Nevertheless, the right to monitor study progress at any reasonable time should be explicitly affirmed in the contract. This right, although perhaps never exercised by the sponsor, should not be relinquished. As a practical matter, unscheduled monitoring visits almost never occur, since the sponsor must recognize that the study staff may be unavailable at the time of the visit, making the trip a wasted one.

Likewise, the contract should explicitly grant the sponsor access to the laboratory's quality assurance (QA) inspection reports of the study. These reports are ordinarily not available to government investigators, and some contract laboratories prefer not to share them. However, a sponsor should ensure that the contract grants access to the QA reports.

VII. IN-PROGRESS MONITORING

As mentioned before, "Compliance Inspection Manuals" which are used by inspectors in their agency laboratory inspection programs are available from EPA and FDA. The manuals offer a systematic and thorough means of reviewing elements of GLP compliance and can serve as guides regarding standardized aspects of laboratories and studies.

Having carefully evaluated the laboratory before contracting the study, the focus of in-progress monitoring changes from general to specific. Whereas initially the animal feed room was inspected for cleanliness, good housekeeping and a rodent-free environment, now the feed should be inspected to see if it is segregated and logged out at suitable times and in amounts proportional to specific study needs.

Likewise, much of the other in-progress monitoring will focus on previously gathered data. In performing this review, notes should be made and a list of items prepared for discussion with facility and study management at an exit conference. In-progress monitoring should also include review of vivarium conditions (temperature, humidity) and animal husbandry records. Although not the most fascinating data to review, the conditions under which the animals are housed can seriously influence the study's outcome, both from a biological point of view as well as relative to the study's acceptability by regulatory agencies.

All data pertaining to clinical observations, blood and clinical chemistry analyses, weights, and feed consumption statistics should be reviewed. Not all of these may apply and some studies will have more complex in-life observations than described here.

The laboratory's QA inspection reports should be reviewed at this time. These reports should demonstrate that QA inspections are being carried out according to QA SOPs. The content of the reports should be reviewed as a means of ensuring adherence to the study protocol and the laboratory's standard operating procedures.

The purpose of an in-progress monitoring visit is to review all the data collected since the last visit in order to ascertain that the study is progressing smoothly and without major problems. The data reviewed should be generally consistent with the sponsor's understanding of study progress derived from previous inspections or reports from the laboratory. If the study appears to be changing in unsuspected ways, the sponsor and the study director should discuss the possibility of alteration of the study design: adding more or different observations, adjusting doses or dosing schedules, inserting an unplanned interim sacrifice. The study protocol is designed to accommodate all reasonably foreseeable events in the study. However, some unexpected events may occur, particularly in a complex study. The monitoring visit allows the opportunity for the sponsor and study director to adapt the study design, if necessary.

If the study design has been changed since the sponsor's last visit, protocol amendments that clearly state the change, its scope, and the reason for the change should be found in the study documentation. If the amendment was authorized by the sponsor during a previous communication, this should be referred to.

The facility's SOPs should again be checked to ensure that relevant procedures are being followed (from cage washing to histological preparation). Most procedures generate some kind of documentation that should be reviewed.

When all available documentation has been reviewed, the sponsor will have a list of items for discussion with study management. Sponsor and study director, together with other pertinent laboratory staff (pathologist, animal care supervisor, quality assurance staff) should meet to resolve these issues.

Generally, the questions can be resolved fairly easily. Sometimes things beyond the control of facility management go wrong, such as temperature or humidity excursions in the animal room. If not numerous, extreme, or cyclical, such excursions are probably of little importance. However, if patterns of consistent difficulties are detected, facility management should be required to improve its control over environmental conditions. This may involve moving the study to a different room for completion or providing the facility maintenance staff with additional instruction and training. Whatever the cause, the desired effect is correction of excessive environmental variation.

Since the laboratory was selected on the basis of a thorough preplacement evaluation, now is the time to ask laboratory management to bring its expertise to bear on whatever problems have arisen in the study.

What if major problems arise that warrant aborting the study and restarting it? A frank discussion with study management (and your own management!) should be the starting point. If the sponsor's judgment to abort comes as the result of in-progress monitoring without any previous idea that such serious deficiencies existed, the sponsor's and the study director's views are apparently far apart. If, on the other hand, the sponsor's inspection is the result of the laboratory's report of problems, then the decision to restart the study may be easily and jointly reached.

The contract confers rights and responsibilities on both parties, and should therefore be consulted if study abortion and restart is contemplated. If the contract clearly permits the sponsor to judge at what point a major problem or a series of minor problems constitutes grounds for aborting the study, the decision to do so should be made expeditiously. Having learned from the experience, sponsor and study director should proceed to restart the study with as little delay as possible.

VIII. THE STUDY REPORT

Most sponsors will want interim reports for major long-term studies. Since the interim reports will form the basis for the final report, they should be read carefully and critically. If misinformation, confidential business information, or poor interpretations of data are presented in the interim reports, they should be corrected at once. Interim reports may also be sought by regulators, so they should be held to the same exacting standards of thoroughness and accuracy as the final report.

The final report should be presented to the sponsor in draft form. Several years ago, this was a contested notion, with many contract laboratories objecting to draft reports. However, the current practice is for contract laboratories to submit drafts for review by sponsors.

The study report should contain all essential elements, generally those covered in GLP regulations. Additional data may be included, for example, information about the test material, interpretative statements by sponsor scientists, references to other studies of the test material, or a host of other information. The sponsor should make such inclusions after receipt of the final report from the testing laboratory. For example, if previous study data are relevant, they might usefully be included in a discussion section.

A great deal of information required by GLPs deals with methodological details that should have been carefully described in the protocol. Appending the protocol to the study report can serve to fulfill these requirements. This saves time and retains the study plan as a historical document. If the protocol was not strictly followed or if it required extensive alterations, a new description of methodology may be preferable.

The final study report should contain in the signatures of all required parties: study director, QA inspector, pathologist, statistician, clinical chemist, and any other scientists who contributed significantly to the work. It is also a good idea to list the study personnel. Such personnel can change frequently, and personnel lists may not be available if there is a need to identify study staff at some time in the future.

The study report should take no more than two drafts in order for sponsor and contract laboratory to agree on a final version. If the sponsor feels that additional drafts are needed, this should be resolved quickly with the contract laboratory. Frequently there is a reluctance to rewrite reports many times, and the zeal with which the perfect report is pursued will diminish with time. A qualified scientist is entitled to disagree with conclusions reached by another in an addendum to the report, although agreeing on the conclusions drawn from the study at the outset is a less awkward means of presenting conclusions in the report. Nevertheless it is not uncommon for a sponsor's final report to include statements of opinion differing from those offered by the contract laboratory.

IX. ANCILLARY SERVICES

The contract laboratory may not have available all the services needed to complete the study. For example, some laboratories use contract pathology services. Archiving of raw data, specimens, samples, and interim and final reports may be done at a commercial archiving operation rather than at the laboratory. Prior to contracting, decisions need to be made concerning services that the laboratory itself will not provide. In the case where pathology is subcontracted, the sponsor should be able to specify a pathology laboratory other than the one the contract laboratory usually uses. Likewise, if the contractor does not have its own archive space, the samples could be retained by the sponsor, rather than having them sent to a commercial archivist or warehouse. These issues should be anticipated and addressed in the contract. If circumstances require a change in the planned provider of these services, sponsor and contract laboratory should keep each other informed.

X. ONGOING CONTRACTS

Having successfully completed a contracted study, an ongoing contract with this laboratory for future work should be considered if the sponsor anticipates a continuing need. Establishing a continuing relationship with one or several laboratories enables the sponsor to familiarize the laboratory thoroughly with the sponsor's study methods as well as with any idiosyncrasies of reporting or data gathering. In addition, economies can usually be effected on the basis of volume and/or regular scheduling. Also, establishing an ongoing relationship with a contract laboratory may improve the turnaround time of "rush" studies, since the laboratory might be able to accommodate such a request more easily for an established than for a onetime customer.

Many sponsors have found it useful to establish such ongoing testing contracts with several laboratories simultaneously. Some advantages of this approach are: expanding the possibilities of squeezing in a "rush" study, extending the standardization of test methodology from the sponsor's perspective, and increasing the objectivity of the overall testing program by bringing several observation and judgment capabilities to bear on similar methods and data sets.

A fourth advantage is that failures of individual contract laboratories will not leave a sponsor's testing program grounded so that the process of finding a suitable laboratory must be begun again.

Some specialties are well practiced in only a handful of laboratories. In these cases, the objective must be to get a good study done each time. More and closer overseeing may be required in such cases than if several laboratories are adept and ready to do the required testing.

REFERENCES AND NOTES

1. Jackson, F.M. (1985). International Directory of Contract Laboratories. New York: Marcel Dekker, Inc.
2. Texas Research Institute. (1986). Directory of Toxicology Testing Institutions. Houston, Texas Research Institute.
3. Freudenthal, R.I. (1997). Directory of Toxicology Laboratories Offering Contract Service, Aribel Books: West Palm Beach, Florida.
4. To obtain inspection reports from FDA, call their FOI office at (301) 443-6310. For EPA reports, the telephone number of their FOI office is (202) 382-4048. The respective addresses are: Department of Health and Human Services, 200 Independence Ave., SW, Washington, DC 20201; FOI Office (A-101), USEPA, 401 M Street, NW, Washington, DC 20460.
5. Code of Federal Regulations, Title 21, Part 58 (Food, Drug and Cosmetic Act).
6. Code of Federal Regulations, Title 40, Part 792 (Toxic Substances Control Act).
7. Code of Federal Regulations, Title 40, Part 160 (Federal Insecticide, Fungicide and Rodenticide Act).
8. Principles of Good Laboratory Practice have been enumerated by the Organization for Economic Cooperation and Development. Other countries (Japan, United Kingdom, The Netherlands) and the European Economic Community have also proposed or finalized GLP guidelines and requirements.
9. Good Laboratory Practice Compliance Inspections of Laboratories Conducting Health Effects Studies, Inspectors' Manual. (1985). Washington, DC: USEPA, Office of Pesticides and Toxic Substances, Office of Compliance Monitoring.
10. Compliance Program Guidance Manual, Chapter 48, Human drugs and biologics: Bioresearch monitoring. (1984). Washington, DC: Food and Drug Administration.
11. MacDougall, I.C. (1981). Some contractual and legal aspects of toxicological research. In Scientific Considerations in Monitoring and Evaluating Toxicological Research. Edited by E.J. Gralla. Washington, DC: Hemisphere Publishing Corporation, p. 193.

ADDITIONAL READING

Drug Information Association, Computerized Data Systems for Non-Clinical Safety Assessments: Current Concepts and Quality Assurance, Maple Glen, PA, September 1988.

Food and Drug Administration's Good Laboratory Practice Regulations original proposal, Fed. Reg. 41:51206–51230 (1976). This details the reasons for the proposed GLPs and includes a catalog of deficiencies found in laboratories which performed studies in support of FDA regulated products.

Gad, S.C. and Taulbee, S.M. (1996). Handbook of Data Recording, Maintenance, and Management for the Biomedical Sciences, CRC Press: Boca Raton, Florida.

Guide for the Care and Use of Laboratory Animals, DHEW Publ. No. (NIH) 78-23, revised 1985.

Guide to the Care and Use of Laboratory Animals, National Institutes of Health, Bethesda, MD, 1985–1986.

Gralla, E.J. (ed.). (1981). Scientific Considerations in Monitoring and Evaluating Toxicological Research. Washington, DC: Hemisphere Publishing Corporation.

Hoover, B.K., Baldwin, J.K., Uelner, A.F., Whitmire, C.E., Davies, C.L., and Bristol, D.W. (eds.). (1986). Managing Conduct and Data Quality of Toxicology Studies. Princeton: Princeton Scientific Publishing Co., Inc.

Institutional Animal Care and Use Committee Guidebook, NIH Pub. No. 92-3415. U.S. Department of Health and Human Services, pp. E33–37.

Jackson, E.M. (1984). How to choose a contract laboratory: Utilizing a laboratory clearance procedure. J. Toxicol. Cut. Ocular Toxicol. 3:83–92.

James, J.W. (1982). Good Laboratory Practice, ChemTech, 1962–1965, March 1982.

Paget, G.E. (1977). Quality Control in Toxicology. Baltimore, MD: University Park Press.

Paget, G.E. (1979). Good Laboratory Practice. Baltimore, MD: University Park Press.

Paget, G.E. and Thompson, R. (eds.). (1979). Standard Operating Procedures in Toxicology. Baltimore, MD: University Park Press.

Paget, G.E. and Thompson, R. (eds.). (1979). Standard Operating Procedures in Pathology. Baltimore, MD: University Park Press.

Sheehan, D.C. and Hrapchak, B.B. (1980). Theory and Practice of Histotechnology, C.V. Mosby: St. Louis.

Taulbee, S.M. and DeWoskin, R.S. (1993). Taulbee's Pocket Companion: U.S. FDA and DPA GLPs in Parallel, Interpharm Press: Buffalo Grove, IL.

U.S. EPA. FIFRA Good Laboratory Practice Standards, Final Rule, Fed. Reg. 54:34052–34074, August 17, 1989.

U.S. EPA. TSCA Good Laboratory Practice Regulations, Final Rule, Fed. Reg. 52: 48933–48946, August 17, 1989.

U.S. FDA. Good Laboratory Practice Regulations, Final Rule, Fed. Reg. 52:33768–33782, September 4, 1987.

U.S. EPA. (1986). Pr Notice 86-5, U.S. EPA, Washington, D.C.

U.S. EPA. Clean Air Act, Fed. Reg. 59, No. 122, June 27, 1994.

U.S. EPA. (1995). Good Automated Laboratory Practices, Office of Information Resources, Research Triangle Park, NC, August.

U.S. EPA. Enforcement Response Policy for the Federal Insecticide, Fungicide, and Rodenticide Good Laboratory Practices (GLP) Pesticide Enforcement Branch, Office of Compliance Monitoring, Office of Pesticides and Toxic Substances, U.S. EPA.

U.S. FDA. Good Clinical Practices: CFR, Title 21, Part 50, 56, 312, April 1, 1993.

U.S. FDA. Guide for Detecting Fraud in Bioresearch Monitoring Inspections, Office of Regulatory Affairs, U.S. FDA, April 1993.

U.S. FDA. Current Good Manufacturing Practices for Finished Pharmaceuticals, CFR, Title 21, Part 211.

U.S. FDA. Current Good Manufacturing Practices for Medical Devices, General, CFR, Title 21, Part 820.

U.S. FDA. Electronic Signatures; Electronic Records; Proposed Rule, Fed. Reg. 59: 13200, August 31, 1994.

15
Hazard and Risk Assessment

Shayne Cox Gad
Gad Consulting Services, Raleigh, North Carolina

I. INTRODUCTION

The problem of understanding the hazards and risks associated with unintentional or coincidental exposures to chemicals is a complex one with multiple uncertainties built into it. All too many members of our society either fail or refuse to understand this fundamental fact. Worse, all too many, including scientists, do not understand that toxicity (the potential of a chemical to cause health effects under a laboratory situation) and hazard (the practical consideration of whether such an adverse health effect could occur in real life) though related, are neither the same nor directly correlated. In toxicology, risk assessment is the act of trying to evaluate and express (as quantitatively as possible) the hazard associated with toxic materials.

It must also be understood that contrary to popular belief, risk assessment in toxicology is not limited to carcinogenesis. Rather, it may be applied to any of the possible deferred catastrophic toxicological consequences of exposure to chemicals or agents where the effect is separated in time from the putative cause, and where the effect (say a birth defect) is also something that occurs at some low baseline incidence level in the human population, that is, those things (such as carcinogenesis, developmental toxicity, or reproductive impairment) that threaten life (either existing or prospective) at a time distant to the actual exposure to the chemical or agent. Because the consequences of these toxic events are extreme, yet are distanced from the actual cause by time (unlike overexposure to an acutely lethal agent, such as carbon monoxide), society is willing to accept only some low-level risk while maintaining the benefits of use of the agent. Though the most familiar (and, to date, best developed) case is that of carcinogenesis, much of what is presented here for risk assessment may also be applied to the other endpoints of concern.

Finally it is necessary to understand that risk management is a multistep process, and each step in the process is subject to varying degrees of uncertainty and calls for sound scientific judgment. There are at least five major steps in the process. These steps and the uncertainties and judgments associated with them are:

1. *Physical, Chemical, and Manufacturing/Use Characteristics.* The starting point for understanding the exposure and subsequent risk associated with a chemical entity and its use is to understand both the innate characteristics of the entity (physical state, vapor pressure, boiling point, flash point, etc.) and its life cycle (how it is made, transported, used, and disposed of). These are crucial points to truly characterize and understand a material—the toxicity and hazard cannot be separated from these factors (particularly how it is used). These factors are also the easiest to characterize with minimal uncertainty.

2. *Data Qualification.* Evaluating available pertinent data sets (such as human epidemiology studies and animals bioassays) for adequacy and suitability, and then selecting which will be used to build a risk assessment model is the initial first step. Data sets of adequate (but not first rate) quality can be used later to "check" the model for accuracy.

3. *Low Dose Extrapolation.* Using the selected mathematical model, the dose–response information from one or more animal studies is extrapolated from the levels at which we have dose–response data to the dose/exposure region of concern (that is, where there is likely human exposure, generally four or more orders of magnitude distant from our actual data).

4. *Cross Species Extrapolation* (*also called scaling*). Now, having a dose–response model for what happens to an animal species at a low dose level, we must relate what happens in the species used in bioassays (usually mice and rats) to human. Methods for doing this will be reviewed toward the end of this chapter. Though they generally have much better biological basis than the low-dose extrapolation methods (which really have no biological basis), the uncertainty associated with them is still generally a couple of orders of magnitude.

5. *Real Life Exposure Estimation.* The last step in the process is estimating human exposure: how many people (and who) are exposed to how much? As we shall see, this final step again has significant uncertainty associated with it.

So we have multiple steps, each with a level of uncertainty attached to it. The objective of the entire process (given the uncertainties involved) is to identify a level of exposure associated with an unacceptable degree of concern as to human health effects. One can then compare this region of exposure which represents unacceptable risk with that which contains human exposure to determine if risk is acceptable.

There are two major approaches to dealing with this uncertainty.

Most Conservative. Based on worst case answer to any element of uncertainty, including

Most sensitive species
Most sensitive strain
Most sensitive sex
Assumption of no threshold
Use of upper confidence limits of vsd (virtually safe dose)

Most Appropriate. Based on judgment, including

Most appropriate route
Best data (i.e., With least uncertainty)
No prima facie acceptance or rejection of a threshold or of linearity (or lack of it) in the dose response at regions beyond our data

Just as it is inappropriate to substitute the term "safe" for "virtually safe" or "having acceptable risk" when describing very low-level exposures to the classes of toxic agents we are speaking of, it is also not correct or acceptable to equate "most conservative" with "best science." The best science approach is that which minimizes the uncertainty associated with each of these steps to the extent possible. In the face of continuing uncertainty, the most conservative approach within the bounds of the data is appropriate and should be selected.

Our challenge then, is to select and utilize those methods that minimize the uncertainty in the entire risk assessment process. This process is presented diagramatically in Figure 1.

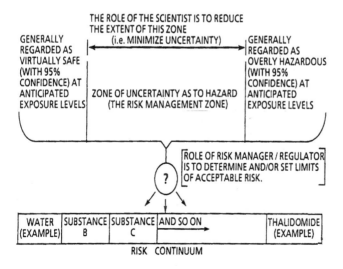

Figure 1 Risk assessment uncertainty and risk management.

II. PHYSICAL, CHEMICAL, AND MANUFACTURING/ USE CHARACTERISTICS

For a chemical entity to cause any of the adverse health effects that are of concern in this chapter, it is first necessary that the material gain entry into the body. Such entry is determined by two sets of requirements. First, exposure must occur. The determinants of such exposure will be looked at in more detail under exposure assessment (Section III). The second, however, is whether such materials will be absorbed. And the major determinants of absorption (and, indeed, of generation of the potential for exposure to a chemical) are its innate chemical and physical characteristics.

There is a long list of chemical and physical factors that may potentially influence exposure and absorption of chemicals. We will only briefly look at four of these here: physical state, vapor pressure, boiling point, and chemical stability.

Physical state (whether a material is a gas, liquid, or solid at room temperature, and if a solid whether it is a powder or gum, for example) is important in that it determines both in what ways a material can be handled and transported and if there is a potential for inhalation exposure. Gases, liquids which can be aerosolized, or solids which are low-density fine powders can all find their way into the atmosphere of the work place, and from there be absorbed.

Likewise, vapor pressures of liquids determine how much of the material will be in the gas phase at room temperatures. In addition, gases possess the greatest potential to be inhaled.

Boiling point is closely related to vapor pressure, and is of interest for similar reasons. The actual temperatures and atmospheric pressures at which a material is handled will determine how much material is vaporized, for vapor pressures are traditionally characterized for "standard" conditions. But not all work places meet such conditions. Some factories may be located in areas where ambient temperatures are higher (the South) or where atmospheric pressure is lower (such as in Denver); both of these conditions would increase the real potential of a nominal liquid to convert to the gas phase.

Chemical stability in industry is of concern for a host of reasons. But one reason which may be overlooked is that working with a chemical of low stability may lead to exposure of a worker to a compound other than the one being manufactured.

Directly interfacing with chemical and physical characteristics are the details of the substance life cycle. This cycle includes the manufacturing process, any formulation that may occur, transportation, use, and finally, the disposal of a material. Chemical and physical properties influence each of these steps, and the details of each step (in conjunction with these same physical and chemical characteristics) determine how much and what kind of worker and population exposure will occur.

III. EXPOSURE IDENTIFICATION AND ASSESSMENT

Determining the significance of any exposure is impossible without consideration of the inherent hazard or toxicity of the material. Similarly, the practical consequences of a material's intrinsic hazard is meaningless without evaluation of the exposure or dose that is delivered to the site of action. The following algorithm illustrates this simple but profound relationship between exposure and hazard in the estimation of risk:

$$Risk = f \text{ (exposure) (hazard)}$$

Risk is directly proportional to the level of exposure and hazard and both must be present for there to be any consequence. These two entities of exposure and hazard are inextricably connected in the risk-assessment process. In practice, the risk assessor usually runs an iterative process weighing his or her knowledge of the one versus the other to help focus attention and actions to arrive at a reasoned conclusion. For example, a situation with a very low exposure potential can tolerate considerable inherent hazard (i.e., toxicity) without resulting in a conclusion of unreasonable risk.

The level of scientific uncertainty with either the nature or the objective level of exposure or hazard color our actions or conclusions in the overall risk assessment. The interfacing of the uncertainties around hazard and exposure has consequences with regard to how far one needs to go in the analysis. Take an example of a low exposure application with a material of unknown but potentially high hazard. If we had a high confidence in the low exposure potential of the use scenarios of the material we could tolerate a high degree of uncertainty in our knowledge of the hazard of the material even though it has an ascribed hazard level that is relatively high. In this case, reasonable and easily defensible worst-case assumptions of hazard render a conclusion of acceptable risk when viewed in the context of the total assessment. This approach precludes the necessity for expending precious resources on sharpening our understanding of the compound's hazard. It's not difficult for the reader to imagine situations where the opposite is true, that is, when one has a high degree of confidence in the material's inherent hazard as being low but much less certainty about its exposure patterns. The challenge comes in the typically intermediate situation where "gray" levels of exposure and hazard exist. Here the assessor needs to decide where the resources should be best spent to render the required decisions.

Since risk assessment is dependent on both exposure and hazard the exposure–assessment process properly involves close iterative interaction with that of the hazard evaluation. In this scheme uncertainty is addressed by using the upper bounds of exposure and hazard from the objective evidence at hand. Each examination of hazard or exposure then drives the other until enough resources are committed to the evaluation and the assessor finds him or herself with a reasonable determination of acceptable or unacceptable risk based on the accumulated data.

With this inseparable interactive relationship of exposure and hazard firmly in mind, we can seek to characterize the elements of each separately.

A. Preliminary Exposure Assessment

1. Chemical and Physical Properties

Characterization of critical chemical and physical properties for compounds with potential adverse health impact establishes a basis for subsequent exposure analysis. An insoluble solid without fines will have virtually no inhalation exposure potential, while a volatile liquid in an open vessel can offer significant inhalation potential. Since it helps to focus attention and activity, property characteristics should be the first task for the investigator. Some critical properties related to exposure potential are listed below:

a. Vapor Pressure-Boiling Point. Assuming a constant area of air–liquid interface, the vapor pressure of the liquid is a direct measure of its exposure potential. Indeed, knowing the vapor pressure allows one to calculate the worse case of vapor exposure:

Saturation Concentration (ppm v/v) = (VP/760) (1,000,000)

where VP is the vapor pressure in torr or mmHg.

A scheme for the reasonable estimation of vapor pressure at various temperatures when the compound's structure and boiling point (at normal or reduced pressure) or its vapor pressure at a prescribed temperature are known is presented in [1].

b. Particle Size Distribution of Bulk Powders. Particles greater than 100 Tm in diameter settle rapidly and thus offer little inhalation potential in most instances. Similarly, particles larger than about 10 μm tend to be removed in the upper respiratory tract and rarely make it to deep lung tissue of humans. Thus, knowledge of the particle size distribution of granular material offers important information relative to its inhalation potential.

c. Solubility and Octanol/Water Coefficient. The solubility of a substance in water (or lipids) can in large measure determine the fate of the material in the environment or in the body. For instance, a material with a high octanol/water coefficient will tend to partition and be found in the organic-rich sediment of a lake or stream rather than in the water column. In another instance, insoluble particulates that reach the deep lung because of small particle size tend to remain in the alveolar region and will not be distributed throughout the systemic circulation.

2. Site-Specific Characteristics

Airborne exposure potential to vapors from liquids is directly related to the ambient use temperature and the surface area of exposed liquid. With all other conditions held steady, the exposure potential of any application will also be proportional to the quantity of material transferred per unit time.

3. Absorbed Versus Available Dose

The most meaningful description of exposure is a quantification of the amount of toxicant per unit time that reaches the site of toxic action in the physiology of the species involved. This is rarely achieved and assessors usually settle for less direct measures of exposure; namely, the dose that is available for absorption by the organism. Thus, human inhalation exposure is gauged by measuring the concentration of the toxicant in the air that might be breathed by an individual. This concentration is multiplied by the individuals' residence time in and their inhalation rate of this air to arrive at an estimate of exposure.

4. Dose

Absorption of the dose is more often not addressed or it is implicitly assumed to be 100% of the available dose. The situation with dermal exposure is even less precise. The simplest schemes estimate the amount of material applied or remaining on the skin and then assume a certain percentage (5–100%) of percutaneous absorption into the systemic circulation (2). More sophisticated approaches attempt to estimate the kinetic transfer rate of toxicant through the skin multiplied by the affected surface area of skin to give a systemically absorbed dose (3–5).

5. Monitoring Versus Modeling

Estimation of available dose from inhalation of air contaminant can be accomplished by analytical sampling of the ambient air. The details of what constitutes statistically valid and reliable sampling are presented elsewhere (6,7). Protocols for the sampling of dermal dosing are also available (8–10). These direct sampling techniques require the development and validation of analytical protocols that are specific to the compound(s) of concern. Assuming proper validation and sampling strategies are employed, these data represent the best (i.e., the most precise and accurate) measure of the exposure potential based on available dose.

A more general approach involves exposure estimation based on physiochemical principles or an empirically derived database or a combination of these two techniques.

The decision whether to monitor or model an exposure is dependent primarily on the precision needs of the analysis and the availability of validated monitoring and modeling tools. If anticipated exposures are close to ascribed exposure limits, then monitoring methods and sampling strategies that render a high level of statistical evaluative power may be necessary. Conversely, in scenarios where exposure potential is low, modeling using conservative (i.e., overestimating) assumptions may show a lack of significant exposure potential visa-vis exposure limits and thus allow a conclusion of relative safety without the need for or the expense of direct measurements. Thus, the first step in any exposure assessment should be the use of conservative models of exposure potential in a preliminary screening. Monitoring or model refinement remain as possible next steps in the process if the worst-case model does not allow a conclusion of relative safety.

The state of development for exposure models for the estimation of inhalation or percutaneous exposure of occupationally exposed workers is relatively crude. Their current value lies in the above mentioned preliminary screening. Assessors who want or need to refine their estimates of exposure beyond this stage can choose either to refine the model or do monitoring. Historically they have almost invariably chosen the latter because it gives a direct answer and in the short run is certainly less expensive. Refined and validated models remain a highly viable but essentially untapped resource for cost-effective exposure assessment. Specific discussion of the research needs in this area are presented later.

Exposure models in the areas of outdoor ambient air and surface and ground water are more highly developed than models developed for occupational exposure indoors. Part of the reason for this is the above mentioned tendency of industrial hygienists to directly monitor exposures. This luxury is often unavailable to the assessor trying the gauge ambient exposure levels in the environment. Direct measurement may be impossible or highly impractical because of the large areas involved or the generally lower (often analytically undetectable concentrations) of toxicants found in the multiple and interacting compartments of the general environment.

B. Distribution of Xenobiotics

The highest concentration of xenobiotic agents available to affect human health are usually found in the workplace. Conditions that enhance the exposure potential are large quantities of chemical toxicants existent in occupational settings as raw materials, intermediates, or products that may be handled in operations which are somewhat "open." Relatively high exposures are also possible in living quarters from direct product use (e.g., pesticides) or incidental contaminants (e.g., formaldehyde from building materials). Recent studies (11) have shown significant levels of indoor air contamination and subsequent health risk in some homes from naturally occurring radon gas seeping into the structures from the ground.

Any contaminant entering the general air volume in the indoor environment will have a comparatively long residence time in that volume because indoor ventilation rates are, for the most part, much lower than those outdoors. This assumes that the incoming ventilatory air is essentially free of the contaminant and thus dilutes and purges it. Overall ventilation rates in private residences are typically much lower than those found in industrial rooms (12).

If the source of the xenobiotic contaminant is not in or directly proximate to the indoor industrial or residential environment then it must travel through time and space to be available for human exposure. Ambient air contamination can come from specific industrial point sources or general and highly disperse "line" or "area" sources such as motor vehicles on a highway or on a congested city. The scale of these contaminant concentrations are measured in fractions of miles to hundreds or even thousands of miles while the scale of indoor exposure fields from proximate sources is measured in feet.

General contamination of the soil or surface water and ground water can allow toxicants to travel to human targets either directly or through possible accumulation or concentration in food. The physical scale of these contaminant soil and surface water fields are also quite large compared to specific local indoor environments and the time scale of these events is usually much longer than those for air contamination. It takes considerably longer to contaminate (or clean up) an aquifer or a lake than it does to foul (or clear) the air.

C. Air Concentration Modeling

Modeling of air concentrations of toxicants like many other exposure models is typically based on the conservation of mass. Contaminant mass is generated, injected into the air, and then accounted for as it disperses, deposits, or transforms with time. The elements can be divided into three areas of characterization:

Source. The strength (mass/time) and location of contaminant release.
Dispersion. A quantitative description of contaminant transport in the air.
Depuration. The time-dependent loss of contaminant form an air volume of interest. Mechanisms of loss include ventilatory dilution and purging from a specified volume of air, deposition losses onto environmental surfaces, and chemical transformation.

The level to which we can identify and quantify each of the above is the extent that our models will be true simulations of reality.

1. Workplace

The following equation describes the conservation of mass in the workroom air:

$VdC = Gdt - QCdt - KCdt$

V = room volume

C = contaminant concentration (weight/volume)

G = contaminant input rate (weight/time)

Q = ventilation rate (volume/time)

K = nonventilatory depuration coefficient (dimensionless)   (1)

This equation simply states that in any "snapshot" of time (dt), the amount of toxicant in the workroom air (VdC) will be equal to the amount that went in (Gdt) minus the amount that comes out by ventilation-purging ($QCdt$) and other clearing mechanisms (KCdt).

This model assumes complete if not perfectly efficient mixing of air and contaminant. As such it predicts there will be a uniform concentration within the volume of the room with no concentration gradient. This assumption has been tested and validated in relatively small industrial rooms (13). However, its ability to predict the maximum exposure potential in larger rooms is questionable.

Recent studies have shown that in some industrial ventilation fields, point sources in large rooms result in essentially spherical or hemispheric diffusion patterns from the source with diatomically decreasing concentration from the source to distal points in the room (14–16). Thus, the maximum concentration and exposure potential in many industrial ventilation fields appear to be concentrated within a relatively short distance from the source.

Adequate treatment of ventilatory purging in the real world requires one to account for the incomplete mixing of the incoming clean air with contaminated air. This is typically expressed as an effective ventilation rate (Q'), which is the nominal ventilation rate (Q) lowered by a mixing factor (m) between 0 (poor) and 1.0 (perfect mixing).

$Q' = (Q)\,(m)$ (2)

Thus, Q' replaces Q in Eq. (1).

Input into the system (Gdt) is estimated by determining how much contaminant is injected into the room volume (V) per unit time. Injection can occur from such operations as spraying, drumming with subsequent displacement of vapors into the workroom air, fugitive emissions from pressure vessels, and simple evaporation. Models for the estimation of input (G) from these types of sources are presented elsewhere (17–20). These source term models use measured or estimated physiochemical properties of the contaminant as a neat material or in solution.

Very little work has been done to measure the effect of nonventilatory depuration (KCdt). Work reported on SO_2, NO_2, and O_3 indicate that these mechanisms could be as effective as typical ventilation rates in lowering contaminant levels (21–23); however, very little work has been done on other gases and vapors and without quantification with objective data, K is usually ignored and the term is dropped. As such, models without ventilatory depuration could seriously overestimate concentration and exposure.

Ignoring K and assuming a constant source and ventilation rate yields a simple solution to the above equation at steady-state equilibrium viz:

$$C_{eq} = G/(m) \ (Q) \tag{3}$$

Thus, inhalation exposure potential estimated by this model is directly proportional to the rate of source generation and inversely proportional to nominal ventilation rate and mixing efficiency.

A simple approach to the problem of modeling maximum exposure potential in a large industrial room is to use the above conservation of mass model but restrict the volume to that in the immediate vicinity of the source (24). The modeler then predicts equilibrium concentration in this "affected volume" around the source by calculating the source strength (G) using one of the above methods, applying a mixing factor between 0.2 and 1, and estimating the general ventilation that is actually entering or leaving this "affected volume." An affected volume of 8,000 ft^3 (a 20-foot cube) around the source has been suggested from theoretical considerations (24). Given a nominal ventilation rate of 3 air changes/hour yields a ventilation rate in this affected volume around the source of 400 cfm. Using a conservatively low mixing factor of 0.3 gives the following simple model for equilibrium concentration estimation:

$$C_{eq} = G/(3)(4) \tag{4}$$

where C_{eq} is estimated workroom air concentration of contaminant in milligrams per cubic meter (mg/m^3) and G is the amount of contaminant entering the affected volume per unit time in milligrams per minute.

The above treatment is valid for systems in which the rate of contaminant generation is relatively constant and essentially continuous. The estimation of concentration averages for short-term activities (i.e., those of a few hours duration or less) requires a more general and computationally complicated solution to the above conservation of mass equation. Integrating Eq. (1) to solve for average concentration C over time ($t - t_0$) with the assumption of constant contaminant release starting at $t = 0$ yields:

$$C_{avg} = G/(Qm + K) - [GV/(t \ (Qm + K)^2)] \ (1 - e^{(-t(Qm + K)/V)})$$

C_{avg} = average concentration

t = elapsed time

e = natural log base number (2.7182 . . .) $\tag{5}$

If one assumes $K = 0$, average concentrations calculated for "long" time intervals (i.e., large values of the quantity (tQm/V) approach the equilibrium concentration presented in Eqs. (3) or (4). However, low ventilation rates, large volumes, and poor mixing will dramatically decrease the actual integrated dose for any person exposed during a batch operation. For example, consider a batch job lasting one hour in a room with poor mixing ($m = 0.1$) and 14,160 1pm (500 cfm) general ventilation in a 6.1 m (20 ft) cube. The one-hour time-weighed exposure or dose is less than 20% of that calculated by using C_{eq}.

It should be noted that the above model inputs are suggested for use in large industrial rooms with ventilation rates of 1–5 air changes per hour and low levels of air turbulence. Rooms with significantly higher levels of air turnover or turbulence (e.g., mixing fans) will not have a strong exposure gradient around sources and a larger "affected volume" with generally higher mixing factors and ventilation rates will render better predictions of exposure.

2. Community

Models used for the estimation of outdoor concentrations and subsequent exposure to toxicant sources also address the basic issues of source strength, dispersion, and extinction; however, instead of conserving mass in a defined "box" of air the approach has been to provide a stochastic description of the dispersion of a plume of contaminant as it diffuses downwind. These models divide the diffusion into vertical and horizontal directions; it assumes the diffusion in each direction will conform to a normal or distribution around the centerline. Downwind concentrations are predicted from the following basic relationship:

$C_c = G/(\sigma y) (\sigma z) (u) (\pi))$

C_c = centerline concentration (with ground level release)

G = contaminant source rate (weight/time)

σy = horizontal dispersion coefficient (length)

φz = vertical dispersion coefficient (length)

u = wind speed (length/time)

The dispersion coefficients are empirically derived and dependent on conditions of atmospheric stability and terrain. Details on this modeling technique are available elsewhere (25). Suffice it to say that these models have been claimed to be accurate to within a factor of 2 or 3 (26).

D. Dermal Exposure Modeling

Biological monitoring for the contaminant or its metabolite(s) can offer a direct indication of the level of percutaneous absorption through dermal exposure. Assuming the opportunities for ingestion and inhalation are relatively low, the monitoring data can reveal the level of toxicant that is most likely entering the body via dermal absorption. A published assessment of wood preservative workers' exposure to pentachlorophenol (27) used this technique to estimate that 93% of the workers' total exposure was from "nonrespiratory routes."

It is important to note that any estimation of worker dosage to a toxicant requires a consideration of the fact that the actual dose is a combination of the equally important factors of toxicant concentration, time of exposure, and fraction of the applied dose that is absorbed. Monitoring the biological levels or effect gives one an integrated endpoint of these factors. Biological monitoring data can be particularly enlightening with regard to percutaneous exposure, which is more difficult to model than inhalation.

In most cases, the exposure limits for inhalation of contaminants are set based on some physical response to an airborne concentration multiplied by a safety factor. Thus the risk-assessment process simply monitors or estimates the level of airborne contamination and compares it with the established exposure limit. The simplicity of this system is not available to the exposure-risk assessor of cutaneous exposure. The relationship between applied dermal exposure subsequent systemic dose is more uncertain and is more tentative, especially when comparing or attempting to predict the response of different species. Thus, if actual direct and quantitative evidence of human percutaneous absorption is available, it is of the utmost value to the risk-assessment process, particularly if it can be related to at least qualitative levels of dermal exposure.

1. Absolute Worst Case: Instantaneous Systemic Absorption

This modeling scenario assumes that liquid splashed or flowed over the skin will remain on the skin as a thin film and then all or a percentage of the toxic compound will be rapidly and completely absorbed into the systemic circulation. Experimental work (28) indicates that the worst case of completely immersing and withdrawing a hand from liquid will result in approximately 3 mg/cm^2 retention of water and 14 mg/cm^2 retention of mineral oil. Using these data, the above assumptions, an estimate of affected surface area(s), and the number of exposures per day will allow one to directly calculate a worst-case dose. This approach can be grossly conservative (depending on the percentage ascribed to the absorbed dose) but usable as a "first-tier" assessment for compounds with low orders of toxic hazard or exposure.

2. Realistic Worst Case: Diffusional Absorption

In addition to having the potential for being too conservative, the total absorption assessment method outlined above is essentially unusable in any exposure scenario in which part or the whole body is totally immersed for extended periods of time. Attempting to use the total absorption technique in these settings will result in the assumption that all or a percentage of the available toxicant in solution is immediately available for absorption. The calculated dose from dissolved compounds in a swimming pool or lake would be massive indeed! Other than being very conservative, this instantaneous absorption model has a critical flaw. In treating dermal exposure as a process independent of time, it is incapable of estimating continuous dermal exposure. As mentioned above, its value lies as a screening tool in those applications where its assumptions and conservativeness are acceptable.

A kinetic approach seeks to determine transport rate of toxicant through the skin in order to estimate the level of systemic absorption per unit of skin area and time of cutaneous exposure [i.e., weight of toxicant absorbed/(skin area) (time of exposure)]. A straightforward model aimed at this determination (3) assumes the uppermost layer of skin, the stratum corneum (SC) is the rate-limiting skin barrier and purely Fickian or passive diffusion in the dominant transport mechanism. These assumptions render a very simple relationship for dermal absorption:

$$J = (K_p) (C_v)$$

J = the absorption rate per unit area and time (mg/cm^2 hr)

K_p = the permeability constant (cm/hr)

C_v = concentration of toxicant (mg/cm^3)

An expanded version is also presented (3):

$$J = \frac{(K_m)(C_v)(D_m)}{(Z)}$$

K_m = the SC:vehicle partition coefficient

D_m = the diffusion constant of the toxicant in the SC layer

Z = the thickness of the SC layer

Measured permeability constants for human skin range (3) from approximately 10^{-6} to 10^{-2} cm/hr. Where necessary, in vitro testing techniques offer expeditions, germane, and relatively inexpensive means of determining these critical permeability constants. It is important to note that a lag time to steady state exists during the transport of the toxicant across the epidermis and this time is often quite long. The lag time represents an important piece of the potential exposure assessment and should be carefully characterized.

A rational approach for the modeling of discreet instances of dermal dosing is contained in a recently proposed biophysically based kinetic model of chemical absorption via human skin (4). This model also assumes passive diffusion of compounds and includes first-order rate expressions for transport first across the SC, then further across viable epidermal tissue to the blood, and finally to the urine. Reverse diffusion from the viable epidermis to the SC, reflecting the compound's relative affinity for the SC over viable tissue is also considered. This non–steady-state model allows one to calculate the percent of the applied compound appearing in the urine as a function of time. The most intriguing aspect of this model is that all but one of the first-order rate constants are calculated from physical properties. Only the rate constant for elimination from blood to urine requires experimental determination.

These kinetic models are still in the developmental stage; however, they exemplify the innovative approaches to dermal exposure modeling that are currently and will continue to be needed to realistically assess risk.

Example.   Consider a person sampling a hypothetical amine in a propylene glycol solution (100 mg amine/g of glycol solution) once per hour. We will assume he/she is quite sloppy and covers both hands with the material for the 5 minutes it takes to sample the material. Given 8 exposures/day, 1300 cm^2 of exposed skin, 5% absorption and 3 mg/cm^2 retained solution per exposure results in a calculated dose of:

$$(8/\text{day}) \ (1300 \ \text{cm}^2) \ (3 \ \text{mg/cm}^2) \ (0.05) \ (0.1) = 156 \ \text{mg/(person) (day)}$$

Estimating the percutaneous dose by diffusion transport modeling requires the determination of the kinetic rate coefficient (K_p) discussed above. Literature values for this coefficient typically range from 10^{-6} to 10^{-2} cm/hr. Assume we tested our solution and the steady-state kinetic transport rate for the amine in propylene glycol is in the middle of this range at 10^{-4} cm/hr. Given unit density for the liquid mixture, the rate of transfer of the amine at steady state is:

$$J = (K_p) \ (C_v) = (10^{-4} \ \text{cm/hr}) \ (100 \ \text{mg/cm}^3)$$
$$= 0.01 \ \text{mg/((cm}^2) \ (\text{hr}))$$

Assuming 40 minutes of total exposure daily to 1300 cm^2 of skin:

$$(1300 \ \text{cm}^2) \ (40/60 \ \text{hr}) \ (0.01 \ \text{mg/((cm}^2) \ (\text{hr})) = 9 \ \text{mg/((person) (day))}$$

Equilibrium or steady-state percutaneous absorption is somewhat analogous to the equilibrium airborne concentration of containment (C_{eq}) in the general ventilation model. Both require a finite period of time to achieve this equilibrium and the time-integrated dose for many batch exposure scenarios will be substantially lower than that calculated assuming steady-state conditions. As such, the above represents a conservative estimate of the percutaneous dose.

E. Demographics and Exposure Profile

As mentioned above, actual human exposure or delivered dose results from the time-weighted integration of contaminant concentration and uptake rate. Obviously, concentration modeling alone will not suffice to completely answer questions of how much toxicant was delivered. Ultimately the models or combination of monitoring/modeling must render an acceptable estimation of dose and be validated against measured data of human exposure in various settings.

Job exposure profiling is a process that seeks to characterize a specific job or worker's exposure. Different approaches are used, one being to use historical personal monitoring data (or observations in the case of dermal exposure) to characterize the exposure for a particular job. Another measures or estimates spatial and temporal contaminant and worker position patterns in an area, which in turn allows estimation of job exposures within this work space. Regardless of the method, job exposure profiling represents a vital piece of the occupational exposure-risk-assessment process. Air concentration measurements and models mean little if the amount of well characterized air inhaled during a work day is unknown. The job-exposure profile is critical because it places and times the worker in the workroom environment and allows a more reasonable estimation of available dose and hopefully a data base for model verification.

A similar concept is available for assessing exposure and subsequent risk to the general population. Combining demographic data with estimated environmental concentrations will allow for an integrated estimation of total risk associated with any release. Recent government publications offer a wealth of specific information for exposure profiling in the general population (29).

F. Future Research

Experimental work designed to refine and validate ventilation and dermal exposure models remains the single most important element in the future success of the exposure assessment process. As mentioned above, the magnitude and form of the extinction factor (K) in the ventilation model will only be available experimentally using a range of representative materials. Similarly, the choice of predictive scheme(s) for the estimation of evaporative generation dates (G) will only be adequately decided with real data.

Before laboratory simulation can properly validate any indoor exposure model, however, a statistical description of ventilation fields or resultant isopleth concentrations typically present in industrial rooms needs to be available in much more detail than is currently available. The indoor ventilation model presented in this chapter assumes random omnidirectional air movement. This assumption needs to be tested by characterizing ventilation field data in a number of representative indoor settings. Once this critical information is in hand, experimental model validation can proceed.

IV. HAZARD IDENTIFICATION

The initial process of identifying which compounds have the potential to be hazardous is, indeed, the process of toxicology testing. Such testing and its proper conduct are the subject of many of the preceding chapters. This testing serves to generate the initial biological information—hopefully, the only biological system data that will be available for most chemicals.

V. DATA QUALIFICATION

Are the studies from which the toxicology data are generated adequate? Some are totally sound, most are somewhat flawed but the data still are usable, and some are such that no data from them may be used in the risk-assessment process. I will not attempt to address evaluation of all the types of studies associated with risk assessment, but rather as an example point out common flaws in animal carcinogenicity studies. These flaws arise from the wrong answers to the following questions.

Is test animal survival sufficient?

Were there enough animals in groups to start with?

Are there both statistical and biological trends associated with the observed evidence of carcinogenesis? Statistical trend is demonstrated by the presence of a dose-responsive increase in tumor incidence. Biological trend is demonstrated by evidence of preoplastic tissue alterations in animals which do not have frank tumors.

Is the target tissue a "null" one? That is, one such that due to high control group incidences of the same tumor a judgment as to either statistical or biological significance cannot be made.

Was the tissue sampling (for histopathology) adequate (both sufficient in number and unbiased)?

Is the target organ a problem tissue? That is, is it one such that the occurrence of a tumor at that site in the test animal is of unclear significance to humans. In such cases, the existence of supporting (or negative) mutagenicity data can help to clarify the issue.

Animal carcinogenicity bioassays are of two types in terms of their objectives: detection screens and dose-response quantifiers. Traditional NCI bioassays and current NTP bioassays were intended as screens; they have high sensitivity, limited discrimination, and do not serve well in estimating risk, but they do very well in serving their objective, which is to detect potentially carcinogenic "bad actors" in an efficient and economical manner. Dose-response quantifiers generally start at a lower high dose (than the MTD), cover a broader range of doses, and use more animals (particularly in the lower dose groups, employing an "unbalanced" design). Properly designed, they should also have at least three dose groups in the response range.

The interpretation of the results of even the best designed carcinogenesis bioassay is a complex statistical and biological problem. In addressing the statistical aspects, we shall have to review some biological points that have statistical implications as we proceed.

First, all such bioassays are evaluated by comparison of the observed results in treatment groups with those in one or more control groups. These control groups always include at least one group that is concurrent, but because of concern about variability in background tumor rates, a historical control "group" is also considered in at least some manner.

The underlying problem in the use of concurrent controls alone is the belief that the selected populations of animals are subject both to an inordinate degree of variability in their spontaneous tumor incidence rates and that the strains maintained at separate breeding facilities are each subject to a slow but significant degree of genetic drift. The first problem raises concern that, by chance, the animals selected to be controls for any particular study will be either "too high" or "too low" in their tumor incidences, leading to either a false positive or false negative statistical test result when test animals are compared to these controls. The second problem leads to concern that, over the years, different laboratories will be using different standards (control groups) against which to compare the outcome of their tests, making any kind of relative comparison between compounds or laboratories impossible.

The last decade has seen at least eight separate publications reporting 5 sets of background tumor incidences in test animals (30). These publications are summarized and compared for B6C3F1 mice and Fischer 344 rats in Gad and Weil (31). The related survival and growth data on control animals (broken out by type of treatment and vehicle) has also been published (32).

Historical control incidences should not be used to generate an "exclusion zone" associated with its range. Such data should be evaluated as to where the mean historical incidence of tumors at a site are and what the density function is and if this historical data represents the same population, i.e., animals in the same laboratory during recent history. But extreme outlier values in a range (either high or low) are not appropriately used to sort out and discard data. The local (concurrent) control group data is generally much more important in any evaluation, and historical control group data (as a general rule) are used primarily as a check to ensure that the statistical evaluations used in comparing treatment groups to concurrent controls have a sound starting point.

Dempster et al. (33) have, however, proposed a method for incorporating historical control data in the actual process of statistical analysis. A variable degree of pooling (combining) of historical with concurrent controls is performed based on the extent to which the historical data fit an assumed normal logistic (log transformed) model.

Having selected which studies to use to develop a model on, that is, those of the highest quality which have the least uncertainty associated with them, risks should then be calculated on the basis of highest tumor incidence rates at any single organ site, and not on combined total incidences of tumors in control animals at only those sites where test animals have higher incidences than control animals.

The decision on which tumor count to use (highest single site or total animals with tumors at those sites showing significant increases in controls) makes minimal difference in some cases, as there are few animals with tumors at other than one site. This, of course, excludes mammary and forestomach tumors as "null" tissues in rats for predicting human effects. More importantly, I believe that competing risks makes the combining of selected tumor sites inappropriate. If we look at more than one site, should we not look at the total incidence of animals with any malignant tumor in each group as a comparator, and then adjust the increased risk (if any) of being in a test group downward for the baseline level of incidence seen in controls? In other words, if we look at total tumor incidences, we must address the question as some investigators have suggested: are we only shifting age-related patterns of tumor incidence?

A. Use of Biomarkers in Quantitative Risk Assessment

Biomarkers provide an important tool to the toxicologist/risk analyst in incorporating biological insights relevant to mechanisms of action into risk assessments. The purpose of this section is to provide a brief overview of the types of biomarkers and to discuss their utility in reducing uncertainty when extrapolating across species. An example is presented to illustrate their use. Biomarkers are broadly defined as indicators of events in biological systems. They can be divided into three types including biomarkers of exposure, effect, and susceptibility (126,127).

A graduation of events often occurs between the uptake of an agent and the ultimate manifestations of impaired health. Confusion often arises over inadequate attention being directed toward clear terminology in distinguishing between external exposure, internal exposure, biologically effective dose, and pharmacodynamic effects (early biological changes and subsequent progression clinical expression). Biomarkers provide a means to elucidate these intermediate events along the casual pathway and thereby quantitatively link exposure and relevant response or effect variables. In providing biologically based insights into the affected damage processes, biomarkers offer a means to reduce the uncertainties inherent in high to low-dose extrapolation and cross-species extrapolation.

Use of biomarkers offers several clear benefits in attempting to provide biologically based risk assessments.

1. They can lead to more complete scientific understanding incorporating more relevant information about causal mechanisms than simple input-output analysis based on external dose and the incidence of end effects.

2. They offer the eventual prospect of a better mechanism-based projection of risk beyond the range of possible observations in terms of dose, rate, duration and species.

3. They offer the possibility of greater sensitivity of detection and quantification of adverse effects. In some cases, biomarkers allow for going from the whole animal to the cellular or subcellular level for the units in which damage is quantified and analyzed (i.e., molecular dosimetry).

4. In some cases (e.g., where effects are detected in the form of long-term changes in higher nervous system functions that may be subject to a number of psychosocial confounding influences which are difficult to control in some exposed groups), biomarkers offer the prospect of confirming exposure-related effects and narrowing the search for causative agents.

Biomarkers have played two principal roles in the study of cancer:

1. They can assist in the interpolation of risk from high doses to low doses by helping sort out pharmacokinetic nonlinearities from nonlinearities that are produced by the central pharmacodynamic processes that lead to cellular transitions along the pathway to cancer. Because of its importance in the cancer risk assessments, an example is presented.

2. They can help in the quantification of comparative dosage and associated risks between different species.

Advances in molecular and cellular biology will continue to shed new light on mechanisms linking exposure and response. Significant reductions in uncertainty are expected as biomarkers clarify events as markers of exposure, effect, and/or susceptibility. While offering many advantages, the toxicologist/risk analyst must consider some limitations when applying biomarkers for the purposes of risk assessment. Biomarkers tend to be "windows" on biological systems that are not completely understood and not directly amenable to complete and definitive observation. In any risk assessment that relies on the use of biomarkers, a critical assumption concerns the choice of the biomarker. Is it the most appropriate predictor of exposure, effect, or susceptibility? Another difficulty for the basic experimental scientist is that a full development of biomarkers of exposure and early effects generally requires the development of dynamic models for (a) the appearance and disappearance/repair of the marker in relation to exposure or toxicant uptake and (b) the production of ultimate effects of concern in relation to the presence or quantitative level of the marker.

VI. STATISTICAL MODELS FOR LOW-DOSE EXTRAPOLATION

Given knowledge of what happens at relatively high doses by one or more routes in one or more animal species, one must next predict what would happen in the same species at much lower dose levels. These doses may be separated by as much as seven orders of magnitude. It should be remembered at this point that risk assessment is not limited to carcinogenesis, but rather is generally applicable to any catastrophic irreversible effect where real human exposures are at much lower levels than those of animals and where the cause (exposure to a chemical) is separated significantly in time from the effect (such as cancer) that also occurs at some background level in the normal course of human events. None of the mathematical models we use has a sound biological basis (in fact, most have no biological basis). They can give vastly different (by five or more orders of magnitude) answers, and have very wide regions of uncertainty (called 95% confidence intervals, which may range from two to as high as five orders of magnitude) associated with them.

A. Estimating Human Exposure

The most toxic material in existence would not have risk associated with it if there weren't any exposure. Having now produced a model that will estimate risk to humans at any given dose (with a noticeable degree of uncertainty already in hand), measurements or estimates of human exposure (both incidence and extent) must be generated.

This remaining step in performing a risk assessment (quantitating the exposure of the human population, both in terms of how many people are exposed, by what routes, and to what quantities of an agent they are exposed) unfortunately, also has uncertainties associated with it.

With the exception of some key points, the process of identifying and quantitating exposure groups within the human population is beyond the scope of this text. Classification methods are again the key tool for identifying and properly delimiting human populations at risk. An investigator must first understand the process involved in making, shipping, using, and disposing of a material. The exposure groups can be very large or relatively small subpopulations, each with a markedly different potential for exposure. For di-(2-ethyl-hexyl)-phthalate (DEHP), for example, the following at-risk populations have been identified:

IV Route	Oral Route
3,000,000 receiving blood transfusions (50 mg/year)	10,800,000 children under 3 years of age (434 mg/year)
50,000 dialysis patients (4,500 mg/year)	220,000,000 adults (dietary contamination of 1.1 mg/year)
10,000 hemophiliacs (760 mg/year)	

Not quantitated were possible inhalation and dermal exposures.

All such estimates of exposure in humans (and of the number of humans exposed), again, are subject to a large degree of uncertainty.

An alternative approach to achieving society's objective for the entire risk assessment procedure, namely protecting the human population from unacceptable levels of known risks, is the classical approach of using safety factors. In 1972, Weil (125) summarized this approach as "In summary, for the evaluation of safety for man, it is necessary to: (1) design and conduct appropriate toxicologic tests, (2) statistically compare the data from treated and control animals, (3) delineate the minimum effect and maximum no ill-effect levels (NIEL) for these animals, and (4) if the material is to be used, apply an appropriate safety factor, e.g., (a) 1/100 (NIEL) or 1/500 (NIEL) for some effects or (b) 1/500 (NIEL), if the effect was a significant increase in cancer in an appropriate test." This approach has served society reasonably well over the years, once the experimental work has identified the potential hazards and quantitated the observable dose–response relationships. The safety factor approach has not generally been accepted or seriously entertained by regulatory agencies. Until such time as the most elegant risk assessment procedures can instill greater public confidence, the use of the safety factor approach should perhaps not be abandoned so readily for more "mathematically precise" methodologies.

As a final sanity check to this multistep process, the datapoints generated by other studies addressing the endpoint of interest should be evaluated to determine if they fall within the 95% confidence bounds of the projection. If we find that real data do not fit our extrapolation model at this point, then as scientists we have no choice but to reject such a model and start anew.

B.   Low Dose Extrapolation

As has been previously discussed, risk assessment, in the sense in which we will consider it in this book (and as it is performed by toxicologists), involves a number of separate steps, each of which involves some form of mathematical model to bridge gaps in biological knowledge. Here we must consider that, given the dose response estimation made (for animals) and exposure estimates for classes of people, we must finally couple the two by some model which translates "mice-to-men." That is, we must perform a species-to-species extrapolation.

C.   Threshold

The process of low dose extrapolation, no matter which method is used, consists of three distinct steps. First, the actual dose–response datapoints available (which, for reasons discussed earlier, are invariably in the high dose and/or high response region) are identified, providing us with a starting point. Second, a mathematical method is selected and employed to extend the dose–response relationship from the region we know to the regions we are interested in or concerned about. Third, we make a basic assumption about the nature of the dose response relationship in the extreme low dose and/or response region, then proceed to develop a model specific to the compound of interest.

This basic assumption about the extreme low-dose region is the question of threshold. For all biological phenomena except carcinogenesis and mutagenesis, it is a basic principle of biology that there is a dose level (threshold) below which no response is evolved. But there is an ongoing controversy as to applicability of the concept of a threshold for these two phenomena. Regulatory bodies in the U.S. have based much of their risk assessment work on the belief (which cannot, of course, be either proved or disproved) that a single molecule of any agent found to be a carcinogen or mutagen at high dose levels will involve some increase in the incidence of that response. Epstein (35), in quoting Umberto Saffiotti, presented one major argument against the concept of the use threshold.

> Certain approaches to the problem of identifying a "safe threshold" for carcinogens are scientifically and economically unsound. I have in mind some proposals to test graded doses of one carcinogen down to extremely low levels, such as those to which a human population may be exposed through, say residues in food. In order to detect possible low incidences of tumors, such a study would use large numbers of mice, of the order of magnitude of 100,000 mice per experiment. This approach seems to assume that such a study would reveal that there is a threshold dose below which the carcinogen is not longer effective, and, therefore, that a "safe dose" can be identified in this manner. Now, there is presently no scientific basis for assuming that such a threshold would appear. Chances are that such a "megamouse experiment" would actually confirm that no threshold can be determined. But let us assume that the results showed a lack of measurable tumor response below a certain dose level in the selected set of experimental conditions and for the single carcinogen under test. In order to base any generalization for safety extrapolations on such a hypothetical finding, one would have to confirm it and extend it to include other carcinogens and other experimental conditions such as variations in diet, in the vehicle used, in the age of the animals, their sex, etc. Each of these tests would then imply other "megamouse experiments." The task would be formidable: suffice it to say that an experiment on 100,000 mice would cost about 15 million dollars: if one did 20 such experiments, it would cost 300 million dollars. All this to try and estimate the possible shape of a dose response curve which would still leave most of our problems in the evaluation of carcinogenesis hazards unsolved. This effort would also block the nation's resources for long term bioassays for years to come and actually prevent the use of such resources for the detection of potent carcinogenic hazards from yet untested environmental chemicals. If two million mice are made available as resources, they can be used effectively to test 4,000 new compounds, each on 500 mice, thereby detecting among them those that are highly carcinogenic in the test conditions.

The argument against the existence of a threshold for carcinogens continues with the following points:

1. In vitro a single molecule of a chemical can achieve an alteration of the genetic elements of a cell, mutating it. Such mutations can be to neoplastic forms, therefore including the process which (in the end) would produce a cancer in vivo. Albert et al. (36) have presented a variation on this theme with initiation promotion in mouse skin as a model.

2. Even if there is a biological threshold for any individual agent of concern due to various defense mechanisms, we cannot rule out the possibility of the presence of other agents in the environment, which may either act as promoters for our agent of concern or saturate the existing defense mechanisms, effectively "humping over" the threshold. Mantel (37) presented this argument in his 1963 review of the concept of threshold in carcinogenesis.

3. The presence of a threshold would preclude the possibility of linear dose response. Mantel and Schneiderman (38) presented this point of view, which is a variation on point one. Of course, the existence of a threshold would actually only mean that a linear (or any other dose–response relationship) would start at some point above zero, being discontinuous only in the extreme lowest dose range.

4. The presence of a background exposure of carcinogens and promoters, and of spontaneously occurring cancers in a population at risk as large and diverse as that of human beings, implies that even if there are thresholds for some or most individuals, there will still remain others who have been "jumped over" their individual thresholds by background events. Crump et al. (39) termed this the existence of a "random threshold" such that there could be no exposure that was absolutely safe for absolutely everyone who might be exposed. Interestingly, Gross et al. (40) presented a similar argument for "absolute safety" in addressing reproductive toxicity data for a food additive.

5. Existing methods of low-dose risk extrapolation implicitly account for the increase in time-to-tumor statistics insofar as they accord for the decrease in tumor incidence, invalidating the pro-threshold argument (to be reviewed later) that at very low doses time-to-tumor would become so long that it would exceed lifespan. Guess and Hoel (41) proposed this argument against thresholds.

All five of these arguments against the existence of a threshold center on the belief that without proof of absolute safety, we must proceed in the most conservative manner possible. Calabrese (42) summarized the essence of this approach as lack of belief in threshold together with six other principles.

1. Use of upper confidence limits on the estimated VSD (Virtually Safe Dose) instead of on the VSD themselves.
2. Use of the most sensitive animal species.
3. Use of the most sensitive sex of that species.

4. Use of the most sensitive strain within a species.
5. Expression of dosage given on a dietary concentration basis rather than on a bodyweight basis when extrapolating from animals to humans; this will result in about a 15-fold lower acceptable exposure for humans as compared to the mouse.
6. The slope of unity by Mantel Bryan (a model for low-dose extrapolation to be discussed later) is almost always less than the observed data, thereby resulting in lower acceptable exposure.

The arguments for the existence of the threshold are as numerous and tend to be more mechanistic. These are summarized as follows:

1. Most (if not all) carcinogens and mutagens exhibit a dose–response relationship, resulting in an apparent or effective threshold for at least some agents. This is the classical toxicology argument, coming from the general case of all other toxic actions and finding no reason or data to support these actions being different (43). Theoretical analysis of the process of carcinogenesis as understood for radiation (the case in which we have the most human data) likewise suggests a lack of linearity at very low doses (44).

2. Toxicity, including carcinogenesis, is a dynamic process which includes absorption of an agent into the body, distribution to various tissues, reversible or irreversible reactions with cellular components, adaptation and repair by molecular and cellular components of the body, and ultimately clearance from the body by metabolism and/or excretion. Such pharmacokinetic processes are generally linear only within prescribed ranges. Gehring et al. (45) have proposed that such pharmacokinetic processes provide a conceptual basis for understanding how metabolic thresholds may lead to a disproportionate increase in toxicity, including carcinogenesis, above certain dose levels. They have also conducted and presented work on vinyl chloride carcinogenesis and pharmacokinetic data to support this proposal.

3. Because an organism as large as either a mouse or a man has a tremendous number of cells, a large number of defense mechanisms of high efficiency, and low probability of a "hit" by a carcinogen being effective in initiating or promoting a neoplasm, there is a biological threshold based on just stochastic or probabilistic grounds. The last aspect (low probability of a "meaningful" reaction) arises from consideration of the fact that the vast majority of molecules that a carcinogen comes in contact with (and reacts with) in a multicellular organism cannot then contribute to the development of a neoplasm; they are, in effect, a multitude of "dummies" acting to block the assassin's shot.

Dinman (46) originally proposed this concept with the following six elements:

a. A cell is estimated to be composed of approximately 10^{14} molecules and atoms with which a xenobiotic substance may interact.

    b.   A major factor influencing activity is molecular specificity, as compared to the mere presence of an atom or molecule in a cell.

    c.   There are lower concentration limits for the occurrence of biologically significant intracellular molecular reactivity. Numerous examples of in vitro studies of specific inhibitors have demonstrated that a lower concentration limit for such inhibition is 10^{-8}M.

    d.   Binding or interaction with proteins or other molecules at sites where there is no resulting functional effect may not happen frequently.

    e.   All chemical components of the cells and cells themselves are in a dynamic flux. The major consideration is that the rate of loss exceeds the rate of normal replacement.

    f.   Cells of different types of tissues have the capacity to induce normal DNA repair mechanisms to repair genetic damage caused by environmental mutagens. In fact, the absence of DNA repair mechanisms in persons with Xeroderma pigmentosum clearly demonstrates the life-saving functional capacity of this process in normal individuals.

    Based on these elements and the estimate that 10^4 molecules per cell is the lower limit for a material to be biologically active, Friedman (47) has calculated threshold levels for a number of materials. The calculations were also based on the assumption that there are 6×10^{13} cells in a 70 kg "average man" therefore requiring a minimum effective dose of 8.6×10^{15} molecules per kilogram of cells. Some of these results are presented in Table 1.

Table 1   Estimated No-Effect Quantities of Some Potent Carcinogens and Toxic Agents

Agent	Molecular weight	Calculated no-effect level (g/kg body weight)	Molarity	Molecules per kilogram body weight
Aflatoxin	312	5×10^{-9}	1.6×10^{-11}	9.6×10^{12}
1,2,5,6-dibenzanthracene (subcutaneous)	278	2.5×10^{-4}	9×10^{-7}	5.4×10^{17}
1,2,5,6-dibenzanthracene (subcutaneous)	278	2.5×10^{-5}	9×10^{-8}	5.4×10^{16}
3-Methylcholanthrene (subcutaneous)	268	2.5×10^{-5}	9.3×10^{-8}	5.6×10^{16}
2,4-Benz-a-pyrene (skin)	252	2.5×10^{-6}	1×10^{-8}	6×10^{16}
Aramite	335	1×10^{-1}	3×10^{-4}	1.8×10^{20}
Tetrachlorodibenzodioxin	320	6×10^{-8}	1.9×10^{-10}	1.1×10^{14}
Botulinum toxin (mouse)	900,000	6.5×10^{-11}	7×10^{-17}	4.2×10^{7}

Source: Friedman (1973).

Several such calculated values (vitamin A, estradiol, and diethylstilbestrol) were also shown to be conservative—below experimentally established effect levels.

4. As dose or exposure to a carcinogenic agent decreases, it is well established that the time it takes for tumors to be expressed gets longer and longer. At some point in the dose time-to-tumor curve, the time necessary for a tumor to develop will exceed the life span of the exposed member of a population. Yanysheva and Antomonov (48) have reported on the dose–time–effect relationship with respect to the carcinogen benzo-(a)-pyrene. They found that the number of animals with tumors decreases as exposure to benzo-(a)-pyrene decreases. Furthermore, the latency period varies inversely with the dose. Based on their results, Yanysheva and Antomonov (48) developed a dose–time–effect relationship as shown in Table 2. Based on the information in Table 2, Yanysheva and Antomonov suggested a dose of benzo-(a)-pyrene that they believed would lead to a carcinogenic effect only after the normal lifespan of the exposed individual. Kraybill (49) combined arguments in 3 (above) and those for a time-to-tumor threshold in suggesting that "the fallacy of considering just singular insults in a biomedical assessment, the traditional approach, can thus be appreciated."

5. There are directly demonstrable physiochemical factors that cause some agents to be carcinogens above certain dose levels and, conversely, cause these particular materials not to be carcinogens (at least by the mechanism operative at the higher levels) at lower levels.

Elizabeth Miller used and presented the case of xylitol as part of her 1977 presidential address to the American Association for Cancer Research (50):

> The recent report on the development of tumors of the urinary bladder in male mice fed the sweetener xylitol as 10–20% of their diets in 2-year tests and its possible implications for the use of xylitol in human foods provide an example of the problems to be resolved. These tumors apparently devel-

Table 2 Calculated Time for Appearance of the First Lung Tumor Following Administration of Various Total Benzo-a-pyrene Doses in 10 Portions, Intratracheally

Benzo-(a)-pyrene dose (mg)	Time of tumor occurrence (months)
0.1	27.0
0.05	38.0
0.02	67.9
0.01	118.9
0.005	221.0
0.002	527.3

oped only in urinary bladders that contained stones (oxalates), a condition long known to predispose rodents to the development of bladder tumors. Neither bladder stones nor bladder tumors were reported in female mice fed the high levels of xylitol or in male mice fed 2% of the sweetener. Since xylitol is a normal intermediate in the metabolism of D-glucuronate, has not shown mutagenic activity and would not be expected to yield strong electrophilic reactants on metabolism, there seems to be little reason for concern of hazard to humans ingesting low levels of xylitol in foods. Yet, strict interpretation of the Delaney amendment to the Pure Food and Drug Act would prohibit the use of xylitol, since the act does not permit addition to food of any chemical that has caused tumors in either humans or animals.

Currently, of course, the Food Safety Protection Act would preclude such an action.

There are numerous cases of data which support (but do not "prove") the concept of a threshold. As early as 1943 Bryan and Shimkin (51) reported skin painting data for three carcinogenic hydrocarbons which at least suggested thresholds. In 1977, Wolfe (52) reported a similar case for radiation exposure and Stokinger presented evidence for the existence of thresholds for seven chemical carcinogens (Table 3).

The ultimate empirical answer to the question of whether or not there are thresholds for carcinogens and mutagens in multicellular organisms would be a massive study with sufficient animals to allow for establishing a dose response curve across the broad dose range. Such a study is both logistically and economically unfeasible, but NCTR conducted a "megamouse" study which was designed to go part way toward this goal. In the ED_{01} study 24, 192 BALB/c female mice were fed 2-acetylaminofluorene (2-AAF), a carcinogen which results in tumors in two different organs (bladder and liver) by unrelated mechanisms. The spontaneous incidence rates for either of these two tumors in any one BALB/c female control was below 0.1% (54). The entire study was initially reported as a complete issue of a journal (55).

The data resulting from this study (Littlefield et al., 1980) strongly suggest a threshold for bladder tumors, but also emphasize the importance of time-to-tumor in the interpretation of results.

VII. MODELS

There are at least eight different models for extrapolating a line or curve across the entire range from a high-dose region to a low-dose region. In this section we will examine each of these models, and compare them in terms of characteristics and outcome. Some of these models are such that they handle only quantal (also called dichotomous) data, while others will also accommodate time-to-tumor information.

Table 3 Evidence for Thresholds in Carcinogenesis

Test substance	Route	Species	Dose levels eliciting tumors	Dose levels not eliciting tumors	Duration
Bis-chloromethyl ether	Inhalation	Rat	$100\ \mu g/M^3$	$10\ \mu g/m^3$ $1\ \mu g/m^3$	6 months/daily
1,4-Dioxane	Oral	Rat	1% in H_2O	0.1% in H_2O 0.01% in H_2O	2 years
Coal tar	Inhalation	Rat	>1000 ppm	111 ppm	2 yrs./daily
	Topical	Mouse	6400 mg 640 mg 64 mg	<0.64 mg	64 weeks twice
β-Napthylamine	Inhalation Topical	Human	>5% in form	<0.5% in	22 years
Hexamethylphosphoramide	Inhalation	Rat	4000 ppm 400 ppm	50 ppm	8 months
Vinyl chloride	Inhalation	Rat	2500 ppm 200 ppm 50 ppm	<50 ppm >10 ppm	7 months
Vinylidene chloride	Inhalation	Human	>200 ppm	1950–1955, 160 ppm average; 30–170 ppm 1960, <50 ppm decreasing to 10 ppm	25 years
Range					

Source: From Ref. 53.

In the models below, certain standard symbols are used. Most of these models express the probability of a response P, as a function, f, of dosage, D, so that $P = f(D)$ and the models differ only with respect to choice of function, f. The nonthreshold models assume that if proportion p of control animals respond to a dose that $f(D) = p$ only for D equal to zero, and that for any nonzero D, $f(D) \to p$ (that is, there is a response). Threshold models assume the existence of a D_0 such that for all $D < D_0$, $f(D) = p$ (that is, that there is some dose below which there is no response). If safety is defined as zero increase over control response, then a nonthreshold model would require that any nonzero dosage be associated with some finite risk.

One Hit. The one-hit model is based on the assumption that cancer initiates from a single cell as a result of a random occurrence or "hit" that causes an irreversible alteration in the DNA of a susceptible cell type. It is also assumed that the likelihood of this hit is proportional to the level of carcinogen exposure. This suggests a direct linear dose response such that if one is to diminish the risk from 10^{-2} to 10^{-8}, then the dose should be divided by 10^6.

Accordingly, the one-hit model is also called the linear model, though a number of the other models also behave in a linear manner at lower doses. Based on the concept that a single receptor molecule of some form responds after an animal has been exposed to some single unit of an agent, the probability of tumor induction by exposure to the agent is then

$$P(d) = 1 - \exp(-1\lambda)D$$

where

$$D \geq 0,\ 0 \leq P(D) \leq 1,$$

λ is an unknown rate constant (or slope) and D is the expected number of hits at dose level D. "Dose" is used in a very general sense. It may mean the total accumulated dose or the dosage rate in terms of body weight, surface area approximations, or concentration in the diet. Computing the one-hit model in terms of the exponential series gives

$$P(D) = \frac{\lambda D}{1} \frac{(\lambda D)^2}{1 \cdot 2} + \frac{(\lambda D)}{1 \cdot 2 \cdot 3} \cdots$$

which, for small values of $P(D)$, is well approximated by

$$P(D) = \lambda D$$

Though Hoel, Gaylor, Kirchstein, Saffiotti, and Schneiderman (56) have argued that this model is consistent with reasonable biological assumptions, there is now almost universal agreement that the model is excessively conservative. The concept of a hit is a metaphor for a variety of possible elementary biochemical events and the model must be considered phenomenologic rather than molecular. This model is essentially equivalent to assuming that the dose–response curve is linear in the low-dose region. Thus, the slope of the one-hit curve at dose D is $\lambda\,[1 - P(D)]$, and for dose levels at which $P(D) < .05$ varies by less than 5%, i.e. is essentially constant and equal to λ. The linear model is one of two models, the other being the probit model, specified by the Environmental Protection Agency (57) in its interim guidelines for assessment of the health risk of suspected carcinogens. The assumption of low-dose linearity will generally lead to a very low, virtually safe dose (VSD), so low as to lead the Food and Drug Administration Advisory Committee (58) to remark that assuming linearity " . . . would lead to few conflicts with the result of applying the Delaney clause." The one-hit model, having only one disposable parameter, λ, will often fail to provide a satisfactory fit to dose-response data in the observable range. Other models described below, by introducing additional parameters, often lead to reasonable fits in the observable range.

An additional degree of conservatism is introduced by extrapolating back to zero from the upper confidence limit (UCL) for the net excess tumor rate (treated minus control rate). The linear model assumes that the tumor rate is proportional to dose, or that $P(D) = \lambda D$. The upper confidence limit for the slope is UCL divided by experimental dosage. Thus an estimate of an upper limit for the proportion of tumor bearing animals, P_u, for a given dose D is

$$P_u = \frac{UCLD}{D_e}$$

where D_e is the experimental dosage. Conversely, the dose D for a given P_u is

$$D = \frac{P_u D_e}{UCL}$$

The linear model may serve as a conservative upper boundary for probit dose–response curves. This upper boundary on the proportion of tumor-bearing animals may not be as conservative as one might imagine. Crump et al. (39), Peto (59), and Guess et al. (60) have shown that the curvilinear dose–response curve resulting from the multistage model is well approximated by the linear model at low dose levels. Gross et al. (40) discussed the statistical aspects of a linear model for extrapolation.

Example 1 illustrates the linear extrapolation model. Examples of subsequent models can be found in Gad (61).

Example 1. A compound is administered as 5% (50,000 ppm) in diet for two years to a group of 100 animals. Twenty-two of these test animals and six of 100 control animals are found to have developed liver tumors at the end of the study.

Thus upper confidence limit on the excess tumor rate is approximately

$$(p_t - p_c) + Z\sqrt{\frac{p_r(1 - p_t)}{n_t} + \frac{p_c(1 - p_c)}{n_c}}$$

where p_t is the proportion of animals with tumors in n_t treated animals, p_c is the proportion of animals with tumors in n_c control animals, and Z is the normal deviate corresponding to the level of confidence desired.

The upper 99% confidence level for this example is thus

$$(0.22) - 0.06) + 2.33\sqrt{\frac{0.22 \times 0.78}{100} + \frac{0.06 \times 0.94}{100}}$$

$$= (0.16) + 2.33\sqrt{0.001716 + 0.000564}$$

$$= 0.16 + 2.33(0.0477493)$$

$$= 0.271256$$

If it is then desired to estimate an upper limit of risk associated with exposure to 10 ppm of the material in diet, this would be

$$= \frac{0.271256}{50,000} \times 10 = 5.43 \times 10^{-5}$$

The Probit Model. This model assumes that the log tolerances have a normal distribution with mean μ and standard deviation σ. The proportion of individuals responding to dose D, say $P(D)$, is then simply

$$P(D) = \Phi\ [(\log D - \mu)/\sigma] = \Phi\ (\alpha + \beta \log D),$$

where $\Phi\ (x)$ is the standard normal integral from $\bar{\chi}$ to X, $\alpha = -\mu/\sigma$ and $\beta = 1/\sigma$. This dose–response curve has $P(D)$ near zero if D is near zero and $P(D)$ increasing to unity as dose increases. A plot of a typical probit dose–response is given by an S-shaped (sigmoid) curve. The quantity above is referred to as the slope of the probit line, where

$$Y = \Phi^{-1}\ [P(D)] = \alpha + \beta \log D$$

and

$$Y + 5 \text{ is the probit of } P.$$

This is the same model we presented earlier in this book for linearizing a special case of quantal response, the data for LD_{50}s. Despite its nonthreshold assumption it is a characteristic of the probit curve that as dose decreases, zero response is approached very rapidly, more rapidly than any power of dose. Other curves to be considered approach zero response more slowly than the probit.

An alternative derivation of the probit model which relates it to time-to-response has been given by Chand and Hoel (62) using the Druckrey observation that median time to tumor, T, is related to dose, D, by the equation $DT^n = C$, where n and C are constants unrelated to D (63). Combining this relation with an assumed lognormal distribution of response time then gives the $P(D)$ as probability of response to any given time, T_0, where α and β are simple function of n, C, T_0, and the standard deviation of the distribution of response times.

The actual method which has the probit model as its basis is the Mantel-Bryan procedure. As originally proposed, this procedure used the probit model but with a preassigned slope of unity. The rationale for this slope was that all observed probit slopes at the time of the proposal exceeded that value, the procedure therefore being considered conservative. An additional conservative feature involves use of the upper 99% confidence limit of the proportion responding at a dose level, rather than the observed proportion. The procedure then extrapolates downward to a response level of 10^{-8}, using each separate dose level in the experiment, or combinations, taking as the virtually safe dose (VSD) the highest of the values obtained. A conservative method of taking account of the response of the control group was also given. An improved version of the procedure, which included several sets of independent data and better methods of handling background response rates and responses at multiple doses, has since been published (64).

A dosage D_0 is said to be virtually safe if $f(D_0) < p + (1 - p)P_0$, where P_0 is some near-zero lifetime risk, such as 10^{-8}, the value proposed by Mantel and Bryan or 10^{-6}, the value adopted by the FDA. The virtually safe-dose (VSD) is then calculated as $f^{-1}[(1 - p)P_0]$. The calculation thus requires choosing a model, f, determining the value of its disposable constants from observations in the observable range and extrapolating down to the unobservable elevation in response, P_0, to determine the VSD.

One of the advantages of the Mantel-Bryan procedure is that it rewards a larger experiment by reducing the upper confidence limit, which results in a larger dose for a selected proportion of tumor-bearing animals. Table 4 shows some dosages for a series of sample sizes; all yield observed tumor rates of 4%, with no tumors in the controls for a predicted tumor probability of less than one in a million.

Some situations, such as cigarette smoking in man and diethylstilbestrol in mice, have indicated slopes on the order of 1. Thus one must be careful to establish that the slope of the dose-response is sufficiently large before applying the Mantel-Bryan procedure, indicating the desirability of multiple-dose experiments.

Table 4 Mantel-Bryan Dosages for Various Sample Sizes with the
Same Proportion of Experimental Animals with Tumors*

Sample size	No. of animals with tumors	Upper 99% confidence limit	Dosage (fraction of experimental dosage)
50	2	0.158	1/5630
100	4	0.112	1/3430
200	8	0.085	1/2400
400	16	0.069	1/1860

*Predicted tumor probability $<10^{-6}$.

According to Mantel and Schneiderman (38), the Mantel-Bryan methodology has several advantages:

1. It does not need an experimental estimate of the slope.
2. Statistical significance is not needed.
3. It takes into account a nonzero spontaneous background tumor incidence.
4. It considers multiple-dose studies.
5. Any arbitrary acceptable risk can be calculated.
6. It avoids categorizing a substance in absolute terms.
7. It permits the investigator flexibility in study design.

Mantel and Bryan (37) provided an example of an actual study in which the carcinogen 3-methylcholanthrene was given to mice as a single injection, with 12 different dose levels used. Table 5 provides the methodology and findings of the Mantel-Bryan procedure.

Some criticisms of the Mantel Bryan procedure are:

1. The normal distribution may not offer as accurate a description in the tails of the distribution as it does in the central parts, especially if one proceeds out to 10^{-6} or 10^{-8}.
2. The use of the arbitrarily low slope of unity for downward extrapolation has been criticized because of the lack of observational support.
3. The argument does not incorporate any of the present understandings of the process of carcinogenesis.
4. The model is insufficiently conservative, because the extrapolated probability approaches zero with decreasing dose more rapidly than any polynomial function of dose, and, in particular, more rapidly than a linear function of dose and hence may underestimate probability at low dose (65).

Table 5 Illustration of Methodology for Determining the "Safe" Dose from Results at Several Dose Levels

Dose per mouse (mg)	Log dose	Result no. of tumors no. of mice	Combined result no. of tumors no. of mice	Maximum P value 99% assurance	Corresponding normal deviate	Calculated "safe" (1/100 million) Log dose (2)−(6) −5.612
(1)	(2)	(3)	(4)	(5)	(6)	(7)
0.000244	6.388-10	0/79	0/158	0.0288	−1.899	2.675-10
0.000975	6.990-10	0/41	0/79	0.0566	−1.584	2.962-10
0.00195	7.291-10	0/19	0/38	0.1141	−1.205	2.884-10
0.0039	7.592-10	0/19	0/19	0.2152	−0.789	2.769-10
0.0078	7.893-10	3/17	3/17	0.480	−0.050	2.331-10
0.0156	8.194-10	6/18	6/18	0.729	+0.610	1.972-10
0.0312	8.495-10	13/20	13/20	0.871	+1.131	1.752-10
0.0625	8.796-10	17/21	17/21	0.958	+1.728	1.456-10
0.125	9.097-10	21/21	—	—	—	—
0.25	9.398-10	21/21	—	—	—	—
0.50	9.699-10	21/21	—	—	—	—
1.0	10.000-10	20/20	—	—	—	—

Source: From Ref. 37.

5. The model is excessively conservative, because it does not postulate a threshold or accommodate time to tumor data.

Multistage. The multistage model (39,66) represents a generalization of the one-hit model and assumes that the carcinogenic process is composed of an unknown number of stages that are needed for cancer expression. Inherent in this model is the additional assumption that the effect of the carcinogenic agent in question is additive to a carcinogenic effect produced by external stimuli at the same stages. Such an assumption generally leads one to expect a linear dose–response curve at low exposure levels.

This assumes that carcinogenesis occurs in a single cell as a point of origin and, according to the multistage model, is the result of several stages that can include somatic mutation. The transitional events are individually assumed to depend linearly on dose rate. This then leads in general to a model in which the probability of tumor approximates a low-order polynomial in dose rate. In the low dose region, which would relate to environmental levels, one find that the responses are well approximated by a linear function of dose rate. The characteristic in which the low dose probability is proportional to the kth power of dose, where k is the number of stages, was considered by Armitage and Doll (1961) to be quite inconsistent with observation. They derived a multistage model, which by assuming that the effect of the agent at some stages was additive to an effect induced by external stimuli at those stages, led to a lower power than k for D. Crump, et al. (39) discussed this model and, by assuming additivity at all stages, have obtained as an expression for the required probability

$$P(D) = 1 - \exp\left\{ -\sigma \sum_{i=0}^{\alpha} \alpha_i D^i \right\} \quad \alpha_i \geq 0$$

where $\alpha = -\mu/\sigma$. Hartley and Sielken (67) combined this model with time to response, obtaining a more general result. For $\alpha_1 > 0$ these models also imply low dose linearity since

$$\lim_{D \to O} P'(D) = \alpha_1 \exp(-\alpha_0)$$

Armitage and Doll cited data relating lung cancer mortality to previous smoking habits as indicating to a linear dose–response curve, but errors in reporting the amount smoked would lead to such a curve even if the true curve were convex. This supports the view that the apparent low-dose linearity in many epidemiologic studies is an artifact of errors in the reporting of dose. Crump et al. (39) stress the crucial nature of the additivity assumption, pointing out that it can make orders of magnitude differences in the estimated risk associated with the low dose exposure.

Crump (68) describes a procedure for low-dose extrapolation in the presence of background which, although based on the generalized model above, reduces (when upper confidence limits are used) to extrapolation using low-dose linearity. This is because the use of upper confidence limits on χ_1 on the model is equivalent to admitting the possibility of a positive value of χ_1, which at lose doses dominates the expression. Once upper confidence limits on the VSD or risk at a given dose are used, there may be little practical difference, therefore, between use of the one-hit model and the generalization given by the Crump et al., (39) equation above.

Hartley and Sielken (67) have developed a procedure based on maximum likelihood for the Armitage-Doll model. Their program is very general and allows for the inclusion of the effect of the time to a tumor.

In practice, these two approaches result in fitting a polynomial model to the dose response curve such that (where t is time):

$$\frac{p(D),t)}{1 - P(D,t)} = gDh(t)$$

where $P(D,t)$ is the probability of the observance of a tumor in an animal by time t at a dosage D,

$$p(D,t) = \frac{DP(D,t)}{Dt}$$

where $g\ (D)$ is a function of dose such that

$$g(\text{dose}) = (a_1 + b_1\ \text{dose})\ (a_2 + b_2\ \text{dose})\cdots$$
$$(a_n + b_n\ \text{dose})$$
$$= c_0 + c_1\ \text{dose} + c_2\ \text{dose}^2 + \cdots$$
$$+ c_n\ \text{dose}^n,$$

where a_i, b_i, $c_i \geq 0$ are parameters that vary from chemical to chemical and $h(t)$ is a function of time. The probability of a tumor by time t and dosage D is

$$P(D,t) = 1 - \exp\left[-g(D)\ H(t)\right]$$

where

$$H(t) = \int_0^t h(t)\ Dt$$

This function generally fits well in the experimental data range but has limited applicability to the estimation of potential risk at low doses. The limitations arise, first, because the model cannot reflect changes in kinetics, metabolism, and mechanisms at low doses and, second, because low dose estimates are highly sensitive to a change of even a few observed tumors at the lowest experimental dose.

A logical statistical approach to account for the random variation in tumor frequencies is to express the results in terms of best estimates and measures of uncertainty.

Important biological mechanisms of activation and detoxification are not usually specifically considered. However, a steady-state kinetic model that incorporates the process of deactivation as well as other pharmacokinetic considerations has been offered by Cornfield (69). He noted that whenever the detoxification response is irreversible, low exposure levels are predicted to be harmless. However, the presence of a reversible response suggests linearity at low-dose exposures. He additionally predicted that when multiple protective responses are sequentially operational, the dose–response relationship will look like a hockey stick "with the striking part flat or nearly flat and the handle rising steeply once the protective mechanisms are saturated." Despite its seemingly greater biological veracity, the Food Safety Council (70) challenged the multistage model general assumption of low-dose linearity on the basis of 1) the general absence of support for dose-wise additivity seen in many studies in which additivity has been evaluated and 2) studies that showed the effects of one carcinogenic agent offset or prevented the carcinogenic effects of another.

Crump (68) has noted that biostatistical models such as the multistage model assume that the quantity of carcinogen finding its way to the critical sites is proportional to the total body exposure, which is clearly not the case across the entire dose range covered by the model.

Criticism of these models are summarized below.

These models do not consider the variation in susceptibility of the members of the population when deriving their dose–response relationships.

Low-dose linearity is not consistently found in experimental systems.

Low-dose linearity is assumed to occur by a mechanism of additivity to background levels; however, there is a lack of data supporting the additivity hypothesis.

They do not sufficiently recognize pharmacokinetic considerations including rates of absorption, tissue distribution, detoxification processes, repair, and excretion. (This would apply to the Mental-Bryan model as well.)

Multihit. This model is also called the K-hit or gamma multihit model. It is a generalization of the one-hit model.

If k hits of a receptor are required to induce cancer, the probability of a tumor as a function of exposure to a dose (D) is given by

$$P(D) = 1 - \sum_{i=0}^{k-1} \frac{(\lambda D)^i e^{-\gamma D}}{i!} \approx \frac{(\gamma D)^k}{k!}$$

For small values of D, the k-hit model may be approximated by

$$P(D) = \gamma D^k$$

or

$$\log P(D) = \log \gamma + k \log D$$

Thus K represents the slope of $\log P(D)$ versus $\log D$. By the same reasoning, if at least k hits are required for a response, then

$$P(D) = P(X \geq k) = \frac{\int_0^{\lambda D} u^{k-\tau} e^{-u} du}{(k-1)!}$$

Because this equation contains an additional parameter, k, it will ordinarily provide a better description of dose–response data than the one-parameter curve. This can be further generalized by allowing k to be any positive number, not necessarily an integer. In this case the above formula can be described as that dose–response curve that assumes a gamma distribution of tolerances with shape parameter k. We note

$$\lim_{D \to 0} [P(D)/D^k] = \text{constant.}$$

Thus, in the low-dose region, the equation is linear for $k = 1$, concave for $k < 1$ and convex for $k > 1$. At higher doses the gamma and the lognormal distributions are hard to distinguish so that the model provides a blend of the probit model at high dose levels and the logit at low ones.

Procedures for estimating the parameters of the k-hit model by nonlinear maximum likelihood estimation have been developed by Rai and Van Ryzin (71). This method has the advantage of permitting the data to determine the number of hits needed to describe the results without introducing more than two parameters. When only one dose level gives responses greater than zero and less than 100%, unique values of the two parameters can no longer be estimated. The background effect in this model is taken care of using Abbott's correction.

The multihit model is discussed in some detail in the Food Safety Council Report (70). One derivation of this model follows from the assumption that k hits or molecular interactions are necessary to induce the formation of a tumor and the distribution of these molecular events over time follows a Poisson process. In practice the model appears to fit some data sets reasonably well and to give low-dose predictions that are similar to the other models. There are cases, however, in which the predicted values are inconsistent with the predictions of other models by many orders of magnitude. For instance, the virtually safe dose as predicted by the multihit model appears to be too high for nitrolotriacetic acid and far too low for vinyl chloride (70).

Pharmacokinetic Models. Pharmacokinetic models have often been used to predict the concentration of the parent compound and metabolites in the blood and at reactive sites, if identifiable. Cornfield (69), Gehring and Blau (45), and Anderson, Hoel, and Kaplan (131) have extended this concept to include rates for macromolecular events (e.g., DNA damage and repair) involved in the carcinogenic process. The addition of statistical distributions for the rate parameters and a stochastic component representing the probabilistic nature of molecular events and selection processes may represent a useful conceptual framework for describing the tumorigenic mechanism of many chemicals. Pharmacokinetic data are presently useful only in specific parts of the risk assessment process. A more complete understanding of the mechanism of chemically induced carcinogenesis would allow a more complete utilization of pharmacokinetic data. Pharmacokinetic comparisons between animals and humans are presently most useful for making species conversions and for understanding qualitative and quantitative species differences. The modeling of blood concentrations and metabolite concentrations identifies the existence of saturated pathways and adds to an understanding of the mechanism of toxicity in many cases.

Taking advantage of the similarity of the probit and pharmacokinetic models in the 5% to 95% range, Cornfield (69) developed an approximate method of estimating its parameters, particularly the value of T, the saturation dose. Risks at dosages below T are crucially dependent on K^*, the relative speed of the reverse, deactivation reaction. This cannot be well estimated from responses at dosages above T. Low-dose assessment using this model may be more dependent on further pharmacokinetic experimentation than on further statistical developments.

This model considers an agent subjected to simultaneous activation and deactivation reactions, both reversible, with the probability of a response being proportional (linearly related) to the amount of active complex. Denoting total amount of substrate in the system by S and deactivating agent by T and the ratios of the rate constants governing the back and forward reactions by K for the activation step and K^* for the deactivation step, the model is, for $D > T$

$$(D) = \frac{D - S[p(D)] - y}{D - S[P(D)] - y + K}$$

where $y = [P(D)]T/\{K\,[P(D)] + K^*\,[1 - P(D)]\}$ and for $D < T$

$$(D) \cong \frac{D}{S + K\left[1 + \dfrac{T}{K}\right]}$$

These equations follow from standard steady state mass action equations. Thus, at low dose levels, $D < T$, the dose–response curve is nearly linear, but for deactivating reactions in which the rate of the back reaction is small compared to that of the forward reaction, the value of K^* will be quite small and the slope will be near zero. In fact, in the limiting case in which $K^* = 0$ the dose–response curve has a threshold at $D = T$, but since the model is steady state and does not depend on the time course of the reaction, it cannot be considered to have established the existence of a threshold. For $K^* > 0$, the dose–response curve is shaped like a hockey stick with the striking part nearly flat and rising sharply once the administered dose exceeds the dose, T, which saturated the system. Because of the great sensitivity of the slope at low doses to the value of K^*/K, and insensitivity at high doses, responses at dose levels above $D = T$ probably cannot be used to predict those below T. This can be considered a limitation of the model, but it can equally well be considered a limitation of high dose experimentation in the absence of detailed pharmacokinetic knowledge of metabolic pathways. The model can be generalized to cover a chain of simultaneous activating and deactivating reactions intervening between the introduction of D and the formation of activated complex, but this does not appear to change its qualitative characteristics. The kinetic constants, S, T, K, and K^* are presumably subject to animal-to-animal variation. This variation is not formally incorporated in the model, so that the possibility of negative estimates of one or more of these constants cannot be excluded.

Weibull. Another generalization of the one-hit model is the Weibull model:

$$(D) = 1 - \exp(\alpha - \beta D^m),$$

where m and β are parameters. Note that

$$\lim \mid [P(D)/D^m =] = \text{constant}$$

as the dose approaches zero.

Thus, in the low-dose region, this last equation is linear for $m = 1$, concave for $m < 1$, and convex for $m > 1$. With a typical set of data, the Weibull model tends to give an estimated risk at a low dose which lies between the estimates for the gamma multi-hit and the Armitage-Doll models. The Weibull distribution for time-to-tumors has been suggested by human cancers (72,73);

$$I = bD^m (t - w)^k$$

where I is the incidence rate of tumors at time t, b is a constant depending on experimental conditions, D is dosage, w the minimum time to the occurrence of an observable tumor, m and k are parameters to be estimated. Also, Day (74), Peto et al. (75), and Peto and Lee (76) have considered the Weibull distribution for time-to-tumor occurrence. Theoretical models of carcinogenesis also predict the Weibull distribution (77). Theoretical arguments and some experimental data suggest the Weibull distribution where tumor incidence is a polynomial in dose multiplied by a function of age. Hartley and Sielken (67) adopted the form

$$(t) = \sum_{i=1} \xi_i t^i$$

where $\xi_i \geq 0$. They noted that this function regarded as a weighted average of Weibull hazard rates with positive weight coefficients, ξ_i. The conventional statistical procedure of weighted least-squares provides one method of fitting the Weibull model to a set of data. With a background response measured by the parameter p, the model, using Abbott's correction is:

$$P = p + (1 - p)(1 - \exp(-\beta D^m)) =$$
$$1 - \exp(-(\alpha + \beta D^m)),$$

where $\alpha + \beta D^m$

With a nonlinear weighted least-squares regression program, one can estimate the three parameters (m, α, β) directly. With only a linear weighted least-squares regression program, one can use trial and error on m to find the values of the three parameters that produce a minimum error sum of squares.

A nonlinear maximum likelihood method to obtain estimates of the parameters in the Weibull model can also be used. The use of the Weibull distribution for time-to-tumor leads to an extreme value distribution relating tumor response to dosage (62). Hoel (78) gives techniques for cases in which adjustments must be made for competing causes of death.

Logit. This model, like the probit model, leads to an S-shaped dose–response curve, symmetric about the 50% response point. Its equation (79) is:

$$P(D) = 1/[1 + \exp\{-(\alpha + \beta \log D)\}]$$

It approaches zero response as D decreases more slowly than the probit curve, since

$$\lim \ |\ [P(D)/D^\beta] = K$$

as dose approaches zero, where K is a constant.

The practical implication of this characteristic is that the logit model leads to lower VSD than the probit model, 1/25th as much in calculations reported by Cornfield et al. (80), even when both models are equally descriptive of the data in the observable range.

Albert and Altshuler (81) have developed a related model for predicting tumor incidence and life shortening based on the work of Blum (82) on skin tumor response and on Druckrey (63) for a variety of chemical carcinogens in rodents. They had investigated cancer in mice exposed to radium. The basic relationship used was $D_t^n = c$, where Di is dosage, t is the median time to occurrence of tumors, n is a parameter greater than I, and c is a constant depending on the given experimental conditions. It is of interest to determine the time it takes for a small proportion of the population to develop tumors. With this formulation, as the dosage is increased, the time to tumor occurrence is shortened. Albert and Altshuler (81) used the log normal distribution to represent time-to-tumor occurrence, assuming the standard deviation to be independent of dosage.

The log normal distribution of tumor times corresponds closely to the probit transformation as employed in the mantel-Bryan procedure.

Log-Probit. The log-probit model assumes that the individual tolerances follow a lognormal distribution. Specific steps in the complex chain of events that lead to carcinogenesis are likely to have lognormal distributions. For example, it is reasonable to assume that the distribution of a population of kinetic rate constants for detoxification, metabolism, elimination, in addition to the distribution of immunosuppression surveillance capacity and DNA repair capacity, can be adequately approximated by normal or lognormal distributions.

Tolerance distribution models have been found to adequately model many types of biological dose–response data, but it is an overly simplistic expectation to represent the entire carcinogenic process by one tolerance distribution. A tolerance distribution model may give a good description of the observed data, but from a mechanistic point of view there is no reason to expect extrapolation to be valid. The probit model extrapolation has, however, fit well in some instances.

The log-probit model has been used extensively in the bioassay of dichotomous responses (83). A distinguishing feature of this model is that it assumes that each animal has its own threshold dose below which no response occurs and above which a tumor is produced by exposure to a chemical. An animal population has a range of thresholds encompassing the individual thresholds. The log-probit model assumes that the distribution of log dose thresholds is normal. This model states that there are relatively few extremely sensitive or extremely resistant animals in a population. For the log-probit model, the probability of a tumor induced by an exposure to a dose D of a chemical is given by

$$P(D) = \Phi \left(\alpha + \beta \log_{10} D \right)$$

where Φ denotes the standard cumulative Gaussian (normal) distribution. Chand and Hoel (62) showed that the log-probit dose response is obtained when the time-to-tumor distribution is log normal under certain conditions.

Miscellaneous. There are a large number of other proposed models for low dose extrapolation, through these others have not gained any large following. Two examples of these are the extreme value and no-effect-level models.

Chand and Hoel (62) showed that if the time-to-tumor distribution is a Weibull distribution, the dose-response model follows an extreme value model under certain conditions, with

$$P (D) = 1 - \exp [- \exp (\alpha + \beta \log D)]$$

Park and Snee (132) made the observation that many biological responses vary linearly with the logarithm of dose and that practical thresholds exist; therefore the responses can be represented by the following model:

Response = B_1 if dose, D^*
Response = $B_1 + B_2$ log (dose/D^*)   if dose $\geq D^*$

This model incorporates a parameter D^* that represents a threshold below which no dose-related response occurs. In this model, B_1 is the constant response level at doses less than D^*, and B_2 is the slope of the log-dose response curve at doses $\geq D^*$. It has been empirically found that many quantitative toxicological end points can be adequately described by the no-effect-level model. This model may, therefore, be useful for establishing thresholds for end points related to the carcinogenic process in situations where information other than the simple presence or absence of a tumor is available. Both the model and predicted threshold are of value when carcinogenicity is a secondary event.

A. Critique and Comparison of Models

None of the models presented here (or any others) can be "proved" on the basis of biological arguments or available experimental data, but some are more attractive than others on these grounds. The multistage model appears to be the most general model according to the values of the parameters. Unfortunately, most of these models fit experimental data equally well for the observable response rates at experimental dosage levels, but they give quite different estimated responses when extrapolated to low dosage levels. There are now numerous sets of data that have been used to compare two or more of the models against each other.

In 1971, the FDA Advisory Committee on Protocols for Safety Evaluation compared three models (probit, logit, and one-hit) using the data presented in Table 6. It should be clear that with any adequately designed and executed study, these three sets of results are indistinguishable. But in Table 7 the extrapolated doses needed to achieve certain incidences of response in a population are presented. They are seen to give values varying by as much as four orders of magnitude.

Table 8 attempts to summarize the major characteristics of the eight models presented here in terms of their operating characteristics. The performance of each model in any one particular case is dependent on the nature of the observed dose-response curve. All fit true linear data well, but respond differently to concave or convex response curves. The actual choice of model must depend on what information is available and on the professional judgment of the investigator. The authors believe that to attempt to use any purely mathemat-

Table 6 Experimentally Determined Actual
Incidences (%) of Animals with Tumor of Interest

Dose	Probit	Logit	One-hit
2	69	70	75
1	50	50	50
0.5	31	30	29
0.25	16	16	16
0.125	7	8	8
0.0625	2	4	4

ical model is wrong—that an understanding of the pharmacokinetics and mechanisms of toxicity across the dose range is an essential step in the risk assessment
of carcinogens. Any mathematical model must utilize such data, and as there is
now significant evidence that many of these actual response curves are multi-
phasic, only models that can accommodate such nonlinear response surfaces
have a chance of being useful.

B. Cross-Species Extrapolation

Tomatis (84) has provided an excellent evaluation of the comparability of carcinogenicity findings between rodents and man, in general finding the former to
be good predictors of the end point in the latter. However, in his 1984 Stokinger
lecture, Weil (85) pointed out that the model species should respond biologically
to the material as similarly as possible to man; that the routes of exposure (actual
and possible) should be the same; and that there are known wide variations in
response to carcinogens. Diechmann (86), for example, has reviewed studies
demonstrating that 2-naphthylamine is a human and dog carcinogen, but not
active in the mouse, rat, guinea pig, or rabbit.

Smith (87) discussed interspecies variations of response to carcinogens,
including N-2-fluorenyl-acetamide, which is potent for the dog, rabbit, hamster
and rat (believed to be due to formation of an active metabolite by N-hydroxyla-

Table 7 Extrapolated Doses for Low Incidences of Tumors

Incidence of animals with tumors	Probit	Units of dose Logit	One-hit
10^{-3}	1.5×10^{-2}	3.1×10^{-3}	1.4×10^{-3}
10^{-6}	1.4×10^{-3}	9.8×10^{-6}	1.4×10^{-6}
10^{-8}	4.1×10^{-4}	1.6×10^{-7}	1.4×10^{-8}

Table 8 Characteristics and Requirements for Use of Major Low Dose Extrapolation Models

	Low dose linearity	Extrapolates low dose levels	Estimates virtual safe dose	Mechanistic or tolerance distribution	Requires metabolic data	Accommo-dates threshold	Takes time-to-tumor into account	Estimate of potential risk of low doses
One-hit (Linear)	X	X	X	M				Highest
Multistage (Armitage-Doll)	X	X	X	M				High
Weibull (Chand and Hoel)	X		X	T		X	X	High
Multi-hit	X	X	X	M				Medium
Logit (Albert and Altshuler)	X		X	T		X	X	Medium
Probit (Mantel-Bryan)	X		X	T				Medium
Log-Probit (Gehring et al.)		X	X	M	X	X	X	Low
Pharmacokinetic (Cornfield)		X	X	M	X	X	X	Lowest

tion), but not in the guinea pig or steppe lemming, which do not form this metabolic derivative.

Table 9 represents an overview of the classes of factors that should be considered in the first step of a species extrapolation. Examples of such actual differences are almost endless.

The absorption of compounds from the gastrointestinal tract and from the lungs is comparable among vertebrate and mammalian species. There are, however, differences between herbivorous animals and omnivorous animals due to differences in stomach structure. The problem of distribution within the body probably relates less to species than to size, and will be discussed later under scaling. Metabolism, xenobiotic metabolism of foreign compounds, metabolic activation, or toxification/detoxification mechanisms (by whatever name) is perhaps the critical factor, and this can differ widely from species to species. The increasing realization that the original compound administered is not necessarily the ultimate carcinogen makes the further study of these metabolic patterns critical.

In terms of excretory rates, the differences between the species are not very great; small animals tend to excrete compounds more rapidly than large ones in a rather systematic way. The various cellular and intercellular barriers

Table 9 Classes of Factors to Be Considered in Species-to-Species Extrapolations in Risk Assessment

Sensitivity of model animal (relative to humans)	Relative population differences	Differences between test and real world environment
pharmacologic	size	physical (temperature, humidity, etc.)
receptor	heterogeneity	
life span	selected "high class" nature of test population	chemical
size		nutritional
metabolic function		
physiological		
anatomic		
nutritional requirements		
reproductive and developmental processes		
diet		
critical reflex and behavioral responses (as emetic reflex)		
behavioral		
rate of cell division		
other defense mechanisms		

seem to be surprisingly constant throughout the vertebrate phylum. In addition, it is beginning to be appreciated that the receptors, such as DNS, are comparable throughout the mammalian species.

There are lifespan (or temporal) differences that have not been considered adequately, either now or in the past. It takes time to develop a tumor, and at least some of that time may be taken up by the actual cell division process. Cell division rates appear to be significantly higher in smaller animals. Mouse and rat cells turn over faster (perhaps at twice the rate) than human cells. On the other hand, the latent period for development of tumors is much shorter in small animals than in large ones (88).

Another problem is that the lifespan of man is about 35 times that of the mouse or rat; thus there is a much longer time for a tumor to appear. These sorts of temporal considerations are of considerable importance.

Body size, irrespective of species, seems to be important in the rate of distribution of foreign compounds throughout the body. A simple example of this is that the cardiac output of the mouse is on the order of 1 mL/minute, and the mouse has a blood volume of about 1 mL. The mouse is turning its blood volume over every minute. In man, the cardiac output per minute is only 1/20 of its blood volume. So the mouse turns its blood over and distributes whatever is in the blood or collects excretory products over 20 times faster than man.

Another aspect of the size difference which should be considered is that the large animal has a very much greater number of susceptible cells that may interact with potential carcinogenic agents, though there is also a proportionately increased number of "dummy" cells.

Rall (89,90) and Borzelleca (91) have published articles reviewing such factors and Calabrese (42) and Gad and Chengelis (92) have published excellent books on the subject.

Having delineated and quantified species differences (even if only having factored in comparative body weights and food consumption rates), we can now proceed to some form of quantitative extrapolation. This process is called scaling.

There are currently three major approaches to scaling in risk assessment. These are by fraction of diet, by body weight, and by body surface area (42,93).

The by "fraction-of-diet" method is based on converting the results in the experimental animal model to man on a mg (of test substance)/kg (diet)/day basis. When the experimental model is the mouse, this leads to an extrapolation factor that is 6-fold lower than on a body weight (mg/kg) basis (94). Fraction-of-diet factors are not considered accurate indices of actual dosages since the latter are influenced not only by voluntary food intake, as affected by palatability and caloric density of the diet and by single or multiple caging, but more particularly by the age of the animal. During the early stages of life, anatomic, physiologic, metabolic and immunologic capabilities are not fully developed.

Moreover, the potential for toxic effect in an animal is a function of the dose ingested, ultimately, of the number of active molecules reaching the target cell. Additionally, many agents of concern do not have ingestion as the major route of intake in man. Both the Environmental Protection Agency (EPA) and the Consumer Product Safety Commission (CPSC) frequently employ a fraction-of-diet scaling factor.

Human diets are generally assumed to be 600–700 g/day, while that in mice is 4 g/day and in rats 25 g/day (the equivalent of 50 g/kg/day).

There are several ways to perform a scaling operation on a body weight basis. The most common is to simply calculate a conversion factor (K) as

$$\frac{\text{Weight of human (70 kg)}}{\text{Weight of test animal (0.4 kg for rat)}} = K$$

More exotic methods for doing this, such as that based on a form of linear regression, are reviewed by Calabrese (1983), who believes that the body weight method is preferable.

A difficulty with this approach is that the body weights of both animals and man change throughout life. And "ideal man" or "ideal rat" weight is therefore utilized.

Finally, there are the body surface area methods, which attempt to factor in differences in metabolic rates based on the principle that these change in proportion with body surface area (since as the ratio of body surface area to body weight increases, the more energy is required to maintain constant body temperature). There are several methods for doing this, each having a ratio of dose to the animal's body weight (in mg/kg) as a starting point, resulting in a conversion factor with mg/m^2 as the units.

The EPA version is generally calculated as:

$(M_{\text{human}}/M_{\text{animal}})^{1/3}$ – surface factor

where M = mass in kilograms. Another form is calculated based on constants that have been developed for a multitude of species of animals by actual surface area measurements (95). The resulting formula for this is:

$A = KW^{2/3}$

where A = surface area in cm^2

K = constant, specific for each species

and W = weight in grams

A scaling factor is then simply calculated as a ratio of the surface area of man over that of the model species.

The "best" scaling factor is not generally agreed upon. Though the majority opinion is that surface area is preferable where a metabolic activation or deactivation is known to be both critical to the risk producing process and present in both the model species and man, these assumptions may not always be valid. Table 10 presents a comparison of the weight and surface area extrapolation methods for eight species. Schneiderman et al. (96) and Dixon (97) have published comparisons of these methods, but Schmidt-Nielsen (93) should be considered the primary source on scaling in interspecies comparisons.

C. Susceptibility Factors

Of increasing concern in recent years is the realization that not all exposed populations are equally at risk. While experimental data in animals is primarily generated using health young adult animals, these are not necessarily representative of the entire populations that are exposed.

In particular, children, the elderly, and individuals with compromised health should at least be considered in exposure and risk assessments. Such populations may have greater degrees of susceptibility due to a range of factors (98,99).

VIII. BENCHMARK DOSE APPROACH

The entire process of risk assessment as discussed to this point is applicable not just to carcinogens, but also to the other classes of toxic agents that result in

Table 10 Extrapolation of a Dose of 100 mg/kg in the Mouse to Other Species

| | | | Extrapolated dose (mg) | | |
| | Weight | Surface area* | Body weight (A) | Body surface area (B) | Ratio A/B |
Species	(grams)	(sq. cm.)			
Mouse	20	46.4	2	2	1.0
Rat	400	516.7	40	22.3	1.79
Guinea Pig	400	564.5	40	24.3	1.65
Rabbit	1500	1272.0	150	54.8	2.74
Dog	12000	5766.0	1200	248.5	4.83
Cat	2000	1381.0	200	59.5	3.46
Monkey	4000	2975.0	400	128.2	3.12
Human	70000	18000.0	7000	775.8	9.02

*Surface area (except in case of man) calculated from formula: Surface Area $(cm^2) - K(W^{2/3})$ where K is a constant for each species and W is body weight (values of K and surface area of man taken from Spector, 1956).

some form of irreversible harm. The only difference is that the concept of a threshold dose level below which no ill effects are evoked is accepted for most of these other classes (the exception being mutagens) (100).

In recent years, a new approach has been proposed by regulatory representatives for the assessment of risk of quantal endpoints in addition to carcinogenicity (128). Initially the focus was on developmental toxicity (101,102,103), but the proposals have now expanded to include reproductive and neurotoxicants (104). This approach has been labeled the "Benchmark Dose."

Common abbreviations used in such discussions include:

BMD	Benchmark dose
BMD/D	Benchmark dose/concentration
BMR	Benchmark response
ED_{10}	Effective dose (10% response)
LED_{10}	Lower bound on dose (ED_{10})
MLE	Maximum likelihood estimate
NOAEL	No observed adverse effect level
LOAEL	Lowest observed adverse effect level
RfD	Reference dose

Currently, human exposure guidelines for developmental toxicants are based on the no observed adverse effect level (NOAEL) derived from laboratory studies. A NOAEL is defined as the highest experimental dose that fails to induce a significant increase in risk in comparison with the unexposed controls. A reference dose or reference concentration (RfD or RfC) is then obtained by dividing the NOAEL by a suitable uncertainty factor (UF) allowing for difference in susceptibility between animals and humans (105,106). The resulting RfD is then used as a guideline for human exposure (107). Guidelines on the magnitude of the UF to be used in specific cases have been discussed by Barnes and Dourson (108). Current U.S. Environmental Protection Agency uncertainty factors can be found in Table 11.

Table 11 U.S. EPA Guidelines for Uncertainty Factors

Guidelines		Factors
Adult $\longrightarrow$	Child	$\leq 10\times$
Average $\longrightarrow$	Sensitive human	$\leq 10\times$
Animal $\longrightarrow$	Human	$\leq 10\times$
LOAEL $\longrightarrow$	NOAEL	$\leq 10\times$
Database inadequacies		$\leq 10\times$
Subchronic $\longrightarrow$	Chronic	$\leq 10\times$
Modifying factors		$0–10\times$

The NOAEL, restricted in value to one of the experimental doses, fails to properly take sample size into account (smaller and less sensitive experiments lead to higher NOAELs than larger studies), and largely ignores the shape of the dose–response curve. The risk associated with doses at or above the NOAEL is not made explicit. However, Gaylor (109) has shown, for a series of 120 developmental toxicity experiments, that the observed risk exceeds 1% in about one-fourth of the cases. Based on the statistical properties of the NOAELs, it has also been found that the NOAEL may identify a dose level associated with unacceptably high risk with a reasonably high probability. Because of the limitations associated with the use of the NOAEL (110,111,112), the EPA (113) is considering the use of the benchmark dose (BMD) method, proposed by Crump (114), as the basis for deriving the RfD for developmental toxicity (108).

The BMD is generally defined as the lower confidence limit (114,115,116) of the effective dose, d_α, that induces α-percent increase in risk (ED$_\alpha$). Although the α-percent increase in risk may refer to the excessive risk $\pi(0) = \alpha$, or relative risk $[\pi(d_\alpha) - \pi(o)]/[1 - \pi(0)] = \alpha$, the latter takes into account the background risk in the absence of exposure, and is more sensitive to high spontaneous risk. If the background risk is $\pi(0) = 0$, then the two measures of risk are equivalent. It can be shown that the relative risk also has additional mathematical properties that facilitate computation and interpretation. The ED$_\alpha$ may be defined as the solution to the equation

$$\frac{\pi(d_\alpha) - \pi(0)}{1 - \pi(0)} = \alpha$$

where $\pi(d)$ represents an appropriate dose-response model for a particular endpoint. Crump (114) discussed the estimating of BMD based on dose-response model for a single endpoint. Allen et al. (117,118) estimated the BMDs using several dose-response models fitted to data from a large database. They found that the BMDs at 5% level are similar to NOAEL in magnitude on the average. Ryan (119) and Krewski and Zhu (120) used joint dose–response models to estimate the BMDs. A summary of such models is presented in Table 12.

Table 12 Models Used in the Study of BMD Approaches for Developmental Toxicity

RVR	$P(d,s) - [1 - esp \quad \{-(\alpha + \beta(d - d_0)^w)\}] * exp\{-s(\theta_1 + \theta_2(d - d0))\}$
NCTR	$P(d,s) = 1 - exp\{-[(\alpha \times \theta_1 s) + (\beta + \theta_2 s)(d - d_0)^w]\}$
Log-Logistic	$P(d,s) = \alpha + \theta_1 s + [1 - \alpha - \theta_1 s]/[1 + exp(\beta + \theta_2 s - \Gamma log(d - d_0)\}]$

Under the Weibull models for either the incidence of prenatal death or the incidence of fetal malformation, the ED_α is given by

$$d_\alpha = \left(\frac{-\log(1-\alpha)}{b} \right)^{1/\gamma}$$

where the subscript k ($k-1,2$) for the parameters (b_k, γ_k) is suppressed for simplicity of notation. Note that the d_α is obtained by evaluating the above equation at ($\hat{d}$, $\hat{\gamma}$). The variance of $\hat{d}_\alpha$ can be approximated by

$$\text{Var}(\hat{d}_\alpha) = \gamma^{-2} d_\alpha^2 C_1^T \Omega_1 C_1$$

using the δ-method, with the unknown parameters involved replaced by ($\hat{b}$, $\hat{\gamma}$). Here, Ω_1 is the covariance matrix for the estimates ($\hat{b}$, $\hat{\gamma}$)^T and

$$C_1 = (b^{-1}, \gamma^{-1} \log\{-b^{-1} \log(1-\alpha)\})^T$$

The ED_α for overall toxicity, based on the trinomial model $\pi_3 = 1 - (1 - \pi_1)$ $(1 - \pi_2)$ is obtained as the solution to the equation

$$b_1 d^\gamma_\alpha b_2{}^\gamma_\alpha = -\log(1-\alpha)$$

The variance of $\hat{d}_\alpha$ based on the δ-method is given by

$$VAR(\hat{d}_\alpha) = \left[b_{1\gamma1} d_\alpha^{\gamma 1 - 1} + b_{2\gamma2} d_\alpha^{\gamma 2 - 1} \right]^{-2} C_2^T \Omega_2 C_2,$$

where Ω_2 is the covariance matrix of the estimates ($\hat{b}_1$, $\hat{\gamma}_1$, $\hat{b}_2$, $\hat{\gamma}_2$)^T and

$$C_2 = (d_\alpha^{\gamma 1}, b_1 d_0^{\gamma 1} \log d_\alpha, d_\alpha^{\gamma 2}, b_2 d_\alpha^{\gamma 2} \log d_\alpha)^T$$

Since the variance estimates based on the δ-method depend on the dose–response models and the estimates of the unknown parameters, alternative methods, such as those based on likelihood ratio (121) for obtaining confidence limits of ED_α may be used.

The ED_α for overall toxicity derived from the multivariate model $\pi_3 = 1 - (1 - \pi_1)(1 - \pi_2)$ is a more sensitive indicator of developmental toxicity than those for fetal malformation and prenatal death, in that the former is always below the minimum of the latter two (119,120). In the absence of a strong dose–response relationship for one of the latter two end points, the ED_α for overall toxicity approximates their minimum. The estimates of the ED_α for overall toxicity-based multivariate dose–response models for the prenatal death rate rim and fetal malformation rate y/s are generally expected to be more efficient than estimates based on the univariate models for the combined rate $(y + r)/m$ (119). In general, risk assessment that is based on multivariate dose–response models is preferred on the ground that it can simultaneously account for each individual source of risk.

The generalized score tests for trend and dose–response modeling of multiple outcomes from developmental toxicity experiments have been discussed by others (133). Conditional on the number of implants per litter, joint analyses of several outcomes are numerically more stable and statistically more efficient than separate analysis of a single outcome. The extramultinomial variation induced by the litter effects maybe characterized using a parametric covariance function, such as the extended Dirichlet-multinomial covariance. Alternatively, the Rao-Scott transformation, based on the concept of generalized design effects, may be used to allow for the approximation of the multinomial mean and covariance functions to the transformed data. Simple dose–response models, the Weibull model, for example, in conjunction with a power transformation for the dose can be used to describe the dose–response relationship in developmental toxicity data.

The method of generalized estimating equations (GEE) has been employed for model fitting (122). GEEs are not only flexible in distributional assumptions, but also computationally simpler than the maximum likelihood estimation based, for example, on the Dirichlet-multinomial distribution. The GEE estimates of the model parameter are nearly as efficient as the maximum likelihood estimates, although estimates of the dispersion parameters that are based on the quadratic estimating equations are less efficient.

Generalized score functions after local orthogonalization can be used to construct a rich class of statistics for testing increasing trends in developmental toxicity data. These generalized score functions unify many of the specific statistics previously proposed in the literature. Further investigation of the behavior of these generalized score tests under various conditions would be useful.

Joint dose–response models can be directly applied to estimate the benchmark doses in risk assessment for developmental toxicity. The BMD, based on a multivariate dose–response model for multiple endpoints, has the advantage that it simultaneously takes into account different sources of risk. For example, the BMD, based on a multivariate dose–response model for multiple end points, has the advantage that it simultaneously takes into account different sources of risk. For example, the BMD for overall toxicity is a more sensitive measure of risk in that it is less than or equal to the minimum of the BMDs for fetal malformation or prenatal death (129,130).

Both public and professional perception of the entire process leading to risk assessments of carcinogens is not good. The wide acceptance and large sales of Efron's The Apocalyptics—Cancer and The Big Lie (123), which presents a broad-based critique on the entire process surrounding our understanding of environmental carcinogenesis, is an all too telling indicator of the public's increase loss of faith. The reverses of regulatory actions on benzene and formaldehyde, in part due to the faulty nature of the risk assessments presented to support these actions, have reinforced public doubts.

Such doubts are not limited to the laity. Gio Gori, formerly a deputy director of NCI, has presented an overview and general critique (124) of the entire process from a regulatory perspective. Hickey (134), addressed the specific case of low-level radiation effects (where we have the most human data) from a statistician's point of view, pointing out that existing epidemiology data does not match EPA's risk assessment. And certainly there is no consensus within toxicology, as the contents of this chapter should make clear. The consensus within the toxicology community is clearly that a more mechanistic and pharmacokinetic based modeling process is call for. Park and Snee (83) present an excellent outline of such an approach.

IX. CONCLUSION

As scientists, we must clearly communicate the uncertainty associated with our extrapolations; to do otherwise is dishonest and only serves to abandon the job to others such as the news media. We must tell others not just what the results are, but also what they mean. Given our degree of uncertainty (with all our real data up in one small corner of the range), maybe we should evaluate and communicate the risks of chemical carcinogens in a rank order manner which would more clearly and honestly convey the quality of our "data" and understanding of its real life meanings.

Figure 1, presented at the beginning of this chapter, should serve to summarize our problem in completing this entire risk-assessment process. Our most vigorous efforts must be focused on those activities that best allow us to address these problems. Such activities should include designing better studies from the perspective of risk assessment (that is, covering a broader range of doses with an unbalanced design and selecting the doses for such studies on a knowledge of the underlying pharmacokinetics of the compound) and developing a better understanding of the underlying mechanisms on a molecular and cellular basis.

REFERENCES

1. Hass, H.B. and Newton, R.F. (1978). Correction of boiling points to standard pressure. In: CRC Handbook of Chemistry and Physics, 59th Edition. West Palm Beach, FL: CRC Press, p. D-228.
2. U.S. Environmental Protection Agency. Office of Toxic Substances. (1984). A Manual for the Preparation of Engineering Assessments. Unpublished draft, Chemical Engineering Branch, Economics and Technology Division. Washington, D.C., September 1, 1984.
3. Dugard, P.H. (1983). Skin permeability theory in relation to measurements of percutaneous absorption in toxicology. In: Dermatotoxicology, 2nd ed. F.N. Marzulli and H.I. Maibach (eds.), New York: Hemisphere Publishing Corp., Chap. 3.
4. Guy, R.H., Hadgraft, J., and Maibach, H.J. (1985). Percutaneous absorption in man: A kinetic approach. Toxicol. Appl. Pharmacol. 78:1213–1129.
5. Gale, R.M. and Shaw, J.E. (1983). Percutaneous Absorption and Pharmacokinetics. Pharmacokinetics and Topically Applied Cosmetics Symposium Proceedings CTFA Scientific Monograph Series No. 1. Washington, D.C.: CTFA, pp. 11–28.

6. Hosey, A.D. (1973). General principles in evaluating the occupational environment. In: Industrial Environment—its Evaluation and Control. USDHEW/NIOSH, Superintendent of Documents, Washington, D.C.: U.S. Government Printing Office, Chap. 10.

7. Bar-Shalom, Y., Budenaers, D., Schainker, R., and Segall, A. (1975). Handbook of Statistical Test for Evaluating Employee Exposure at Air Contaminants. USDHEW/NIOSH, Contract No. HSM 99–73-78, Superintendent of Documents, Washington, D.C.: U.S. Government Printing Office, April.

8. Davis, J.E. (1980). Minimizing occupational exposure to pesticides: Personal monitoring. Residue Rev. 75:33–50.

9. Durham, W.F. and Wolfe, H.R. (1962). Measurement of the exposure of workers to pesticides. Bull. WHO 26:75–91.

10. Wolfe, H.R. (1976). Field exposure to airborne pesticides. In: Air Pollution from Pesticides and Agricultural Processes. R.E. Lee, Jr. (ed.). Cleveland, OH: CRC Press, pp. 137–161.

11. Colle, R. and McNeil, Jr., P.E. (eds.). (1980). Radon in Buildings. Proceedings of a Roundtable Discussion, NBS SP-581, Library of Congress Catalog Card Number: 80:600069, June.

12. Handley, T.H. and Barton, C.J. (1973). Home Ventilation Rates: A Literature Survey. Atomic Energy Commission Report ORNL-TM-4318.

13. Drivas, P.J., Simmonds, P.G., and Shair, F.H. (1972). Experimental characterization of ventilation systems in buildings. Environ. Sci. Technol. Curr. Res. 6(7): 609–614.

14. Jones, B. and Harris, R.L. (1983). Calculation of time-weighted average concentrations: A computer mapping application. Am. Ind. Hyg. J. 44:795–801.

15. Franke, J.R. and Wadden, R.A. (1985). Eddy diffusivities measured inside a light industrial building, Poster #107. American Industrial Hygiene Conference, Las Vegas, Nevada, May 23, 1985.

16. Cooper, D.W. and Horowitz, M. (1986). Exposures from indoor powder releases: Models and experiments. Am. Ind. Hyg. J. 47:214–218.

17. Berman, D.W. (1982). Methods for Estimating Workplace Exposure to PMN Substances. EPA Contract No. 68-01-6065 (for the USEPA Economics and Technology Division). Arlington, VA: Clements Associates, Inc., October 5, 1982.

18. Kunkel, B.A. (1983). A comparison of evaporative source strength models for toxic chemical spills. Air Force Surveys in Geophysics, No. 446. Atmospheric Sciences Division Project 6670, Hanscom AFB, MA: Air Force Geophysics Laboratory, November 16, 1983.

19. Astelford, W.J., Morrow, T.B., Magott, R.J., Prevost, R.J., Kaplan, H.L., Bass, R.L., and Buckingham, J.C. (1983). Investigation of the Hazards Posed by Chemical Vapors Released in Marine Operations—Phase II. DOT/U.S. Coast Guard, National Technical Information Service, Springfield, VA, January, 1983.

20. Wu, J. and Schroy, J. (1979). Emissions from spills. Paper presented at conference sponsored by Air Pollution Control Association, Gainesville, Florida, February, 1979.

21. Sutton, D.J., Nodolf, K.M., and Makino, K.K. (1976). Predicting ozone concentrations in residential structures. ASHRAE J. 21–26.

22. Wade, W.A., Cote, W.A., and Yocum, J.E. (1975). A study of indoor air pollution. J. Air Pollut. Control Assoc. 25:933–939.

23. Walsh, M.A., Black, A., and Morgan, A. (1977). Sorption of S02 by typical indoor surfaces including wool carpets, wallpaper, and paint. Atmos. Environ. J. 11: 1107–1111.

24. Jayjock, M.A. (1986). Assessment of inhalation exposure and health risk from organic vapors. Paper presented at the American Industrial Hygiene Conference (AIHA), Dallas, Texas, May, 1986.

25. Schulze, R.H. (1977). Notes on Dispersion Modeling. Dallas: Trinity Consultants.

26. Turner, D.B. (1970). Workshop of Atmospheric Dispersion Estimates, U.S. EPA, 1970.

27. U.S. Department of Agriculture. (1980). The Biological and Economic Assessment of Penachlorophenol—Inorganic Arsenicals—Creosote Volume 1: Wood Preservatives. Technical Bulletin No. 1658-I, p. 78, Washington, D.C., November 4, 1980.

28. Anonymous: Draft Report-Exposure Assessment for Retention of Chemical Liquids on Hands. Contract No. 68-01-6271, Task No. 56. Prepared for USEPA, Exposure Evaluation Division, by Vesar Inc., Springfield, VA, February 8, 1984.

29. USEPA. (1985). Methods for Assessing Exposure to Chemical Substances, Vols. 1–9. EPA 560/5-85-004, Washington, D.C.: Office of Toxic Substances.

30. Chu, K. (1977). Percent Spontaneous Primary Tumors in Untreated Species Used at NCI for Carcinogen Bioassays. NCI Clearing House.

31. Gad, S.C. and Weil, C.S. (1986). Statistics and Experimental Design for Toxicologists. Caldwell, NJ: Telford Press, 380 pp.

32. Cameron, T.P., Hickman, R.L., Korneich, M.R., and Tarone, R.E. (1985). History survival and growth patterns of B6C3F1 mice and F344 rats in the National Cancer Institute Carcinogenesis Testing Program. Gund. Appl. Toxicol. 5:526–538.

33. Dempster, A.P., Selwyn, M.R., and Weeks, B.J. (1983). Combining historical and randomized controls for assessing trends in proportions. J. Am. Stat. Assoc. 78: 221–227.

34. Salsburg, D. (1980). The effects of lifetime feeding studies on patterns of senile lesions in mice and rats. Drug Chem. Toxicol. 3:1–33.

35. Epstein, S.S. (1973). The Delaney Amendment. Ecologist 3:424–430.

36. Albert, R.E., Burns, F.J., and Altshuler, B. (1979). Reinterpretation of the Linear Non-Threshold Dose-Response Model in Terms of the Initiation—Promotion Mouse Skin Tumorigenesis, In: New Concepts in Safety Evaluation (M.A. Mehlman, R.E. Shapiro, and H. Blumenthal, eds.). New York: Hemisphere Publishing, pp. 88–95.

37. Mantel, N. and Bryan, W.R. (1961). Safety testing of carcinogenic agents. J. Natl. Canc. Inst. 27:455–470.

38. Mantel, N. and Schneiderman, M.A. (1975). Estimating "Safe" Levels, A Hazardous Undertaking. Cancer Res. 35:1379–1386.

39. Crump, K.S., Hoel, D.G., Langley, C.H., and Peto, R. (1976). Fundamental carcin-

ogenic processes and their implications for low dose risk assessment. Cancer Res. 36:2973.

40. Gross, M.A., Fitzhugh, O.G., and Mantel, N. (1970). Evaluation of safety for food additives: An illustration involving the influence of methylsalicylate on rat reproduction. Biometrics 26:181–194.

41. Guess, H.A. and Hoel, D.G. (1977). The Effect of Dose On Cancer Latency Period. J. Env. Path. Toxicol. 1:279–286.

42. Calabrese, E.J. (1983). Principles of Animal Extrapolation, John Wiley, New York.

43. Klaassen, C.D. and Doull, J. (1980). Evaluation of Safety: Toxicology Evaluation. In: Casarett and Doull's Toxicology (J. Doull, C.D. Klaassen, and M.O. Amdur, eds.). New York: Macmillan Publishing Company, p. 26.

44. Arley, N. (1961). Theoretical Analysis of Carcinogenesis. In: Proceedings of the Fourth Berkeley Symposium on Mathematical Statistics and Probability (J. Neyman, ed.). University of California Press, Berkeley, pp. 1–18.

45. Gehring, P.J. and Blau, G.E. (1977). Mechanisms of Carcinogenicity: Dose Response. J. Env. Path. Toxicol. 1:163–179.

46. Dinman, B.D. (1972). "Non-concept" of "Non-threshold" chemicals in the environment. Science 175:495–497.

47. Friedman, L. (1973). Problems of evaluating the health significance of the chemicals present in foods. In: Pharmacology and the Future of Man Vol. 2, Karger, Basel, pp. 30–41.

48. Yanysheva, N. Ya., and Antomonov, G. Yu. (1976). Predicting the risk of tumor-occurrence under the effect of small doses of carcinogens. Environ. Health Perspect. 13:95–99.

49. Kraybill, H.E. (1977). Newer approaches in assessment of Environmental Carcinogenesis. In: Mycotoxins In Human and Animal Health, Pathotox Publishers, Park Forest South, Illinois, pp. 675–686.

50. Miller, E.C. (1978). Some Current Perspectives on Chemical Carcinogens in Humans and Experimental Animals: Presidential Address. Cancer Res. 38:1471.

51. Bryan, W.R. and Shimkin, M.B. (1943). Quantitative Analysis of Dose-Response Data Obtained with Three Carcinogenic Hydrocarbons in Strain C3H Male Mice. J. Natl. Canc. Inst. 3:503–531.

52. Wolfe, B. (1977). Low-Level Radiation: Predicting the Effects. Science 196:1387–1389.

53. Stokinger, H.E. (1977). Toxicology and drinking water contaminants. J. Am. Water Works Assoc., July, pp. 399–402.

54. Cairnes, T. (1980). The ED_{01} Study: Introduction, Objectives, and Overview. Environ. Path. Toxicol. 3(3):1–7.

55. Staffa, J.A. and Mehlman, M.A. (1980). Innovations in Cancer Risk Assessment (ED_{01} Study). J. Env. Path. Toxicol. 3:1–246.

56. Hoel, D.G., Gaylor, D.W., Kirschstein, R.L., Saffiotti, V., and Schneiderman, M.A. (1975). Estimation of risks of irreversible delayed toxicity. J. Toxicol. Environ. Health 1:133.

57. Environmental Protection Agency. (1976). Federal Register, 41:21402, 42:10412.

58. FDA Advisory Committee on Protocols for Safety Evaluation. (1971). Panel on

carcinogenesis report on cancer testing in the safety evaluation of food additives and pesticides. Toxicol. Appl. Pharmacol. 20:419–438.

59. Peto, R. (1978). The carcinogenic effects of chronic exposure to very low levels of toxic substances. Environ. Health Perspectives 22:155–159.

60. Guess, H.A., Crump, K.S., and Peto, R. (1977). Uncertainty estimates for low-dose-rate extrapolations of animal carcinogenicity data. Cancer Res. 37:3475–3483.

61. Gad, S.C. (1998). Statistics and Experimental Design for Toxicologists, 3rd ed., Boca Raton, Florida: CRC Press.

62. Chand, N. and Hoel, D.G. (1974). A Comparison of Models for Determining Safe Levels of Environmental Agents. In: Reliability and Biometry Statistical Analysis of Lifelength, F. Proschan and R.J. Serfling (ed.), SIAM, Philadelphia.

63. Druckrey, H. (1967). Quantitative aspects in chemical carcinogenesis. In: Potential Carcinogenic Hazards from Drugs, UICC Monograph Series, Vol. 7. R. Truhaut (ed.), Springer-Verlag, Berlin, p. 60.

64. Mantel, N., Bohidar, N.R., Brown, C.C., Cimenera, J.L., and Tukey, J.W. (1975). An improved Mantel-Bryan procedure for "safety" testing of carcinogens. Cancer Res. 35:865–872.

66. Armitage, P. and Doll, R. (1961). Stochastic Models for Carcinogenesis From the Berkeley Symposium on Mathematical Statistics and Probability, Berkeley: University of California Press, pp. 19–38.

67. Hartley, H.O. and Sielken, R.L. (1977). Estimation of "safe doses" in carcinogenic experiments. Biometric 33:1–30.

68. Crump, K.W. (1979). Dose response problems in carcinogenesis. Biometrics 35: 157–167.

69. Cornfield, J. (1977). Carcinogenic Risk Assessment. Science 198:693–699.

70. Food Safety Council. (1980). Quantitative Risk Assessment. Fd. Cosmet. Toxicol. 18:711–734.

71. Rai, K. and Van Ryzin, J. (1979). Risk assessment of toxic environmental substances based on a generalized multihit model. Energy and Health, Philadelphia: SIAM Press, pp. 99–177.

72. Cook, P.J., Doll, R., and Fellingham, S.A. (1969). A Mathematical Model for the Age Distribution of Cancer in Man. Inst. J. Cancer 4:93–112.

73. Lee, P.N. and O'Neill, J.A. (1971). The effect of both time and dose applied on tumor incidence rate in benzopyrene skin painting experiments. Br. J. Cancer 25: 759–770.

74. Day, T.D. (1967). Carcinogenic action of cigarette smoke condensate on mouse skin. Br. J. Cancer 21:56–81.

75. Peto, R., Lee, P.N., and Paige, W.S. (1972). Statistical analysis of the bioassay of continuous carcinogens. Roy J. Cancer 26:258–261.

76. Peto, R. and Lee, P.N. (1973). Weibull distributions for continuous carcinogenesis experiments. Biometrics 29:457–470.

77. Pike, M.C. (1966). A method of analysis of a certain class of experiments in carcinogenesis. Biometrics 22:142–161.

78. Hoel, D.G. (1972). A representation of mortality data by competing risks. Biometrics 28:475–488.

79. Berkson, J. (1944). Application of the logistic function to bio-assay. J. Amer. Stat. Assoc. 39:357–365.

80. Cornfield, J., Carlborg, F.W., and Van Ryzin, J. (1978). Setting Tolerance on the Basis of Mathematical Treatment of Dose-response Data Extrapolated to Low Doses. Proc. Of the Fist Internat. Toxicol. Congress, New York: Academic Press, pp. 143–164.

81. Albert, R.E. and Altshuler, B. (1973). Considerations relating to the formulation of limits for unavoidable population exposures to environmental carcinogens. In: Radionuclide Carcinogenesis (J.E. Ballou et al., eds.). AEC Symposium Series, CONF-72050. NTIS Springfield, pp. 233–253.

82. Blum, H.F. (1959). Carcinogenesis by Ultraviolet Light. Princeton: Princeton University Press.

83. Finney, D.J. (1952). Statistical Methods in Biological Assay. New York: Hafner.

84. Tomatis, L. (1979). The Predictive Value of Rodent Carcinogenicity Tests In the Evaluation of Human Risks. Ann. Rev. Pharmacol. Toxicology 19:511–530.

85. Weil, C.S. (1984). Some Questions and Opinions: Issues In Toxicology and Risk Assessment. Am. Ind. Hyg. Assoc. J. 45:663–670.

86. Deichmann, W.B. (1975). Cummings Memorial Lecture—1975: The Market Basket: Food for Thought. Am. Ind. Hyg. Assoc. J. 36:411.

87. Smith, R.L. (1974). The Problem of Species Variations. Ann. Nutr. Alim. 28:335.

88. Hammond, E.C., Garfinkel, L., and Lew, E.A. (1978). Longevity, Selective Mortality, and Competitive Risks in Relation to Chemical Carcinogenesis. Env. Res. 16:153–173.

89. Rall, D.P. (1977). Species Differences in Carcinogenicity Testing, in Origins of Human Cancer (H.H. Hiatt, J.D. Watson, and J.A. Winsten, eds.). Cold Spring Harbor Laboratories: Cold Spring Harbor, New York, pp. 1283–1290.

90. Rall, D.P. (1979). Relevance of animal experiments to humans. Environ. Health Perspect. 32:297–300.

91. Borzelleca, J.F. (1984). Extrapolation of Animal Data to Man. In: Concepts in Toxicology Vol. I (A.S. Tegeris, ed.). New York: Karger, pp. 294–304.

92. Gad, S.C. and Chengelis, C.P. (1988). Animal Models in Toxicology, Marcel Dekker, Inc.: New York.

93. Schmidt-Nielsen, K. (1984). Scaling: Why Is Animal Size So Important. New York: Cambridge University Press.

94. Association of Food and Drug Officials of the U.S. (1959). Appraisal of the safety of chemicals in foods, drugs and cosmetics. Washington, D.C.

95. Spector, W.S. (1956). Handbook of Biological Data. Philadelphia: W.B. Saunders.

96. Schneiderman, M.A., Mantel, N., and Brown, C.C. (1975). Ann. N.Y. Acad. Sci. 246:237–248.

97. Dixon, R.L. (1976). Problems in Extrapolating Toxicity Data from Laboratory Animals to Man. Envir. Hlth. Perspect. 13:43–50.

98. Guzelian, P.S., Henby, C.J., and Olin, S.S. (1992). Similarities and Differences Between Children and Adults: Implications for Risk Assessment. Washington, D.C.: ILSI Press.

99. Perera, F. (1977). Environment and Cancer: Who are Susceptible. Science 278: 1068–1073.

100. Olin, G., Farland, W., Park, C., Rhomberg, L., Schenplein, R., Starr, T., and Wilson, J. (1995). Low-Dose Extrapolation of Cancer Risks, ILSI Press, Washington, D.C.

101. Auton, T.R. (1994). Calculation of benchmark doses from teratology data. Regul. Toxicol. Pharmacol. 19(2):152–67, April 1994.

102. Barnes, D.G., Daston, G.P., Evans, T.S., Jarabek, A.M., Kavlock, R.J., and Kimmel, C.A. (1995). Park C. Spitzer Benchmark dose workshop: criteria for use of a benchmark dose to estimate a reference dose. Regulatory Toxicology and Pharmacol.

103. National Research Council. (1994). Science and Judgment in Risk Assessment. Washington, D.C.: National Academy Press.

104. USEPA. (1995). Proposed Guidelines for Neurotoxicity Risk Assessment. Federal Register 60:52032–52056.

105. Nair, R.S., Stevens, M.S., Martens, M.A., and Ekuta, J. (1995). Comparisons of BMD with NOAEL and LOAEL values derived from subchronic toxicity studies. Arch. Toxicol. Suppl. 17:44–54.

106. Slob, W. and Pieters, M.N. (1995). Probabilistic Approach to Assess Human RfDs and Human Health Risks from Toxicological Animal Studies. Proceedings for the Annual Meeting of the Society for Risk Analysis and the Japan Section of SRA, Abstract D8.04-A;60.

107. Jarabek, A.M., Menache, M.G., Overton, J.H. Jr., Dourson, M.L., and Miller, F.J. (1990). The U.S. Environmental Protection Agency's inhalation RfD methodology: risk assessment for air toxics. Toxicol. Ind. Health 6:279–301.

108. Barnes, D.G. and Dourson, M. (1988). Reference Dose (RfD): Description and use in health risk assessments. Regulatory Toxicology and Pharm. 8:471–486.

109. Gaylor, D.W. (1992). Incidence of developmental defects at the no observed adverse effects (NOAEL). Regul. Toxicol. Pharmacol. 15:151–160.

110. Gaylor, D.W. (1983). The use of safety factors for controlling risk. J. Toxicol. Environ. Health 11:329–336.

111. Gaylor, D.W. (1989). Quantitative risk analysis for quantal reproductive and developmental effects. Environ. Health Perspect. 79:243–246.

112. Kimmel, C.A. and D.W. Gaylor (1988). Issues in qualitative and quantitative risk analysis for developmental toxicity. Risk Anal. 8:15–20.

113. EPA (Environmental Protection Agency). (1991). Guidelines for developmental toxicity risk assessment. Fed. Regist. 56:63797–63826.

114. Crump, K.S. (1984). A new method for determining allowable daily intakes. Fundam. Appl. Toxicol. 4:854–871.

115. Crump, K. (1995). Calculation of benchmark doses from continuous data. Risk Analysis 15:79–85.

116. Crump, K., Allen, B., Faustman, E., Donison, M., Kimmel, C., and Zenich, H. (1995). The Use of the Benchmark Dose Approach in Health Risk Assessment. Risk Assessment Forum, EPA/630/R-94/007, February 1995.

117. Allen, B.C., Kavlock, R.J., Kimmell, C.A., Faustman, E.M. (1994a). Dose-response assessment for developmental toxicity. II. Comparison of generic benchmark dose estimates with NOAELs. Fundam. Appl. Toxicol. 23:487–495.

118. Allen, B.C., Kavlock, R.J., Kimmell, C.A., and Faustman, E.M. (1994b). Dose-

response assessment for developmental toxicity. III. Statistical models. Fundam. Appl. Toxicol. 23:496–509.

119. Ryan, L. (1992). Quantitative risk assessment for developmental toxicity. Biometrics 48:163–174.

120. Krewski, D. and Zhu, Y. (1995). A simple data transformation for estimating benchmark doses in developmental toxicity experiments. Risk Analysis 15(1):29–39, Feb. 1995.

121. Chen, J.J. and Kodell, R.L. (1989). Quantitative risk assessment for teratological effects. J. Am. Stat. Assoc. 84:966–971.

122. Fan, A.M. and Chang, L.W. (1996). *Toxicology and Risk Assessment*. New York: Marcel Dekker, Inc.

123. Efron, E. (1984). The Apocalyptics. New York: Simon and Schuster.

124. Gori, G.B. (1982). Regulation of Cancer-Causing Substances: Utopia or Reality. Chem. Eng. News (September 6, 1982) 25–32.

125. Weil, C.S. (1972). Statistics vs. safety factors and scientific judgment in the evaluation of safety for man. Toxicol. Appl. Pharmacol. 21:459.

126. National Research Council. (1989). Biologic Markers in Pulmonary Toxicology. Washington, D.C.: National Academy Press.

127. National Research Council. (1989). Biologic Markers in Reproductive Toxicology. Washington, D.C.: National Academy Press.

128. Glowa, J. (1991). Dose-effect approaches to risk assessment. Neusci. Biobehav. Rev. 15(1):153–158.

129. Starr, T.B. (1995a). Concerns with the benchmark dose concept. Toxicology Summer Forum, Aspen, CO, July 14, 1995.

130. Starr, T.B. (1995b). The Benchmark Dose Concept: Questionable Utility for Risk Assessment? Proceedings of the Annual Meeting of the Society for Risk Analysis and the Japan Section of SRA, Abstract H2.03:86-7. Waikiki, Hawaii, Dec. 3–6, 1995.

131. Anderson, M.W., Hoel, D.G., and Kaplan, N.L. (1980). A General Scheme for the Incorporation of Pharmacokinetics in Low-Dose Risk Estimation for Chemical Carcinogenesis: Example-Vinyl Chloride. Toxicol. Appl. Pharmacol. 55:154–161.

132. Park, C.N. and Snee, R.D. (1983). Quantitative Risk Assessment. State-of-the-Art for Carcinogenesis. Amer. Stat. 37:427–441.

133. Kavlock, R.J., Allen, B.C., Faustman, E.M., and Mimmel, C.A. (1995). Dose-response assessments for developmental toxicity. IV. Benchmark doses for fetal weight changes. Fundam. Appl. Toxicol. 26:211–222.

134. Hickey, R.J. (1984). Low-level radiation effects: Extrapolation as "science". Chem. Eng. News (January 16, 1984).

16

Toxicokinetic Studies in the Commercial Development of Agricultural and Industrial Chemical Products

Shayne Cox Gad
Gad Consulting Services, Raleigh, North Carolina

Christopher P. Chengelis
WIL Research Laboratories, Inc., Ashland, Ohio

I. INTRODUCTION

Among the cardinal principles of both toxicology and pharmacology is that the means by which an agent comes in contact with or enters the body (i.e., the route of exposure or administration) does much to determine the nature and magnitude of an effect. Accordingly, an understanding of routes and their implications for absorption is essential. Also, in the day-to-day operations of performing studies in animals or evaluating exposures in humans, such an understanding of routes, their manipulation, means and pitfalls of achieving them, and the art and science of vehicles and formulations is essential to the sound and efficient conduct of any study.

Toxicity studies usually involve a control group of animals (untreated and/ or formulation treated) and at least three treated groups receiving "low," "mid-" and "high" dose levels of the chemical entity of interest. Occasionally a positive control group(s) treated with a known related compound is included for reference purposes and there may be recovery groups. In most instances the high dose level is expected to elicit some toxic effects in the animals, often expressed as decreased food consumption and/or below-normal body weight gain, and has been selected after consideration of earlier data, perhaps from dose range-finding studies. The other two dose levels are anticipated not to cause toxic effects. Generally, but not always (e.g., based on all available evidence, rats and guinea pigs are more sensitive to 2,3,7,8-Tetrachlorodibenzo-p-dioxin (TCDD) than are larger animal species, including human beings), the "low" dose level is a several-fold multiple of the expected human exposure level. However, without knowing the true relationship of these dose levels to each other with respect to the absorption, distribution, and elimination of the new chemical entity as reflected by its toxicokinetics, it is difficult to see how meaningful extrapolations concerning safety margins can be made from the toxicity data obtained. Also, without toxicokinetic data from the positive control group, its inclusion is of limited value and the results obtained could lead to erroneous conclusions.

Toxicokinetic studies can provide information on several aspects, knowledge of which greatly facilitates assessment of safety of the chemical entity. Six such aspects can be mentioned.

1. Relationship between the dose levels used and the relative extent of absorption of the test chemical
2. Relationship between the protein-binding of the test compound and the dose levels used
3. Relationship between pharmacological or toxicological effects and the kinetics of the test compound
4. Effect of repeated doses on the kinetics of the test compound
5. Relationship between the age of the animal and the kinetics of the test compound
6. Relationship between the dose regimens of the test compound used in the toxicity studies and those to which humans will be exposed

There are at least 26 potential routes of administration or exposure to xenobiotics as shown in Table 1. For most agricultural and industrial chemicals, however, the oral, dermal, and inhalation routes are of the greatest concern.

If toxicology can be described as being the study of the effects of a chemical on an organism, metabolism can be described as the opposite—the effects of the organism on the chemical. Metabolism refers to a process by which a chemical (xenobiotic) is chemically modified by an organism. It is part of the overall process of disposition of xenobiotic ADME—the process by which a chemical gains access to the inner working of an organism (Absorption), how it moves around inside an organism (Distribution), how it is changed by the organism (Metabolism), and how it is eventually eliminated from the organism (Elimination). The EPA definition of biotransformation or metabolism is " . . . the sum of processes by which a xenobiotic (foreign chemical) is handled by a living organism." The mathematical formulae used to describe and quantify these processes are collectively known as pharmacokinetics. The EPA definition of pharmacokinetics is " . . . quantitation and determination of the time course

Table 1 Potential Routes of Exposure/Administration

Oral routes
  oral (po)
    Active dosing, e.g. gavage
    Passive dosing, e.g. in diet
  inhalation
  sublingual
  buccal
Respiratory routes
  inhalation (passive)-either whole body or nose only
  intranasal
  intratracheal
Place into other natural orifices in the body
  intranasal
  intraauricular
  rectal
  intravaginal
  intrauterine
  intraurethral
Parentheral (injected into the body or placed under the skin)
  intravenous (i.v.)
  subcutaneous (sc)
  intramuscular (im)
  intraarterial
  intradermal (id)
  intralesional
  epidural
  intrathecal
  intracisternal
  intracardial
  intraventricular
  intraocular
  intraperitoneal (ip)
Topical routes
  cutaneous
  transdermal (also called percutaneous)
  ophthalmic

and dose dependency of the absorption, distribution, biotransformation and excretion of chemicals." The acronym ADME has been used to describe this multifaceted biological process. The term metabolism has also come into common jargon to describe the entire process. This science has long played a central role in pharmaceutical development, but has played a lesser role in the development of other types of products. The purpose of this chapter is to introduce the basic concepts of ADME and practices of studies conducted to study it, as described the regulations under U.S. Environmental Protection Agency (EPA) and Organization for Economic Cooperation and Development (OECD) which require such data for nonpharmaceutical products and to give some real world examples.

II. REGULATIONS

From a regulatory perspective there are three sets of guidelines covering ADME and/or pharmacokinetics for products not covered by the FDA. In the U.S., these would be for products covered under Toxic Substance and Control Act (TSCA) and Federal Insecticide, Fungicide, and Rodenticide Act (FIFRA) (Table 2). As of yet, there are no Occupational Safety and Health Administration (OSHA) or Federal Hazardous Substance Control Act (FHSCA) regulations requiring ADME or pharmacokinetics. In the international arena, there are also requirements under the OECD and Japanese Ministry of Agriculture, Forestry, and Fisheries (MAFF). With regard to FIFRA and TSCA, both these laws are administered by the EPA, but there have traditionally been slight differences in the guidelines between the two agencies. In addition, TSCA requirements were pub-

Table 2

FIFRA Guideline	TSCA Guidelines	OECD	OPPTS Guideline	Title
85-1	798.7485	417	870.7485	Metabolism and Pharmacokinetics
85-3	NA	NA	870.7600	Dermal Penetration
NA	795.235	NA	870.8500	Toxicokinetic Test
NA	795.230	NA	870.830	Oral and Inhalation Pharmacokinetic Test
NA	795.228	NA	870.8320	Oral/Dermal Pharmacokinetics
NA	795.226	NA	870.8300	Dermal Absorption for Compounds that are Volatile and Metabolized to Carbon Dioxide
NA	795.223	NA	870.8223	Pharmacokinetic Test

NA = Not applicable, no comparable guideline published.

lished in the Code of Federal Regulations (CFR) while FIFRA requirements were published as separate guideline documents. (The term guideline, as used here, may be a little misleading, as one is expected to follow the guidelines, or be able to present persuasive arguments as to why they did not apply in a specific circumstance.) In 1996, the Agency moved to harmonize these guidelines, so that one set of guidelines can be used for all studies (whether conducted under TSCA or FIFRA) submitted to the EPA. These harmonized guidelines were published as drafts in 1996 with a request for comments. Final guidelines were released as this chapter was being prepared (August, 1998) for Office of Prevention, Pesticides, and Toxic Substances (OPPTS) 870.7600 and OPPTS 870.7485. For the sake of completeness, we note that two of the proposed OPPTS guidelines (870.8245: Dermal Pharmacokinetics of DGBE and DGBA, and 870.8380: Inhalation and Dermal Pharmacokinetics of Commercial Hexane) were for specific chemicals. Because these may lack general interest and appeal, they will not be discussed further here.

FIFRA/TSCA/OPPTS guidelines are outlined in Table 3, and discussed under study designs. It is of interest that there is only one OECD guideline for ADME work, that being OECD Guideline 417, "Toxicokinetics" It is in no way as specific as EPA guidelines. For example, route, species, numbers of animals, single vs. multiple dose, and use of radiolabelled vs. nonradiolabelled material are not specified in the OECD guidelines.

Essentially, one is expected to select the appropriate species, route and methods to address

Absorption
amount of material in excreta
comparison of biologic response
comparison of amounts renally excreted
comparison of areas under the curve
Distribution
whole body chromatography
qualitative determination in various
organs

Excretion
Metabolism
Structure of the metabolites should be elucidated and the metabolic pathways-proposed in relation to the need to answer questions.

Thus, one would be expected to customize the ADME studies submitted under OECD on the basis of what was discussed in the toxicology studies.

In contrast, all pesticides submitted to the EPA for registration are expected to be the subject of a study conducted according to guidelines—exactly according to guideline OPPTS 870.7485. Studies conducted in accordance with OPPTS 870.7600 ("Dermal Penetration") are not routinely required. They will, however, be requested for chemicals that have significant toxicity and for which dermal exposure is likely, yet there is insufficient information to determine if there is adequate margin of exposure.

Table 3 Comparison of the Different OPPTS Guidelines

Guideline	Purpose	Animals	Design
870.7485 Metabolism and Pharmacokinetics	Absorption, distribution biotransformation, and excretion. Potential for bioaccumulation. Induction of biotransformation (route not given).	Rats (same strain as used of tox studies)	Tier 1—dose 4 rats, single low dose Tier 2—design based on findings from Tier 1
870.8223 Pharmacokinetic Test	Dermal Bioavailability Oral vs. dermal differences in biotransformation Changes in metabolism with repeat dosing	Fischer 344 rats (females)	4 groups of 8 rats each (low and high dose oral and dermal. 1 groups treated i.v. One 1 group treated (unlabelled) po 14 days, then dosed with labeled material. (6 groups total)
870.7600 Dermal Penetration	Assesses dermal absorption for chemicals having serious systemic toxicity	Young adult male rats—same strain as used in toxicity study	24 rats/dose level, at least three dose levels. Doses should be at log intervals. Exposure time points of 0.5, 1, 2, 4, 10 and 24 hr.
8700.8300 Dermal Absorption for Compounds That are Volatile and Metabolized to Carbon Dioxide	Absorption after dermal exposure	Fischer 344 Rat Guinea Pig	5 groups (4/sex group) for each species. Low dose i.v., low dose dermal, high dose dermal.

870.8320 Oral/Dermal Pharmacokinetics	Oral vs. dermal bioavailability Oral vs. dermal metabolism and metabolism Changes in metabolism with repeat dosing	Sprague-Dawley Rat Minipigs (both sexes)	5 groups (4/sex group) for each species. Low dose i.v., low dose dermal, high dose dermal. 1 group of rats treated (unlabelled) po 7 days, then dosed with labeled material (9 groups total)
870.8340 Oral and Inhalation Pharmacokinetics Test	Oral vs. inhalation bioavailability Oral vs. inhalation metabolism Changes in metabolism with repeat dosing	Fischer 344 Rats (both sexes)	7 groups of 4 rats/sex/group: Oral 2 groups (low and high). Inhalation 5 groups nonlabeled, (low mid and high) and 2 groups labeled (low and high) single 6 hour exposures.
870.8500 Toxicokinetics Test	Dermal oral and dermal bioavailability Oral vs. dermal differences in metabolites Effects of multiple oral dosing on metabolism	Fischer 344 Rats (both sexes)	Five groups of 4 rats/sex/group: one low dose oral, one high dose oral, one high dose dermal and one group treated orally for 14 days (non-labelled) with a final dose being with labeled chemical.

Note that all guidelines require the use of radiolabeled chemicals.

Under TSCA, metabolism data is not required in the filing of a Premanu-facturing Notification (PMN). The agency may review the data that is submitted under a PMN and subsequently request (or require under a consent decree) such data, but for the vast majority of chemicals this is not the case.

In Japan, agricultural chemicals are regulated by JMAFF, while industrial chemicals are regulated by MITI under the Japanese chemical substance law. The respective guidelines are very similar to each other, and fall between the OECD and the EPA guidelines with respect to complexity and specificity. The Japanese law is not specific as to when such data would be expected, however. The fact that these guidelines exist should be taken as tacit expectation that these studies should be conducted and reported for products registered in or exported to Japan.

III. PRINCIPLES

An understanding of the design and analysis of toxicokinetic studies requires a broad understanding of the underlying concepts and principles inherent in the ADME process and in our current technology for studying such. Each of these four principal areas is overviewed in this section from a practical basis as it relates to toxicology. First, however, one should consider the fundamental termi-nology used in toxicokinetic studies (Table 4).

A. Absorption

Absorption describes the process by which a chemical crosses a biological mem-brane to gain access to the inner workings of an organism. For mammals, this process results in the entry of the chemical into the blood stream, or systemic circulation. In this case the process is also called systemic absorption. Pharma-ceutical products, procedures and devices, such as hypodermic needles, can be used to bypass biological barriers. Such devices are rarely, if ever, used with consumer products, agricultural, and industrial chemicals. These chemicals gen-erally gain access to the systemic circulation after either oral, dermal, or inhala-tory exposure.

Our working definition of toxicity is the production of target organ dam-age remote from the site of administartion of the chemical. For a material to be toxic (local effects are largely not true toxicities by this definition), the first requirement is that it be absorbed into the organism (for which purpose being in the cavity of the gastrointestinal [GI] tract does not qualify).

There are characteristics that influence absorption by the different routes, and these need to be understood by any person trying to evaluate and/or predict the toxicities of different moieties. Some key characteristics and considerations are summarized below by route.

Table 4 Fundamental Terms Used in Toxicokinetic Studies

Absolute bioavailability	The bioavailability of a dosage form relative to an intravenous administration (see bioavailability below).
Absorption	The process by which a xenobiotic and its metabolites are transferred from the site of absorption to the blood circulation.
Accumulation	The progressive increase of chemical and/or metabolites in the body. Accumulation is influenced by the dosing interval and half-life of the chemical. The process can be characterized by an "accumulation factor," which is the ratio of the plasma concentration at steady state to that following the first dose in a multiple dosing regimen.
Area under curve (AUC)	The concentration of chemical and/or metabolites in the blood (or plasma/serum) integrated over time. This is typically considered the best indicator of exposure.
Bioavailability	The rate and extent to which a xenobiotic entity enters the systemic circulation intact, following oral or dermal administration. Also known as the comparative bioavailability.
Biotransformation	The process by which a xenobiotic is structurally and/or chemically changed in the body by either enzymatic or nonenzymatic reactions. The product of the reaction is a different composition of matter or different configuration than the original compound.
Clearance	The volume of biological fluid that is totally cleared of xenobiotic in a unit time.
C_{max}	The maximum mean concentration of the chemical in the plasma. Also known as the peak plasma concentration.
Disposition	All processes and factors which are involved from the time a chemical enters the body to the time when it is eliminated from the body, either intact or in metabolite form.
Distribution	The process by which an absorbed xenobiotic and/or its metabolites partition between blood and various tissues/organs in the body.
Dosage form	The formulation (diet, lotion, capsule, solution, etc.) administered to animals or man.
Dose proportionality	The relationship between doses of a chemical and bioavailability, usually including tests for linearity.

Table 4 Continued

Enterohepatic circulation	The process by which xenobiotics are emptied via the bile into the small intestine and then reabsorbed into the hepatic circulation.
Enzyme induction	The increase in enzyme content (activity and/or amount) due to xenobiotic challenge, which may result in more rapid metabolism of a chemical.
Enzyme inhibition	The decrease in enzymatic activity due to the effect of xenobiotic challenge.
Excretion	The process by which the administered compound and/or its biotransformation product(s) are eliminated from the body.
First-order kinetics	Kinetic processes, the rate of which is directly proportional to the concentration.
First-pass effect	The phenomenon whereby xenobiotics may be extracted or metabolized by the liver following enteral absorption before reaching the systemic circulation.
Flux	Term (that takes area into consideration) used to describe the movement of a chemical across a barrier. Most typically used to describe the absorption of a chemical across the skin as $ug/cm^2/hr$.
Half-life	The time elapsed for a given chemical entity concentration or amount to be reduced by a factor of two.
Hepatic clearance	The rate of total body clearance accounted for by the liver.
Kel	The elimination constant for a chemical in plasma. Typically calculated using the formula $Kel = -\ln[10] \times b$ where b is the slope of the linear regression line of the log of the mean plasma concentrations vs. time from the t_{max} to 24 hr.
Lag time	The interval between compound administration and when the compound concentration is measurable in blood.
Metabolite characterization	The determination of physiochemical characteristics of the biotransformation product(s).
Metabolite identification	The structural elucidation of the biotransformation product(s).
Metabolite profile	The chromatographic pattern and/or aqueous/nonaqueous partitioning of the biotransformation products of the administered compound.
Nonlinear kinetics (saturation kinetics)	Kinetic processes, the rate of which is not directly proportional to the concentration. Also known as "0" order kinetics. The rate of disappearance of a chemical from the plasma remains constant across time.

Table 4 Continued

Presystemic elimination	The loss of that portion of the dose that is not bioavailable. This would include, among others, loss through intestinal and gut-wall metabolism, lack of absorption, and first-pass hepatic metabolism.
Protein binding	The complexation of a xenobiotic and/or its metabolite(s) with plasma or tissue proteins.
Relative bioavailability	The bioavailability relative to a reference or standard formulation or agent.
Renal clearance	The rate of total body clearance accounted for by the kidney. Its magnitude is determined by the net effects of glomerular filtration, tubular secretion and reabsorption, renal blood flow, and protein binding.
Steady state	An equilibrium state where the rate of chemical input is equal to the rate of elimination during a given dose interval.
T_{max}	The sampling time point at which C_{max} occurs.
Total clearance	The volume of biological fluid totally cleared of xenobiotic per unit time and usually includes hepatic clearance and renal clearance.
Toxicokinetics	The study of the kinetics of absorption, distribution, metabolism, and excretion of toxic or potentially toxic chemicals.
Volume of distribution (V_d)	A hypothetical volume of body fluid into which the chemical distributes. It is not a "real" volume, but is a proportionality constant relating the amount of chemical in the body to the measured concentration in blood or plasma.

A. Oral and rectal routes (gastrointestinal tract)
  1. Lipid-soluble compounds (nonionized) are more readily absorbed than water-soluble compounds (ionized).
     a. Weak organic bases are in the nonionized, lipid-soluble form in the intestine and tend to be absorbed there.
     b. Weak organic acids are in the nonionized, lipid-soluble form in the stomach and one would suspect they would be absorbed there, but the intestine is more important because of time and area of exposure.
  2. Specialized transport systems exist for some moieties: sugars, amino acids, pyrimidines, calcium, and sodium.
  3. Almost everything is absorbed—at least to a small extent (if it has a molecular weight below 10,000).

    4. Digestive fluids may modify the structure of a chemical.

    5. Dilution increases toxicity because of more rapid absorption from the intestine, unless stomach contents bind the moiety.

    6. Physical properties are important—for example, dissolution of metallic mercury is essential to allow absorption.

    7. Age—neonates have a poor intestinal barrier.

    8. Effect of fasting on absorption depends on the properties of the chemical of interest.

B. Inhalation (lungs)

    1. Aerosol deposition

        a. Nasopharyngeal—5 μm or larger in man, less in common laboratory animals.

        b. Tracheobronchiolar—1–5 μm

        c. Alveolar—1 μm

    2. If a solid, mucociliary transport may serve to clear from lungs to GI tract.

    3. Lungs are anatomically good for absorption.

        a. Large surface area (50–100 m^2).

        b. Blood flow is high.

        c. Close to blood (10 μm between gas media and blood).

    4. Absorption of gases is dependent on solubility of the gas in blood.

        a. Chloroform, for example, has high solubility and is all absorbed; respiration rate is the limiting factor.

        b. Ethylene has low solubility and only a small percentage is absorbed—blood flow limited absorption.

C. Parenteral routes.

    1. Not typically of concern for agricultural or industrial chemicals. Mayoccassionally need i.v. pharmacokinetic data for comparative purposes.

D. Dermal route

    1. Most common route of exposure to agricultural and industrial chemical.

    2. Highly dependent on the chemical nature of the test article. Hydrophobicchemicals tend to be more highly absorbed.

    3. Highly dependent on the nature of the vehicle (if in a formulation). Somevehicles will enhance, others impede absorption.

    4. Surface area and concentration are also important considerations (4).

It is still not commonly the case in toxicology study of agricultural or industrial chemicals for the absorption and bioavailability of a compound by any particular route to be extensively studied or determined. However, as a generalization, there is a pattern of relative absorption rates that extends between the different routes that are commonly of interest for these classes. This order of absorption (by rate from fastest to slowest and from most to least) is i.v. > inhalation > im > ip > sc > oral > id > other dermal.

In general, chemicals cross biological barriers by one of three mechanisms: active transport, facilitative transport, and passive transport. In active transport, the chemical is specifically recognized by the organism, which then expends energy to take the chemical up, even against a concentration gradient. In facilitative transport, the organism produces a carrier molecule that reacts with the target molecule to form a complex that more easily traverses the membrane, but no energy is expended to take up the complex. Such complexes do not flow against a concentration barrier. The simplest mechanism is passive transfer or diffusion. Here, a chemical flows down a concentration gradient (from high concentration to a lower concentration) and must passively (no energy expended by organism) cross a biological membrane. Passive transfer or diffusion is the most common (if not the only) mechanism involved in the absorption of the vast majority of chemicals in commerce. Thus, other mechanisms involved in absorption will not be further discussed here.

Chemicals in solution have a natural tendency (more rigorously defined by the laws of thermodynamics) to move down a concentration gradient. That is to say, the individual molecules of solute tend to move from a region of high concentration toward regions of lower concentration. Also, the movement of a chemical across a permeable barrier, such as a biological membrane, is a process called diffusion, as illustrated by Figure 1. For most products, these biological barriers are either the wall of the gastrointestinal tract, the lining of the pulmonary system, and/or the skin.

Absorption from the GI tract is controlled by a variety of factors. These

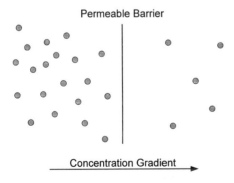

Permeable Barrier

Concentration Gradient

Figure 1 The diffusion process.

include the acid/base characteristics of the chemical (described as the pKa), the solubility, the nature of the delivery (e.g., diet vs. gavage), the nature of any vehicle (suspensions vs. solution, or aqueous vs. nonaqueous), and the gastrointestinal tract of the species under study.

Ionized or charged organic moieties do not readily pass through the lipophilic cell membranes of the epithelial cells that line the GI tract. Thus, more acidic molecules tend to be more readily absorbed from the stomach while more alkaline materials tend to be absorbed from the small intestine. This is because at the acidic pH of the stomach (1–2 in most species), acidic chemicals tend to be nonionized. The pH of the small intestine tends to be 5.5–6.5 in most species, so more alkaline chemicals tend to be more ionized in the stomach and less ionized in the gut. The equilibrium reaction for acidic dissociation can be represented by this equation

$$X-\underset{\underset{O}{\|}}{C}-OH + H_2O == X-\underset{\underset{O}{\|}}{C}-O^- + H_3O^+$$

Like all chemical equations, this one has an equilibrium constant. The discussion of basic chemistry is outside the purview of this book. Readers who may need a refresher are referred to Tse and Jaffe [3]. For every organic chemical, a pKa can be calculated, based on the equilibrium constant, which represents the proportion of ionized and unionized material in solution. The lower the pKa of a chemical the more likely it is to be nonionized in the stomach.

Surface area and transit time will also be factors in absorption from the GI tract. The stomach emptying time for most experimental animals will range from 30–90 minutes. After being expelled from the stomach into the duodenum, an acidic compound will still be absorbed, just more slowly. However, residance time in the small intestine may be several hours and the surface area available for absorption is enormous when compared to that of the stomach.

Solubility, lipophilicity, and the nature of the vehicle/solvent will all interplay to influence absorption. Materials must be in solution to pass through the the GI wall by passive diffusion. Solids will not be absorped until they go into solution. Also, the more lipophillic a chemical, the more readily it will pass through the gut wall. However, the more lipophillic a material, the less water soluble it is. Thus, for many materials a nonaqueous vehicle such as corn oil is used. Oils must be used as vehicles with caution as they may be diarrheagenic and the test substance may thus "shoot through" the GI tract without having a significant oppurtunity to be absorbed.

1. Absorption from the Pulmonary System

Of the three routes discussed here, absorption from the pulmonary system is perhaps the most rapid. Systemic absorption of inhaled materials is highly dependent on the physical properties of the inhaled materials which dictate how easily the materials reach the alveoli of the deep lung. Gases and vapors easily penetrate into the deep lung. For mists and dusts, absorption will be highly dependent on particle size. Materials that reach the lungs are more readily absorbed because of surface area, short diffusion distances, and the richness of the available blood supply. In general, the larger the particles, the less deeply they will penetrate the pulmonary system. (For a more complete review of the various physical forces involved in deposition, the reader is referred to [4,5]. The term impaction describes the deposition of particles in the respiratory tract. Particles of less than 0.2 µm are preferentially deposited in the pulmonary portion of the respiratory system and particles over 2 µm do not reach the alveolar epithelium in great number. Particles from 1–4 µm tend to be distributed over the length of the system and particles over 4 µm tend to be deposited in the nasal region. (In 1991, the Inhalation Specialty Section of the Society of Toxicology published a commentary on particle size. They noted that the USEPA recommended that 25% of the aerosolized particles in an exposure study be 1 µm or less in diameter. The commentary suggested that the remainder of the aerosol be between 1–4 µm as that would provide deposition and exposure along the entire length of the rodent pulmonary system.) Aerosolized particles of greater than 20 µ do not commonly occur in nature. Tidal volume will also influence impaction. In general, the larger the tidal volume, and thus the more forceful the inhalatory process, the more deeply particles of all sizes tend to be driven into the lung.

Once deposited, materials must be in solution before they can be absorbed. Hence, materials in an aerosolized solution will be more readily absorbed than materials that are delivered as solid (e.g., dusts) particles. Solid materials must be able to go into solution in situ in order to be absorbed. Particle size influences dissolution rate. Large particles dissolve more slowly (for any given material) than small particles due to the differences in surface area. Once in solution, the same laws of passive diffusion apply to materials in the lung as apply to material in the GI tract. The large surface area and the rich blood flow at the alveoli make for ideal conditions for rapid absorption into the systemic circulation. Absorption across the mucosa lining the upper airways is less rapid. Materials that do not dissolve are ingested by pulmonary macrophages and either broken down there or moved out of the lungs by the upward movement of the bronchociliary tree. If not expectorated, these particles are typically swallowed and enter the GI tract.

For gases and vapors, the amount absorbed is highly dependent on the partial pressure of the gas and the solubility of the gas in blood. Let's take the simple case of a gas that is not metabolized and is excreted by exhalation (e.g., an anesthetic gas or a CFC type fire extinguishing agent). At any given concentration (or partial pressure) in the atmosphere, the concentration in the blood will reach a steady state in the blood. Accordingly, prolonged exposure does not lead to continual buildup.

At equilibrium, the concentration in the blood is depicted by the formula (also known as the Ostwald coefficient) $X_b/X_a = S$, where X_b is the concentration in the blood and X_a is the concentration in the inspired air. Thus, if one knows the S for a given chemical and the target concentration for a given exposure, one can predict what the resulting concentration may be at equilibrium. Additionally, the lower the S value (i.e., the lower the solubility in blood) the more rapidly the chemical will achieve equilibrium.

2. Absorption Across the Skin

An aqueous carrier may be used for a variety of dermal products. In fact, carriers can be designed to limit the transportation of the penetration of the active ingredient (such as an insect repellent), if the desired effect is to keep the active on the surface of the skin. Once again, however, only those materials that are dissolved will be available for penetration across the skin to gain access to the systemic circulation. For almost all chemicals in or about to enter commerce, dermal penetration is a passive process. The relative thickness of the skin makes absorption (into the systemic circulation) slower than the absorption across the GI or pulmonary barriers. This is compounded by the fact that the stratum corneum function is to be impervious to the environment, as one of the skin's major functions is protection from infection. Once a chemical penetrates into the dermis, it may partition into the subcutaneous fat. Essentially, absorption across the skin is a two step process with the first being penetration and deposition into the skin and the second being release from the skin into the systemic circulation. The pattern of blood levels obtained via dermal penetration is generally one with a delayed absorption, slow buildup to more of a plateau than a peak. Blood levels of chemicals absorbed via the dermal route are generally low.

Given the overwhelming influence of the physical properties of skin in determining bioavailabilities via the dermal route, assessment of dermal penetration is one area in metabolism and toxicology where the use of in vitro methods can be effectively used to predict in vivo results and to screen chemicals. Apparatus and equipment exist that one can use to maintain sections of skin (obtained from euthanized animals or from human cadavers or surgical discard) for such experiments (for examples, see [6]). These apparatus are set up to maintain the metabolic integrity of the skin sample between two reservoirs: the one on the stratum corneum side, called the application reservoir and the one on the subcutaneous side, called the receptor reservoir. One simply places radiolabeled test material in the application reservoir and collects samples at various time points from the receptor fluid.

In general, penetration of most chemicals tends to follow first order kinetics, as presented by $C = C'e^{K_{pen}T}$, where C is the concentration or amount on the skin at the beginning of the time period, C' is the concentration or amount at the end of the time period, e is the natural log constant, K_{pen} is the penetration constant (in μm/hr) and T is the time period of exposure. K_{pen} can be calculated from observed data and/or modeled on the basis of physicochemical characteristics of the chemical. For example, Garner and Mathews (18) demonstrated that the penetration constant for a series of polychlorinated biphenyls followed the formula

$$K_{pen} = -0.0399 \ (\log k_{ow}) + 0.295$$

where k_{ow} is the octanol/water penetration coefficent.

The three major considerations in determining the quantity of material that is absorbed into the skin, and eventually released into the systemic circulation, is primarily dependent upon three factors: the surface area exposed, the volume of material applied, and the concentration of the material applied and the nature of the vehicle.

Surface area: all things being equal, it is clear that the greater the surface exposed, the higher the achieved internal dose.

Volume: the volume of material will obviously play a role in total dose, but it is not as straightforward as the relationship to surface area. Theoretically, the maximum absorption is obtained when the material is spread as thinly and uniformly as possible; piling material on so that it is literally rolling off the animal serves no practical purpose. In face, it is not a sound practice when dealing with an in vivo animal experiment as it makes it more likely for the material to be available for oral ingestion.

3. Parameters Controlling Absorption

The rate of diffusion is proportional to the concentration of molecule in the vehicle. The relationship is linear only at low molecule concentrations and only applies to soluble molecules in the vehicle. The latter factor may explain the variable therapeutic effects of different formulations of the same drug molecule. The partition coefficient is a measure of the molecule's ability to escape from the vehicle and is defined as the equilibrium solubility of molecule in the surface of the stratum corneum relative to its solubility in the vehicle. Increased lipid solubility favors penetration of molecule through the skin by increasing the solubility in the relatively lipophilic stratum corneum. The diffusion coefficient indicates the extent to which the matrix of the barrier restricts the mobility of the molecule. Increases in molecular size of the molecule will increase frictional resistance and decrease the diffusion coefficient (7); molecules over 1,000 daltons usually will not be absorbed easily into normal adult skin.

Finally, intact stratum corneum is an excellent barrier, but in disease states, or if the integrity of the stratum is breached by abrasion, wounding, or stripping, the resistance to absorption is rapidly lost and absorption will be facilitated.

B. Distribution

Once the chemical gains access to the body, it is carried by the bloodstream and distributed to the different organs. The preferential organ of deposition is determined by a variety of factors: the two most important are blood flow to the organ and the affinity of the chemical for that organ. Affinity is governed by two general characteristics. First, the product may be designed to have a specific affinity for a specific molecular entity in a target cell. For example, an anticholinesterase insecticide will tend to accumulate in the cells that have the highest concentration of cholinesterase. Second, the product may have a nonspecific or general chemical attraction for a specific cell type. The more highly lipophilic a chemical, the more likely it is to distribute and remain in adipose tissue. Blood flow will also have a major impact on distribution, as chemicals will be distributed more readily to those organs that are more highly perfused. A highly lipophilic chemical may first be deposited in the brain due to the fact that it is richly perfused, and then be distributed to body fat with time.

Once a material is absorbed, distribution of a compound in most toxicology studies has traditionally been of limited interest. This is beginning to change somewhat, as there is increasing interest in the relationship between target organ toxicity and the tendency, if any, for the chemical to accumulate in that organ. OPPTS guideline 870.7485, which is generally required to support pesticide registration, requires collection of liver, fat, GI tract, kidney, spleen, whole blood, and residual carcass. It further specifies that additional tissues should be collected if a target organ is identified in subchronic or chronic toxicity studies. Some factors which can serve to alter distribution are listed in Table 5.

For most chemicals, the rate of disposition or loss from the biological system is independent of rate and input, once the agent is absorbed. Disposition is defined as what happens to the active molecule after it reaches a site in the blood circulation where concentration measurements can be made (the systemic circulations, generally). Although disposition processes may be independent of input, the inverse is not necessarily true, because disposition can markedly affect the extent of availability. Agents absorbed from the stomach and the intestine must first pass through the liver before reaching the general circulation (Figure 2). Thus, if a compound is metabolized in the liver or excreted in bile, some of the active molecule absorbed from the gastrointestinal tract will be inactivated by hepatic processes before it can reach the systemic circulation and be distributed to its sites of action. If the metabolizing or biliary excreting capacity of the liver is great, the effect on the extent of availability will be substantial. Thus, if the hepatic blood clearance for the chemical is large, relative to hepatic blood

Table 5 Selected Factors that May Affect Chemical Distribution to Various Tissues

Factors relating to the chemical and its administration

    degree of binding of chemical to plasma proteins (i.e., agent affinity for proteins) and tissues

    chelation to calcium, which is deposited in growing bones and teeth (e.g., tetracyclines in young children)

    whether the chemical distributes evenly throughout the body (one compartment model) or differentially between different compartments (two or more compartment model)

    ability of chemical to cross the blood-brain barrier

    diffusion of chemical into the tissues or organs and degree of binding to receptors that are and are not specific for the compound's desired effects

    quantity of chemical given

    route of administration/exposure

    partition coefficients (nonpolar chemicals are distributed more readily to fat tissues than are polar chemicals)

    interactions with other chemicals that may occupy receptors and prevent the drug from attaching to the receptor, inhibit active transport, or otherwise interfere with a drug's activity

    molecular weight of the chemical

Factors relating to the test subject

    body size

    fat content (e.g., obesity affects the distribution of drugs that are highly soluble in fats)

    permeability of membranes

    active transport for chemicals carried across cell membranes by active processes

    amount of proteins in blood, especially albumin

    pathology or altered homeostasis that affects any of the other factors (e.g., cardiac failure and renal failure)

    the presence of competitive binding substances (e.g., specific sites in tissues bind drugs)

    pH of blood and body tissues

    pH of urine[a]

    development of immune response, leading to the production of neutralizing antibodies

    complexation without metabolism (amphophilic chemicals, for example, form complexes with phospholipids and accumulate in lysozomes)

    blood flow to various tissues or organs (e.g., well-perfused organs usually tend to accumulate more chemical than less well-perfused organs)

[a]The pH of urine is usually more important than the pH of blood.

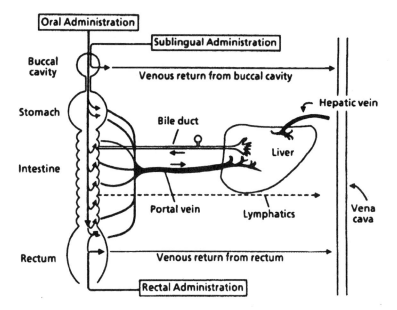

Figure 2 Passage of chemical moieties from the gastrointestinal tract into the bloodstream, shown in a diagrammatic fashion.

flow, the extent of availability for this chemical will be low when it is given by a route that yields first-pass metabolic effects.

First pass effects are primarily a concern with orally administered chemicals. Because of the arrangements of the circulatory system, inhaled or dermally absorbed compounds enter the full range of systemic circulation without any "first pass" metabolism by the liver. The reader is refered to Keberle (8) and O'Reilly (9) whose published reviews of absorption, distribution, and metabolism in toxicology remain relevant. While metabolism in the GI tract, lung, or skin may have some effect on disposition, generally these organs do not have the metabolic capacity of the liver and thus have only a slight effect on absorption and distribution.

1. Protein Binding

The degree to which a chemical binds to plasma proteins will highly influence its distribution. Albumin is the most prominent of the many proteins found in mammalian plasma (accounting for almost half of the total), and at a size of 64–70 kd carries both positive and negative charges with which a polar compound can associate by electrostatic attraction, hydrogen bonding, ion pairing, etc. At plasma pH, albumin has a net negative charge. The more avidly bound the material, the less will be distributed to surrounding fluids as part of a solution and only that portion that is free in solution will be available for diffusion into the tissues.

2. Water Solubility

The solubility of a chemical has a direct bearing on its distribution. Recall that only molecules that are in solution will be available for absorption.

As mentioned above, only that portion that is free in solution will be available for diffusion into the tissues. Hence, the more material that is in solution the more that will be available for diffusion.

3. Volume of Distribution

The interplay between plasma protein binding and water solubility are described by the volume of distribution. If one takes the dose administered (mgs) and divides it by the plasma concentration of the test material (mg/ml), the result is a volume number.

$$\frac{\text{Dose}}{\text{Concentration}} = \text{Volume}$$

One can take this process a step further and extrapolate back from a plasma time curve to the y axis. This is theoretically the plasma concentration (C_0) that would occur if, upon being administered, the material is instantly distributed throughout the body. The volume number obtained with the above equation becomes:

$$\frac{\text{Dose}}{C_0} = V_D$$

Where V_D represents the apparent volume of distribution, a proportionality constant that reflects the relation of the concentration of a xenobiotic in plasma to the total amount of the entity in the body. The V_D is a parameter that is simple to calculate yet gives one important information about the distribution of the chemical under investigation.

If the apparent volume of distribution is determined from the analysis of the total plasma concentration curves, the volume of distribution will tell one a great deal about the chemicals distribution in the body. The lower the V_{el} (Volume of Elimination), the less the chemical has diffused out of the blood. A V_D of 12 l can generally be interpreted that the chemical can distribute through the extracellular fluid, but not enter the cells. A small V_D may mean that the chemical is seqestered in a specific organ, such as the depot fat.

C. Metabolism/Biotransformation

Metabolism describes the process by which chemicals are changed by the body. In fact, very few foreign chemicals that come to enter the body are excreted unchanged. Most are chemically modified. In general, metabolism results in chemicals that are more polar and water soluble, and more easily excreted. Examples of more common metabolic conversions are shown in Table 6. In general, the majority of lipophilic chemicals are first oxidized via the cytochrome P-450 dependent mixed function oxidase system of the liver. The basic biochemical mechanisms involved in the system have been known for some time (19) and will not be reviewed here. This is the process classically called Phase I metabolism. Cytochrome P-450 exists as a family of isozymes (the CYP gene superfamily) with varying but overlapping substrate affinity and responses to different inducing agents. For a review of the molecular biology of the CYP gene superfamily the reader is referred to Meyer (10). Induction is the process whereby exposure to a chemical leads to increased activity of the MMFO due to an increase in a specific cytochrome P-450 isozymes. The isoenzymes induced by a variety of different chemicals are given in Table 7. Many chemicals can induce their own metabolism. Hence, repeated dosing with a chemical may lead to lower blood levels at the end, for example, of a thirteen week study than at the beginning. There could also be alterations in the spectrum of metabolites produced, such that an agent could become more, or less, toxic with repeated dosing depending on the nature of the metabolites. It is not unusual during a subchronic or chronic toxicity test for metabolic tolerance to occur. There may be signs of toxicity early in the study but even with continued daily dosing, the signs abate. This phenomenon, particularly in rodents, is frequently due to microsomal induction, whereby the chemical has induced its own metabolism, and more rapid clearance of the parent chemical occurs.

After the chemical has been metabolically oxidized, it can in fact be further metabolized. In fact, it is possible for the metabolites to also be substrates of the MMFO and to be metabolized themselves. The route of metabolic activation of the classic carcinogen benzo[a]pyrene is due to such a mechanism. The biology of these reactive intermediates has been extensively studied, and does not have to be reviewed here. After a chemical is activated to an electrophilic reactive intermediate it must be deactivated. The most common protective nucleophile is glutithione.Glutathione is among the most common organic intracellular chemical in all mammalian species, being present at a concentration of up to 10 mmol and when glutathione S-transferase is very active. Glutathione is a tripeptide (glutamine-cysteine-glycine). The sulfhydryl group of cysteiyn residue is the business end of the molecule where the reaction with the nucleophilic reactive intermediate takes place. After that, the glutahione conjugate are further metabolized to N-acetyl cysteine conjugates collectively called mercapturic acids, which are generally excreted in the urine. The relative predominance of mercapturic acid over other metabolites may be considered a rough indication

Table 6 Summary of Prominent Phase I Biotransformation Reactions

Reaction	Enzyme	Location	Example/Comments
Hydrolysis	Carboxylesterase	Ubiquitous	Vinyl acetate to acetate and acetaldehyde
	Peptidase	Blood, lysomesq	Amino-, carboxy- and endo peptidase which cleave peptides at specific amino acid linkages
Reductions	Epoxide hydroplase	Microsomes, cytosol	Conversion of styrene 7,8 epoxide to styrene 7,8 glycol
	Azo and nitro reduction	Gut microflora	Sequential conversion of nitrobenzene to aniline
	Carbonyl reductase	Cytosol	Conversion of haloperidol to reduced haloperidol (a secondary alcohol)
	Disulfide reduction	Cytosol	Glutathine dependent reduction of disulfiram to deithyldithiocarbamate
	Sulfoxide reduction	Cytosol	Thioredoxin dependent of sulindac to sulindac sulfide
	Quinone reduction	Cytosol, microsomes	DT diaphorase reduction of menadione to hydroquinone
	Reductive dehalogenation	Microsomes	Conversion of pentabromoethane to tetra bromoethane (releasing free bromide ion)
Oxidation	Alcohol dehydrogenase	Cytosol	Conversion of ethanol to acetaldehyde (DAD/DADH dependent reversible reaction)
	Aldehyde dehydrogenase	Mitochondria/Cytosol	Conversion of acetaldehyde to acetate
	Aldehyde oxidase	Liver cytosol	FAD dependent metalloenzyme, oxidation of benzaldehyde to benzoic acid
	Xanthene oxidase	Cytosol	Oxidation of purine derivative, conversion of allopurinol to alloxanthene
	Monamine oxidase	Mitochondria	FAD dependent oxidative deamination of monoamines, e.g. primaquine
	Diamine oxidase	Cytosol	Pyridoxal dependent, copper containing enzyme. Conversion of allylamine to acrolein
	Prostaglandin oxidase	Microsomes	Cooxidation reaction, can activate chemical in tissues low in cytochrome P-450, e.g. nephrotoxicity of acetaminophen, oxidation of phenylbutazone
	Favin-mono-oxygenase	Microsomes	FAD dependent oxidation of nucleophilic nitrogen, sulfur and phosphorus heteroatoms, e.g. conversion of nicotine to nicotine 1'-N-oxide, cimetidine to cimetidine S-oxide
	Cytochrome P-450	Microsomes	NADPH dependent heme protein requires reduction by microsomal NADPH dependent cytochrome c reductase.

Source: adapted from Ref. 24.

Table 7 Examples of Xenobiotics Activated by Human Cytochrome P450 Isozymes

CYP1A1	CYP2D6
Benzo[a]pyrene and other polycyclic	buforolol
aromatic hydrocarbons	codeine
CYP1A2	timolol
acetaminophen	metoprolol
2-Acetylaminofluorene	CYP2E1
4-Aminobiphenyl	acetaminophen
2-Aminofluorene	acrylonitrile
2-Naphthylamine	benzene
CYP2A6	carbon tetrachloride
N-nitrosodiethylamine	chloroform
butadiene	dichloromethane
coumarin	1,2-dichloropropane
CYP2B6	ethylene dibromide
6-Aminochrysene	ethylene dichloride
Cyclophosphamide	ethyl carbamate
ifosphamine	N-Nitrosodimethylamine
	styrene
CYP2C8	trichloroethylene
taxol	Vinyl chloride
	CYP3A4
CYP2C9	acetaminophen
diclofenac	aflatoxin B_1 and G_1
phenytoin	6-aminochrysene
piroxicam	benzo[a]pyrene 7,8-dihydrodiol
tolbutamide	cyclophosphamide
	Ifosphamide
CYP2C19	1-Nitropyrene
diazepam	sterigmatocystin
diphenylhydantoin	senecionine
hexabarbitol	tris(2,3-dibromopropyl) phosphate
propanolol	CYP4A9/11
	none known

Source: adapted in part from Parkinson Ref. 24.

of how "reactive" the intermediates may have been. Teleological, it is tempting to speculate that it is a very well-designed protective mechanism. So long as intracellular glutathione concentrations remain above a critical level (10% of normal) the destructive actions of active metabolites can be held in check. Thus, a small dose of a chemical (bromo-benzene is a good example) may cause no liver damage while a large dose does. This is also a good example of one of the aspects of toxicokinetics versus pharmacokinetics where a high dose of a chemical will become toxic due to saturation of a detoxification pathway.

The glutathione S-transferase pathway is sometimes in biochemical competition with the epoxide hydralase pathway, in that both deactivate intermediates of the MMFO. Epoxide hydralase is a microsomal enzyme that acts specifically to deactivate epoxide intermediates, by the addition of water across the C—O bond to form a diol. As a very broad generality, the glutathione S-transferase pathway tends to be more prominent in rodents, while the epoxide hydratase pathway tends to be more dominant in nonrodents.

Glutathione conjugation is an example of Phase II (synthetic) reactions. "Unreactive" metabolites can also be conjugated. The hydroxyl or diol containing metabolites of the MMFO can be further metabolized by phase II metabolism whereby they are conjugated to form glucuronides and/or sulfates (so called etherial sulfates). Amines can also be substrates. The net effect of phase II reactions is to create a more polar molecule that is more readily excretable. While there are species differences, glucuronides are actively transported and excreted in the bile into the GI tract. Sulfates are excreted more predominantly in the urine. Both glucuronides and sulfates, however, can be found in both the urine and the feces. Like the MMFO pathway, glutathione S-transferase, UDP-glucuronyl transferase and eopoxide hydratase are inducible, i.e., treatment with exogenous chemicals will increase the amount of enzyme protein present.

Outside of the MMFO mediated (Phase I) reactions there are a few other major reactions that are worthy of note. The two major ones involve ester hydrolysis and alcohol and aldehyde oxidation. All mammalian species have an extensive ability to hydrolyze the ester bond. The products of the reactions then can go on to be further metabolized. In the pharmaceutical industry, this property has been utilized to synthesize pro-drugs; i.e., chemicals that have desirable pharmaceutical properties (generally increased water solubility) that are not converted to their active moiety until hydrolyzed in the body.

The activity of alcohol dehydrogenase is one with which we should all be familiar. It oxidizes alcohols to aldehydes. The aldehydes produced by this reaction can go on to be further metabolized to a carbocylic acid, if they are not sterically hindered. Sidechain constituents of aromatic compounds can also be a substrate for this reaction sequence, producing sidechain carboxylates. The oxidation of alcohols to aldehydhydes can also be a form of metabolic activation as aldehydes can have potent physiological actions. Fortunately, aldehydhyde dehydrogenase has a very high activity when compared to alcohol dehydrogenase, so that the aldehydhydes do not accumulate. Inhibition of aldehyde dehydrogenase by disulfiram (Antabuse^{TM}) leads to the accumulation of acetaldehyde, causing nausea, dizziness, and flushing. Like disulfiram, some pesticides contain dithiocarbamates and have the potential of causing this type of reaction.

Hopefully, this little description of the major metabolic pathways has given one some appreciation of the richness of the processes. The different sites of oxidation, the possibility of additional oxidative metabolism of metabolites, and differences in Phase II reactions all lead to a multiplicity of possible metabolites. Over 100 different metabolites of the human pharmaceutical chlorpromazine have been isolated and identified. When analyzed by HPLC, for example, the parent chemical and the different (detectable) metabolites will form a pattern of different peaks. This is referred to as the metabolic fingerprint or profile of a chemical. Different species will have different profiles. Ideally, in doing a risk assessment, one would like to know the similarity in this pattern between the animals used in the toxicology studies and that produced by human beings. This is only infrequently available for most nonpharmaceutical products, as pesticides (for example) are rarely given intentionally to human subjects for the purposes of study. The technology now exists, however, to address this potential problem. Cell lines with human cytochrome P-450 have been developed that can provide some indication of the similarities of human metabolism of a chemical to that of experimental animals. At least they may be able to assist in identifying the major oxidative metabolite. For nonpharmaceutical products, it may be an unusual circumstance that would require one to identify potential human metabolites as part of a marketing application; however, it may be useful for one to know that the technology exists to do so.

Suffice it to say that the processes of metabolic conversion are frequently involved in the mechanisms of toxicity and carcinogenicity.

1. Metabolic Activation

As mentioned, most nonnutritive chemicals pass through the GI tract by passive absorption, and then enter the mesenteric circulation. The venous circulation from the mesentery flows through the portal vein into the liver. The metabolic action of the liver literally sits between the GI tract and the general systemic circulation. Thus, even chemicals that may be highly absorbed from the GI tract could appear only sparingly in systemic circulation if they are highly metabolized by the liver. The combination of absorption from the GI tract and metabolism from the liver leads to what is called the first pass effect. An extension of this is the fact that the gut flora contain glucuronidases, that can cleave glucuronides of chemicals and/or metabolites that are then available to be reabsorbed. This process is called enterohepatic circulation.

2. Induction of P-450 Metabolism and Isoenzymes

When organisms are exposed to certain xenobiotics their ability to metabolize a variety of chemicals is increased. This phenomenon produces a transitory resistance to the toxicity of many compounds. However, this may not be the case with compounds that require metabolic activation. The exact toxicological outcome of such increased metabolism is dependent on the specific xenobiotic and its specific metabolic pathway. Since the outcome of a xenobiotic exposure can depend on the balance between those reactions that represent detoxication and those that represent activation, increases in metabolic capacity may at times produce unpredictable results.

The ability of different chemicals to differentially inhibit and/or induce different cytochrome P450 is gaining increased importance for a regulatory and risk assessment point of view. These type of effects are typically investigated by examining the actions of a test material on the metabolism of model substrates for specific cytochrome P450 isozymes. Draper et al. have published on the use of human liver microsomes for determining the levels of activity or inhibition a chemical has on the formation of 6-alpha-testosterone as a model for CYP3A activity (1) and chlorzoxazone for CYP2E1 activity (2). If, for example, a chemical under study competitively inhibits the metabolism of these model substrates in these systems, then it is a substrate for that human isozyme. Using these more recently available in vitro systems, it is much easier to perform cross species comparisons with regard to biotransformation. It is now easier to determine how similar the routes of metabolism are in the experimental animals with comparison to that in man without having to administer the chemical to human subjects.

3. Species Differences

Species differences in metabolism are among the most prominent reasons that there are species differences in toxicity. Differences in cytochrome P450 is one of the most common reason for differences in metabolism. For example, Monostory et al. (11) recently published a paper comparing the metabolism of panomifene (a tamoxifen analog) in four different species, summarized in Table 8.

Table 8 Examples of Species Differences in Microsomal Metabolism of Panomifene

Metabolite	Mouse (%)	Rat (%)	Dog (%)	Human (%)
M1	—	—	25	—
M2	39	23	—	—
M3	—	—	43	—
M4	—	—	18	—
M5	—	29	8	51
M6	27	27	6	49
M7	34	21	—	—
Total rate (pmol/min/mg)	9.33	22.1	49.6	4.11

Source: adapted from Monostory et al. (Ref. 11).

These data demonstrate that the rates of metabolism in the nonhuman species was most rapid in the dog and slowest in the mouse. Thus, one should not a priori make any assumptions about which species will have the more rapid metabolism. Also note that of the seven metabolites, only one was produced in all four species. Both the rat and the dog produced the two metabolites (M5 and M6) produced by human microsomes. So how does one decide which species best represents man? One needs to consider the chemical structure of the metabolites and the rates at which they are produced. In this particular case, M5 and M6 were relatively minor metabolites in the dog, which produced three other metabolites in larger proportion. The rat produced the same metabolites at a higher proportion, with fewer other metabolites than the dog. Thus, in this particular instance the rat, rather than the dog, was a better model for human metabolism.

A more thorough review on species differences in pharmacokinetics has been prepared by Smith (12).

4. Sex-Related Differences in Rodents

Not only are there differences in biotransformation and metabolism between species, there may also be differences between sexes within a species. Griffin et al. (13) has demonstrated sex-related differences in the metabolism of 2,4-dichlorophenoxyacetic acid (Table 9). They noted that while there were differences between sexes, they tended to be quantitative (rates), not qualitative (metabolites). Differences between species were greater than sex-related differences. With regard to sex-related differences, it is noteworthy that males do not always have the higher rates, as Griffin et al. have shown; in hamsters, the female metabolizes 2,4-D more rapidly than males. In general, male rats tend to have higher activity than female rats, especially with regard to CYP dependent activ-

Table 9 Differences in the Disposition of 2,4-dichlorophenoxyacetic Acid

Species	Sex	Urine	Feces
Rat	M	31.2	2.7
	F	16.5	1.1
Mouse	M	12.7	2.8
	F	26.8	6.7
Hamster	M	4.9	2.5
	F	33.9	14.5

All animals dosed orally with radiolabeled 2.4-D, 200 mg/ kg. Results are expressed as percent of 14C dose recovered. Urine was collected for 8 hr and feces for 24 hr.

ity. In the case of 2,4-D, the only urinary metabolite is 2,4-D glucuronide, but the half life of 2,4-D was 138 min in males and 382 in females.

For a more complete review of the biochemical differences that lead to differences between gender, the reader is referred to Mugford and Kidderis (20).

a. Stereoisomerism. Stereoisomerism will influence metabolism and toxicity, but it is rarely considered in the assessment of agricultural and industrial chemicals. For example, Lu (16) reported a comparison of (S)-(−)Ifosfamide and (R)-(+)-Ifosfamide. They demonstrated that there were significant differences between the two stereoisomers with regard to pharmacokinetic behavior and major metabolite formation, as shown in Table 10.

In addition, treatment of animals with phenobarbital not only increased overall rates of metabolism and clearance, but also shifted the metabolite patterns. One of the more common methods used for determining an exposure to (or the amount of a metabolite produced) is to determine an area under the curve (AUC) for the metabolite. Further, one of the more common methods for representing a racemically preferred metabolite is to calculate the ratio of the R to the S. For example, the 3-decholoro metabolite of ifosfamide was produced in higher amounts from the R enantiomer while the 2-decholorometabolite was the major metabolite produced from the R enantiomer in naive animals. Treatment with phenobarbital shifted the metabolism so that the 3-dechloro metabolite was no longer the major metabolite for the S enantiomer.

D. Excretion

Excretion encompasses the process by which chemicals or their metabolites are transported out of the body. There are three possible major routes of excretion,

Table 10 Example of Stereoselective Differences in Metabolism (R) vs (S) Ifosfamide

Parameter	Phenobarb	R	S	R/S
Term half life	—	34.3	41.8	.820
(min)	+	19.8	19.41	1.02
AUC	—	4853	6259	.820
(uM*min)	+	1479	1356	1.03
2-dehloro metabolite	—	799	2794	.287
AUC	+	229	1205	.186
3-dehloro metabolite	—	1380	996	1.41
AUC	+	192	1175	.159

Adapted from Lu et al. (Ref. 16).
Animals were pretreated with phenobarbital (80 mg/kg) for four days.

and a handful of minor ones. The major routes of excretion for chemicals, and in particular their metabolites, are:

1. Urine

The kidneys filter the entire cardiac output multiple times each day, and thus provide a large opportunity for the removal of chemicals from the bloodstream. How much of a xenobiotic is actually excreted is dependent on three factors or processes.

1. The glomerular membrane has pores of 70–80 Å; and under the positive hydrostatic conditions in the glomerulus, all molecules smaller than about 20,000 D are filtered. Proteins and protein-bound compounds thus remain in the plasma, and about 20% of the nonbound entity is carried with 20% of the plasma water into the glomular filtrate.
2. Because the glomerular filtrate contains many important body constituents (e.g., glucose), there are specific active re-uptake processes for them. Also, lipid-soluble chemicals diffuse back from the tubule into the blood, especially as the urine becomes more concentrated because of water reabsorption. The pH of the urine is generally lower than that of the plasma, and therefore pH partitioning tends to increase the reabsorption of weak acids. The pH of the urine can be altered appreciably by treatment with ammonium chloride (decreases pH) or sodium carbonate (increases pH); the buffered plasma shows little change.
3. Xenobiotics may be secreted actively into the renal tubule against a concentration gradient by anion and cation carrier processes. These processes are saturable and of relatively low specificity; many basic or acidic compounds and their metabolites (especially conjugation products) are removed by them. Because the dissociation rate for the chemical-albumin complex is rapid, it is possible for highly protein-bound compounds to be almost completely cleared at a single passage through the kidney.

2. Feces

The most important mechanism allowing circulating foreign compounds to enter the gut is in the bile. The biological aspects of this mechanism have been reviewed, and certain pertinent points have emerged. The bile may be regarded as a complementary pathway to the urine, with small molecules being eliminated by the kidney and large molecules in the bile. Thus the bile becomes the principal excretory route for many drug conjugates. Species differences exist in the molecular weight requirement for significant biliary excretion, which has been estimated as 325 ± 50 in the rat, 440 ± 50 in the guinea pig, and 475 ± 50 in the rabbit. In the rat, small molecules (less than 350 D) are not eliminated in the bile or large molecules (more than 450 D) in the urine, even if the principal excretory mechanism is blocked by ligation of the renal pedicles or bile duct, respectively. Compounds of intermediate molecular weight (350–450 D) are excreted by both routes, and ligation of one pathway results in increased use of the other.

Foreign compounds may also enter the gut by direct diffusion or secretion across the gut wall, elimination in the saliva, pH partitioning of bases into the low pH of the stomach, and elimination in the pancreatic juice.

3. Expired Air

Volatile compounds or metabolites can be extensively excreted by passage across pulmonary membranes into the airspace of the lungs, then expulsion from the lungs in expired air.

Minor routes for excretion can include tears, saliva, sweat, exfoliated keratinocytes, hair, and nasal discharge. These are of concern or significance only in rare cases. Accordingly, quantitation of excretion typically requires collection of urine and feces (and occasionally expired air) over a period of time.

E. Pharmacokinetics

The interplay of the processes of absorption, distribution, metabolism, and excretion result in changes in concentration of the test chemical in different organs with time. With regard to the practical concerns of monitoring human exposure, the organ of interest is the blood. Blood can be considered a central compartment. Determining the concentration of the chemical in plasma gives one an assessment of exposure. Mathematical formulas are used to quantitatively describe this exposure.

The relevant questions with regard to the use of pharmacokinetic data include:

How much of the dose was absorbed?
What are the plasma levels associated with toxicity?
What was total systemic exposure?
How fast is the material cleared from the body?
Is there evidence of accumulation?

Some of the pharmacokinetic parameters that are of value in answering these questions include:

To what extent is there dose/exposure proportionality?
Peak plasma and t_{max}

Half-life and k_d
Increases in auc with repeated exposures

Chemicals that bioaccumulate have an increased hazard potential as toxic levels may slowly develop. Elimination rates dictate bioaccumulation. The longer the half-life, the more likely it is that bioaccumulation will occur. If a chemical is administered (or exposure occurs) on a regular basis, as a rule steady state will be achieved in five half-lives.

IV. LABORATORY METHODS

The actual means by which toxicokinetic information is collected is through the conduct of one or more specific studies. Through the application of available analytical techniques, xenobiotics can be identified and quantified in relevant samples collected in accordance with carefully designed and executed protocols.

A. Analytical Methods

There are three broad categories of analytical techniques now available—instrumental (cold chemical), radiolabeled, and immunological. Each of these has advantages and disadvantages. Only an overview of these techniques will be given here—detailed explanations are beyond the scope of this text. These methodologies are all directed at being able to identify and/or quantify a chemical (and/or its metabolites) in various biological matrices.

1. Instrumental Methods

These bioanalytical methods are also sometimes called cold chemistry methods. These generally start from a place of isolating the compound or compounds of interest, for which the workhorse methodology is high pressure liquid chromatography (HPLC). A wide variety of specialized columns are used to achieve desired separation. At the end of the column, where separation of molecular entities has been achieved, the outflow of the column can be directed to any of a wide variety of detection instruments, including various forms of detectors intrinsic to the HPLC. In general, traditional cold chemistry methodologies have less sensitivity (higher detection limits) than do radiochemical or immunological methods. The most recent advances in HPLC/MS technologies now have sensitivity limits that surpass those of radiolabelled techniques.

Mass spectrometry (MS), nuclear magnetic resonance (NMR) spectrography, electron skin resonance (ESR) spectrography, ultraviolet, infrared, and visible spectrography and raman spectroscopy are all well-established detection methodologies (see [14] for a more thorough discussion of these).

2. Radiochemical Methods

The massive expansion of our understanding of toxicokinetics since the late 1970s is to a large degree a reflection of the wide use of radioactive isotopes as tracers of chemical and biological processes. Appropriately radiolabeled test compounds are commonly used in toxicokinetic studies, providing a simple means of following the administered dose in the body. This is particularly important when specific analytical methods are unavailable or too insensitive. The use of total radioactivity measurements allows an estimation of the total exposure to drug-related material and facilitates the achievement of material balance.

The most commonly used radionuclides in drug metabolism and disposition studies are carbon-14 (^{14}C) and tritium (^{3}H), both of which are referred to as beta emitters. Since these beta-emitting isotopes have relatively long half-lives (see Table 11), their radioactive decay during an experiment is insignificant. Additionally, they provide sufficient emission energy for measurement and are relatively safe to use, as indicated by the data in Table 11. Although individual beta particles can have any energy up to the maximum, E_{max}, the basic quantity in determining the energy imparted to tissues by beta emitters is the average energy, E_β. The range is the maximum thickness the beta particles can penetrate. Beta particles present virtually no hazard when they originate outside the body (15). This is not the case with the gamma emitters such as chromium-51 (^{51}Cr) and iodine-125 (^{125}I), which see use in radioimmunoassays precisely due th their higher energies.

During the synthesis of radiolabeled compounds, the label is usually introduced as part of the molecular skeleton in a metabolically stable and, with tritium, nonexchangeable position. The in vivo stability of ^{14}C labels is often reflected by the extent of [^{14}C] carbon dioxide formation. The biologic stability of ^{3}H labels can be estimated by the extent of tritiated water formation. The tritiated water concentration (dpm/ml) in urine samples collected during a designated time interval after dosing, assumedly after equilibrium is reached between

Table 11 Properties of Tritium, Carbon-14, Chromium-51, and Iodine 125

Property	^{3}H	^{51}Cr	^{14}C	^{125}I
Half-life (yr)	12.3	27.8 (d)	5730	13 (d)
Maximum beta energy (MeV)	0.0186	0.752	0.156	2.150
Average beta energy (MeV)	0.006	NA	0.049	NA
Range in air (mm)	6		300	
Range in unit density material (mm)	0.0052		0.29	

urine and the body water pool, is determined. This value is extrapolated from the midpoint of the collection interval to zero time, based on the known half-life of tritiated water in the given species. The percentage of the radioactive dose that is transformed to tritiated water ($\%^3H_2O$) can be calculated using the following equation:

$$\%^3H_2O = \frac{^3H_2O \text{ concentration at zero time} \times \text{exchangeable body water volume}}{\text{radioactivity dose}} \times 100\%$$

Values for the exchangeable body water content as well as the half-life of triti-ated water in some mammalian species that can be applied to the above equation are shown in Table 12. If the molecule is likely to or is known to fragment into two major portions, it may be desirable to monitor both fragments by differential labeling (^3H and ^{14}C).

The chemical and radiochemical purity of the labeled compound must be ascertained prior to use. In practice a value of $\geq 95\%$ is usually acceptable. The desired specific activity of the administered radioactive compound depends on the dose to be used as well as the species studied. Doses of ^{14}C on the order of 5 µCi/kg for the dog and 20 µCi/kg for the rat have been found adequate in most studies, while doses of ^3H are usually two to three times higher owing to lower counting efficiency of this isotope.

Liquid scintillation counting is the most popular technique for the detec-tion and measurement of radioactivity. In order to count a liquid specimen such as plasma, urine, or digested blood or tissues directly in a liquid-scintillation spectrometer, an aliquot of the specimen is first mixed with a liquid scintillant. Aliquots of blood, feces, or tissue homogenates are air-dried and ash-free filter papers and combusted in a sample oxidizer provided with an appropriate absorp-tion medium and a liquid scintillant prior to counting. The liquid scintillant plays the role of an energy transducer, converting energy from nuclear decay

Table 12 Volume and Half-Life of Body Water in Selected Species

Species	Sex	Exchangeable body water (% of body weight)	Half-life (days)
Mouse	F	58.5	1.13
Rat	M	59.6	2.53
Rabbit	F	58.4	3.87
Dog	M	66.0	5.14
Cynomolgus monkey	F	64.2	7.23
Rhesus monkey	M	61.6	7.80
Man	M,F	55.3	9.46

into light. The light generates electrical signal pulses which are analyzed according to their timing and amplitude, and are subsequently recorded as a count rate, e.g., counts per minute (cpm). Based on the counting efficiency of the radionuclide used, the count rate is then converted to the rate of disintegration, e.g., disintegrations per minute (dpm), which is a representation of the amount of radioactivity present in the sample.

3. Immunoassay Methods

Radioimmunoassay (RIA) allows measurement of biologically active materials which are not detectable by traditional cold chemistry techniques. RIAs can be used to measure molecules that cannot be radiolabeled to detectable levels in vivo. They also are used for molecules unable to fix complement when bound to antibodies, or they can be used to identify cross-reacting antigens that compete and bind with the antibody.

Competitive inhibition of radiolabeled hormone antibody binding by unlabeled hormone (either as a standard or an unknown mixture) is the principle of most RIAs. A standard curve for measuring antigen (hormone) binding to antibody is constructed by placing known amounts of radiolabeled antigen and the antibody into a set of test tubes. Varying amounts of unlabeled antigen are added to the test tubes. Antigen–antibody complexes are separated from the antigen and the amount of radioactivity from each sample is measured to detect how much unlabeled antigen is bound to the antibody. Smaller amounts of radiolabeled antigen-antibody complexes are present in the fractions containing higher amounts of unlabeled antigen. A standard curve must be constructed to correlate the percentage of radiolabeled antigen bound with the concentration of unlabeled antigen present.

Two methods are commonly employed in RIAs to separate antigen–antibody complexes. The first, the double-antibody technique, precipitates antigen–antibody complexes out of solution by utilizing a second antibody, which binds to the first antibody. The second most commonly used method is the dextran-coated activated charcoal technique. Addition of dextran-coated activated charcoal to the sample followed immediately by centrifugation absorbs free antigen and leaves antigen-antibody complexes in the supernatant fraction. This technique works best when the molecular weight of the antigen is 30 kilodaltons (kDa) or less. Also, sufficient carrier protein must be present to prevent adsorption of unbound antibody.

Once a standard curve has been constructed, the RIA can determine the concentration of hormone in a sample (usually plasma or urine). The values of hormone levels are usually accurate using the RIA, but certain factors (e.g., pH or ionic strength) can affect antigen binding to the antibody. Thus similar conditions must be used for the standard and the sample.

Problems of RIAs include lack of specificity. This problem is usually due to nonspecific cross-reactivity of the antibody. Unlike assays that often require large amounts of tissue (or blood), the greater sensitivity of the RIAs or monoclonal antibody techniques can be achieved using small samples of biological fluids. Some of these RIA methodologies are more useful than others and to some extent depend on the degree of hormonal cross-reactions or, in the case of monoclonal antibody methods, their degree of sensitivity.

Enzyme-linked immunosorbent assay (ELISA) is comparable to the immunoradiometric assay, except that an enzyme tag is attached to the antibody instead of a radioactive label. ELISAs have the advantage of no radioactive materials and produce an end product that can be assessed with a spectrophotometer. The molecule of interest is bound to the enzyme-labeled antibody, and the excess antibody is removed for immunoradiometric assays. After excess antibody has been removed or the second antibody containing the enzyme has been added (two-site assay), the substrate and cofactors necessary are added in order to visualize and record enzyme activity. The level of molecule of interest present is directly related to the level of enzymatic activity. The sensitivity of the ELISAs can be enhanced by increasing the incubation time for producing substrate.

Immunoradiometric assays (IRMAs) are like RIAs in that a radiolabeled substance is used in an antibody–antigen reaction, except that the radioactive label is attached to the antibody instead of the hormone. Furthermore, excess of antibody, rather than limited quantity, is present in the assay. All the unknown antigen becomes bound in an IRMA rather than just a portion, as in a RIA; IRMAs are more sensitive. In the one-site assay, the excess antibody that is not bound to the sample is removed by addition of a precipitating binder. In a two-site assay, a molecule with at least two antibody-binding sites is adsorbed onto a solid phase, to which one of the antibodies is attached. After binding to this antibody is completed, a second antibody labeled with ^{125}I is added to the assay. This antibody reacts with the second antibody-binding site to form a "sandwich," composed to antibody-hormone-labeled antibody. The amount of hormone present is proportional to the amount of radioactivity measured in the assay.

With enzyme-multiplied immunoassay technique (EMIT) assays, enzyme tags are used instead of radiolabels. The antibody binding alters the enzyme characteristics, allowing for measurement of target molecules without separating the bound and free components (i.e., homogeneous assay). The enzyme is attached to the molecule being tested. This enzyme-labeled antigen is incubated with the sample and with antibody to the molecule. Binding of the antibody to the enzyme-linked molecule either physically blocks the active site of the enzyme or changes the protein conformation so that the enzyme is no longer active. After antibody binding occurs, the enzyme substrate and cofactor are added, and enzyme activity is measured. If the sample contains subject molecules, it will compete with enzyme-linked molecules for antibody binding, enzyme will not be blocked by the antibody, and more enzyme activity will be measurable.

Most chemical entities can now be assessed using monoclonal antibody (MAb) techniques. It is possible to produce antisera containing a variety of polyclonal antibodies that recognize and bind many parts of the molecule. Polyclonal antisera can create some nonspecificity problems such as cross-reactivity and variation in binding affinity. Therefore it is oftentimes desirable to produce a group of antibodies that selectively bind to a specific region of the molecule (i.e., antigenic determinant). In the past, investigators produced antisera to antigenic determinants of the molecule by cleaving the molecule and immunizing an animal with the fragment of the hormone containing the antigenic determinant of interest. This approach solved some problems with cross-reactivity of antisera with other similar antigenic determinants, but problems were still associated with the heterogeneous collection of antibodies found in polyclonal antisera.

The production of MAbs offers investigators a homogenous collection of antibodies that could bind selectively to a specific antigenic determinant with the same affinity. In addition to protein isolation and diagnostic techniques, MAbs have contributed greatly to RIAs.

While MAbs offer a highly sensitive, specific method for detecting antigen, sometimes increasing MAb specificity compromises affinity of the antibody for the antigen. In addition, there is usually decreased complement fixation, and costs are usually high for preparing and maintaining hybridomas that produce MAbs (Table 13).

The monoclonal antibody techniques provide a means of producing a specific antibody for binding antigen. This technique is useful for studying protein structure relations (or alterations) and has been used for devising specific RIAs.

Table 13 Advantages and Disadvantages of Monoclonal Antibodies Compared to Polyclonal Antisera

Advantages	Disadvantages
Sensitivity	Overly specific
Quantities available	Decreased affinity
Immunologically defined	Diminished complement fixation
Detection of neoantigens on cell membrane	Labor intensive; high cost

Modified from Stites et al.

B. Sampling Methods and Intervals

Methodology is presented here for the case of use in the rat, the most commonly utilized species, as a prototypical example. Similar methodology exists for other model species (17).

Blood. Since blood (plasma and serum) is the most easily accessible body compartment, the blood concentration profile is most commonly used to describe the time course of drug disposition in the animal. With the development of sensitive analytical methods that require small volumes (100–200 µl) of blood, ADME data from individual rats can be obtained by serial sample collection. Numerous cannulation techniques have been utilized to facilitate repeated blood collection, but the animal preparation procedures are elaborate and tedious and are incompatible with prolonged sampling periods in studies involving a large number of animals. In contrast, noncannulation methods such as collection from the tail vein, orbital sinus, or jugular vein are most practical. Significant volumes of blood can be obtained from the intact rat by cardiac puncture, although this method can cause shock to the animal system and subsequent death.

Blood collection from the tail vein is a simple and rapid, nonsurgical method that does not require anesthesia. A relatively large number of serial samples can be obtained within a short period of time. However, this method is limited to relatively small sample volumes (≤250 µl per sample). Although larger volumes can be obtained by placing the rat in a warming chamber, this procedure could significantly influence the disposition of the test compound and therefore is not recommended for routine studies. Blood collected from the cut tail has been shown to provide valid concentration data for numerous compounds.

The rat is placed in a suitable restrainer with the tail hanging freely. The tail is immersed in a beaker of warm water (37–40°C) for 1–2 min to increase the blood flow. Using surgical scissors or a scalpel, the tail is completely transected approximately 5 mm above the tip. The tail is then gently "milked" by sliding the fingers down the tail from its base. It should be noted that excessive "milking" could cause damage to the blood capillaries or increase the white cell count in the blood. A heparinized micropipet of desired capacity (25–250 µl) is held at a 30–45° downward angle in contact with the cut end of the tail. This allows blood to fill the micropipet by capillary action. Application of gentle pressure with a gauze pad for approximately 15 sec is sufficient to stop bleeding. A sufficient number of serial blood samples may be obtained to adequately describe the blood level profile of a compound.

If plasma is required, the blood is centrifuged after sealing one end of the filled micropipet and placing it in a padded centrifuge tube. The volume of plasma is determined by measuring the length of plasma as a fraction of the length of the micropipet, multiplied by the total capacity of the pipet. The tube is then broken at the plasma/red blood cell interface and the sample is expelled using a small bulb. If serum is needed, the blood should be collected without using anticoagulants in the sampling tube.

Serial blood samples can also be collected from the orbital sinus, permitting rapid collection of larger (1–3 ml) samples.

Excreta. Excretion samples commonly collected from the rat include urine, feces, bile, and expired air. By using properly designed cages and techniques, the samples can be completely collected so that the mass balance is readily determined. These samples also serve to elucidate the biotransformation characteristics of the compound.

These samples can be easily collected through the use of suitable metabolism cages. Since rodents are coprophagic, the cage must be designed to prevent the animal from ingesting the feces as it is passed. Other main features of the cage should include the ability to effectively separate urine from feces with minimal cross-contamination, a feed and water system that prevents spillage and subsequent contamination of collected samples, and collection containers that can be easily removed without disturbing the animal. Also, the cage should be designed so that it can be easily disassembled for cleaning or autoclaving.

Following dose administration, rats are placed in individual cages. The urine and feces that collect in containers are removed at predetermined intervals. The volume of urine and the weight of feces are measured. After the final collection, the cage is rinsed, normally with ethanol or water, to assure complete recovery of excreta. If the rats are also used for serial blood sampling, it is important that bleeding be performed inside the cage to avoid possible loss of urine or feces.

Bile. As previously mentioned, systemically absorbed chemicals and their metabolites are excreted largely in the urine and feces. Analysis of feces, however, is problematic when the animals have been dosed orally. The presence of the parent chemical in the feces may be due to either the presence of unabsorbed materials or excreted, unmetabolized materials. This difficulty in analysis can be overcome by analysis of the bile.

The bile is the pathway through which an absorbed compound is excreted in the feces. In order to collect this sample, surgical cannulation of the animal is necessary (21), and the animals must be carefully maintained. Surgically prepared animals can be purchased from most of the major suppliers.

Expired Air. For ^{14}C-labeled chemicals, the tracer carbon may be incorporated in vivo into carbon dioxide, a possible metabolic product. Therefore, when the position of the radiolabel indicates the potential for biological instability, a pilot study to collect expired air and monitor its radioactivity content should be conducted prior to initiating a full-scale study. Expired air studies should also be performed in situations where the radiolabel has been postulated to be stable, but analyses of urine and feces from the toxicokinetic study fail to yield complete recovery (mass balance) of the dose.

Following drug administration, the rat is placed in a special metabolism cage. Using a vacuum pump, a constant flow of room air (approx. 500 ml/min) is drawn through a drying column containing anhydrous calcium sulfate impregnated with a moisture indicator (cobalt chloride), and passed into a second column containing Ascarite® II, where it is rendered carbon dioxide free. The air is then drawn in through the top of the metabolism cage. Exhaled breath exiting the metabolism cage is passed through a carbon dioxide adsorption tower, where the expired $^{14}CO_2$ is trapped in a solution, such as a mixture of 2-ethoxyethanol and 2-aminoethanol $(2:1)$. The trapping solution is collected, replaced with fresh solution, and assayed at designated times postdose so that the total amount of radioactivity expired as labeled carbon dioxide can be determined.

Milk. The study of passage of a xenobiotic into milk serves to assess the potential risk to breast-fed infants in the absence of human data. The passage into milk can be estimated as the milk-plasma ratio of drug concentrations at each sampling time or that of the AUC values. Approximately 30 rats in their first lactation are used. The litter size is adjusted to about 10 within 1–2 days following parturition. The test compound is administered to the mothers 8–10 days after parturition. The rats are then divided into groups for milk and blood collection at designated times postdose. All sucklings are removed from the mother rats several hours before milking. Oxytocin, 1 IU per rat, is given intramuscularly 10–15 min before each collection of milk to stimulate milk ejection. The usual yield of milk is about 1 ml from each rat. Blood is obtained immediately after milking. In order to minimize the number of animals used, the sucklings can be returned to the mother rat which can then be milked again 8–12 hr later.

In all the fluid sampling techniques above, the limitations of availability should be kept in mind. Table 14 presents a summary of such availability for the principle model species.

Table 14 Approximate Volumes of Pertient Biological Fluids in Adult Laboratory Animals

Fluid	Rat	Mouse	Dog	Rabbit	Monkey
Blood (ml/kg)	75	75	70	60	75
Plasma (ml/kg)	40	45	40	30	45
Urine (ml/kg/day)	60	50	30	60	75
Bile (ml/kg/day)	90	100	12	120	25

For topical exposures, determining absorption (into the skin and into the systemic circulation) requires a different set of techniques. For determining how much material is left, skin washing is required. There are two components to skin washing in the recovery of chemicals. The first component may involve the physical rubbing and removal from the skin surface. The second component is the surfactant action of soap and water. However, the addition of soap effects the partitioning. Some chemicals may require multiple successive washing with soap and water applications for removal from skin. OPPTS guideline 870.7600 provides very specific directions on how the application site is to be washed.

Skin tape stripping can be used to determine the concentration of chemical in the stratum corneum at the end of a short application period (30 min) and by linear extrapolation predicts the percutaneous absorption of that chemical for longer application periods. The chemical is applied to skin of animals or humans, and after a 30-min skin contact application time, the stratum corneum is blotted and then removed by successive tape applications. The tape-strippings are assayed for chemical content. There is a linear relationship between this stratum corneum reservoir content and percutaneous absorption. The major advantages of this method are 1) the elimination of urinary and fecal excretion to determine absorption and 2) the applicability to nonradiolabeled determination of percutaneous absorption, because the skin strippings contain adequate chemical concentrations for nonlabeled assay methodology.

Finally, a complete determination of the distribution and potential departing of a chemical and its metabolites requires some form of measurement or sampling of tissues/organs. Autoradiography provides a nonquantitative means of doing such, but quantitation requires actual collection and sampling of tissues. Table 15 provides guidance as to the relative percentage of total body mass that the organs constitute in the common model species.

Table 15 Typical Organ Weights in Adult Laboratory Animals

Organ	Percent of body weight				
	Rat	Mouse	Dog	Rabbit	Monkey
Liver	3.5	6	3.5	3	2.5
Kidney	0.8	1.6	0.5	0.8	0.5
Heart	0.4	0.4	0.8	0.3	0.4
Spleen	0.3	0.5	0.3	0.04	0.1
Brain	0.5	0.6	0.8	0.4	3
Adrenals	0.02	0.01	0.01	0.02	0.03
Lung	0.6	0.6	1	0.6	0.7

1. Sampling Interval

To be able to perform valid toxicokinetic analysis, it is not only necessary to properly collect samples of appropriate biological fluids, but also to collect a sufficient number of samples at the current intervals. Both of these variables are determined by the nature of the answers sought. Useful parameters in toxicokinetic studies are C_{max} (peak plasma test compound concentration), T_{max} (time at which the peak plasma test compound concentration occurs), C_{min} (plasma test compound concentration immediately before the next dose is administered), AUC (area under the plasma test compound concentration-time curve during a dosage interval), and $t_{1/2}$ (half-life for the decline of test compound concentrations in plasma). The samples required to obtain these parameters are shown in Table 16. C_{min} requires one blood sample immediately before a dose is given and provides information on accumulation. If there is no accumulation in plasma, the test compound may not be detected in this sample.

Several C_{min} samples are required at intervals during the toxicity study to check whether accumulation is occurring. CT is a blood sample taken at a chosen time after dosing and provides proof of absorption as required by the GLP regulations, but little else. C_{max} requires several blood samples to be taken for its accurate definition as does T_{max}: these two parameters provide information on rate of absorption. AUC also requires several blood samples to be taken so that it can be calculated: it provides information on extent of absorption. $t_{1/2}$, the half-life, requires several samples to be taken during the terminal decline phase of the test compound concentration-time curve: this parameter provides information on various aspects such as any change in the kinetics of the test compound during repeated doses or at different dose levels. Depending on the other parameters obtained, the accumulation ratio can be calculated from C_{min}, C_{max} and/or AUC when these are available after the first dose and after several doses to steady-state.

Table 16 Blood Samples Required so that Certain Toxicokinetic Parameters Can Be Obtained and Calculated

Parameter	Blood sample required	Information obtained
C_{min} (C_{24})	24-h	Accumulation
CT	T-h	Proof of absorption
C_{max} (C peak)	Several*	Rate of absorption
T_{max} (T peak)	Several*	Rate of absorption
AUC	Several*	Extent of absorption
$t_{1/2}$	Several*	Various
Accumulation ratio	Several after first and repeated doses	Extent of accumulation

*Several samples to define concentration-time profile.

Operational and metabolic considerations generally make urine sampling and assay of limited value for toxicokinetic purposes.

2. Study Type

The design of rodent metabolism studies is defined in some detail in the U.S. Environmental Protection Agency (EPA) guidelines for pesticide registration. The basic EPA experimental package is as follows:

1. Single low oral dose
2. Single high oral dose
3. Single intravenous dose
4. Multiple low oral dose

It sets out to determine absorption, distribution, biotransformation and excretion, as well as dose-dependency of metabolism and the effects of the chemical on its own metabolism. No data on the rates of accumulation and depletion of residues are obtained (though the accumulation phase is requested by JMAFF).

Dosing is usually by gavage. The possible effects of dose formulation on absorption and first-pass metabolism have been reviewed in some detail in an earlier paper and will be discussed further below. Administration by gavage dosing and by dietary inclusion can afford some spectacular differences in both the toxicity and the metabolism of a test chemical. Clearly, formulation and dose presentation are important aspects which, unless carefully controlled, tend to isolate metabolism studies from toxicity studies.

The EPA pesticide registration guidelines are currently under review. One aspect which is receiving attention from EPA scientists is that of making metabolism studies more relevant to toxicity testing. The appetite of the industry is for fewer mandatory "guidelines" and for more flexibility. This is undoubtedly the scientifically correct route to take, but could involve much expensive and lengthy discussion and reiteration between industry and the Agency. However, two types of study under discussion are of interest:

1. Repeated oral dosing studies when unusual toxicity is observed in conjunction with slow rates of biotransformation and excretion
2. Evaluation of the saturation of metabolic processes using multiple dosing studies for the purposes of dose selection and dose justification for chronic toxicity studies

The results of the preliminary biotransformation/kinetic study, together with the current regulatory metabolism studies and the 28- and 90-day studies should allow the selection of a relatively small number of appropriate tissues and/or fluids for monitoring purposes. Satellite groups of animals will provide the material for analysis. Methods must be developed to analyze nonradioactive test chemicals. Obviously it is important to monitor blood. It is accessible, convenient and, in certain circumstances, sequential sampling from the same animal may be important. The most useful aspect of blood is that the results can be compared with those obtained in man (see below). It is important, however, not to be constrained by this aspect. The most relevant tissues and body fluids should also be analyzed. These are target organs (if known) and indicator organs, tissues or fluids; i.e. those in which the concentration of pesticide or metabolite is a measure of that in the whole animal. In cases where distribution varies with dose (if shown in the preliminary study), a larger number of organs/tissues would be chosen for monitoring.

Whether the parent chemical or metabolite (or both) is chosen for analysis depends on the preliminary study. In principle, analysis for the parent compound should always be carried out; however, there are situations (e.g., rapid metabolism) when this is quite futile and a major retained metabolite should be used. Covalently bound metabolites are addressed below.

Four occasions may be adequate for monitoring:

1. One month (equilibrium between intake of chemical and elimination of metabolites should be established; the time relates to the 28-day preliminary study)
2. Three months (confirmation of results at one month; relates to the 90-day study)
3. One year (coincides with the interim kill)
4. Two years (effects of age; coincides with termination of study)

Consideration should be given to the analysis of moribund animals.

V. PHYSIOLOGICALLY-BASED PHARMACOKINETIC (PBK) MODELING

Pharmacokinetic parameters are descriptive in nature. They quantitatively describe the manner in which a test material is absorbed and excreted, such that a specific blood or tissue level is achieved or maintained. In the past, experiments had to be done by every route of administration to gather the data appropriate for describing the pharmacokinetic behavior of a chemical administered by different routes. The development of more sophisticated and readily accessible computers has led to the development of a different approach, that of pharmacokinetic modeling. In this computerized model, different compartments are represented as shown in boxes and the movement of the material in and out of the compartments is defined by the rate constants. These can be determined either in vivo or in vitro. Other physiological parameters are brought into play as well, such as octanol/water partition coefficient, blood flow through an organ, respiration rate (for the inhalation route of exposure), rate of microsomal metabolism, etc.

Pharmacokinetic modeling is the process of developing mathematical explanations of absorption, distribution, metabolism, and excretion of chemicals in organisms. Two commonly used types of compartmental pharmacokinetic models are (a) data-based and (b) physiologically based. The data-based pharmacokinetic models correspond to mathematical descriptions of the temporal change in the blood/tissue level of a xenobiotic in the animal species of interest. This procedure considers the organism as a single homogeneous compartment or as a multicompartmental system with elimination occurring in specific compartments of the model. The number, behavior, and volume of these hypothetical compartments are estimated by the type of equation chosen to describe the data, and not necessarily by the physiological characteristics of the model species in which the blood/tissue concentration data were acquired.

Whereas these data-based pharmacokinetic models can be used for interpolation, they should not be used for extrapolation outside the range of doses, dose routes, and species used in the study on which they were based. In order to use the data-based models to describe the pharmacokinetic behavior of a chemical administered at various doses by different routes, extensive animal experimentation would be required to generate similar blood-time course data under respective conditions. Even within the same species of animal, the time-dependent nature of critical biological determinants of the disposition (e.g., tissue glutathione depletion and resynthesis) cannot easily be included or evaluated with the data-based pharmacokinetic modeling approach. Further, due to the lack of actual anatomical, physiological, and biochemical realism, these data-based compartmental models cannot easily be used in interspecies extrapolation, particularly to predict pharmacokinetic behavior of chemicals in humans. These various extrapolations, which are essential for the conduct of dose-response assessment of chemicals, can be performed more confidently with a physiologically based pharmacokinetic modeling approach. This chapter presents the principles and methods of physiologically based pharmacokinetic modeling as applied to the study of toxicologically important chemicals.

PBPK/modeling is the development of mathematical descriptions of the uptake and disposition of chemicals based on quantitative interrelationships among the critical biological determinants of these processes. For a thorough review, the reader is refered to Conally and Anderson (22). These determinants include partition coefficients, rates of biochemical reactions, and physiological characteristics of the animal species. The biological and mechanistic basis of the PBPK models enable them to be used, with limited animal experimentation, for extrapolation of the kinetic behavior of chemicals from high dose to low dose, from one exposure route to another, and from test animal species to people.

The development of PBPK models is performed in four interconnected steps: model representation, model parameterization, model stimulation, and model validation. Model representation involves the development of conceptual, functional, and computational descriptions of the relevant compartments of the animal as well as the exposure and metabolic pathways of the chemical. Model parameterization involves obtaining independent measures of the mechanistic determinants, such as physiological, physicochemical, and biochemical parameters, which are included in one or more of the PBPK model equations. Model simulation involves the prediction of the uptake and disposition of a chemical for defined exposure scenarios, using a numerical integration algorithm, simulation software, and a computer. Finally, the model validation step involves the comparison of the a priori predictions of the PBPK model with experimental data to refute, validate, or refine the model description, and the characterization of the sensitivity of tissue dose to changes in model parameter values. PBPK models, after appropriate testing and validation, can be used to conduct extrapolations of the pharmacokinetic behavior of chemicals from one exposure route/ scenario to another, from high dose to low dose, and from one species to another.

The PBPK model development for a chemical is preceded by the definition of the problem, which in toxicology may often be related to the apparent complex nature of toxicity. Examples of such apparent complex toxic responses include nonlinearity in dose-response, sex/species differences in tissue response, differential response of tissues to chemical exposure, qualitatively and/or quantitatively difference responses for the same cumulative dose administered by different routes/scenarios, etc. In these instances, PBPK modeling studies can be utilized to evaluate the pharmacokinetic basis of the apparent complex nature of toxicity induced by the chemical. One of the values of PBPK modeling, in fact, is that accurate description of target tissue dose often resolves behavior that appears complex at the administered dose level.

The principal application of PBPK models is in the prediction of the target tissue dose of the toxic parent chemical or its reactive metabolite. Use of the target tissue dose of the toxic moiety of a chemical in risk assessment calculations provides a better basis of relating to the observed toxic effects than the external or exposure concentration of the parent chemical. Because PBPK models facilitate the prediction of target tissue dose for various exposure scenarios, routes, doses, and species, they can help reduce the uncertainty associated with the conventional extrapolation approaches. Direct application of modeling includes:

- High-dose/low-dose extrapolation
- Route-route extrapolation
- Exposure scenario extrapolation
- Interspecies extrapolation

Despite the utility of PBPK modeling in using existing data to make objective projections, only recently has the use of these techniques come to the attention of regulatory authorities. It is of interest that in OPPTS guideline 870.7485 there is a section on physiologically based modeling that addresses circumstances as to when PBPK modeling may be used to address specific issues relating to biotransformation.

An example of a current use of PBPK modeling was published by Vinegar and Jepson (23). They examined the time course required for blood levels of halon replacements associated with cardiac sensitization to be achieved under different exposure scenarios. They were attempting to predict the time required for a human being to exit an area in which a halon replacement fire extinguisher had discharged before potential toxic levels of gas could be achieved in the plasma.

REFERENCES

1. Draper, A., Madan, A., Smith, K., and Parkinson, A. (1998). Development of a non-high pressure liquid chromatography assay to determine testosterone hydroxylase (CYP3A) activity in human liver microsomes. Drug Metab. Dispo. 26:299–304.

2. Draper, A., Madan, A., Latham, J., and Parkinson, A. (1998). Development of a non-high pressure liquid chromatography assay to determine [^{14}C]chlorzoxazone 6-hydroxylase (CYP2E1) activity in human liver microsomes. Drug Metab. Dispo. 26:305–312.

3. Tse, F.L.S. and Jaffe, J.M. (1991). Preclinical Drug Disposition, Marcel Dekker, Inc., New York.

4. Gad, S.C. and Chengelis, C.P. (1997). Acute Toxicology Testing, 2nd ed, San Diego, CA: Academic Press.

5. Goldstein, A., Aronow, L., and Kalman, S. (1974). Principles of Drug Action: The Basis of Pharmacology, New York: John Wiley & Sons.

6. Holland, J., Kao, M., and Whitaker, M.J. (1984). A multisample apparatus for kinetic evaluation of skin penetration in vitro: The influence and metabolic status of the skin. Toxicol. Appl. Pharmacol. 72:272–280.

7. Branaugh, R.L. (1998). Methods for in Vitro Percutaneous Absorption in Dermatotoxicology Methods (F.N. Marzulli and H.I. Maibach, eds.), Philadelphia: Taylor & Francis.

8. O'Reilly, W.J. (1972). Pharmacokinetics in drug metabolism and toxicology. Can. J. Pharm. Sci. 7:66–77.

9. Keberle, G., Brindle, S.D., and Greengard, P. (1971). The route of absorption of intraperitoneally administered compounds. J. Pharmacol. Exp. Ther. 178:562–566.

10. Meyer, U.A. (1994). The molecular basis of genetic polymorphisms of drug metabolism. J. Pharm. Pharmacol. (Suppl 1):409–415.

11. Monostory, K., Jemnitz, K., Vereczkey, L., and Czira, G. (1997). Species differences in metabolism of panomifene, an analogue of tamoxifen. Drug Metab. Dispo. 25:1370–1378.

12. Smith, D. (1991). Species differences in metabolism and pharmacokinetics: are we close to an understanding? Drug Metab. Rev. 23:355–373.

13. Griffin, R., Godfrey, V., Kim, Y., and Burka, L. (1997). Sex-dependent differences

in the disposition of 2,4-dichlorophenoxyacetic acid in Sprague-Dawley rats, B6C3F1 mice and Syrian hamsters. Drug Metab. Dispo. 25:1065–1071.

14. Caldwell, W.S., Byrd, C.D., DeBethizz, J.D., and Brooks, P.A. (1994). Modern Instrumental Methods for Studying Mechanisms of Toxicity in Principles and Methods of Toxicology (A.W. Hayes, ed.), New York: Raven Press.

15. Shapiro, J. (1981). Radiation Protection, 2nd ed., Cambridge, MA: Harvard University Press, pp. 12–18.

16. Lu, H., Wang, J., Chan, K., and Young, D. (1998). Effects of phenobarbital of stereoselective metabolism of ifosfamide in rats. Drug Metab. Disp. 26:476–482.

17. Gad, S.C. and Chengelis, C.P. (eds.) (1992). Animal Models in Toxicology. Marcel Dekker Inc., New York. 884 pages.

18. Garner, C. and Mathews, H. (1998). The effect of chlorine substitution on the dermal absoption of polychlorinated biphenyls. Toxicol. Appl. Pharmacol. 149: 150–158.

19. La Du, B., Mandel, H., and Way, E. (1972). Fundamentals of Drug Metabolism and Drug Disposition, Baltimore, MD: The Williams & Wilkins Co.

20. Mugfor, C. and Kidderis, G. (1998). Sex-Dependent Metabolism of Xenobiotics, Drug Metab. Reviews, pp. 441–498.

21. Wang, Y.M. and Reuning, R. (1994). A comparison of two surgical techniques for the preparation of rats with chronic bile duct canulae for the investigation of enterohepatic circulation. Lab. Animal Sci. 44:479–485.

22. Conally, R. and Anderson, M. (1991). Biologically based pharmacokinetic models: Tools for toxicological research and risk assessment. Annu. Rev. Pharmacol. Toxicol. 31:503–523.

23. Vinegar, A. and Jepson, G. (1996). Cardiac sensitization thresholds of halon replacement chemicals in humans by physiologically based pharmacokinetic modeling. Risk Analysis 16:571–579.

24. Parkinson, A. (1996). Biotransformation of Xenobiotics. In: Casarett & Doull's Toxicology: The basic science of poisons, 5th Ed. (C. Klaassen, ed.), New York: McGraw-Hill, Inc., pp. 113–186.

Index